As more and more
people are ...

Total fat, saturated fat, trans fat—how do you tell the difference? Which is the most dangerous? Are there any good fats? *The Fat Counter,* 7th Edition, answers these questions and much more. Fat can be part of a healthy diet if you choose wisely. This comprehensive, easy-to-understand guide will help readers decide how much and what kind of fat to eat.

In the seventh edition of their popular nutrition guide *The Fat Counter,* Annette B. Natow, Ph.D., and Jo Ann Heslin, M.A., R.D., C.D.N.—nationally recognized professional nutrition educators—demystify fats and offer helpful tips for healthy eating. This one-of-a-kind resource features reliable fat, saturated fat, and trans fat counts for over 21,000 foods in a convenient, easy-to-use format. Before you take another bite, make you sure you're getting the most out of your meal.

THE FAT COUNTER, 7th Edition

More than one million copies sold!

***Turn the page for more essential titles from
nutrition experts Natow and Heslin—
available now from Pocket Books!***

THE COMPLETE FOOD COUNTER
3rd Edition

Eat healthier—start today!

Updated, revised, and expanded, *The Complete Food Counter*, 3rd Edition, is the most reliable resource available for nutrition information about the foods you eat. This easy-to-understand, easy-to-use comprehensive guide from nationally recognized nutrition experts Annette Natow and Jo-Ann Heslin will tell you everything you need to know to eat a healthy diet. . . .

- Thousands of brand name, generic, regional, vegetarian, international, and organic foods—and more.
- Helpful tips, shopping suggestions, and the latest research findings.
- Simple guidelines to consuming the right amounts of calories, fat, cholesterol, protein, carbohydrates, fiber, and sodium for you.

THE HEALTHY WHOLEFOODS COUNTER

Good food that's good for you—
and good for the earth!

America is going "green." Organic, natural, sustainable, free-range, vegetarian, whole grain, antibiotic-free, eco-friendly—what does it all mean? Marketing hype and media headlines can blur the facts, and you want answers about which are the best foods to buy and eat. In an easy-to-read Question and Answer format, nationally known nutrition experts Annette Natow and Jo-Ann Heslin provide a guide to choosing wholesome foods. Here you'll find:

- Easy-to-understand explanations that demystify antioxidants, phytochemicals, probiotics, trans fats—and more.
- The real scoop on calorie-burning drinks, satiety-enhancing products, immunity-boosting foods, and superfruits.
- Information on planet-friendly farming and food processing to help you buy the healthiest foods.
- How to become a label-reading expert to make the best choices when you shop.

Making the naturally delicious,
wholesome choice has never been easier!

Books by Annette B. Natow and Jo-Ann Heslin

The Calorie Counter
(*Fourth Edition*)

The Cholesterol Counter
(*Seventh Edition*)

The Complete Food Counter
(*Third Edition*)

The Diabetes Carbohydrate and Calorie Counter
(*Third Edition*)

Eating Out Food Counter

The Fat Counter
(*Seventh Edition*)

The Healthy Heart Food Counter

The Healthy Wholefoods Counter

The Most Complete Food Counter
(*Second Edition*)

The Protein Counter
(*Second Edition*)

The Ultimate Carbohydrate Counter

The Vitamin and Mineral Food Counter

Published by POCKET BOOKS

THE
FAT COUNTER

Seventh Edition

20th Anniversary Edition

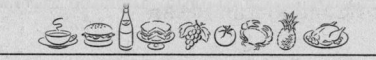

Annette B. Natow, Ph.D.
Jo-Ann Heslin, M.A., R.D.
With the Assistance of Karen J. Nolan, Ph.D.

POCKET BOOKS
New York   London   Toronto   Sydney

Pocket Books
A Division of Simon & Schuster, Inc.
1230 Avenue of the Americas
New York, NY 10020

Copyright © 1989, 1993, 1995, 1998, 2000, 2005, 2009 by Annette B. Natow and Jo-Ann Heslin

First Pocket Books paperback edition January 2009

POCKET and colophon are registered trademarks of Simon & Schuster, Inc.

For information about special discounts for bulk purchases, please contact Simon & Schuster Special Sales at 1-800-456-6798 or business@simonandschuster.com.

Cover photo by Getty Images

Manufactured in the United States of America

10 9 8 7 6 5 4 3 2 1

ISBN-13: 978-1-4165-0986-8
ISBN-10:   1-4165-0986-0

*To our families, who support us
through every project:*

*Harry, Allen, Irene, Sarah, Meryl, Marty, Laura, George,
Emily, Steven, Rebecca, Joseph, Kristen,
Brian, Karen, and John.*

ACKNOWLEDGMENTS

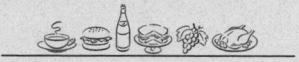

For graciously sharing her knowledge, Karen J. Nolan, Ph.D.

For all her continuous support and help, our agent, Nancy Trichter.

For her suggestions and editing skills, Sara Clemence.

Without the tireless cooperation of Stephen Llano and the production department at Pocket Books, *The Fat Counter, 7th Edition* would never have been completed.

A special thank you to our editor, Micki Nuding.

And we'd like to thank all of our readers for their suggestions and questions. Your input helps us to provide you with the most useful information.

"From hundreds of digestion experiments we have learned ... that an ounce of pure carbohydrate or pure protein will yield 113 Calories ... an ounce of fat, 255 Calories ... the more fat a food contains, the higher its energy value."

Mary Swartz Rose, Ph.D.
Feeding the Family
The MacMillan Company, 1919

CONTENTS

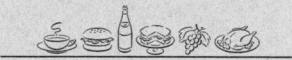

Just the Fats   1

Fats—A Simple Science Lesson   4

Fats—Why Your Body Needs Them   15

Fat—How Much Should You Eat?   18

Finding Fats in Food   26

Tracking Fat   34

Using Your Fat Counter   38

  Definitions   41

  Abbreviations   42

  Notes   43

PART ONE

Brand Name, Nonbranded (Generic),
and Take-Out Foods

45

PART TWO

Restaurant Chains

575

THE
FAT COUNTER

JUST THE FATS

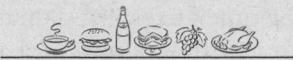

If you are like most people, you just want to know, "Are fats good for me or bad for me?" A simple question—too bad the answer is anything but.

The Fat Counter, 7th Edition, is celebrating its twentieth year in print. Over the last two decades, the book has changed to reflect the most current information and recommendations about fat. Both have changed considerably as scientific information has evolved.

In the 1970s, researchers were looking at the effects on health of moderate to high fat intake versus low fat intake. With the release of the first Dietary Guidelines for Americans in 1980, low fat took the spotlight. This led to the all-you-can-eat low fat era.

When health professionals recommend low fat eating plans, they mean meals high in fruits, vegetables, beans, grains, and lean protein choices. That advice didn't stand a chance against the food manufacturers who were churning out low fat and no fat cookies, candy, chips, ice cream, and salad dressing. Americans stuffed themselves with low fat choices, and got fatter and fatter because low fat foods aren't always low in calories.

Too much of any food, even low fat choices,
promotes weight gain.

When the high fat gurus, like Dr. Atkins, came along during the mid 1990s, it was back to eating bacon and whipped cream. We felt fuller longer, our cholesterol went down, and we lost weight. Though high fat diets were shown to be quick fixes that didn't last in the long haul, they did give birth to a new idea about fats—you can eat them and not be unhealthy.

The concept that eating moderate amounts of the right fat can be healthy—and possibly even healthier than low fat intake—was born.

Where does that leave us today? Researchers would say we are seeing a shift in the basic paradigm of healthy eating. In simpler terms, we now understand that some fats are good for us, some are bad for us, and some should be avoided altogether.

Experts redirected eating recommendations from a low fat to a moderate fat message. We've looked at cultures that eat more fat and examined the fat choices they've made. Though a low fat diet is still used successfully by many, we now know there are other healthy eating options.

Both low fat and moderate fat intakes are options for healthy eating.

The simplistic view that all fats are bad and you should eat less fat is no longer accurate. The more accurate message is:

- Not all fats are bad for you.
- The type of fat you eat may be more important than how much you eat.
- A moderate fat intake can be healthy.

Yes, it was easier when we told you that all fats were bad and that you should simply eat less fat. But as our knowledge gets more sophisticated, so does our advice about eating well. In *The Fat Counter,* 7th edition, we'll do what we have always done: we'll help you sort out the research and unravel the information so you can make the healthiest food choices.

There are still many good reasons to keep track of the fat you eat, because:

- Too much fat puts you at risk for health problems.
- Too much fat causes you to gain weight.
- Too much saturated fat and trans fat increases your risk for heart disease.

FATS—A SIMPLE SCIENCE LESSON

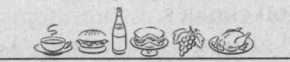

Fats mystify people. They have big-sounding names that are hard to wrap your tongue around and even harder to understand—triglycerides, saturated, monounsaturated, and polyunsaturated. But the information doesn't have to be hard, and we'll help you make sense of it all.

Basic Fat Facts

Fats are also called *lipids*. All fats are similar: your body fat and the fat you eat.

Triglycerides are the most typical fat compound, made up of smaller fat fragments called *fatty acids*. The term *triglyceride* describes the chemical structure of the fat. Triglycerides in food are used to meet part of your daily need for calories. Triglycerides in food can be in solid, "butters," or liquid, "oils." Triglycerides can also be stored in your body as fat for future use as energy.

Fatty acids are the building blocks that make up triglycerides. They can be saturated, monounsaturated, or polyunsaturated fatty acids. This is important because each type of fatty acids affects your health.

Every food with fat contains a mixture of different

fatty acids, but we classify the food by the predominant fatty acid present. For example: butter is high in saturated fatty acids; olives are high in monounsaturated fatty acids; corn oil is high in polyunsaturated fatty acids. Each of these foods contains other types of fatty acids as well, but to a lesser amount.

Every fatty acid contains carbon atoms with hydrogen atoms attached. You can think of these as necklaces that vary in the number of beads in each strand and in the way the beads are hooked together. This chemical structure affects how the fats look and how they act in your body.

FAT FACT

The type of fat you eat may be more important to your health than the amount you eat.

Saturated Fats—*eat less of this type of fat*

Animal fats are high in saturated fats and are usually solid at room temperature.

Saturated Fatty Acid

A saturated fatty acid looks like the chain above, with the maximum number of hydrogen atoms attached to each carbon atom. Saturated fats are very stable because the bonds between the carbon and hydrogen are strong. Saturated fats have a very high melting point and are good

FOOD HIGH IN SATURATED FATS	HEALTH EFFECTS OF ALL SATURATED FATS
Meat	Raises cholesterol levels.
Whole milk	Raises LDL (bad) cholesterol.
Cheese	Increases heart disease risk.
Cream	Increases risk for stroke.
Ice cream	May increase risk for cancer.
Butter	
Lard	
Poultry	
Palm oil	
Palm kernel oil	
Coconut and coconut oil	
Cocoa butter	
Bacon	
Sour cream	
Pies	
Pastries	

for frying and making flaky pastries. In your body they are very potent at raising your blood cholesterol levels, which puts you at risk for a blocked artery that could lead to a heart attack or stroke.

You can't eliminate all saturated fats from your diet, and you really don't have to, but it is important to limit them. That's easy when it comes to milk, cream, sour cream, and cheese. Simply choose the nonfat or lower fat versions. When it comes to meat, choose leaner cuts and smaller portions. Trim fat and skin from poultry, and don't use bacon grease or lard for cooking. When you eat food naturally high in saturated fat—butter, bacon, coconut—keep portions small.

There are good reasons to include some saturated fat

in your diet. Many of the foods with saturated fats—milk, meat, poultry—contain important nutrients we need for good health. In addition, not all saturated fats are bad for you. A good example is a saturated fat called *stearic acid,* found in beef and chocolate, which does not raise cholesterol levels.

FAT FACT

Foods high in saturated fat should be eaten in moderation. Keep portions small.

Vegetable fats, better known as oils, are high in monounsaturated fats and polyunsaturated fats and are liquid at room temperature.

Monounsaturated Fats—
use these fats to replace some saturated fats

FOOD HIGH IN MONOUNSATURATED FATS	HEALTH EFFECTS OF ALL MONOUNSATURATED FATS
Olives and olive oil	Reduces cholesterol levels.
Canola oil	Reduces triglycerides levels.
Peanuts and peanut oil	Reduces LDL (bad)
Almonds and almond oil	cholesterol levels.
Avocados	Maintains or raises HDL
Cashews	(good) cholesterol levels.
Hazelnuts	May lower blood pressure.
Macadamia nuts	Reduces risk for diabetes.
Pine nuts	
Pistachios	
Chicken fat	

$$H - C-C-C-C-C = C-C-C-C - COOH$$

with hydrogen atoms shown as H bonded above and below each carbon in the chain.

Monounsaturated Fatty Acid

A monounsaturated fatty acid looks like the chain above, and has one double bond. This is a place on the molecule where there is a weaker link and more hydrogen atoms could be attached or the chain could be broken. The addition of one double bond on the fatty acid structure lowers the melting point of the fat and it becomes oil. That's why monounsaturated fats, like olive oil, are not good for frying at high temperatures—heat breaks the double bond and the fat begins to smoke. But using monounsaturated fats in foods, like salad dressing, is a healthy option.

Research shows that when you substitute foods high in monounsaturated fat for foods high in saturated fat, your risk for heart disease goes down. Monounsaturated fats—olive oil, nuts, avocados, and olives—are the major fats eaten by people who follow the much-praised Mediterranean diet. But you can't simply dunk Italian bread in olive oil and expect to be healthy. The Mediterranean lifestyle also includes plenty of fruits and vegetables, less whole milk, cheeses and meats, and a lot of activity.

FAT FACT

A Handful, Not a Canful

Nuts and seeds have gone from high fat forbidden foods to healthy choices.

We now know that a small serving of nuts daily is a healthy eating habit because they are rich in healthy monounsaturated fats.

Polyunsaturated Fats—*eat more of these fats*

$$H - C\!-\!C\!-\!C = C\!-\!C = C\!=\!C\!-\!C\!-\!C - COOH$$

Polyunsaturated Fatty Acid

Polyunsaturated fatty acids look like the chain above, with 2 or more double bonds in the chain. Now the fatty acid chain has many places where the chain can be broken and more hydrogen can be added. Most of the oils we eat are polyunsaturated fats and they are considered heart healthy.

FAT FACT

Soft, whipped, and squeeze margarines have more polyunsaturated fats.

Stick margarines have more saturated fats.

There are two main groups of polyunsaturated fats: omega-6 and omega-3. Think of them as two different strands of beads, similar in shape but different in color sequence. Each is important to good health, so eating foods with both is important.

Most types of vegetable oils are high in omega-6 fats. More than 80% of the vegetable oil used in the U.S. is soybean oil. Even if you don't use soybean oil at home, it's the preferred oil used by food manufacturers and restaurants, so you are probably eating more than you realize. Based on that, it may be wise to select another type of

FOOD HIGH IN OMEGA-6 FATS	HEALTH EFFECTS OF ALL OMEGA-6 FATS
Safflower oil	Reduces cholesterol levels.
Sesame oil	Reduces LDL (bad)
Soybean oil	cholesterol.
Soybeans	Improves blood pressure.
Corn oil	Reduces inflammation.
Sunflower oil	Reduces blood clots.
Grapeseed oil	Reduces heart disease risk.
Nuts	May protect against cancer.
Seeds	
Soft margarine	
Wheat germ	

vegetable oil for home use, to vary the types of fatty acids you eat—all have benefits.

FAT FACT

The most commonly used oils in the U.S. are soybean, corn, and cottonseed; all are high in omega-6 fatty acids.

Omega-3 fats are in shorter supply in our diets. It's been estimated that the ratio of omega-6 fats to omega-3 fats should range from 5:1 to 10:1 for health benefits. In typical American diets the ratio is about 20:1. So make an effort to eat foods higher in omega-3 fats—fish, olive oil, canola oil. Research is showing that this imbalance in the polyunsaturated fats we eat may be contributing to higher risks for cancer, heart disease, and arthritis. The good news is that eating as little as 2 servings of fish a week, a rich source of omega-3 fats, can lower your risks.

FOOD HIGH IN OMEGA-3 FATS	HEALTH EFFECTS OF ALL OMEGA-3 FATS
Canola oil	Reduces triglyceride levels.
Flaxseeds	Improves immune function.
Olives and olive oil	Reduces inflammatory
Walnuts and walnut oil	diseases.
Hempseeds	Protects against sudden
Herring	death from heart disease.
Mackerel	Reduces tumor growth.
Tuna	Reduces formation of plaque
Trout	in arteries.
Sardines	Reduces blood pressure.
Salmon	Reduces blood clots.
Bluefish	May help regulate mood.
Oysters	May protect against dementia.

FAT FACT

To protect yourself from "sudden cardiac death,"
which causes half of all heart disease deaths,
eat more fish rich in omega-3 fats.

Trans Fats—*eat as little as possible of these fats*

Many experts feel that eating foods containing trans fats is a greater health risk than eating foods rich in saturated fats. The good news is that you can easily cut down on trans fats.

Almost all the trans fat found in our foods is created artificially by passing hydrogen gas through vegetable oil, a process called *hydrogenation*. The double bonds in the polyunsaturated fats above are broken and more hydrogen is added to the chain to make the oil solid.

If oil is completely hydrogenated—filled up with hy-

FOOD HIGH IN TRANS FATS	HEALTH EFFECTS OF ALL TRANS FATS
Cookies	Raises cholesterol levels.
Crackers	Lowers HDL (good) cholesterol.
Cakes	Raises LDL (bad) cholesterol.
Pastries	Raises triglyceride levels.
Shortening	Increases heart disease risk.
Stick margarine	May increase the risk for
Deep-fried foods	Alzheimer's disease and
Doughnuts	Parkinson's disease.
Muffins	Increases the risk for type 2
Breaded and deep-fried fish and chicken nuggets	diabetes.
	May increase the risk for infertility.
Processed cheese foods	May increase the risk for
Partially hydrogenated oil	blood clots.

drogen—it becomes hard and waxy like candle wax and is not useful in cooking. Most vegetable oils are partially hydrogenated—filling up some but not all of the double bonds—resulting in stick margarines, shortenings, and oils that are more stable during frying. This creates a type of fatty acid referred to as the "trans" form, which has many negative effects on your health. But we didn't always understand that trans fat was bad. In fact, when first used, it was thought to be a healthy option.

Hydrogenated fats became popular during World War II, when butter was scarce. They were used extensively by the food industry to produce light and flaky pastries and crunchy crackers. Hydrogenated fats do not spoil easily, giving foods like cookies a long shelf life. They have a high smoking point, which makes them ideal for deep fat frying.

Hydrogenated fats—high in trans fatty acids—were used

initially to replace saturated fats such as lard and butter. As our knowledge about fats expanded, we learned that eating trans fat was as bad for our health, and maybe even worse, than eating saturated fat. Food manufacturers and restaurants have been working to correct this problem by reformulating products to cut down or eliminate trans fats.

You will be seeing even more trans fat free products as time goes on. Food consumption surveys are already showing a small but steady decline in the amount of trans fats we eat. Cutting down on or eliminating foods with trans fats will not eliminate any important nutrients from your diet. In fact, it may help you cut back on less healthy choices like French fries and cakes.

FAT FACT

Trans Fat vs. Saturated Fat

Many scientific studies show that eating some saturated fats offers beneficial effects. Eating small amounts is okay.

Eating artificially produced trans fats offers no health benefits—avoid them.

As with most scientific findings, the story of trans fat is not all bad. If a fat is totally hydrogenated, it does not contain trans fats. The trans fat structure only occurs when fats are partially hydrogenated, which jumbles up the normal placement of hydrogen atoms on the carbon chain. Companies are using the process of total hydrogenation to produce new trans fat free shortenings for use in commercial baking. They harden the fat and then add back oil to get the desired consistency. If you see "fully hydrogenated" or "totally hydrogenated" fat listed on a food label, the ingredient is trans fat free.

There are also small amounts of naturally occurring

trans fat in meat, butter, milk, cheese, and cabbage. These natural trans fats have a different structure then those artificially produced and they may have health benefits. Two natural trans fats—CLA (conjugated linoleic acid) and VA (vaccenic acid)—may play a role in preventing cancer, heart disease, and diabetes.

FAT FACT

Labeling Loophole

The value for trans fat listed on the nutrition label includes both artificially produced and natural trans fat. This can be confusing because only artificial trans fat needs to be limited.

What the Future Holds

The fat story is still evolving and we still have much to learn. What we know so far is:

- Too much fat is not a healthy eating option.
- Eating moderate amounts of the right fats can provide health benefits.
- Artificially produced trans fat should be avoided.
- Natural trans fats—this story is still unfolding, but it looks promising.

FAT FACT

Exercise helps you burn fat. A study showed that your body burns more polyunsaturated fats than saturated fats after exercising. Saturated fats were more likely to be stored; just another reason to eat them in moderation.

FATS—WHY YOUR BODY NEEDS THEM

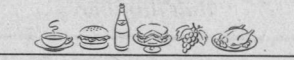

Fat gets no respect. Fat in food is considered bad for you. Fat on your body is considered unattractive. But you need fat—both in your food and on your body.

Fat in Food

Fat is the most concentrated source of energy you can eat, providing 9 calories per gram—more than double the calories found in the same amount of carbohydrate or protein. Fat enhances the flavor of food, contributes to its enjoyment, provides a pleasurable mouth feel, and makes you feel fuller longer.

We used to think that people like fatty foods because of the textural appeal, but recent research has shown that there are chemical receptors for fat in our taste buds. These receptors signal both the brain and the digestive tract when fat—whether it's in French fries, whipped cream or salad dressing—is eaten. Some people seem to have a stronger taste perception for fat than others, and they tend to crave fatty foods more often. This ability to taste fat vividly may be one reason for weight gain.

Fat on Your Body

FAT FACT

A lean adult has about 40 billion fat cells.
An overweight adult can have two to three times
that number.

Everyone wants to get rid of fat and it's true that most of us carry too much on our bodies. But having a certain proportion of fat on your frame is vital to your health. That's because fat:

Provides energy reserves. Stored fat is a concentrated source of reserve energy that your body draws upon when you eat too little, get sick, or need to recover from an injury. The human body has an almost limitless capacity to store extra fat.

Provides important vitamins. Fat helps the absorption of the fat-soluble vitamins A, D, E, and K.

Provides essential fatty acids. Your body is able to make some fats, but others must be provided through food. Omega-6 and omega-3 fatty acids are called "essential" because they can't be made in the body and therefore must be provided by the fat you eat.

Provides padding. Vital organs such as your eyes and kidneys are supported and protected from mechanical shocks by fat pads.

Provides insulation. Lose weight, and the next winter you'll feel colder than normal. Fat layers insulate your body against both high and low temperatures, and the fatty sheath surrounding nerve fibers helps transmit impulses.

Provides lubrication. Your body manufactures its own internal lubricant that slows the loss of water from tissues and keeps the body parts moving smoothly.

FAT FACT

Researchers used to think that fat cells were nothing more than storage compartments, but they now recognize that fat cells are potent chemical factories that produce hormones and other substances.

FAT—HOW MUCH
SHOULD YOU EAT?

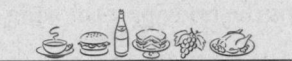

Let's set the record straight. Even though the current research suggests that a moderate fat intake may be healthier, no one is suggesting a *high* fat intake is good for you.

Eating too much fat puts you at risk for:

- Heart disease
- Stroke
- High blood pressure
- High cholesterol
- Cancer
- Obesity
- Diabetes
- Arthritis
- Gout
- Age-related macular degeneration (ARMD),
    a leading cause of blindness
- Alzheimer's disease, a leading cause of dementia

A high fat diet may even disrupt your body's clock. We all operate on a 24-hour circadian cycle that regulates sleeping, waking, fluid balance, body temperature, heart output, oxygen use, and gland functions. When the body's clock is disrupted it throws our internal signals off, including appetite control. Researchers have found that a misaligned body clock can increase the risk for obesity and diabetes. More recent research on animals confirmed that a high fat diet disrupts normal circadian rhythms—another good reason to eat a moderate amount of fat.

Total Fat—
should be 20% to 35% of total calories

Americans have gotten the message that too much fat is not good for them. Current consumption studies show we eat about 33% of our daily calories as fat. That is close to the upper end of the recommended 20% to 35% of total calories each day.

The following table will help you set your own daily target fat intake. First, select the number of calories you eat each day. Next, select the percentage of fat calories you wish to eat, and the chart will give you the grams of fat to aim for daily. This means if you regularly eat 1,800 calories a day, you should eat somewhere between 40 grams (20%) and 70 grams (35%) of fat each day.

If you aim for 20% to 25% of your daily calories to come from fat, you will be eating a low fat intake. Thirty to 35% is considered a moderate fat intake.

DAILY TARGET FAT INTAKE				
CALORIES PER DAY	**PERCENTAGE OF FAT CALORIES EACH DAY IN GRAMS**			
	20%	**25%**	**30%**	**35%**
1,000	22	28	33	39
1,100	24	31	37	43
1,200	27	33	40	47

DAILY TARGET FAT INTAKE (*cont.*)			
CALORIES PER DAY	**PERCENTAGE OF FAT CALORIES EACH DAY IN GRAMS**		
	20%	**25%**	**30%**	**35%**
1,300	29	36	43	51
1,400	31	39	47	54
1,500	33	42	50	58
1,600	36	44	53	62
1,700	38	47	57	66
1,800	40	50	60	70
1,900	42	53	63	74
2,000	44	56	67	78
2,100	47	58	70	82
2,200	49	61	73	86
2,300	51	64	77	89
2,400	53	67	80	93
2,500	56	69	83	97
2,600	58	72	87	101
2,700	60	75	90	105
2,800	62	78	93	109
2,900	64	81	97	113
3,000	67	83	100	117

FAT FACT

When you eat less total fat, you automatically eat less saturated fat and less trans fat.

Saturated Fat—
should be less than 10% of total calories

Americans get approximately 11% to 14% of their daily calories from saturated fat. The current Dietary Guidelines for Americans recommends eating less than 10% of daily calories from saturated fat, while the American Heart Association and others recommend less than 7% daily. Using common sense, and knowing that we currently eat between 11% and 14% of our daily calories as saturated fat, anything under 10% would be a significant reduction and provide health benefits.

The following table will help you set your own daily target saturated fat intake. First, select the number of calories you eat each day. Next, select the percentage of saturated fat calories you wish to eat, and the chart will give you the grams of saturated fat to aim for daily. This means if you regularly eat 1,800 calories a day, you should eat less than 14 grams (7%) or less than 20 grams (10%) of saturated fat each day.

Aiming for 7%, if you ordered a large cheeseburger for lunch, you would use up all your saturated fat for the day.

DAILY TARGET SATURATED FAT INTAKE		
CALORIES PER DAY	PERCENTAGE OF SATURATED FAT CALORIES EACH DAY IN GRAMS	
	7%	10%
1,000	8	11
1,100	9	12
1,200	9	13
1,300	10	14
1,400	11	16

DAILY TARGET SATURATED FAT INTAKE (*cont.*)		
CALORIES PER DAY	**PERCENTAGE OF SATURATED FAT CALORIES EACH DAY IN GRAMS**	
	7%	**10%**
1,500	12	17
1,600	12	18
1,700	13	19
1,800	14	20
1,900	15	21
2,000	16	22
2,100	16	23
2,200	17	24
2,300	18	26
2,400	19	27
2,500	19	28
2,600	20	29
2,700	21	30
2,800	22	31
2,900	23	32
3,000	23	33

At 10%, you have a few grams left over for the remainder of the day. That is why we encourage people to aim for lean and low fat protein choices, such as lowfat milk, as often as possible. When you want to indulge in a higher fat choice, like a hamburger, order small and skip the cheese. Both changes reduce the saturated fat in a serving.

Trans Fat—*should be as low as possible, less than 1% of total calories daily*

Most experts recommend eliminating *all* artificially produced trans fat. This means eliminating all foods made with partially hydrogenated oils. The latest USDA Dietary Guidelines for Americans recommends keeping trans fat intake to less than 1% of total daily calories.

Food consumption studies report that Americans regularly eat between 2% and 7% of total calories as trans fat. This intake will go down as food manufacturers and restaurants begin to remove trans fat from their products. Deep-fried foods, such as French fries and chicken nuggets, and cakes, cookies, and pies are our largest source of trans fats.

The following table will help you see how many grams of trans fat make up 1% of your total daily calories. This means if you regularly eat 1,800 calories a day, you should eat less than 2 grams (1%) of trans fat each day. At all calorie levels, the recommended intake of trans fat is very low.

DAILY TARGET TRANS FAT INTAKE	
CALORIES PER DAY	PERCENTAGE OF TRANS FAT CALORIES EACH DAY IN GRAMS
1,000	1
1,100	1
1,200	1
1,300	1
1,400	1–2
1,500	1–2
1,600	1–2

DAILY TARGET TRANS FAT INTAKE *(cont.)*	
CALORIES PER DAY	**PERCENTAGE OF TRANS FAT CALORIES EACH DAY IN GRAMS**
1,700	1–2
1,800	2
1,900	2
2,000	2
2,100	2
2,200	2
2,300	2–3
2,400	2–3
2,500	2–3
2,600	2–3
2,700	3
2,800	3
2,900	3
3,000	3

FAT FACT

The total amount of fat in a food is most important. There's little health benefit in choosing a food low in trans fat but high in saturated fat.

Keep in mind that just because a food is reformulated to remove trans fats, it does not automatically become a healthier choice. Trans fat free French fries are still high in fat. And cookies containing zero grams of trans fat doesn't give you license to eat the whole box: the cookies are still high in calories.

YOUR DAILY TARGETS

Daily calories = _____

_____% *Total Fat =* _____ *grams total fat per day*

_____% *Saturated Fat =* _____ *grams saturated fat per day*

1 % trans fat = _____ *grams trans fat per day*

FINDING FATS IN FOOD

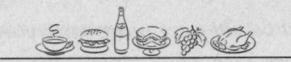

We may be eating more poultry and fish than red meat, but each year we still eat 57 pounds per person more of all types of meat than we did in the 1950's. Meanwhile, our consumption of cheese, high in saturated fat, has nearly quadrupled. And, the use of fats and shortenings has climbed to slightly more than 35 pounds per person per year.

In other words, instead of eating less fat, people are trading fats. Less red meat but more poultry and cheese. Less butter but more salad dressing.

These same studies show us that most people are not good at recognizing hidden fats in foods—in pastries, pizza, casseroles, sandwiches, drinks. We need to upgrade our fat-finding skills.

More importantly, we need to eat less food. Today, we eat 300 more calories every day than we did 20 years ago. By eating more of everything, we wind up eating more fat. This creates an interesting statistical picture. The percentage of calories we eat as fat each day has gone down, but the actual amount of fat we eat has gone up. Why? Because we are eating more food and we are eating more convenience food that has a lot of hidden fat.

> **FAT FACT**
>
> *It's been shown over and over again that people have trouble sticking with a low fat eating plan.*
>
> *Moderate fat intakes are more satisfying and people find them easier to adopt for the long haul.*

Keeping Your Fat Intake Moderate

- Choose lean cuts of meat and poultry.
- Eat less red meat and fewer fatty cuts of meats—use more poultry, fish and plant proteins, like beans and tofu.
- Eat fish—all varieties contain less saturated fat than meat and are richer in omega-3 heart healthy fats.
- Eat fried, battered, and breaded foods infrequently.
- Eat lower fat versions of milk, yogurt, sour cream, heavy cream, cheese, and ice cream.
- Use whipped cream cheese, butter, and margarine with less fat than the regular varieties.
- Measure fats you add on, such as butter, margarine, sour cream, cream cheese, and peanut butter, to keep portions reasonable.
- Eat nuts and seeds by the handful, not the canful.
- Broil, roast, grill, and steam to avoid adding extra fat when cooking.
- Eat tuna packed in water, and sardines packed in water, mustard, or tomato sauce, rather than oil.
- Avoid self-basting turkeys.

- Eat small portions of cookies, cakes, candies, and pastries.
- Trade pasta in cheese sauce for pasta in tomato sauce.

FAT FACT

A Moderate Fat Serving Is:

Red meat = 3 to 4 ounces
Stick butter or margarine = 2 teaspoons
Whipped butter or margarine = 1 tablespoon
Salad dressing = 2 tablespoons
Sour cream = 2 tablespoons
Whipped cream cheese = 2 tablespoons
Peanut and other nut butters = 2 tablespoons
Cream = 1 tablespoon
Whipped cream = ¼ cup
Ice cream = ½ cup

Even lowfat and reduced fat varieties have calories—keep servings moderate.

What's on the Label?

Food labels offer a lot of information about fat and are worth reading.

LABEL CLAIMS FOR FAT

IF THE LABEL SAYS:	THAT MEANS:
Fat Free	One serving of food has 0.5 grams of fat or less. Foods in this group can also be called "nonfat."
Low Fat	One serving of food has 3 grams of fat or less.

LABEL CLAIMS FOR FAT

IF THE LABEL SAYS:	THAT MEANS:
Reduced Fat	One serving of food has 25% less fat than the traditional product. Foods in this group can also be called "lower fat."
Light	One serving of food has at least 33% fewer calories or 50% less fat than the traditional product. Foods in this group may also be called "lite."
Extra Lean	One serving of food has less than 5 grams of total fat, less than 2 grams of saturated fat, and less than 95 milligrams of cholesterol.
Lean	One serving of food has less than 10 grams of total fat, less than 4.5 grams of saturated fat, and less than 95 milligrams of cholesterol.

FAT FACT

Food Labels—Understanding Fat Values

Total fat equals the amount of fat in one serving of food.

The saturated fat and trans fat values listed are part of the total fat value.

If you subtract the amount of saturated fat and trans fat from the total fat, what remains is the combined amount of monounsaturated and polyunsaturated fat in one serving.

Ingredient Listing

The ingredient listings on food labels tell you all the ingredients in that food, in order of amount. The ingredient listed first will be found in the largest amount. If fat, butter, or oil is close to the beginning of the list, you can be fairly confident there is a good deal of fat in each serving. The ingredient listing can also help you find "hidden fats." All of the following ingredients add fat to food.

Butter	Hydrogenated fat*
Cheese	Hydrogenated oil*
Chicken fat	Fully hydrogenated oil
Cocoa butter	Lard
Cream	Margarine**
Cream cheese**	Monoglycerides
Diglycerides	Oil
Fat	Partially hydrogenated oil*
Peanut butter**	Tropical oil
Shortening**	Vegetable fat
Sour cream	Vegetable shortening**
Suet	Whipped cream
	Whole milk

* Contains trans fat   ** May contain trans fat

FAT FACT

Meatless Mondays

To help Americans reduce their saturated fat intake, the Johns Hopkins Bloomberg School of Public Health has initiated Meatless Monday.

Every Monday, keep your saturated fat intake as low as possible. Plan meals without meat or high fat dairy foods.

What's on Your Plate?

Many fats you eat are visible—the fat around a steak, butter, or oil. Others are not that easy to see—fat baked into a muffin or used to fry potato chips—but it still adds up because the fat is part of the food. In other cases, it is easy to overdo—like pouring dressing on a salad or heaping grated cheese on pasta.

Though a moderate amount of fat can make you feel fuller after a meal, and many fats have health benefits, all fats are loaded with calories. Snacking on walnuts, rich in omega-3 polyunsaturated fats, is a good idea. Adding olive oil–rich salad dressing to your greens is healthy and tastes good. Just remember: 2 tablespoons is a serving. Because all fats pack a caloric wallop in a small amount, it's easy to eat too much.

FAT FACT

1 teaspoon of fat = 45 calories
1 teaspoon of carbohydrate (starch and sugar) = 20 calories
1 teaspoon of protein = 20 calories

When cooking, use nonstick cooking sprays to coat pans. Some brands offer butter or olive oil varieties that can add a punch of flavor to cooked pasta, rice, or potatoes. Measure, don't pour, when you add oil to a frying pan, dressing to a salad, gravy to meat, or sour cream to a potato. A tablespoon or 2 is fine; more starts to pack on calories.

There are now reduced fat versions of old high-fat favorites, including whipped cream, half-and-half, sour cream, ice cream, cream cheese, and peanut butter. Switching could save you thousands of calories in a year. If you prefer the full fat versions, that's fine; just keep portions moderate.

FAT FACT

*To find out if a food has hidden fat, place it on
a napkin or blot the top:
greasy napkin = hidden fat.*

Choosing the Best Oil

You may feel like you need a chemistry degree to select
the right oil from the ever-growing selection in the gro-
cery store! Let's try to make this simple.

- All oils have approximately 120 calories and 14
  grams of fat per tablespoon.
- All salad or cooking oils are made from
  vegetable, nut, or seed sources; unidentified
  vegetable oils are usually from soybeans.
- Oils are low in unhealthy saturated fats—
  exceptions are coconut, palm kernel, and palm
  oil, also called tropical oils.
- Many oils are high in healthy polyunsaturated
  fats—corn, cottonseed, grapeseed, poppyseed,
  safflower, soybean, sunflower, walnut, and
  wheat germ oil.
- Many oils are high in healthy monounsaturated
  fats—almond, avocado, canola, hazelnut, and
  olive oil.
- Some oils have an almost equal amount of
  polyunsaturated and monounsaturated fats—
  peanut, rice bran, and sesame.
- All liquid oils are trans fat free.

FAT FACT

*Most nonstick cooking sprays list "0" calories for a
⅓-second spray, but it takes 1 second or longer
to cover a 10-inch pan.*

*A 1-second spray = 5 to 7 calories, much less than
1 tablespoon of oil with 120 calories, but still,
seconds count.*

TRACKING FAT

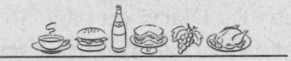

Too much fat puts you at risk for health problems.
Too much fat causes you to gain weight.
Too much saturated fat and trans fat increases
your risk for heart disease.
Keep your total fat intake moderate.
Keep your saturated and trans fat intake low.

Eating the right amount of fat may help you lose weight, control risks for heart disease, and manage diabetes. When you make the effort to write down what you eat, you learn a lot about how you eat, why you eat, and when you eat. Many of us eat on the go, substituting meals with a snatch-and-grab lifestyle, giving little thought to what we're eating. If you pay closer attention to what and how much you eat, we guarantee you'll see positive results.

FAST FACT

People cut calories by 10% when they
write down what they eat:
30% to 50% of those who keep food records make
positive changes in their eating habits.

The Fat Counter, 7th edition, is the best source you can use to keep track of fat, saturated fat, and trans fat. With more than 21,000 foods listed, values for everything you eat are at your fingertips. To determine how much fat you should eat, refer to the charts on pages 19, 21, and 23 to decide your target daily fat intake, see page 25.

Use "Your Daily Fat Diary" on page 36 to keep track of the fats and calories you eat. You don't have to track your saturated fat or trans fat intake daily, but it's a good thing to do once in a while to see if you're meeting the recommendations.

"Your Daily Fat Diary" will tell you a lot about how you eat, why you eat, and what you eat. Everyone under-reports how much they really eat—men more so than women—but no one will ever see what you write down, so be honest.

We suggest you note the day and date, because you may eat differently on different days of the week. Some people eat more on weekends or days off; others eat more at work. If you keep track, you may begin to see patterns.

We appreciate that many people eat on a crazy schedule, so the day is broken into 3 periods. That will help you figure out when you do the most eating.

"A.M." is from midnight till noon. Many people eat in the middle of the night, so this includes middle-of-the-night noshing, breakfast, coffee break, or morning snack.

"Midday" is from noon until dinner. It includes lunch and any afternoon or pre-dinner snack, like a drink after work.

"P.M." is dinnertime through midnight. It includes your evening meal and after-dinner, TV, and bedtime snacks.

By subtotaling your fats and calories 3 times during the day, you can make adjustments for unexpected situations. For example, if you had a big lunch at work, you can eat a lighter dinner or skip snacks to compensate for the extra calories.

YOUR DAILY FAT DIARY

Your Target Daily calories ____

Your Target Fat grams ____

Your Target Saturated Fat grams ____

Your Target Trans Far grams ____

Day _____

Date _____

FOOD	PORTION	CALORIES	TOTAL FAT	SATURATED FAT	TRANS FAT
AM					
AM Totals		____	____	____	____
MIDDAY					
Midday Totals		____	____	____	____
PM					
PM Totals		____	____	____	____
Daily Totals		____	____	____	____

FAT FACT

After you eat a high fat meal, your blood vessels are unable to properly expand and contract to regulate blood pressure correctly for up to 6 hours.

A brisk walk or other vigorous exercise within 2 hours of eating the high fat meal will fix the problem.

USING YOUR FAT COUNTER

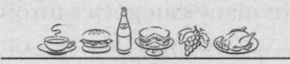

The Fat Counter, 7th edition, lists the portion size, calories, total fat, saturated fat, and trans fat for more than 21,000 foods. Now you can compare the values in your favorite foods and, when necessary, choose substitutes *before* you go out to shop or eat. This will save you time and help you decide what to buy.

The counter section of the book is divided into two parts: Part One: Brand Name, Nonbranded (Generic), and Take-Out Foods (page 45); and Part Two: Restaurant Chains (page 575). Each part lists foods or restaurant chains alphabetically.

In Part One, for each category you will find non-branded (generic) foods listed first, in alphabetical order, followed by an alphabetical listing of brand name foods. The nonbranded listing will help you estimate the calorie, total fat, saturated fat, and trans fat values when you don't see your favorite brand. They can also help you to evaluate store brands. Large categories are divided into subcategories, such as canned, fresh, frozen, and ready-to-eat, to make it easier to find what you're looking for. Some categories have "see" and "see also" references, to help you find related items.

When a dash (–) appears, it means that no analysis was done for saturated fat or trans fat for that food. It is not the same as a "0," which means there is no fat, saturated fat, or trans fat in the food.

Because we eat out so often, more than 600 take-out foods are listed in Part One. These are found in the take-out subcategory in many categories throughout this section. Look there for foods you take out or order in, since they are not nutrition labeled.

Most foods are listed alphabetically. In some cases, though, foods are grouped by category. For example, a tuna sandwich is found in the SANDWICH category. Other group categories include:

ASIAN FOOD: **Page 54**
　　Includes all types of Asian foods
　　except egg rolls and sushi,
　　which are found in the Egg Rolls
　　and Sushi categories.

DELI MEATS/COLD CUTS: **Page 223**
　　Includes all sandwich meats
　　except chicken, ham, and
　　turkey, which are found in
　　separate categories.

DINNER: **Page 225**
　　Includes all by brand name,
　　except pasta dinners, which
　　are found in the Pasta Dinner
　　category.

LIQUOR/LIQUEUR: **Page 339**
　　Includes all alcoholic beverages
　　and mixed drinks except beer,
　　champagne, and wine, which
　　are found in separate categories.

NUTRITION SUPPLEMENTS: **Page 369**
Includes all dieting aids, meal
replacements, and drinks,
except energy bars and energy
drinks, which are found in
separate categories.

SANDWICHES: **Page 464**
Includes popular sandwich,
calzone, and panini choices.

SNACKS: **Page 487**
Includes a variety of
miscellaneous snack items such
as pork rinds and cheese puffs.

SPANISH FOOD: **Page 515**
Includes all types of Spanish
and Mexican foods except salsa
and tortillas, which are found in
separate categories

In Part Two, Restaurant Chains, 124 national and regional restaurant, candy, coffee, doughnut, ice cream,
pizza, and sandwich chains are listed. Brand name foods
are required by federal law to have nutrition information
on labels, but in most areas of the country, restaurants
only provide this information voluntarily.

With *The Fat Counter* as your guide, you will never
again wonder how much fat, saturated fat, or trans fat is
in the food you eat. You will always be able to tell if a food
is high, moderate, or low in fat.

DEFINITIONS

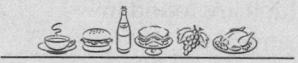

as prep (as prepared)—refers to food that has been prepared according to package directions

lean and fat—describes meat with some fat on its edges that is not cut away before cooking, or poultry prepared with skin and fat as purchased

lean only—refers to lean meat that is trimmed of all visible fat, or poultry without skin

not prep (not prepared)—refers to food that has not been cooked and may require the addition of other ingredients

shelf stable—refers to prepared products found on the supermarket shelf that are not canned but are packaged and ready-to-eat, or are ready to be heated but do not require refrigeration

take-out—describes prepared dishes that you purchase ready-to-eat; those included serve as a guide to the calories, fat, saturated fat, and trans fat in products you may purchase.

ABBREVIATIONS

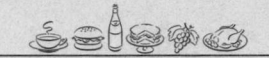

avg	=	average
diam	=	diameter
fl	=	fluid
frzn	=	frozen
g	=	gram
in	=	inch
lb	=	pound
lg	=	large
med	=	medium
mg	=	milligram
oz	=	ounce
pkg	=	package
pt	=	pint
prep	=	prepared
qt	=	quart
reg	=	regular
sec	=	second
serv	=	serving
sm	=	small
sq	=	square
tbsp	=	tablespoon
tr	=	trace
tsp	=	teaspoon
w/	=	with
w/o	=	without
<	=	less than

NOTES

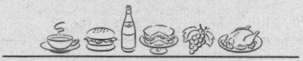

Cals = Calories
Fat = Total fat
   All fat values are given in grams (g)
   All values have been rounded to the nearest gram
Sat Fat = Saturated Fat
   All saturated fat values are given in grams (g)
   All values have been rounded to the nearest gram
Trans Fat = Trans Fat
   All trans fat values are given in grams (g)
   All values have been rounded to the nearest gram
tr (trace) = less than 0.5 gram of total fat, saturated fat, or
   trans fat
– (dash) indicates data was not available
0 (zero) indicates there are no calories, total fat, saturated
   fat, or trans fat in that food

Discrepancies in figures are due to rounding of values, product reformulation, and reevaluation. The current labeling law allows rounding. Much of the data listed is analysis data, obtained directly from manufacturers, not from labels; therefore, some values may differ slightly from labels because they have not been rounded.

PART ONE

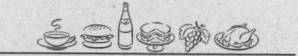

Brand Name, Nonbranded (Generic), and Take-Out Foods

FOOD	PORTION	CALS	FAT	SAT FAT	TRANS FAT
ABALONE					
breaded & fried	1 serv (3 oz)	162	6	1	–
steamed	1 serv (3 oz)	127	3	1	0
ACAI JUICE					
Zola					
100% Juice	1 box (11 oz)	170	2	1	0
ACEROLA					
fresh	1 (5 g)	2	tr	tr	–
ACEROLA JUICE					
juice	1 cup	56	1	tr	–
ADZUKI BEANS					
canned sweetened	½ cup	351	tr	tr	–
dried cooked w/o salt	½ cup	147	tr	tr	–
Arrowhead Mills					
Organic Dried not prep	¼ cup	130	0	0	0
AKEE					
fresh	3.5 oz	223	20	–	–
ALCOHOL (see BEER AND ALE, CHAMPAGNE, LIQUOR/LIQUEUR, MALT, WINE)					
ALE (see BEER AND ALE)					
ALFALFA					
sprouts	½ cup	40	tr	tr	–
ALLIGATOR					
cooked	3 oz	126	2	–	–
ALLSPICE					
ground	1 tsp	5	tr	tr	0
ALMONDS					
almond butter w/ salt	2 tbsp	203	19	2	–
almond butter w/o salt	2 tbsp	203	19	2	–
almond extract	1 tsp	38	tr	–	–
almond paste	¼ cup	260	16	1	–
chocolate covered	6 pieces (0.6 oz)	102	8	1	–
dry roasted w/ salt	¼ cup	206	18	1	–
dry roasted w/o salt	¼ cup	206	18	1	–
honey roasted	¼ cup	214	18	2	–

FOOD	PORTION	CALS	FAT	SAT FAT	TRANS FAT
jordan almonds	6 (0.7 oz)	99	4	tr	–
oil roasted w/ salt	¼ cup	238	22	2	–
oil roasted w/o salt	¼ cup	238	22	2	–
praline	17 pieces (1.4 oz)	210	12	1	–
yogurt covered	6 pieces (0.8 oz)	122	8	3	–
American Almond					
Marzipan	2 tbsp	130	5	0	–
Arrowhead Mills					
Organic Almond Butter Creamy	2 tbsp	200	17	2	0
Blue Diamond					
Almond Roca Buttercrunch	3 pieces (1.3 oz)	210	14	8	–
Honey Roasted	¼ cup	170	14	1	–
Jalapeno Smokehouse	28 pieces (1 oz)	170	15	1	0
Jordon Pastels	15 pieces (1.4 oz)	180	8	5	–
Lime 'N Chili	28 pieces (1 oz)	170	16	1	0
Maui Onion & Garlic	28 pieces (1 oz)	170	15	1	0
Milk Chocolate Covered	9 pieces (1.4 oz)	230	14	5	–
Salted	¼ cup	170	16	1	–
Smokehouse	28 pieces (1.3 oz)	170	16	1	–
Wasabi & Soy Sauce	28 pieces (1 oz)	170	15	1	0
Whole Natural	¼ cup	180	14	1	–
Yogurt Covered	12 pieces (1.4 oz)	210	14	8	–
Brach's					
Chocolate Coated	11 pieces	220	13	6	–
Eden					
Tamari	3 tbsp (1 oz)	160	11	1	0
Good Sense					
Hickory Smoked	¼ cup	180	16	1	0
Raw Whole	¼ cup	180	15	1	–
Judy's					
Sugar Free Coconut Almond Brittle	¼ piece (1 oz)	90	5	2	–
Keto					
Chocolatey Covered	1 oz	169	13	6	–
Kettle					
Butter Salted	2 tbsp	180	17	2	0
Butter Unsalted	2 tbsp	180	17	2	0
Love'n Bake					
Almond Paste	2 tbsp	140	9	1	–

FOOD	PORTION	CALS	FAT	SAT FAT	TRANS FAT
Almond Schmear	2 tbsp	140	8	0	–
Roasted Butter	2 tbsp	180	16	2	–
Low Carb Creations					
Soft Almond Brittle	2 pieces (1 oz)	170	12	2	–
Maisie Jane's					
Almond Butter	1 oz	184	16	2	0
Cappuccino	9 pieces (1.4 oz)	220	15	6	0
Chocolate Toffee	9 pieces (1.4 oz)	210	13	5	0
Coffee Glazed	2 tbsp (1 oz)	150	12	1	0
Cowboy BBQ	2 tbsp (1 oz)	140	11	0	0
Mint Chocolate	9 pieces (1.4 oz)	210	15	7	0
Organic Honey Glazed	2 tbsp (1 oz)	160	14	1	0
Tamari	2 tbsp (1 oz)	160	14	2	0
Mama Mellace's					
Butter Rum	1 oz	150	10	1	–
Cinnamon Roasted	1 oz	140	9	1	–
Maranatha					
Almond Butter	2 tbsp	220	18	1	–
Tamari Almonds	¼ cup	160	14	2	–
Mrs. May's					
Almond Crunch	1 oz	156	13	1	0
Odense					
Almond Paste	2 tbsp (1.4 oz)	170	7	1	–
Planters					
Chocolate Lovers Dark Chocolate	11 pieces (1.4 oz)	220	17	6	0
Dry Roasted	23 pieces (1 oz)	160	14	1	0
Sunkist					
Accents Italian Parmesan	1 tbsp	40	4	0	0
Accents Original Oven Roasted	1 tbsp	40	4	0	0
Sweet Delights					
Almond Roasters	⅓ pkg (1 oz)	190	14	–	–
AMARANTH					
leaves cooked	½ cup	14	tr	tr	–
uncooked	½ cup (3.4 oz)	365	6	2	–
Arrowhead Mills					
Organic Whole Grain not prep	¼ cup	180	3	1	0
ANCHOVY					
boneless	1 oz	60	3	1	–

FOOD	PORTION	CALS	FAT	SAT FAT	TRANS FAT
canned in oil drained	1 can (2 oz)	94	4	1	–
fresh	1 (4 g)	8	tr	tr	–
fresh fillets	3 (0.4 oz)	21	1	–	–
Brunswick					
Flat Fillets	1 can (2 oz)	25	2	0	–

ANGLERFISH
raw	3.5 oz	72	1	–	–

ANISE
seed	1 tsp	7	tr	tr	0

ANTELOPE
roasted	4 oz	215	4	2	–

APPLE
CANNED

sliced sweetened	½ cup	68	1	tr	–
Glory					
Fried Apples	½ cup	80	0	0	0
DRIED					
chopped	½ cup	104	tr	tr	–
cooked w/o sugar	½ cup	73	tr	tr	–
rings	5	78	tr	tr	–
Bare Fruit					
Chips Cinnamon	1 pkg (0.6 oz)	43	0	0	0
Crispy Green					
Crispy Apples	1 pkg (0.36 oz)	35	0	0	0
Del Monte					
Dried Apples	¼ cup	110	0	0	0
Fruit Ripples					
Cinnamon Apple	1 pkg	50	0	0	0
Strawberry Apple	1 pkg	50	0	0	0
Mrs. May's					
Fruit Chips	1 pkg	35	0	0	0
FRESH					
apple	1 sm	55	tr	tr	–
apple	1 med	72	tr	tr	–
apple	1 lg	110	tr	tr	–
candied	1 sm (4.9 oz)	179	3	2	–
candied	1 med (6.5 oz)	234	4	3	–
candied	1 lg (9.8 oz)	357	6	4	–

FOOD	PORTION	CALS	FAT	SAT FAT	TRANS FAT
w/ skin sliced	1 cup	57	tr	tr	–
w/o skin sliced	1 cup	53	tr	tr	–
Chiquita					
Apple	1 med (5.4 oz)	80	0	0	0
Earthbound Farm					
Organic Slices	1 pkg (2 oz)	30	0	0	0
Mrs. Prindable's					
Caramel Triple Chocolate	¼ apple (1.7 oz)	120	6	4	0
Caramel Walnut	¼ apple (2 oz)	160	10	4	0
Rainier					
Apple	1 med (5.5 oz)	80	0	0	0
Sullivan					
McIntosh	1 (5.4 oz)	80	1	–	0
TreeTop					
Slices Red or Green	1 pkg (2 oz)	35	0	0	0
FROZEN					
sliced w/o sugar	½ cup	42	tr	tr	–
Roast Works					
Flame Roasted Fuji	1 serv (5 oz)	90	0	0	0
TAKE-OUT					
baked	1 (6 oz)	128	tr	tr	–
baked no sugar	1 (5.6 oz)	136	tr	tr	–
fried apple rings	1 serv (2.7 oz)	91	4	1	–
APPLE JUICE					
cider	1 cup	117	tr	tr	–
juice + vitamin C & calcium	1 cup	117	tr	tr	–
mulled cider	1 pkg	265	1	tr	–
unsweetened w/o vitamin C	1 cup	117	tr	tr	–
After The Fall					
Organic	8 oz	90	0	0	0
Apple & Eve					
100% Juice	8 oz	110	0	0	0
Celestial Seasonings					
Cider Apple Caramel Kiss as prep	1 cup	80	0	0	0
Eden					
Organic Juice	8 oz	90	0	0	0
Fizz Ed.					
Green Apple	1 can (8.4 oz)	100	0	0	0

FOOD	PORTION	CALS	FAT	SAT FAT	TRANS FAT
Hansen's					
100% Juice	8 oz	120	0	0	0
Hood					
100% Juice	1 cup	120	0	0	0
Izze					
Sparkling Apple	12 oz	138	0	0	0
Kedem					
100% Juice	8 oz	110	0	0	0
Langers					
Diet Cocktail 50% Juice	8 oz	60	0	0	0
Harvest Apple 100% Juice	8 oz	120	0	0	0
Low Carb Creations					
Apple Cider as prep	1 pkg	10	0	0	0
Minute Maid					
100% Juice	8 oz	100	0	0	0
Mott's					
Hot Spiced Cider All Flavors as prep	1 pkg	80	0	0	0
Naked Juice					
Just Apple	8 oz	120	0	0	0
Ocean Spray					
100% Juice	8 oz	110	0	0	0
Old Orchard					
Cider 100%	8 oz	120	0	0	0
Healthy Balance Apple	8 oz	30	0	0	0
Organic 100% Juice	8 oz	128	0	0	0
Phat Phruit					
Green Apple	8 oz	40	0	0	0
Red Cheek					
100% Juice	8 oz	120	0	0	0
Robert & James					
100% Juice	8 oz	110	0	0	0
Seneca					
100% Juice	8 oz	110	0	0	0
Snapple					
Diet	8 oz	15	0	0	0
Tree Ripe					
Organic 100% Juice	6 oz	80	0	0	0
TreeTop					
100% Juice	8 oz	120	0	0	0

FOOD	PORTION	CALS	FAT	SAT FAT	TRANS FAT
Cider 100% Juice No Sugar Added	8 oz	120	0	0	0
Tropicana					
Orchard Style	14 oz	200	0	0	0
Walnut Acres					
Organic Juice	8 oz	110	0	0	0
Zeigler's					
Old Fashioned Cider	8 oz	110	0	0	0

APPLESAUCE

FOOD	PORTION	CALS	FAT	SAT FAT	TRANS FAT
sweetened	½ cup	97	tr	tr	–
unsweetened	½ cup	52	tr	tr	–
Eden					
Organic	½ cup	60	0	0	0
Organic Apple Cherry	½ cup	70	0	0	0
Organic Apple Strawberry	½ cup	60	0	0	0
Organic Cinnamon	1 pkg (4 oz)	70	0	0	0
Jok'n'Al					
Low Carb	1 tbsp	10	0	0	0
Langers					
Unsweetened	½ cup	50	0	0	0
Mott's					
Original	½ cup	110	0	0	0
Single-Serve Cinnamon	1 pkg (4 oz)	100	0	0	0
Single-Serve Natural	1 pkg (4 oz)	50	0	0	0
Musselman's					
Apple Sauce	1 pkg (4 oz)	80	0	0	0
Lite	1 pkg (4 oz)	50	0	0	0
Vermont Village					
Organic Unsweetened	½ cup	80	0	0	0
White House					
Apple Sauce	1 pkg (4 oz)	90	0	0	0

APRICOT JUICE

FOOD	PORTION	CALS	FAT	SAT FAT	TRANS FAT
nectar	6 oz	106	tr	tr	–
Ceres					
Apricot	8 oz	120	0	0	0

APRICOTS

FOOD	PORTION	CALS	FAT	SAT FAT	TRANS FAT
canned in heavy syrup	½ cup	91	tr	tr	0

FOOD	PORTION	CALS	FAT	SAT FAT	TRANS FAT
canned in juice	½ cup	59	tr	tr	0
canned in water	½ cup	33	tr	tr	0
canned in light syrup	½ cup	80	tr	tr	0
dried halves	6	51	tr	tr	0
dried halves cooked w/o sugar	½ cup	106	tr	tr	0
fresh	1	17	tr	tr	0
fresh sliced	½ cup	40	tr	tr	0
frozen sweetened	½ cup	119	tr	tr	0
Chiquita					
Fresh	3 med (4 oz)	60	1	0	–
Crispy Green					
Crispy Dried	1 pkg (0.36 oz)	40	0	0	0
Del Monte					
Halves In Heavy Syrup	½ cup	100	0	0	0
Orchard Select Halves	½ cup	80	0	0	0
Harvest Bay					
Dried	5 (1.4 oz)	60	0	0	0
Mariani					
Ultimate Dried	¼ cup (1.4 oz)	100	0	0	0
Sunsweet					
Dried	6 (1.4 oz)	100	0	0	0

ARROWHEAD

FOOD	PORTION	CALS	FAT	SAT FAT	TRANS FAT
corm boiled	1 med	9	tr	–	–

ARROWROOT

FOOD	PORTION	CALS	FAT	SAT FAT	TRANS FAT
raw	1 root (1.2 oz)	21	tr	tr	–
raw root sliced	1 cup	78	tr	tr	–
Bob's Red Mill					
Starch	¼ cup	110	0	0	0

ARTICHOKE
CANNED

FOOD	PORTION	CALS	FAT	SAT FAT	TRANS FAT
hearts in oil	1 serv (3 oz)	100	7	1	–
Gertie's Finest					
Tapenade	2 tbsp	29	3	tr	0
Native Forest					
Organic Hearts Quartered	1 serv (4 oz)	35	0	0	0
Progresso					
Hearts	1	15	0	0	0

FOOD	PORTION	CALS	FAT	SAT FAT	TRANS FAT
FRESH					
cooked	1 med	60	tr	tr	–
hearts cooked	½ cup	42	tr	tr	–
FROZEN					
cooked	1 cup	42	tr	tr	–
cooked w/o salt	1 pkg (9 oz)	108	1	0	–
C&W					
Hearts	12 (3 oz)	40	1	0	0
TAKE-OUT					
stuffed	1 (8.8 oz)	397	14	3	–

ARUGULA

FOOD	PORTION	CALS	FAT	SAT FAT	TRANS FAT
fresh	1 cup	3	tr	tr	–

ASIAN FOOD (see also DINNER, EGG ROLLS, SAUCE, SOY SAUCE, SUSHI)

FOOD	PORTION	CALS	FAT	SAT FAT	TRANS FAT
CANNED					
chow mein chicken w/o noodles	1 cup	194	8	2	–
FRESH					
wonton wrappers	1	23	tr	tr	–
Azumaya					
Round Wraps	10	160	1	0	–
Wrappers Large Square	8	160	1	0	–
Frieda's					
Won Ton Wrappers	4 (1 oz)	80	0	0	0
Nasoya					
Won Ton Wrappers	8	160	1	0	–
FROZEN					
Amy's					
Skillet Meals Teriyaki Stir Fry	1 cup	320	3	0	–
Contessa					
Chow Mein Chicken w/ Sauce not prep	1¾ cups	320	3	1	0
Curry Chicken w/ Sauce not prep	1¾ cups	240	8	4	0
Fried Rice Chicken w/ Sauce not prep	1¾ cups	260	4	1	0
General Tsao Shrimp w/ Sauce not prep	1¾ cups	270	4	1	0
Kung Pao Shrimp w/ Sauce not prep	1¾ cups	200	4	1	0

FOOD	PORTION	CALS	FAT	SAT FAT	TRANS FAT
Low Mein Shrimp w/ Sauce not prep	1¾ cups	250	10	2	0
Stir-Fry Beef w/ sauce not prep	1¾ cup	190	3	1	0
Stir-Fry Chicken w/ Sauce not prep	1¾ cups	160	3	1	0
Stir-Fry Shrimp w/ Sauce not prep	1¾ cups	120	3	1	0
Sweet & Sour Shrimp w/ Sauce not prep	1½ cups	180	0	0	0
Tandoori Chicken w/ Sauce not prep	1⅓ cups	200	4	1	0
Glutino					
Gluten Free Chicken Pad Thai Peach	1 pkg (7 oz)	370	5	1	0
Helen's Kitchen					
Thai Yellow Curry w/ Tofu Steaks & Vegetables & Basmati Rice	1 pkg (9 oz)	280	5	1	0
Kahiki					
Beef & Broccoli	1 pkg (10.9 oz)	360	10	4	0
Chicken Fried Rice	1 pkg (10.9 oz)	460	10	2	0
General Tso's Chicken	1 pkg (10 oz)	400	10	2	0
Naturals General Tso's Chicken	1 pkg (10 oz)	330	5	1	0
Naturals Mandarin Orange Chicken	1 pkg (10 oz)	340	5	1	0
Naturals Szechuan Peppercorn Beef	1 pkg (10 oz)	350	14	5	0
Naturals Teriyaki Mixed Vegetables	1 pkg (10 oz)	260	2	0	0
Sesame Orange Chicken	1 pkg (10.9 oz)	420	12	2	0
Soothing Lettuce Wraps	4 tbsp (2 oz)	90	4	1	0
Tempura Chicken Nuggets	¾ cup (3.5 oz)	230	14	3	0
Tropical Sweet & Sour Chicken	1 pkg (10.9 oz)	490	11	2	0
Lean Cuisine					
Cafe Classics Asian Style Beef w/ Ginger & Soy	1 pkg (9.25 oz)	210	4	4	0
Cafe Classics Bowl Chicken Fried Rice	1 pkg (10 oz)	310	7	2	0

FOOD	PORTION	CALS	FAT	SAT FAT	TRANS FAT
Cafe Classics Bowl Chicken Teriyaki	1 pkg (11 oz)	320	3	1	0
Cafe Classics Bowl Teriyaki Steak	1 pkg (10.5 oz)	340	7	3	0
Cafe Classics Chicken Teriyaki Stir Fry	1 pkg (10 oz)	300	5	1	0
Cafe Classics Hunan Beef & Broccoli	1 pkg (8.5 oz)	230	4	2	0
Cafe Classics Thai-Style Chicken	1 pkg (9 oz)	230	4	2	0
One Dish Favorites Asian Style Pot Stickers	1 pkg (9 oz)	320	6	2	0
One Dish Favorites Chicken Chow Mein	1 pkg (9 oz)	200	3	1	0
Skillet Asian Style Chicken & Vegetables	1 serv	160	3	1	0
Organic Classics					
Thai Chicken Curry	1 pkg (10 oz)	420	17	6	0
Seeds Of Change					
Asian Stir-Fry Noodles	1 pkg (11 oz)	290	4	1	0
Spicy Peanut Noodles	1 pkg (11 oz)	370	12	5	0
Teriyaki Stir Fried Rice	1 pkg (11 oz)	340	8	1	0
Tyson					
Meal Kit Chicken Fried Rice	2½ cups	440	6	2	0
MIX					
Annie Chun's					
Meal Kit Chow Mein Noodles w/ Garlic Black Bean Sauce	⅓ pkg	230	3	0	–
Meal Kit Chow Mein Noodles w/ Peanut Sesame Sauce	⅓ pkg	270	7	1	–
Meal Kit Chow Mein Noodles w/ Scallion Sauce	⅓ pkg	240	5	1	–
Meal Kit Chow Mein Noodles w/ Teriyaki Sauce	⅓ box	210	1	0	–
Meal Kit Pad Thai Noodles w/ Pad Thai Sauce	⅓ pkg	210	1	0	–
Meal Kit Soba Noodles w/ Soy Ginger Sauce	⅓ pkg	210	2	0	–
Nissin					
Chow Mein Chicken as prep	½ pkg (2 oz)	240	9	5	0

FOOD	PORTION	CALS	FAT	SAT FAT	TRANS FAT
Chow Mein Thai Peanut as prep	½ pkg (2 oz)	270	12	4	0
SHELF-STABLE					
Fantastic					
Pad Thai w/ Rice Noodles	1 pkg (7 oz)	400	11	3	–
Thai Lemon Grass w/ Rice Noodles	1 pkg (7.4 oz)	340	10	4	–
TAKE-OUT					
beef & broccoli	1 cup	221	12	3	–
buddha's delight w/ cellophane noodles fat choi jai	1 serv (7.6 oz)	211	4	1	–
cha siu bao steamed buns w/ chicken filling	1 (2.3 oz)	160	3	1	–
chinese style fried egg noodles w/ seafood & lettuce	1 serv (14 oz)	694	37	14	–
chow mein beef w/o noodles	1 cup	271	15	4	–
chow mein noodles	1 cup	237	14	2	–
chow mein pork w/o noodles	1 cup	284	16	4	–
chow mein shrimp w/o noodles	1 cup	154	5	1	–
chow mein vegetable w/o noodles	1 cup	224	15	2	0
dim sum meat filled	3 pieces (4 oz)	124	3	1	–
egg foo yung beef	1 patty (6 oz)	243	16	4	–
egg foo yung chicken	1 patty (3 oz)	121	8	2	–
egg foo yung pork	1 patty (3 oz)	125	8	2	–
egg foo yung shrimp	1 patty (3 oz)	153	12	3	–
filipino chicken adobo	1 serv (15 oz)	555	26	7	–
foochow fish ball	1 (1 oz)	36	2	1	–
fried rice	1 cup	333	12	2	–
fried rice beef	1 cup	346	14	3	–
fried rice chicken	1 cup	329	12	2	0
fried rice pork	1 cup	335	13	3	–
fried rice shrimp	1 cup	323	12	2	–
general tsao's chicken	1 cup	296	17	4	–
green beans szechuan style	1 cup	176	12	2	–
indian style fried egg noodles w/ eggs tomato sauce & lime	1 serv (15 oz)	721	31	13	–
kung pao beef	1 cup	410	30	8	–
kung pao chicken	1 cup	434	31	5	–

FOOD	PORTION	CALS	FAT	SAT FAT	TRANS FAT
kung pao pork	1 cup	460	34	7	–
kung pao shrimp	1 cup	345	20	3	–
lo mein beef	1 cup	286	11	3	–
lo mein chicken	1 cup	262	9	2	–
lo mein meatless	1 cup	234	6	1	–
lo mein pork	1 cup	314	14	4	–
lo mein shrimp	1 cup	236	7	1	–
moo goo gai pan chicken	1 cup	272	19	4	–
moo shu pork w/o pancake	1 cup	512	46	7	–
phad thai	1 serv (9.2 oz)	232	9	1	–
sesame seed paste bun	1 (2.5 oz)	220	6	1	–
shrimp chips banh phong tom	6 med	214	14	2	–
shrimp w/ lobster sauce	1 cup	298	12	2	–
shu mai chicken & vegetable dumplings	6 (3.6 oz)	160	5	1	–
spring roll	1 (3.5 oz)	112	2	–	–
sukiyaki beef	1 cup	165	7	3	–
sweet & sour chicken w/o rice	1 cup	670	37	9	–
sweet & sour pork w/ rice	1 cup	268	6	2	–
sweet & sour pork w/o rice	1 cup	231	8	2	–
sweet & sour shrimp	1 cup	480	30	4	–
sweet red bean bun	1 (2.5 oz)	130	1	0	–
szechuan chicken	1 cup	190	9	2	–
szechuan shrimp & vegetables	1 cup	159	7	1	–
tempura vegetable	8 pieces	90	6	1	–
tempura hawaiian fish tofu vegetable	2 cups	285	22	4	–
teriyaki beef	1 cup	454	19	6	–
teriyaki chicken plain	¾ cup	399	27	6	–
teriyaki chicken w/ rice	1 serv (11 oz)	430	6	1	–
teriyaki shrimp	1 cup	271	3	1	–
thai style pineapple rice w/ ham & pork floss	1 serv (7.7 oz)	408	14	6	–
wonton fried meat filled	1 (0.7 oz)	54	3	1	–
wonton meat & shrimp boiled	1 (0.5 oz)	19	1	tr	–

ASPARAGUS
CANNED

FOOD	PORTION	CALS	FAT	SAT FAT	TRANS FAT
spears	1	3	tr	tr	0
spears	1 cup	46	2	tr	–

FOOD	PORTION	CALS	FAT	SAT FAT	TRANS FAT
Del Monte					
Cuts & Tips	½ cup	20	0	0	0
Spears	½ cup	20	0	0	0
Tips	½ cup	20	0	0	0
Gertie's Finest					
White	1 oz	15	0	0	0
Green Giant					
Spears Extra Long	5	20	0	0	0
Native Forest					
White	1 serv (4 oz)	20	0	0	0
S&W					
Green	6 (4.5 oz)	15	0	0	0
Tillen Farms					
Crispy Asparagus Pickled	3 spears	10	0	0	0
FRESH					
cooked	½ cup	20	tr	tr	–
cooked	4 spears	13	tr	tr	–
spears raw	4	10	tr	tr	–
Alpine Fresh					
Fresh Green	5 spears (3.3 oz)	20	0	0	0
Frieda's					
White	⅔ cup	20	0	0	0
FROZEN					
cooked	1 pkg (10 oz)	53	1	tr	–
cooked	4 spears	11	tr	tr	–
C&W					
Spears	7 (3 oz)	20	0	0	0
Europe's Best					
Spears	7 spears	15	1	0	0
ATEMOYA					
fresh	½ cup	94	1	–	–
AVOCADO					
california mashed	¼ cup	96	9	1	–
california peeled & pitted	1	289	27	4	–
florida mashed	¼ cup	69	6	1	–
florida peeled & pitted	1	365	31	6	–
Brooks Tropical					
Lite SlimCado	1 tbsp	35	3	1	–

FOOD	PORTION	CALS	FAT	SAT FAT	TRANS FAT
Calavo					
Fresh	⅕ med (1 oz)	55	5	1	–
Chiquita					
Fresh	⅓ med (1 oz)	55	5	1	–
Earthbound Farm					
Organic Fresh	⅕ med (1 oz)	55	5	1	0
Frieda's					
Fresh Cocktail	1 (1.4 oz)	60	6	1	–
TAKE-OUT					
guacamole	1 serv (2.2 oz)	105	10	1	–
BACON					
bacon grease	1 tbsp	116	13	5	–
beef breakfast strips cooked	3 strips	153	12	5	–
gammon lean & fat grilled	4.2 oz	274	15	–	–
pan fried	3 strips	109	9	3	–
turkey	2 (0.8 oz)	84	6	6	–
Boar's Head					
Fully Cooked Slices	3 (0.5 oz)	70	6	2	0
Jennie-O					
Turkey Bacon	1 slice (0.5 oz)	35	3	1	–
Oscar Mayer					
Bacon Bits	1 tbsp (7 g)	25	2	1	0
Center Cut cooked	2 slices (0.4 oz)	50	4	2	–
Hardwood Smoked	2 slices (0.5 oz)	70	6	2	–
Lower Sodium	3 slices (0.5 oz)	70	6	3	0
Ready To Serve	3 slices	70	5	2	0
Uncured	3 slices (0.5 oz)	60	5	3	0
Tyson					
Hickory Thick Cut	2 pieces (0.8 oz)	140	11	4	–
Wellshire					
Beef Uncured	2 oz	114	3	1	–
Panchetta Sliced	1 slice (0.4 oz)	60	3	2	–
Pork Range Sliced Dry Rubbed	2 slices	30	3	2	–
Uncured Turkey	1 slice (1 oz)	20	1	0	0
BACON SUBSTITUTES					
bacon bits meatless	1 tbsp	33	2	tr	–
meatless	1 strip	16	1	tr	–
Bob's Red Mill					
Bac'Ums	4 tsp	25	1	0	0

FOOD	PORTION	CALS	FAT	SAT FAT	TRANS FAT
Lightlife					
Organic Tempeh Smokey Strips	3 slices (2 oz)	80	3	1	–
Smart Bacon	2 strips (0.8 oz)	45	2	0	–
Worthington					
Stripples	2 strips (0.5 oz)	60	5	1	0
BAGEL					
cinnamon raisin	1 mini	71	tr	tr	–
cinnamon raisin	1 lg (4 in)	244	2	tr	–
egg	1 lg (4.5 in)	364	3	1	–
low carb	1 (4 oz)	216	0	0	0
mini onion	1 (1.4 oz)	100	0	0	0
oat bran	1 lg (4 in)	227	1	tr	–
plain	1 sm (3 in)	190	1	tr	–
plain	1 med (3.5 in)	289	2	tr	–
plain	1 lg (4.5 in)	360	2	tr	–
Alvarado Street Bakery					
Sprouted Wheat Cinnamon Raisin	1 (3.3 oz)	280	1	0	0
David's					
Deli Bagels	1 (2.8 oz)	230	1	0	0
Enjoy Life					
Nut Gluten Free Classic Original	1 (3 oz)	270	7	0	0
Natural Ovens					
Blueberry	1 (3 oz)	190	2	0	–
Brainy	1 (3 oz)	170	2	0	–
Cinnamon Raisin	1 (3 oz)	180	1	0	–
Golden Crunch	1 (3 oz)	190	11	0	–
Hearty Grains & Onion	1 (3 oz)	190	4	1	–
Raspberry	1 (3 oz)	180	2	0	–
Whole Grain	1 (3 oz)	170	3	0	–
New York Style					
Crisps Natural Whole Wheat	6	120	6	3	0
Crisps Plain	7	140	6	3	0
Pepperidge Farm					
100% Whole Wheat	1	250	2	0	0
Everything	1	260	2	1	0
Mini 100% Whole Wheat	1	100	1	0	0
Mini Plain	1	110	1	0	0

FOOD	PORTION	CALS	FAT	SAT FAT	TRANS FAT
Sara Lee					
Apple Cinnamon	1 (4 oz)	310	2	0	–
Banana Walnut	1 (4 oz)	350	7	2	–
Blueberry Deluxe	1 (3.3 oz)	260	1	0	–
Blueberry Junior	1 (1 oz)	70	0	0	0
Blueberry Toaster Size	1 (2.1 oz)	160	1	0	–
Cinnamon Raisin Deluxe	1 (3.3 oz)	260	1	0	–
Heart Healthy 100% Whole Wheat	1 (3.3 oz)	220	2	1	0
Heart Healthy Cinnamon Raisin	1 (3.3 oz)	250	2	1	0
Plain	1 (2.1 oz)	160	1	0	–
Sundried Tomato & Basil	1 (4 oz)	300	2	0	–
Whole Grain Plain	1 (3.3 oz)	240	1	1	0
Thomas'					
Bagelbread Mini Squares 100% Whole Wheat	1 (2 oz)	150	1	0	0
Carb Consider Plain	1	150	3	1	–
Carb Consider Whole Wheat	1	140	3	1	–
Weight Watchers					
Original	1 (2.8 oz)	190	2	1	–
BAKING POWDER					
baking powder	1 tsp	2	0	0	0
low sodium	1 tsp	5	tr	tr	0
Bob's Red Mills					
Baking Powder	1 tsp	5	0	0	0
Calumet					
Double Acting	⅛ tsp	0	0	0	0
Clabber Girl					
Baking Powder	1 tsp	0	0	0	0
Davis					
Baking Powder	1 tsp	0	0	0	0
Rumford					
Aluminum Free	⅛ tsp	0	0	0	0
BAKING SODA					
baking soda	1 tsp	0	0	0	0
Bob's Red Mill					
Baking Soda	¼ tsp	0	0	0	0

FOOD	PORTION	CALS	FAT	SAT FAT	TRANS FAT
BALSAM PEAR (BITTER GOURD)					
leafy tips cooked w/o salt	1 cup	20	tr	tr	–
leafy tips raw	1 cup	14	tr	–	–
pods raw sliced	1 cup	16	tr	–	–
pods sliced cooked w/ salt	1 cup	24	tr	–	–
BAMBOO SHOOTS					
canned sliced	½ cup	12	tr	tr	–
fresh sliced cooked w/ salt	½ cup	7	tr	tr	–
raw sliced	½ cup	20	tr	tr	–
BANANA					
banana chips	1 oz	147	10	8	–
fresh	1 sm (6 in)	90	tr	tr	–
fresh	1 med (7 in)	105	tr	tr	–
fresh	1 lg (8 in)	121	tr	tr	–
fresh baby	1 extra sm (<6 in)	72	tr	tr	0
fresh mashed	½ cup	100	tr	tr	–
fresh sliced	1 cup	134	1	tr	–
powder	1 tbsp	21	tr	tr	–
whole dried	1 piece (1.2 oz)	130	1	0	–
Bob's Red Mill					
Chips	25 (1.4 oz)	210	11	1	0
Frieda's					
Burro	1 (3 oz)	80	0	0	0
Dried	1 piece (1.2 oz)	130	1	0	0
Goodniks					
Nutty Bananas Crunchy Snack	⅔ cup	230	16	13	0
TAKE-OUT					
fritter	1 (2.3 oz)	197	5	3	1
BARBECUE SAUCE					
barbecue	2 tbsp	52	tr	0	0
low sodium	2 tbsp	52	tr	0	0
Annie's Naturals					
Organic Orignal	2 tbsp	45	1	–	–
Bone Suckin'					
Sauce	2 tbsp	40	0	0	0
Carb Options					
Original	2 tbsp	10	0	0	0

FOOD	PORTION	CALS	FAT	SAT FAT	TRANS FAT
Cattlemen's					
Classic	2 tbsp	60	0	0	0
Honey	2 tbsp	70	0	0	0
Smokehouse	2 tbsp	60	0	0	0
Consorzio					
Organic Original	1 tbsp	50	0	0	0
Organic Spicy	1 tbsp	50	0	0	0
David Burke					
Flavor Spray Memphis BBQ	2 sprays	0	0	0	0
Emeril's					
Original BBQ	2 tbsp	45	0	0	0
Hunt's					
Hickory	2 tbsp	45	0	0	0
Hickory & Brown Sugar	2 tbsp	70	0	0	0
Honey Hickory	2 tbsp	50	0	0	0
Honey Mustard	2 tbsp	50	0	0	0
Hot & Spicy	2 tbsp	45	0	0	0
Mesquite	2 tbsp	40	0	0	0
Original	2 tbsp	50	0	0	0
Original Bold	2 tbsp	45	0	0	0
Nando's					
Barbecue	1 tbsp	7	0	0	0
San-J					
Asian BBQ	2 tbsp	40	0	0	0
Steel's					
Sugar Free	2 tbsp	15	0	0	0
Wellshire					
Original	2 tbsp	39	0	0	0
BARLEY					
flour	1 cup	511	2	tr	–
pearled cooked	1 cup (5.5 oz)	193	1	tr	–
pearled uncooked	¼ cup	176	1	tr	–
Arrowhead Mills					
Organic Pearled not prep	¼ cup	160	1	0	0
Mother's					
Quick Cooking	⅓ cup	170	1	0	–
Robinsons					
Barley Water Lemon as prep	9 oz	48	5	–	–

FOOD	PORTION	CALS	FAT	SAT FAT	TRANS FAT
BARRACUDA					
broiled	4 oz	239	14	4	–
cooked flaked	1 cup	287	16	4	–
poached	4 oz	227	11	3	–
TAKE-OUT					
breaded & fried	4 oz	282	17	4	–
BASIL					
fresh chopped	2 tbsp	1	tr	tr	0
ground	1 tsp	4	tr	tr	0
leaves fresh	5	1	tr	tr	0
Dorot					
Chopped Cube frzn	1 cube (4 g)	5	tr	tr	0
Eden					
Shiso Leaf Powder	1 tsp	0	0	0	0
BASS					
breaded baked	4 oz	205	7	1	0
pickled mero en escabeche	2 oz	156	14	2	0
striped baked	3 oz	105	3	1	0
striped bass farm raised	4 oz	110	3	1	–
BAY LEAF					
crumbled	1 tsp	2	tr	tr	0
BEAN SPROUTS (see ALFALFA SPROUTS)					
BEANS (see also individual names)					
CANNED					
baked beans plain	½ cup	119	tr	tr	–
baked beans vegetarian	½ cup	119	tr	tr	–
baked beans w/ franks	½ cup	184	9	3	–
baked beans w/ pork	½ cup	134	2	1	–
baked beans w/ pork & tomato sauce	½ cup	119	1	tr	–
refried beans	½ cup	134	1	1	–
Amy's					
Vegetarian Baked	½ cup	120	5	1	–
B&M					
Bacon & Onion	½ cup	190	2	1	0
Maple Baked	½ cup	150	1	0	–
Vegetarian 99% Fat Free	½ cup	150	1	0	–

FOOD	PORTION	CALS	FAT	SAT FAT	TRANS FAT
Bush's					
Barbecue	½ cup	150	1	0	0
Boston Recipe	½ cup	150	1	0	0
Country Style	½ cup	170	1	0	–
Homestyle	½ cup	140	1	0	0
Maple Cured Bacon	½ cup	150	1	1	–
Onion 98% Fat Free	½ cup	140	1	0	0
Original	½ cup	150	1	0	–
Vegetarian Fat Free	½ cup	130	0	0	0
Campbell's					
Pork & Beans	½ cup	140	2	1	0
Eden					
Organic Baked w/ Sorghum	½ cup	150	0	0	0
Green Giant					
Three Bean Salad	½ cup	80	0	0	0
Heinz					
Vegetarian	1 cup	250	1	0	–
Las Palmas					
Refried	½ cup	150	3	1	0
Old El Paso					
Refried Fat Free	½ cup	100	0	0	0
Refried Fat Free Spicy	½ cup	100	0	0	0
Pace					
Refried Salsa	½ cup	70	0	0	0
Ranch Style					
Original Texas	½ cup	138	3	1	–
Read					
3 Bean Salad	½ cup	60	0	0	0
Rosarita					
Refried No Fat	½ cup	90	0	0	0
Refried Traditional 98% Fat Free	½ cup	100	2	1	–
Van Camp's					
Baked Beans w/ Chicken	1 cup	360	2	0	0
Baked Original	½ cup	140	1	0	–
Pork And Beans	½ cup	110	1	0	0
FROZEN					
Lean Cuisine					
Cafe Classics Sante Fe Style Rice & Beans	1 pkg (10.4 oz)	290	5	2	0

FOOD	PORTION	CALS	FAT	SAT FAT	TRANS FAT
MIX					
Fantastic					
Instant Black Beans not prep	⅓ cup	160	2	0	–
Instant Refried Beans not prep	¼ cup	130	2	0	–
TAKE-OUT					
baked beans	½ cup	191	7	2	–
barbecue beans	3.5 oz	120	tr	tr	–
frijolas a la charra w/ pork tomatoes & chili peppers	1 cup	341	22	8	–
refried beans	½ cup	43	2	1	–
three bean salad	1 cup	114	5	1	–
BEAR					
simmered	3 oz	220	11	3	0
BEAVER					
roasted	4 oz	240	8	2	0
BEECHNUTS					
dried	1 oz	163	14	2	0
BEEF (see also BEEF DISHES, MEAT STICKS, MEATBALLS, VEAL)					
CANNED					
corned beef	1 oz	71	4	2	–
FRESH					
arm pot roast trim 0 fat braised	3.5 oz	297	19	8	–
arm pot roast trim ⅛ in fat braised	3.5 oz	302	19	8	–
beef crumbles 70% lean pan browned	3 oz	230	15	6	–
bottom round roast trim 0 in fat braised	4 oz	253	10	4	–
bottom round roast trim 0 in fat roasted	3.5 oz	187	8	3	–
bottom round roast trim ½ in fat braised	4 oz	337	22	8	–
bottom round roast trim ⅛ in fat braised	4 oz	280	13	5	–
bottom round roast trim ⅛ in fat roasted	4 oz	247	13	5	–

FOOD	PORTION	CALS	FAT	SAT FAT	TRANS FAT
bottom sirloin butt roast trim 0 in roasted	3.5 oz	182	8	3	–
brisket flat half trim 1/8 in fat braised	3.5 oz	298	19	8	–
brisket flat trim 0 fat braised	3.5 oz	221	9	4	–
brisket point half trim 0 fat braised	3.5 oz	358	29	11	–
brisket point half trim 1/4 in fat braised	3.5 oz	404	22	14	–
brisket point half trim 1/8 in fat braised	3.5 oz	349	27	11	–
chuck boston cut roast trim 0 fat roasted	3.5 oz	207	11	4	–
chuck boston cut roast trim 1/4 in fat roasted	3.5 oz	242	15	6	–
chuck bottom roast trim 0 fat braised	3.5 oz	334	24	10	–
chuck bottom roast trim 1/4 in fat braised	3.5 oz	345	26	10	–
chuck fillet steak trim 0 fat broiled	4 oz	181	6	2	–
chuck top roast trim 0 fat broiled	4 oz	245	13	4	–
club steak trim 1/2 in fat broiled	4 oz	384	29	12	–
corned beef brisket cooked	3 oz	213	16	5	–
crosscut shank trim 1/4 in fat stewed	1 serv (6.8 oz)	510	28	11	–
delmonico steak trim 1/4 in fat broiled	4 oz	409	33	13	–
entrecote steak trim 1/2 in fat broiled	4 oz	413	33	14	–
eye round roast trim 0 in fat roasted	4 oz	190	5	2	–
eye round roast trim 1/4 in fat roasted	4 oz	283	17	7	–
eye round roast trim 1/8 in fat roasted	4 oz	236	11	4	–
filet mignon roast trim 1/4 in fat roasted	4 oz	376	29	11	–

FOOD	PORTION	CALS	FAT	SAT FAT	TRANS FAT
filet mignon roast trim ⅛ in fat roasted	4 oz	367	28	11	–
filet mignon trim 0 in fat broiled	4 oz	247	13	5	–
filet mignon trim ⅛ in fat broiled	4 oz	303	19	8	–
ground 70% lean broiled	3.5 oz	273	18	7	–
ground 75% lean broiled	2.5 oz	195	13	5	–
ground 80% lean broiled	3 oz	234	15	6	–
ground 85% lean pan fried	3 oz	197	12	5	–
ground 90% lean pan fried	3 oz	173	9	4	–
ground 95% lean pan fried	3 oz	139	5	2	–
ground 97% fat free irradiated	4 oz	160	8	3	–
ground low-fat w/ carrageenan raw	4 oz	160	7	4	–
london broil trim 0 fat broiled	3.5 oz	188	8	3	–
london broil trim ¼ in fat broiled	4 oz	260	12	4	–
new york strip steak trim 0 fat broiled	4 oz	219	9	3	–
oxtails cooked	6 pieces (6.3 oz)	472	26	10	0
porterhouse steak trim 0 in fat broiled	1 lb	1252	87	33	–
porterhouse steak trim ¼ in fat broiled	1 lb	1492	117	46	–
porterhouse steak trim ⅛ in fat broiled	1 lb	1324	99	38	–
porterhouse steak trim ⅛ in fat broiled	4 oz	337	25	10	–
rib eye roast trim ¼ in fat roasted	3.5 oz	365	30	12	–
rib eye steak trim ⅛ in fat broiled	4 oz	221	9	3	–
rib roast trim ¼ in fat roasted	4 oz	406	33	13	–
rib steak trim ¼ in fat broiled	4 oz	388	31	13	–
round tip roast trim 0 in fat roasted	4 oz	213	9	3	–
sandwich steaks thinly sliced	1 serv (2 oz)	173	15	6	–
shell steak trim ¼ in fat broiled	4 oz	366	27	11	–

FOOD	PORTION	CALS	FAT	SAT FAT	TRANS FAT
shortribs lean & fat braised	1 serv (7.8 oz)	1060	94	40	–
skirt steak trim 0 fat broiled	4 oz	289	19	8	–
t-bone steak trim 0 fat broiled	4 oz	280	18	7	–
t-bone steak trim ¼ in fat broiled	1 lb	1388	103	40	–
t-bone steak trim ⅛ in fat broiled	1 lb	804	56	22	–
tip round roast trim ⅛ in fat roasted	4 oz	248	13	5	–
top loin steak boneless trim ⅛ in fat broiled	4 oz	299	19	7	–
top round roast trim 0 fat braised	4 oz	237	7	3	–
top round roast trim ¼ in fat braised	4 oz	281	13	5	–
top round roast trim ¼ in fat roasted	4 oz	265	15	6	–
top round steak trim ¼ in fat pan fried	4 oz	314	17	6	–
top sirloin steak trim ⅛ in fat broiled	4 oz	275	16	6	–
top sirloin steak trim ⅛ in fat pan fried	4 oz	355	24	9	–
tri-tip roast trim 0 fat roasted	3.5 oz	218	12	5	–
tri-tip steak trim 0 fat broiled	4 oz	300	17	6	–
Laura's Lean					
Eye Of Round	4 oz	135	4	2	–
Flank Steak	4 oz	140	5	2	–
Ground Beef 92% Lean	4 oz	160	9	4	–
Ground Beef Patties	1 (4 oz)	160	9	4	–
Ground Round 96% Lean	4 oz	140	5	2	–
Ribeye Steak	4 oz	175	9	4	–
Sirloin Steak	4 oz	145	5	2	–
Sirloin Tip	4 oz	130	4	2	–
Strip Steak	4 oz	150	5	2	–
Tenderloin Filet	4 oz	145	5	2	–
Top Round	4 oz	135	4	2	–
Maverick Ranch					
Filet Mignon	4 oz	120	4	2	–
Ground	4 oz	130	5	2	–

FOOD	PORTION	CALS	FAT	SAT FAT	TRANS FAT
Ground Round	4 oz	130	4	2	–
Ground Sirloin & Chuck	4 oz	130	5	2	–
NY Strip Steak	4 oz	150	7	3	–
Rib Eye Steak	4 oz	170	10	4	–
Top Round Steak & Roast	4 oz	110	4	2	–
Top Sirloin	4 oz	160	8	3	–
Organic Prairie					
90% Lean Ground	4 oz	250	13	5	0
Shady Brook					
Tri-Tip Roast Rosemary Garlic & Chardonnay	4 oz	180	9	4	–
Tri-Tip Roast Sizzling Ginger	4 oz	210	10	4	–
FROZEN					
patty broiled medium	3 oz	240	17	7	–
Organic Prairie					
Rib Eye Steak	1 (6 oz)	470	31	12	–
Soy Lean					
Beef Patty	1 (2.5 oz)	90	4	2	–
READY-TO-EAT					
dried beef smoked chopped	1 oz	37	1	1	–
roast beef spread	¼ cup	127	9	4	–
smoked beef cooked	1 sausage (1.4 oz)	134	12	–	–
Boar's Head					
Corned Beef Brisket	2 oz	80	4	2	–
Top Round Deluxe	2 oz	80	2	1	–
Top Round Oven Roasted No Salt Added	2 oz	90	3	2	–
Healthy Ones					
Deli Roast Beef	2 oz	70	2	1	0
Laura's Lean					
Beef Pot Roast Au Jus	3 oz	110	4	2	–
Oscar Mayer					
Slow Roasted Shaved	¼ pkg (1.8 oz)	60	3	1	0
Sara Lee					
Roast Beef Medium or Rare	2 oz	60	2	1	–
Tyson					
Beef Strips Seasoned	1 serv (3 oz)	130	6	2	–
TAKE-OUT					
roast beef rare	2 oz	70	2	1	–

FOOD	PORTION	CALS	FAT	SAT FAT	TRANS FAT
BEEF DISHES					
CANNED					
corned beef hash	3 oz	155	10	5	–
Hormel					
Corned Beef Hash 50% Reduced Fat	1 cup	290	12	5	1
Libby's					
Hash Corned Beef	1 cup	420	24	11	–
FROZEN					
Quaker Maid					
Sandwich Steaks Pure Beef	1 serv (1.8 oz)	120	10	4	0
Tyson					
Steak Country Fried	1 (3.2 oz)	310	23	7	–
REFRIGERATED					
Chi Chi's					
For Tacos! Ground Beef	¼ cup	90	4	2	1
Hormel					
Beef Roast Au Jus	1 serv (5 oz)	200	9	4	–
Beef Tips w/ Gravy	½ cup	170	8	3	0
Huxtable's					
Shepherds Pie Beef	1 pkg (10 oz)	270	11	3	0
Laura's Lean					
Meatloaf w/ Tomato Sauce	1 serv (5 oz)	230	8	4	–
Shredded Beef w/ Barbecue Sauce	1 serv (5 oz)	245	5	2	–
Morton's Of Omaha					
Beef Pot Roast w/ Gravy	1 serv (3 oz)	160	5	2	–
Smithfield					
Beef Tips w/ Gravy	½ cup	170	5	2	–
Tyson					
Chuck Roast w/ Vegetables	1 serv (4 oz)	320	21	9	–
Seasoned Meatloaf	1 serv (5 oz)	320	23	10	–
Steak Tips In Burbon Sauce	1 serv (5 oz)	180	5	2	0
TAKE-OUT					
beef bourguignonne	1 cup	339	12	3	–
beef satay + peanut sauce	2 skewers	253	16	8	0
bool kogi korean marinated beef ribs	4 oz	190	10	4	–
bracciola	1 roll (4.7 oz)	276	14	5	–
bubble & squeak	5 oz	186	13	–	–

FOOD	PORTION	CALS	FAT	SAT FAT	TRANS FAT
bulgoghi korean grilled beef	1 serv (5.2 oz)	256	15	5	–
chipped beef on toast	1 slice (5 oz)	226	10	3	–
cornish pasty	1 (8 oz)	847	52	–	–
goulash w/ potatoes	1 cup	298	12	4	–
greek moussaka	1 serv (8.5 oz)	450	33	14	–
irish stew	1 cup (7 oz)	280	16	9	–
kebab indian	1 (5.4 oz)	553	40	–	–
kheena	6.7 oz	781	71	–	–
koftas	5	280	22	–	–
meatloaf	1 lg slice (5 oz)	294	17	6	–
pepper steak	1 cup	317	20	4	–
pot roast w/ gravy	1 serv (6 oz)	320	10	4	–
samosa	2 (4 oz)	652	62	–	–
shepherds pie	1 serv (7 oz)	282	16	6	–
sloppy joes	1 serv (9 oz)	398	6	2	–
steak & kidney pie w/ top crust	1 slice (5 oz)	400	26	–	–
stew w/ potatoes & vegetables	1 cup	199	5	1	–
stroganoff	1 cup	394	25	10	–
swiss steak w/ sauce	1 serv (8 oz)	234	10	2	–
toad in the hole	1 (4.7 oz)	383	29	–	–
BEEFALO					
roasted	4 oz	213	7	3	–
BEER AND ALE					
alcohol free beer	7 oz	50	tr	–	–
ale brown	10 oz	77	0	0	0
ale pale	10 oz	88	0	0	0
beer light	12 oz	103	0	0	0
beer regular	12 oz	153	0	0	0
black & tan	12 oz	146	0	0	0
boilermaker	1 serv	216	0	0	0
lager	10 oz	80	0	0	0
mead	1 serv	250	0	0	0
pilsener lager	7 oz	85	tr	–	–
shandy	1 serv	125	0	0	0
stout	10 oz	102	0	0	0
Amstel					
Light	12 oz	95	0	0	0
Anchor					
Liberty Ale	12 oz	188	0	0	0

FOOD	PORTION	CALS	FAT	SAT FAT	TRANS FAT
Porter	12 oz	205	0	0	0
Steam	12 oz	152	0	0	0
Beck's					
Beer	12 oz	143	0	0	0
Premium Light	12 oz	64	0	0	0
Blue Moon					
White	12 oz	171	0	0	0
Bud					
Ice Light	12 oz	110	0	0	0
Budweiser					
Beer	12 oz	143	0	0	0
Ice	12 oz	148	0	0	0
Light	12 oz	110	0	0	0
Busch					
Beer	12 oz	133	0	0	0
Ice	12 oz	173	0	0	0
Light	12 oz	110	0	0	0
Clausthaler					
Beer	12 oz	96	0	0	0
Colt 45					
Malt Liquor	12 oz	172	0	0	0
Coors					
Extra Gold	12 oz	147	0	0	0
Light	12 oz	102	0	0	0
Nonalcoholic	12 oz	73	0	0	0
Original	12 oz	148	0	0	0
Corona					
Extra	12 oz	148	0	0	0
Light	12 oz	109	0	0	0
Deschutes					
Bachelor ESB	12 oz	180	0	0	0
Black Butt Porter	12 oz	185	0	0	0
Cascade Ale	12 oz	140	0	0	0
Mirror Pond Pale	12 oz	175	0	0	0
Edison					
Light	12 oz	109	0	0	0
Genessee					
12 Horse	12 oz	152	0	0	0
Genny Light	12 oz	96	0	0	0

FOOD	PORTION	CALS	FAT	SAT FAT	TRANS FAT
Guiness					
Draught	12 oz	125	0	0	0
Foreign Extra Stout	12 oz	176	0	0	0
Hamm's					
Beer	12 oz	144	0	0	0
Light	12 oz	110	0	0	0
Heineken					
Beer	12 oz	166	0	0	0
I.C.					
Light	12 oz	96	0	0	0
Icehouse					
5.0	12 oz	132	0	0	0
5.5	12 oz	149	0	0	0
J.W. Dundee					
Honey Brown	12 oz	150	0	0	0
Keystone					
Light	12 oz	100	0	0	0
Kilarney's					
Red Lager	12 oz	197	0	0	0
Killian's					
Beer	12 oz	163	0	0	0
Lowenbrau					
Beer	12 oz	160	0	0	0
Michelob					
Ultra Low Carbohydrate	12 oz	95	0	0	0
Weinhard's					
Ale	12 oz	147	0	0	0
Amber Ale	12 oz	169	0	0	0
Dark	12 oz	150	0	0	0
Hefeweizen	12 oz	128	0	0	0
BEET JUICE					
juice	7 oz	72	0	0	0
BEETS					
CANNED					
harvard	½ cup	90	tr	tr	–
pickled	½ cup	74	tr	tr	–
sliced	½ cup	37	tr	tr	–

FOOD	PORTION	CALS	FAT	SAT FAT	TRANS FAT
Del Monte					
Pickled Sliced	½ cup	35	0	0	0
Sliced	½ cup	35	0	0	0
Greenwood					
Harvard	1 serv (4.4 oz)	100	0	0	0
Pickled	1 oz	25	0	0	0
S&W					
Sliced	½ cup (4.3 oz)	30	0	0	0
FRESH					
greens cooked w/o salt	½ cup	19	tr	tr	–
sliced cooked	½ cup	37	tr	tr	–
whole cooked	2 med (3.5 oz)	44	tr	tr	–
Frieda's					
Beets	½ cup	35	0	0	0

BEVERAGES (see BEER AND ALE, CHAMPAGNE, COFFEE, DRINK MIXERS, ENERGY DRINKS, FRUIT DRINKS, ICED TEA, LIQUOR/LIQUEUR, MALT, MILKSHAKE, SMOOTHIES, SODA, TEA/HERBAL TEA, WATER, WINE, YOGURT DRINKS)

BISCUIT

FOOD	PORTION	CALS	FAT	SAT FAT	TRANS FAT
MIX					
plain as prep	1 (2 oz)	190	7	2	–
Bisquick					
Cheese Garlic	½ cup	160	7	2	–
Heart Smart	⅓ cup	140	3	0	0
Mix	⅓ cup (1.4 oz)	160	6	2	–
Jiffy					
Buttermilk as prep	1	170	4	2	–
King Arthur					
Whole Grain Buttermilk not prep	¼ cup	100	1	0	0
MiniCarb					
Buttery as prep	1	255	21	12	–
REFRIGERATED					
plain baked	1 (1 oz)	93	4	1	–
TAKE-OUT					
buttermilk	1 lg (2.7 oz)	280	13	2	–
oatcakes	2 (4 oz)	115	5	–	–
plain	1 sm (1.2 oz)	127	6	1	–
tea biscuit	1 (3 oz)	210	3	2	–
w/ egg	1 (4.8 oz)	373	22	5	–

FOOD	PORTION	CALS	FAT	SAT FAT	TRANS FAT
w/ egg & bacon	1 (5.3 oz)	458	31	8	–
w/ egg & ham	1 (6.7 oz)	442	27	6	–
w/ egg & sausage	1 (6.3 oz)	581	39	15	–
w/ egg & steak	1 (5.2 oz)	410	28	9	–
w/ egg cheese & bacon	1 (5.1 oz)	477	31	11	–
w/ ham	1 (4 oz)	386	18	11	–
w/ sausage	1 (4.4 oz)	485	32	14	–

BITTERMELON
Frieda's
Foo Qua	1 cup	15	0	0	0

BLACK BEANS
dried cooked	1 cup	227	1	tr	–

Eden
Organic Caribbean	½ cup	90	1	0	0
Organic Refried	½ cup	110	2	0	0

BLACKBERRIES
canned in heavy syrup	½ cup	118	tr	tr	–
fresh	½ cup	31	tr	tr	–
unsweetened frzn	½ cup	48	tr	tr	–

Cascadian Farm
Organic frzn	1 cup	80	1	0	0

Oregon
In Light Syrup	½ cup	120	0	0	0

BLACKBERRY JUICE
canned	6 oz	65	1	tr	–

Izze
Sparkling Blackberry	8 oz	140	0	0	0

BLACKEYE PEAS
catjang dried cooked	1 cup (2.9 oz)	200	1	tr	–
cowpeas canned	1 cup	184	1	tr	–
cowpeas frozen cooked	½ cup	112	tr	tr	–
cowpeas leafy tips chopped cooked	1 cup	12	tr	tr	–
cowpeas leafy tips raw chopped	1 cup	10	tr	tr	–

CANNED
w/pork	½ cup	199	4	1	–

FOOD	PORTION	CALS	FAT	SAT FAT	TRANS FAT
Eden					
Organic	½ cup	90	1	0	0
DRIED					
cooked	1 cup	198	1	tr	–
FROZEN					
McKenzie					
Blackeye Peas	1 serv (2.8 oz)	110	1	0	–
TAKE-OUT					
blackeye peas & pork	1 cup	236	5	2	–
BLINTZE					
Cohen's & Wilton					
Cheese	1	80	3	1	–
Golden					
Cheese	1 (2.1 oz)	80	2	1	0
Potato	1	90	4	1	–
Vegetable	1	110	5	1	–
Ratner's					
Cheese	1 (2.2 oz)	100	2	1	0
TAKE-OUT					
cheese	1 (2.7 oz)	160	9	4	–
BLUEBERRIES					
canned in heavy syrup	½ cup	113	tr	tr	–
fresh	1 pt	229	1	tr	–
fresh	½ cup	41	tr	tr	–
frzn unsweetened	½ cup	40	1	tr	–
A&L Farms					
Bleuets Fresh	1 pt	80	0	0	0
C&W					
Ultimate	¾ cup	70	0	0	0
De-Lite					
Dried Sweetened	1 oz	86	1	tr	0
Eden					
Organic Dried Wild	¼ cup	150	0	0	0
Europe's Best					
Woodland frzn	¾ cup	70	1	0	0
Frieda's					
Dried	¼ cup (1.4 oz)	140	0	0	0
Hodgson Mill					
Dried Wild	¼ cup	120	1	0	–

FOOD	PORTION	CALS	FAT	SAT FAT	TRANS FAT
Marie's					
Glaze	2 tbsp	40	0	0	0
Oregon					
In Light Syrup	½ cup	110	0	0	0
Sunsweet					
Dried	¼ cup (1.4 oz)	140	0	0	0
BLUEBERRY JUICE					
Izze					
Sparkling Blueberry	8 oz	100	0	0	0
Van Dyk's					
100% Juice	6 oz	74	0	0	0
Walnut Acres					
Organic	8 oz	130	0	0	0
BLUEFIN					
fillet baked	4.1 oz	186	6	1	–
BLUEFISH					
fresh baked	3 oz	135	5	1	–
BOAR					
wild roasted	3 oz	136	4	1	–
BOK CHOY (see CABBAGE)					
BONITO					
dried	1 oz	50	2	tr	0
fresh	3 oz	117	4	–	–
BORAGE					
fresh chopped	1 cup	19	tr	tr	–
BOTTLED WATER (see WATER)					
BOYSENBERRIES					
frzn unsweetened	½ cup	33	tr	tr	–
in heavy syrup	½ cup	113	tr	tr	–
BRAINS					
beef pan-fried	3 oz	167	13	3	–
beef simmered	3 oz	123	9	3	–
lamb braised	3 oz	123	9	2	–
lamb fried	3 oz	232	19	5	0
pork braised	3 oz	117	8	2	–

FOOD	PORTION	CALS	FAT	SAT FAT	TRANS FAT
veal braised	3 oz	116	8	2	0
veal fried	3 oz	181	14	3	0

BRAN

FOOD	PORTION	CALS	FAT	SAT FAT	TRANS FAT
corn	1 cup (2.7 oz)	170	1	tr	–
oat	½ cup (1.6 oz)	116	3	1	–
oat cooked	½ cup (3.8 oz)	44	1	tr	–
rice	½ cup (2.1 oz)	187	12	2	–
wheat	½ cup (2 oz)	63	1	tr	–
Bob's Red Mill					
Rice Bran	2 tbsp	60	3	1	0

BRAZIL NUTS

FOOD	PORTION	CALS	FAT	SAT FAT	TRANS FAT
dried unblanched	1 oz	186	19	5	–

BREAD
CANNED

FOOD	PORTION	CALS	FAT	SAT FAT	TRANS FAT
boston brown	1 slice (1.6 oz)	88	1	tr	–
FROZEN					
Alexia					
Baguette Garlic	2 pieces (1.6 oz)	130	5	3	0
Cedarlane					
Organic Mediterranean Stuffed Focaccia	1 piece (4 oz)	295	10	6	0
Corbi's					
Chee-Zee Bread Original	½ piece (1.8 oz)	180	8	4	1
Marie Callender's					
Cornbread & Honey Butter	1 piece + butter	210	11	5	–
Parmesan & Romano Garlic	1 piece	200	10	3	–
Pepperidge Farm					
Garlic	1 slice (2.5 in)	170	7	3	3
Texas Toast Five Cheese	1 slice	150	7	2	1
Whole Grain Texas Toast	1 slice	150	8	3	0
MIX					
cornbread	1 piece (2 oz)	188	6	2	–
Buitoni					
Focaccia Italian Herb & Cheese	1 slice	110	2	1	–
Focaccia Rosemary & Garlic	1 piece (1 oz)	110	1	0	–
Carbolite					
Bread Mix as prep	1 slice	45	5	1	–

FOOD	PORTION	CALS	FAT	SAT FAT	TRANS FAT
Keto					
Quick Bread All Flavors as prep	1 slice	55	0	0	0
MiniCarb					
Country White as prep	1 slice	80	3	0	–
Sassafras					
12 Grain & Sunflower	1 slice (1.4 oz)	150	2	0	–
READY-TO-EAT					
anadama	1 (1.1 oz)	87	1	tr	–
baguette whole wheat	2 oz	140	0	0	0
challah	1 slice (1.4 oz)	115	2	1	–
cinnamon	1 slice (0.9 oz)	69	1	tr	–
cracked wheat	1 slice (1.1 oz)	78	1	tr	–
cuban bread	1 slice (1.1 oz)	83	1	tr	–
french	1 slice (1.1 oz)	88	1	tr	–
italian	1 loaf (1 lb)	1255	4	1	–
jewish rye	1 slice	90	2	0	0
navajo fry	1 piece	281	10	4	–
oat bran	1 slice (1.1 oz)	71	1	tr	–
oatmeal	1 slice (0.9 oz)	73	1	tr	–
pan criollo	1 piece (0.9 oz)	69	1	tr	–
pannetone	1 slice (0.9 oz)	86	2	1	–
pita	1 lg (2 oz)	165	1	tr	–
pita	1 sm (1 oz)	77	tr	tr	–
pita whole wheat	1 lg (2.2 oz)	170	2	tr	–
pita whole wheat	1 sm (1 oz)	74	1	tr	–
potato scallion	1 slice (2 oz)	120	1	0	–
pumpernickel	1 slice (0.9 oz)	65	1	tr	–
raisin	1 slice (1.1 oz)	88	1	tr	–
rye	1 slice (1.1 oz)	83	1	tr	–
seven grain	1 slice (1.1 oz)	80	1	tr	–
wheat berry	1 slice (0.9 oz)	65	1	tr	–
wheat bran	1 slice (1.3 oz)	89	1	tr	–
wheat germ	1 slice (1 oz)	73	1	tr	–
white cubed	1 cup	93	1	tr	–
whole wheat	1 slice (1 oz)	69	1	tr	–
Alvarado Street Bakery					
Sprouted Whole Wheat	1 slice	90	1	0	0
Arnold					
Bakery Light	1 slice	80	1	0	–
100% Whole Wheat					

FOOD	PORTION	CALS	FAT	SAT FAT	TRANS FAT
Country Classics Wheat	1 slice	100	2	0	0
Raisin Cinnamon	1 slice (1 oz)	80	2	0	–
Smart & Healthy Omega-3 100% Whole Wheat	1 slice	80	1	0	0
Smart & Healthy Sugar Free 100% Whole Wheat	1 slice	80	1	0	0
Whole Grains 12 Grain	1 slice	110	2	0	0
Whole Grains 7 Grain	1 slice	110	2	0	0
Baker's Inn					
9 Grain	1 slice	100	2	0	0
Cracked Wheat	1 slice	100	2	0	0
Honey White Made w/ Whole Grain	1 slice	110	2	0	0
Honey Whole Wheat	1 slice	100	2	0	0
Potato Made w/ Whole Grain	1 slice	100	2	0	0
Beefsteak					
Rye Soft	1 slice	70	1	0	–
Cedar's					
Wraps Whole Wheat	1 (2 oz)	180	4	1	–
Damascus					
Roll-Up Flax	1 (2 oz)	110	3	1	0
Roll-Up Whole Wheat	1 (2 oz)	110	3	1	0
Wraps Honey Wheat	½ wrap (2 oz)	130	0	0	0
Wraps Spinach	1 (4 oz)	280	0	0	0
Earth Grains					
100% Multi Grain Extra Fiber	1 slice	110	2	0	0
Oat & Nut	1 slice	120	3	1	0
Potato	1 slice	110	1	0	0
Whole Grain Honey	1 slice	110	2	0	0
Whole Wheat Honey	1 slice	110	2	0	0
Ecce Panis					
Country Wheat	1 slice (2 oz)	150	0	0	0
European Baguette	2 oz	150	0	0	0
Food For Life					
Brown Rice Bread Yeast Free	1 slice	100	1	0	0
Rice Bread Fruit & Seed Yeast Free	1 slice	140	1	0	0
Rice Bread Multi Seed Yeast Free	1 slice	120	1	0	0
White Rice Bread Yeast Free	1 slice	100	0	0	0

FOOD	PORTION	CALS	FAT	SAT FAT	TRANS FAT
Freihofer's					
100% Whole Wheat	1 slice	90	2	0	–
Whole Wheat Light	2 slices	80	1	0	–
French Meadow Bakery					
Healthy Hemp	1 slice	110	3	0	0
Organic Men's Bread	1 slice	120	5	1	0
Gold Medal					
100% Whole Wheat	1 slice	70	2	0	–
Home Pride					
Wheat	1 slice (1 oz)	80	1	0	–
Kangaroo					
Bread Wraps	1 (2.6 oz)	140	3	0	–
Greek Pita Flat	1 (2.6 oz)	200	2	0	–
Greek Pita Flat Wheat	1 (2.4 oz)	145	2	0	–
Pita Pockets Onion	½ (1.2 oz)	90	0	0	0
Pita Pockets Wheat N'Honey	½ (1.2 oz)	90	0	0	0
Pita Pockets White	½ (1.2 oz)	90	0	0	0
Salad Pockets	1 (1.2 oz)	90	0	0	0
Sandwich Pockets Whole Grain	1 (1.2 oz)	80	1	0	–
La Tortilla Factory					
Wraps Smart & Delicious Gluten Free Dark Teff	1 (2.3 oz)	180	5	1	0
Wraps Smart & Delicious Gluten Free Ivory Teff	1 (2.3 oz)	180	5	1	0
Matthew's					
All Natural Cinnamon Raisin	1 slice	80	1	0	–
Milton's					
100% Whole Wheat	1 slice	110	1	0	0
Buttermilk	1 slice	90	1	0	–
Gourmet White	1 slice	110	1	0	0
Original Multi-Grain	1 slice	120	1	0	–
Potato	1 slice	90	1	0	–
Whole Grain	1 slice	90	1	0	–
Natural Ovens					
100% Whole Grain	1 slice	60	1	0	–
7 Grain Herb	1 slice	70	1	0	–
Better White	1 slice	80	1	0	–
Cracked Wheat	1 slice	80	1	0	–
English Muffin Bread	1 slice	80	1	0	–
Glorious Cinnamon Raisin	1 slice	70	1	0	–

FOOD	PORTION	CALS	FAT	SAT FAT	TRANS FAT
Happiness Raisin Pecan	1 slice	70	1	0	–
Health Max	1 slice	80	1	0	–
Hunger Filler	1 slice	60	1	0	–
Lo Carb Golden Crunch	1 slice	70	4	0	–
Lo Carb Original	1 slice	60	2	0	–
Mild Rye	1 slice	70	1	0	–
Multi-Grain Stay Slim	1 slice	60	1	0	–
Nutty Natural	1 slice	70	1	0	–
Right Wheat	1 slice	60	1	0	–
Soft Wheat	1 slice	70	1	0	–
Sunny Millet	1 slice	60	1	0	–
Nature's Own					
100% Whole Wheat	1 slice	50	1	0	0
9 Grain	1 slice	120	2	0	0
Hearty Oatmeal	1 slice	100	2	1	0
Wheat Double Fiber	1 slice	10	1	0	0
Wheat Light	2 slices	80	1	0	0
Wheat N' Fiber	1 slice	60	1	0	0
Whole Wheat w/ Organic Flour	1 slice	100	2	0	0
Nature's Path					
Manna Carrot Raisin	1 slice	130	0	0	0
Manna Millet Rice	1 slice	130	0	0	0
Manna SunSeed	1 slice	160	2	0	–
Pepperidge Farm					
100% Natural Whole Grain Germain Dark Wheat	1 slice	100	2	0	0
Canadian White	1 slice	100	2	0	0
Carb Style 7 Grain	1 slice	60	2	0	0
Farmhouse Hearty White	1 slice	120	2	1	0
Farmhouse Honey Wheatberry	1 slice	120	2	0	0
Farmhouse Soft 100% Whole Wheat	1 slice	110	2	1	0
Farmhouse Soft Oatmeal	1 slice	120	2	1	0
Farmhouse Whole Grain White	1 slice	110	2	1	0
Hot & Crusty Italian	1 slice (2 in thick)	150	2	1	0
Jewish Rye Seeded	1 slice	80	1	0	0
Light Style Oatmeal	3 slices	140	1	0	0
Party Pumpernickel	5 slices	130	2	0	0
Very Thin White	3 slices	120	1	0	0
Whole Grain Honey Oat	1 slice	110	2	1	0

FOOD	PORTION	CALS	FAT	SAT FAT	TRANS FAT
Whole Grain Honey Whole Wheat	1 slice	110	2	1	0
Whole Grain Swirl Cinnamon	1 slice	100	2	0	0
Whole Grain Swirl Cinnamon Raisin	1 slice	100	2	0	0
Rudi's Organic Bakery					
100% Whole Wheat	1 slice	100	1	0	–
14 Grain	1 slice	90	1	0	0
Artisan Country French	1 slice	100	1	0	0
Artisan Rosemary Olive Oil	1 slice	100	1	0	0
Low Carb Right Choice	1 slice	45	1	0	0
Spelt Ancient Grain	1 slice	120	3	0	0
Whole Grain Apple N Spice	1 slice	110	1	0	0
Sara Lee					
100% Whole Wheat	1 slice	70	1	0	0
Blueberry Crumble	1 slice	180	3	1	0
Cinnamon Raisin	1 slice	190	4	2	0
Classic Wheat	1 slice	70	1	0	–
Delightful Wheat	1 slice	45	0	0	0
Delightful White	1 slice	90	1	0	0
Heart Healthy 100% Whole Wheat Essentials	1 slice	80	1	0	0
Heart Healthy Multigrain	1 slice	100	1	0	–
Honey Wheat	1 slice	70	1	0	–
Honey White	1 slice	100	1	0	–
Multigrain	1 slice	100	2	0	0
Soft & Smooth 100% Whole Wheat	1 slice	70	1	0	0
Soft & Smooth Whole Grain White	2 slices	150	2	1	0
Sonoma					
Wraps Organic Multi Grain	1 (2.4 oz)	180	7	1	0
Wraps Organic Wheat	1 (2.4 oz)	190	7	1	0
Wraps Original White Whole Wheat	1 (2.4 oz)	200	5	1	0
Stroehmann					
100% Whole Wheat	1 slice	90	2	0	0
Family Grains Twisted Bread	1 slice	70	1	0	–
Honey Cracked Wheat	1 slice	90	1	0	–
New York Rye	1 slice (1 oz)	80	1	0	–

FOOD	PORTION	CALS	FAT	SAT FAT	TRANS FAT
Potato	1 slice	100	2	0	0
Soft Rye Seeded	1 slice	90	2	0	0
Super Bakery					
Athlete's Formula	1 slice (1.5 oz)	100	4	0	–
Fitness Formula	1 slice (1.5 oz)	90	3	0	–
Wrap Organic	1 (4 oz)	340	8	0	0
The Baker					
Yoga Bread	1 slice	70	1	0	0
Thomas'					
Breakfast Original	1 slice	90	1	0	0
Corn	1 slice	110	2	0	0
Swirl Whole Grain Cinnamon Raisin	1 slice	110	3	1	0
Toasting Cinnamon	1 slice	130	5	2	–
Toufayan					
Wraps Sundried Tomato Basil	1 (2 oz)	183	5	1	–
Wraps Wheat	1 (2 oz)	183	5	1	–
Tumaro's					
Wraps Chipotle Chili & Peppers	1 (2.3 oz)	170	2	0	–
Wraps Sun Dried Tomato & Basil	1 (2.3 oz)	170	2	0	–
TAKE-OUT					
banana	1 slice (2 oz)	196	6	1	–
chapatis as prep w/ fat	1 (1.6 oz)	95	2	1	–
chapatis as prep w/o fat	1 (2.5 oz)	141	1	–	–
cornbread	1 piece (2.3 oz)	183	6	1	–
cornstick	1 (1.4 oz)	118	4	1	–
focaccia onion	1 piece (4.6 oz)	282	10	1	–
focaccia rosemary	1 piece (3.5 oz)	251	7	1	–
focaccia tomato olive	1 piece (4.7 oz)	270	8	1	–
garlic bread	1 slice (1 oz)	96	4	1	–
irish soda bread	1 slice (3 oz)	247	4	1	–
italian garlic	1 loaf (11 oz)	990	38	7	–
naan	1 bread (3.5 oz)	286	9	5	–
papadums fried	2 (1.5 oz)	81	4	–	–
paratha	1 bread (2.1 oz)	201	10	7	–
poori indian puffed bread	1 piece (1.3 oz)	112	4	2	–
zucchini	1 slice (1.4 oz)	150	7	1	–

FOOD	PORTION	CALS	FAT	SAT FAT	TRANS FAT
BREAD COATING					
Don's Chuck Wagon					
Chicken Baking Mix	¼ cup	95	0	0	0
Fish Mix	¼ cup	95	0	0	0
Onion Ring Mix	¼ cup	100	0	0	0
Fryin' Magic					
Cornmeal	1 tbsp	30	0	0	0
Hodgson Mill					
Vidalia Sweet Onion Mix not prep	¼ cup	100	0	0	0
Luzianne					
Cajun Chicken Coating Mix	2 tbsp (1 oz)	100	1	0	–
BREAD MACHINE MIX					
Betty Crocker					
Harvest Wheat	1/11 loaf	140	3	1	–
Home-Style White	1/11 loaf	130	2	0	–
Carbsense					
Harvest Wheat as prep	1 slice	60	0	0	0
Keto					
Cinnamon Raisin as prep	1 slice	79	0	0	0
French Loaf as prep	1 slice	79	0	0	0
Sourdough Rye as prep	1 slice	79	1	–	–
Ketogenics					
Low Carb Honey Wheat as prep	1 slice	80	1	1	–
Low Carb Original White as prep	1 slice	62	0	0	0
Low Carb Pumpernickel Rye as prep	1 slice	80	2	1	–
BREADCRUMBS					
dry seasoned	¼ cup	115	2	tr	–
fresh	¼ cup	30	tr	tr	–
plain	¼ cup	107	1	tr	–
4C					
Carb Careful Seasoned	⅓ cup	110	1	0	0
Salt Free Seasoned	⅓ cup	110	1	0	0
Arnold					
Italian	¼ cup	110	2	0	–

FOOD	PORTION	CALS	FAT	SAT FAT	TRANS FAT
Edward & Sons					
Organic Lightly Salted	⅓ cup	110	1	0	0
Organic Panko	⅓ cup	110	1	0	0
Ian's					
Panko Italian	¼ cup	70	1	0	0
Panko Original	¼ cup	71	0	0	0
Panko Whole Wheat	¼ cup	70	1	0	0
Keto					
Low Carb Cajun	½ cup	185	1	–	–
Low Carb Italian	½ cup	185	1	–	–
Low Carb Original	½ cup	185	1	–	–
Progresso					
Italian Style	¼ cup	110	2	1	0
Rienzi					
Italian Style	¼ cup	120	2	1	–
Ronzoni					
Italian Flavored	¼ cup	120	2	1	–

BREADFRUIT

FOOD	PORTION	CALS	FAT	SAT FAT	TRANS FAT
fresh	1 sm (13.5 oz)	396	1	tr	–
fried	1 cup	379	21	3	–
raw	1 cup	227	1	tr	–

BREADNUTTREE SEEDS

FOOD	PORTION	CALS	FAT	SAT FAT	TRANS FAT
dried	1 oz	104	tr	tr	–

BREADSTICKS

FOOD	PORTION	CALS	FAT	SAT FAT	TRANS FAT
plain	1 lg	41	1	tr	–
plain	1 sm	21	tr	tr	–
Angonoa					
Deli Style Sesame	3 (0.5 oz)	730	3	0	–
Fattorie & Pandea					
Grissini Sesame	3	70	2	0	0
John Wm Macy's					
CheeseSticks Original Cheddar	3 (1 oz)	130	6	3	–
Pepperidge Farm					
Garlic frzn	1	160	5	1	1
Stella D'Oro					
Mini Cracked Pepper	4 (0.5 oz)	70	2	0	0
Original	1 (0.3 oz)	40	1	0	0
Roasted Garlic	1	45	1	0	0

FOOD	PORTION	CALS	FAT	SAT FAT	TRANS FAT
Sesame	1 (0.4 oz)	50	3	0	0
Sodium Free	1 (0.3 oz)	40	1	0	0

BREAKFAST BARS (see CEREAL BARS, ENERGY BARS)

BREAKFAST DRINKS
Carnation

FOOD	PORTION	CALS	FAT	SAT FAT	TRANS FAT
Instant Breakfast Chocolate Malt as prep w/ fat free milk	1 serv	220	1	1	–
Instant Breakfast Classic French Vanilla as prep w/ fat free milk	1 serv	220	1	tr	–
Instant Breakfast Milk Chocolate as prep w/ fat free milk	1 serv	220	1	1	–
Instant Breakfast Ready-To-Drink Carb Conscious French Vanilla	1 pkg	150	5	1	0
Instant Breakfast Ready-To-Drink Carb Conscious Milk Chocolate	1 pkg	150	5	2	0
Instant Breakfast Ready-To-Drink Creamy Milk Chocolate	1 pkg	250	5	2	0
Instant Breakfast Ready-To-Drink French Vanilla	1 pkg	240	5	1	0
Instant Breakfast Ready-To-Drink Strawberry Creme	1 pkg	250	5	1	0
Instant Breakfast Strawberry as prep w/ fat free milk	1 serv	220	6	tr	–
Instant Breakfast Junior Vanilla	1 box (8.8 oz)	250	12	–	–
Instant Breakfast No Sugar Added Vanilla as prep w/ fat free milk	1 serv	150	1	tr	–

BROAD BEANS

FOOD	PORTION	CALS	FAT	SAT FAT	TRANS FAT
canned	½ cup	91	tr	tr	–
fava fresh cooked	½ cup	94	tr	tr	–

BROCCOFLOWER

FOOD	PORTION	CALS	FAT	SAT FAT	TRANS FAT
fresh raw	½ cup (1.8 oz)	16	tr	tr	–

FOOD	PORTION	CALS	FAT	SAT FAT	TRANS FAT
BROCCOLI					
FRESH					
chinese broccoli (gai lan) cooked	½ cup	10	tr	tr	–
raab cooked	½ cup	28	tr	tr	–
raw	1 bunch (1.3 lbs)	207	2	tr	–
raw flower	1 piece	3	tr	tr	–
raw flowers	1 cup	20	tr	tr	–
BroccoSprouts					
Broccoli Sprouts	½ cup	16	0	0	0
River Ranch					
Broccoli Slaw	1 cup	25	0	0	0
Florets	1¼ cups	25	0	0	0
FROZEN					
chopped cooked	½ cup	26	tr	tr	–
spears cooked	1 pkg (10 oz)	70	tr	tr	–
spears cooked	½ cup	26	tr	tr	–
Birds Eye					
Broccoli & Cheese Sauce	½ cup	90	5	3	0
Steamfresh Cuts	1 cup	30	0	0	0
C&W					
Broccoli & Cheddar Cheese Sauce	1⅓ cups	70	3	1	0
Florets	1 cup	30	0	0	0
Cascadian Farm					
Organic Florets	⅔ cup	20	0	0	0
Fresh Like					
Spear	3.5 oz	26	tr	–	–
Green Giant					
Broccoli & Cheese Sauce	⅔ cup	60	3	1	0
Butter Sauce Low Fat	3 spears (4 oz)	40	2	1	0
Cuts as prep	⅔ cup	25	0	0	0
Pasta Broccoli & Alfredo Sauce as prep	1 cup	210	4	1	1
TAKE-OUT					
batter dipped & fried	4 pieces	77	5	1	–
w/ cheese sauce	1 cup	242	15	7	–

FOOD	PORTION	CALS	FAT	SAT FAT	TRANS FAT
BROWNIE					
brownie	1 (2 oz)	227	9	2	–
butterscotch	1 (1.2 oz)	151	8	1	–
Arrowhead Mills					
Gluten Free as prep	1	160	8	2	0
Aunt Paula's					
Low Carb Chef Fudge Brownie as prep	1 (2.5 in)	89	5	2	–
Betty Crocker					
Chocolate Chunk as prep	1	180	9	2	–
Dark Chocolate Fudge as prep	1	170	7	1	–
Dark Chocolate w/ Syrup as prep	1	170	7	1	–
Fudge as prep	1	170	7	1	–
German Chocolate Coconut Pecan Filling as prep	1	200	8	2	–
Hot Fudge as prep	1	170	8	2	–
Original as prep	1	180	6	1	–
Peanut Butter as prep	1	180	8	3	–
Stir'n Bake w/ Mini Kisses as prep	1 serv	220	7	3	–
Turtle w/ Caramel & Pecans as prep	1	170	8	1	–
Walnut as prep	1	180	9	1	–
Big Train					
Low Carb Chocolate Chip as prep	1 (2 in)	140	9	5	–
Bob's Red Mill					
Gluten Free as prep	1	140	5	1	0
Foxy's Bake Shop					
Milk Chocolate	½ (1.7 oz)	200	11	5	0
White Chocolate	½ (1.7 oz)	200	12	6	0
French Meadow Bakery					
Gluten Free Fudge	1 (1.3 oz)	150	5	1	0
Glenny's					
100 Calorie 75% Organic	1 (1.45 oz)	100	4	2	0
Jiffy					
Fudge as prep	1	160	5	1	–
Joseph's					
Sugar Free	1 (1.5 oz)	150	7	2	0

FOOD	PORTION	CALS	FAT	SAT FAT	TRANS FAT
Keto					
Chocolate Fudge as prep	1	59	3	–	–
Laura's Wholesome Junk Food					
Gluten Free Better Brownie	2	120	6	2	0
MiniCarb					
Chocolate Brownie as prep	1	220	17	4	–
Nature's Path					
Organic Double Fudge	1/10 pkg	150	3	2	0
Organic HempPlus	1/10 pkg	140	2	0	0
No Pudge!					
All Flavors as prep	1	100	0	0	0
Sara Lee					
Brownie Bites Chocolate Dipped	1 (0.7 oz)	90	4	2	–
Sweet Rewards					
Low Fat Fudge as prep	1	130	3	1	–
Reduced Fat Supreme as prep	1	140	3	1	–
VitaBrownie					
Dark Chocolate Pomegranate	1 (2 oz)	100	2	1	0
Deep Velvety Chocolate	1 (2 oz)	100	3	1	0
BRUSSELS SPROUTS					
FRESH					
cooked	6 pieces	45	1	tr	–
Select Gourmet					
Fresh	½ cup	35	0	0	0
FROZEN					
cooked	1 cup	65	1	tr	–
C&W					
Petite	10 (3 oz)	45	0	0	0
Green Giant					
Baby & Butter Sauce as prep	½ cup	60	1	1	0
BUCKWHEAT					
groats roasted cooked	½ cup	323	1	tr	–
groats roasted uncooked	½ cup	292	3	1	–
Bob's Red Mill					
Organic Kernels	¼ cup	142	1	0	0
BUFFALO (see also MEAT STICKS)					
burger	3 oz	202	13	5	0

FOOD	PORTION	CALS	FAT	SAT FAT	TRANS FAT
chuck braised	4 oz	205	6	2	0
top round steak broiled	3 oz	313	9	4	0
water buffalo roasted	3 oz	111	2	1	–
BULGUR					
cooked	½ cup	76	tr	tr	0
uncooked	½ cup	239	1	tr	0
Bob's Red Mill					
From Soft White Wheat	¼ cup	150	1	0	0
Fantastic					
Tabouli Mix not prep	2 tbsp	70	0	0	0
Sabra					
Black Bean & Wheat Pilaf	2 oz	45	2	0	–
Cracked Wheat Salad	2 oz	80	3	0	–
Tabouli	2 oz	70	4	1	–
TAKE-OUT					
tabbouleh	1 cup	198	15	2	–
BURBOT (FISH)					
fresh baked	3 oz	98	1	tr	–
BURDOCK ROOT					
cooked w/o salt	1 cup	110	tr	tr	–
cooked w/o salt	1 root (5.8 oz)	146	tr	tr	–
Frieda's					
Gobo Root	¾ cup	60	0	0	0
BUTTER					
clarified butter	3.5 oz	876	99	62	–
ghee cow's milk	1 tbsp	126	14	–	–
ghee vegetable oil	1 tbsp	126	14	–	–
stick	1 pat (5 g)	36	4	3	–
stick	1 stick (4 oz)	813	92	57	–
whipped	1 pat (4 g)	27	3	2	–
whipped	1 tbsp	70	7	5	–
whipped	4 oz	542	61	38	–
Cabot					
Salted	1 tbsp	100	11	7	0
Unsalted	1 tbsp	100	11	7	0
Crystal Farms					
Butter	1 tbsp	100	11	7	0
Whipped	1 tbsp	70	7	5	0

FOOD	PORTION	CALS	FAT	SAT FAT	TRANS FAT
Deerfield					
Creamy	1 tbsp	100	11	7	0
Horizon Organic					
European	1 tbsp	100	12	7	0
Land O Lakes					
Unsalted	1 tbsp	100	11	7	0
Organic Valley					
European Style	1 tbsp	110	12	8	0

BUTTER SUBSTITUTES

stick	1 stick	811	91	32	–
Butter Buds					
Granules	1 pkg (2 g)	5	0	0	0
Keto					
Butta	1 tsp	43	5	5	–
Molly McButter					
Natural Butter	1 tsp	5	0	0	0
Natural Cheese	1 tsp	5	0	0	0
Roasted Garlic	1 tsp	5	0	0	0
Sunsweet					
Lighter Bake	1 tbsp	35	0	0	0

BUTTERBUR

canned fuki chopped	1 cup	3	tr	–	–
fresh fuki	1 cup	13	tr	–	–

BUTTERFISH

baked	3 oz	159	9	–	–
fillet baked	1 oz	47	3	–	–

BUTTERNUTS

dried	1 oz	174	16	tr	–

BUTTERSCOTCH (see also CANDY)

E. Guittard					
Baking Chips	33 (0.5 oz)	80	5	4	0
Hershey's					
Chips	1 tbsp	80	4	4	–

CABBAGE (see also COLESLAW)

chinese bok choy shredded cooked w/o salt	1 cup	20	tr	tr	0

FOOD	PORTION	CALS	FAT	SAT FAT	TRANS FAT
chinese pe-tsai shredded cooked w/o salt	1 cup	17	tr	tr	0
green raw shredded	1 cup	19	tr	tr	0
green shredded cooked w/o salt	1 cup	34	tr	tr	0
japanese pickled	½ cup	22	tr	tr	0
red raw shredded	1 cup	22	tr	tr	0
red shredded cooked w/o salt	1 cup	44	tr	tr	0
savoy shredded cooked w/o salt	1 cup	35	tr	tr	0
Aunt Nellie's					
Sweet & Sour Red	¼ cup	40	0	0	0
Frieda's					
Baby Bok Choy	⅔ cup	10	0	0	0
Bok Choy	1 cup	10	0	0	0
Gai Choy	1 cup (3 oz)	20	0	0	0
Napa	1 cup (3 oz)	15	0	0	0
Salad Savoy	⅔ cup (3 oz)	25	0	0	0
Tuscan	⅔ cup (3 oz)	20	0	0	0
Glory					
Country Cabbage	½ cup	25	0	0	0
Greenwood					
Red	½ cup	100	0	0	0
Lohmann					
Red Cabbage Sweet & Sour	¼ cup	40	0	0	0
River Ranch					
Angel Hair	1½ cups	20	0	0	0
TAKE-OUT					
creamed	1 cup	158	10	3	–
kimchee	1 cup	32	tr	tr	0
stuffed cabbage w/ rice & beef	1 (3.6 oz)	117	5	2	–
sweet & sour red cabbage	4 oz	61	3	–	–

CACAO
Navitas Naturals

Butter	1 tbsp	120	14	8	0
Nibs	1 oz	130	12	7	0
Powder	1 oz	120	3	2	0

FOOD	PORTION	CALS	FAT	SAT FAT	TRANS FAT
CACTUS					
fresh cooked w/ fat	1 pad (1 oz)	11	1	tr	0
fresh cooked w/o fat	1 cup (5.2 oz)	22	tr	tr	0
prickly pear fresh	1 cup (5.3 oz)	56	1	–	–
Frieda's					
Cactus Pads	¾ cup (3 oz)	20	0	0	0
CAKE (see also CAKE MIX)					
battenburg cake	1 slice (2 oz)	204	10	–	–
cream puff shell	1 (2.3 oz)	239	17	4	–
crumpet	1 (2.3 oz)	131	1	–	–
eccles cake	1 slice (2 oz)	285	16	–	–
madeira cake	1 slice (1 oz)	98	4	–	–
sponge	1 piece (1.3 oz)	110	1	tr	0
sponge cake dessert shell	1 (0.8 oz)	70	2	1	–
treacle tart	1 slice (2.5 oz)	258	10	–	–
Amy's					
Toaster Pops Apple	1	140	3	0	–
Toaster Pops Strawberry	1	140	3	0	–
Arnold					
Date Nut Loaf	1 slice (2 oz)	190	5	1	0
Aunt Trudy's					
Organic Baklava Soy Nut	1 (1.8 oz)	190	6	1	0
Balocco					
Il Panettone	1 serv (3.5 oz)	380	15	8	0
Boboli					
Mini Eclairs Custard Filled	4 (2.3 oz)	224	12	8	–
Chudleigh's					
Apple Blossoms	1 (4 oz)	350	19	10	0
Drake's					
Coffee Cake Low Fat	2 (2.3 oz)	210	2	1	0
Coffee Cakes	1 (1.2 oz)	140	6	2	–
Entenmann's					
All Butter French Crumb	⅛ cake (1.8 oz)	210	10	5	0
Cheese Cake Deluxe French	⅙ cake (3.8 oz)	390	24	13	0
Coffee Cake Cheese Filled Crumb	1 serv (1.9 oz)	200	10	3	–
Coffee Cake Crumb	1 serv (2 oz)	260	12	5	0
Danish Twist Raspberry	⅛ cake	220	11	5	0
Fudge Iced Golden Cake	⅛ cake	290	13	5	0

FOOD	PORTION	CALS	FAT	SAT FAT	TRANS FAT
Light Loaf Cake Fat Free	⅛ cake (1.7 oz)	120	0	0	0
Loaf All Butter	⅙ cake (2.4 oz)	220	9	6	0
Louisiana Crunch	⅑ cake (2.9 oz)	330	14	4	–
Marble Loaf	⅛ cake	190	8	2	0
Marshmallow Iced Devil's Food	⅛ cake	280	14	5	0
Mini's Carrot Cake	1 (1.4 oz)	160	7	2	0
Strawberry Cheese Buns	1 (3 oz)	320	14	6	0
Fillo Factory					
Organic Apple Strudel	1 (4.4 oz)	290	10	1	0
Organic Apple Turnovers	1 (3 oz)	180	6	1	0
Glenny's					
Blondie 100 Calorie 75% Organic	1 (1.45 oz)	100	3	1	0
Goody Man					
Happy Birthday Cupcake Chocolate	1 (1.75 oz)	200	6	3	–
Happy Birthday Cupcake White	1 (1.75 oz)	190	5	2	–
Gourmet Pastries					
Baklava Walnut	1 piece (1.8 oz)	240	11	3	0
Guiltless Gourmet					
Dessert Bowl Bananas Foster Cake	1 pkg (2 oz)	200	2	1	0
Dessert Bowl Black Velvet Cake	1 pkg (2 oz)	200	3	2	0
Hostess					
100 Calorie Pack Carrot Cake Mini	1 pkg (1.2 oz)	100	3	1	0
100 Calorie Pack Golden Cake w/ Creamy Filling	1 pkg (1.2 oz)	100	3	1	0
Crumb Cake Light	1 (1 oz)	100	2	0	–
Shortcake Dessert Cups	1 (1.1 oz)	100	1	0	–
Kellogg's					
Pop-Tarts Apple Cinnamon	1 (1.8 oz)	210	6	3	0
Pop-Tarts French Toast	1	220	8	3	0
Pop-Tarts Frosted Cookies & Cream	1	200	5	2	0
Pop-Tarts Low Fat Frosted Brown Sugar Cinnamon	1 (1.8 oz)	190	3	2	0
Pop-Tarts Yogurt Blast Strawberry	1 (1.8 oz)	210	6	3	0

FOOD	PORTION	CALS	FAT	SAT FAT	TRANS FAT
Low Carb Creations					
Cheesecake Blueberry Swirl	1 slice (3 oz)	220	16	10	–
Cheesecake Chocolate	1 slice (3 oz)	250	20	12	–
Cheesecake Key Lime	1 slice (3 oz)	250	20	12	–
Cheesecake New York	1 slice (3 oz)	250	15	9	–
Cheesecake Pumpkin Swirl	1 slice (3 oz)	220	16	10	–
Marie Callender's					
Cobbler Apple	1 serv (4.25 oz)	370	20	9	–
Cobbler Berry	1 serv (4.25 oz)	370	21	5	–
Cobbler Cherry	1 serv (4.25 oz)	380	19	8	–
Cobbler Peach	1 serv (4.25 oz)	380	18	6	–
Mrs. Smith's					
Carrot	⅛ cake (2.9 oz)	300	16	3	2
Cobbler Blackberry	1 serv (4 oz)	260	10	5	0
Nature's Path					
Organic Toaster Pastry Apple Cinnamon	1 (2 oz)	210	5	2	0
Organic Toaster Pastry Blueberry	1 (2 oz)	210	5	2	0
Organic Toaster Pastry Frosted Apple Cinnamon	1 (2 oz)	210	5	2	0
Organic Toaster Pastry Frosted Blueberry	1 (2 oz)	200	4	2	0
Organic Toaster Pastry Frosted Strawberry	1 (2 oz)	210	4	2	0
Neuman's					
Date Nut Bread	1 oz	90	2	tr	0
Pepperidge Farm					
Chocolate Coconut 3 Layer	⅛ cake	240	10	3	2
Devil's Food 3 Layer	⅛ cake	220	9	2	2
Golden 3 Layers	⅛ cake	230	9	2	2
Lemon 3 Layer	⅛ cake	240	11	3	3
Peach Turnover	1	290	15	4	5
Turnover Apple	1	290	15	4	5
Philadelphia					
Snack Bars Classic Cheesecake	1 (1.5 oz)	190	11	3	–
Snack Bars Strawberry Cheesecake	1 (1.5 oz)	190	9	3	–
Sara Lee					
Cheesecake Classic French	1 piece (4.7 oz)	410	25	16	–

FOOD	PORTION	CALS	FAT	SAT FAT	TRANS FAT
Cheesecake French Strawberry	1 piece (4.3 oz)	320	14	9	–
Cheesecake French Chocolate	1 piece (4.2 oz)	430	22	8	4
Cheesecake Strawberry Swirl	1 piece (2.9 oz)	290	11	3	–
Cobbler Anytime Apple	1 (4 oz)	350	17	4	–
Coffee Cake Butter Streusel	1 piece (2 oz)	190	9	5	–
Coffee Cake Crumb	1 serv (2 oz)	190	8	2	–
Layer Cake Coconut	1 slice (2.8 oz)	260	14	10	–
Layer Cake Double Chocolate	1 slice (2.8 oz)	260	13	9	–
Layer Cake Fudge Golden	1 slice (2.8 oz)	260	13	10	–
Layer Cake Vanilla	1 slice (2.8 oz)	260	14	10	–
Pound Cake All Butter	1 slice (0.6 oz)	240	16	9	–
Pound Cake Free & Light	1 slice (2.5 oz)	200	4	1	–
Snack & Smile					
Mini Loaf Apple Cinnamon	1 loaf (2 oz)	190	8	2	–
Mini Loaf Banana	1 loaf (2 oz)	200	8	2	–
Mini Loaf Blueberry	1 loaf (2 oz)	190	8	2	–
Mini Loaf Carrot	1 loaf (2 oz)	200	8	2	–
Tastykake					
Koffee Kake Cream Filled	2 (2 oz)	240	10	2	–
Koffee Kakes	1 (2 oz)	210	7	1	–
Krimpets Butterscotch Iced	2 (2 oz)	210	5	1	–
Weight Watchers					
Lemon w/ Lemon Icing	1 (1 oz)	80	3	1	0
TAKE-OUT					
angelfood	1 slice (2 oz)	143	tr	tr	0
apple crisp	1 serv (8.6 oz)	384	8	1	0
baklava	1 piece (2.7 oz)	334	23	10	0
basbousa namoura	1 piece (1 oz)	60	3	0	–
bean cake	1 cake (1.1 oz)	130	7	1	0
black forest chocolate cherry	1 piece (2.5 oz)	187	9	4	0
boston cream pie	1 slice (3.2 oz)	232	8	2	0
cannoli w/ cannoli cream	1	369	21	–	–
carrot w/ icing	1 slice (4.7 oz)	543	28	5	0
cheesecake	1 slice (4.5 oz)	410	25	10	0
cheesecake chocolate	1 slice (4.5 oz)	489	32	15	0
chinese moon cake	1 (4.8 oz)	458	6	1	0
coconut mochiko filipino cake	1 piece (2.7 oz)	252	12	10	0
coffeecake iced	1 piece (1.6 oz)	175	8	1	0
cream puff custard filled chocolate frosted	1 (3.9 oz)	293	18	5	0

FOOD	PORTION	CALS	FAT	SAT FAT	TRANS FAT
dutch honey cake	1 slice (0.8 oz)	70	0	0	0
eclair	1 (3.5 oz)	262	16	4	0
french apple tart	1 (3.5 oz)	302	15	9	–
fruitcake	1 slice (1.5 oz)	139	4	tr	0
funnel cake	1 (3.2 oz)	276	14	3	0
gingerbread	1 piece (2.4 oz)	213	7	2	0
jelly roll	1 slice (1.8 oz)	146	2	1	0
jelly roll lemon filled	1 slice (3 oz)	210	2	1	–
napoleon	1 (3 oz)	348	25	7	0
napoleon	1 mini (1 oz)	123	9	2	0
panettone	1/12 cake (2.9 oz)	300	12	9	–
petit fours	2 (0.9 oz)	120	7	3	–
pineapple upside down	1 piece (4.2 oz)	387	15	4	0
pound	1 slice (1 oz)	120	5	1	–
pound fat free	1 slice (2 oz)	160	1	tr	0
sacher torte	1 slice (2.2 oz)	240	11	5	–
sacher torte chocolate + apricot jam	1 serv	430	12	–	–
strawberry shortcake	1 serv (4.1 oz)	211	5	2	0
strudel apple	1 piece (2.2 oz)	175	7	1	0
strudel cheese	1 piece (2.2 oz)	195	8	4	0
strudel cherry	1 piece (2.2 oz)	179	6	1	0
tiramisu	1 cake (4.4 lbs)	5732	421	217	–
tiramisu	1 piece (5.1 oz)	409	30	15	–
torte chocolate ganache	1 slice (3.5 oz)	400	26	10	–
trifle w/ cream	6 oz	291	16	–	–
white w/ coconut icing	1 slice (3.9 oz)	399	12	4	–
zucchini bread	1 slice (1.4 oz)	150	7	1	0

CAKE ICING

chocolate	1/4 cup	269	7	2	0
vanilla	1/4 cup	322	8	2	0
Betty Crocker					
HomeStyle Mix Coconut Pecan as prep	2 tbsp	160	2	3	–
HomeStyle Mix White Fluffy as prep	6 tbsp	100	0	0	–
Party Frosting Chocolate w/ Stars	2 tbsp (1.2 oz)	140	5	2	–
Rich & Creamy Butter Cream	2 tbsp (1.3 oz)	140	5	2	–

FOOD	PORTION	CALS	FAT	SAT FAT	TRANS FAT
Rich & Creamy Cherry	2 tbsp (1.2 oz)	140	5	2	–
Rich & Creamy Chocolate	2 tbsp (1.2 oz)	130	5	2	–
Rich & Creamy Cream Cheese	2 tbsp (1.2 oz)	140	5	2	–
Rich & Creamy Dark Chocolate	2 tbsp (1.3 oz)	130	6	2	–
Rich & Creamy French Vanilla	2 tbsp (1.2 oz)	140	5	2	–
Rich & Creamy Milk Chocolate	2 tbsp (1.3 oz)	130	5	2	–
Rich & Creamy Rainbow Chip	2 tbsp (1.2 oz)	140	5	2	–
Rich & Creamy Vanilla	2 tbsp (1.2 oz)	140	5	2	–
Toppers Milk Chocolate	2 tbsp (1.2 oz)	130	5	2	–
Toppers Vanilla	2 tbsp (1.2 oz)	140	5	2	–
Jiffy					
Fudge Frosting	¼ cup	150	4	2	–
White Frosting	¼ cup	150	5	1	–
Sweet Rewards					
Ready-To-Spread Reduced Fat Chocolate	2 tbsp (1.2 oz)	120	2	1	–
Ready-To-Spread Reduced Fat Vanilla	2 tbsp (1.2 oz)	130	2	1	–

CAKE MIX
Betty Crocker

FOOD	PORTION	CALS	FAT	SAT FAT	TRANS FAT
Angel Food Fat Free	1/12 cake	140	0	0	0
Cheesecake Chocolate Chip as prep	⅛ cake	410	28	13	–
Cheesecake Original as prep	⅛ cake	400	27	12	–
Cheesecake Strawberry Swirl as prep	⅛ cake	380	25	11	–
Pineapple Upside Down as prep	⅙ cake	420	14	3	–
Quick Bread Banana	1/12 cake	170	7	1	–
Quick Bread Cinnamon Streusel as prep	1/14 cake	180	7	2	–
Quick Bread Cranberry Orange as prep	1/12 cake	170	6	2	–
Quick Bread Lemon Poppy Seed as prep	1/12 cake	170	7	1	–
Stir'n Bake Carrot Cake w/ Cream Cheese Frosting as prep	⅙ cake	260	7	2	–

FOOD	PORTION	CALS	FAT	SAT FAT	TRANS FAT
Stir'n Bake Coffee Cake w/ Cinnamon Streusel as prep	⅙ cake	230	2	1	–
Stir'n Bake Devils Food w/ Chocolate Frosting as prep	⅙ cake	240	7	2	–
Stir'n Bake Yellow w/ Chocolate Frosting as prep	⅛ cake	240	7	2	–
SuperMoist Butter Pecan as prep	1/12 cake	240	10	2	–
SuperMoist Butter Yellow as prep	1/12 cake	260	11	6	–
SuperMoist Carrot as prep	1/10 cake	320	15	3	–
SuperMoist Cherry Chip	1/10 cake	300	13	3	–
SuperMoist Chocolate Fudge as prep	1/12 cake	270	12	3	–
SuperMoist Golden Vanilla as prep	1/12 cake	240	10	2	–
SuperMoist Lemon as prep	1/12 cake	240	10	2	–
SuperMoist Milk Chocolate as prep	1/12 cake	240	10	2	–
SuperMoist Pineapple as prep	1/12 cake	250	7	2	–
SuperMoist Spice as prep	1/12 cake	240	10	2	–
SuperMoist Strawberry as prep	1/12 cake	250	10	2	–
SuperMoist White as prep	1/12 cake	230	14	2	–
SuperMoist White Light as prep	1/10 cake	210	3	1	–
Bisquick					
Heart Smart	⅓ cup	140	3	0	0
Carbolite					
Cheesecake Chocolate as prep	⅛ cake	260	25	–	–
Carbsense					
Zero Carb Baking Mix	1 oz	110	1	1	–
Don's Chuck Wagon					
All Purpose Batter Mix	¼ cup	100	0	0	0
Jiffy					
Devil's Food as prep	⅕ cake	220	6	2	–
Golden Yellow as prep	⅕ cake	220	5	1	–
White Cake as prep	⅕ cake	210	5	1	–
King Arthur					
Cinnamon Buns Kit not prep	½ cup	240	1	0	0

FOOD	PORTION	CALS	FAT	SAT FAT	TRANS FAT
MiniCarb					
Carrot as prep	1 slice	280	20	3	–
Chocolate as prep	1 slice	230	18	4	–
Zero Carb Baking Mix not prep	½ cup	55	1	0	–
Sweet Rewards					
Reduced Fat White as prep	¹/₁₂ cake	180	3	1	–
Reduced Fat Yellow as prep as prep	¹/₁₂ cake	200	5	1	–

CALABAZA
fresh	½ cup	32	tr	–	–

CALZONE (see SANDWICHES)

CANADIAN BACON
grilled	2 slices (1.6 oz)	87	4	1	0
Boar's Head					
Canadian Bacon	2 oz	70	2	1	–
Celebrity					
98% Fat Free	3 slices (1.8 oz)	60	1	1	–
Jones					
Slices	3	70	3	1	–
Organic Prairie					
Hardwood Smoked	1 oz	40	1	1	–
Real Canadian Bacon					
Peameal	4 oz	130	5	2	–
Wellshire					
Sliced	2 oz	20	3	1	0

CANADIAN BACON SUBSTITUTES
Yves					
Meatless Canadian Bacon	2 slices (2 oz)	80	1	0	0

CANDY
butterscotch	1 piece (6 g)	24	tr	tr	–
candied cherries	1 (4 g)	12	tr	tr	–
candied citron	1 oz	89	tr	–	–
candied lemon peel	1 oz	90	tr	–	–
candied orange peel	1 oz	90	tr	–	–
candied pineapple slice	1 slice (2 oz)	179	tr	tr	–
candy corn	1 oz	105	0	0	0
caramels	1 piece (8 g)	31	1	1	–

FOOD	PORTION	CALS	FAT	SAT FAT	TRANS FAT
caramels chocolate	1 piece (6 g)	22	tr	tr	–
carob bar	1 (3.1 oz)	453	28	7	–
crisped rice bar almond	1 bar (1 oz)	130	6	1	–
crisped rice bar chocolate chip	1 bar (1 oz)	115	4	1	–
dark chocolate	1 oz	150	10	6	–
fondant	1 piece (0.6 oz)	57	0	–	0
fondant chocolate coated	1 piece (0.4 oz)	40	1	1	–
fondant mint	1 oz	105	0	0	0
fruit pastilles	1 tube (1.4 oz)	101	0	–	0
fudge brown sugar w/ nuts	1 piece (0.5 oz)	56	1	tr	–
fudge chocolate marshmallow	1 piece (0.7 oz)	84	3	2	–
fudge chocolate marshmallow w/ nuts	1 piece (0.8 oz)	96	4	2	–
fudge chocolate w/ nuts	1 piece (0.7 oz)	81	3	1	–
fudge peanut butter	1 piece (0.6 oz)	59	1	tr	–
fudge vanilla w/ nuts	1 piece (0.5 oz)	62	2	1	–
gumdrops	10 lg (3.8 oz)	420	0	0	0
gumdrops	10 sm (0.4 oz)	135	0	0	0
hard candy	1 oz	106	0	0	0
jelly beans	10 lg (1 oz)	104	tr	–	–
jelly beans	10 sm (0.4 oz)	40	tr	–	–
lollipop	1 (6 g)	22	0	0	0
marzipan	1 oz	128	7	1	–
milk chocolate	1 bar (1.55 oz)	226	14	8	–
milk chocolate crisp	1 bar (1.45 oz)	203	11	7	–
milk chocolate w/ almonds	1 bar (1.45 oz)	215	14	7	–
nougat nut cream	0.5 oz	49	4	–	–
organic dark chocolate w/ raisins & pecans	1.4 oz	220	14	7	–
peanut bar	1 (1.4 oz)	209	14	2	–
peanut brittle	1 oz	128	5	1	–
peanuts chocolate covered	1 cup (5.2 oz)	773	50	22	–
peanuts chocolate covered	10 (1.4 oz)	208	13	6	–
praline	1 piece (1.4 oz)	177	10	1	–
pretzels chocolate covered	1 (0.4 oz)	50	2	1	–
pretzels chocolate covered	1 oz	130	5	2	–
sesame crunch	20 pieces (1.2 oz)	181	12	2	–
sweet chocolate	1 bar (1.45 oz)	201	14	8	–
sweet chocolate	1 oz	143	10	6	–
taffy	1 piece (0.5 oz)	56	1	tr	–

FOOD	PORTION	CALS	FAT	SAT FAT	TRANS FAT
toffee	1 piece (0.4 oz)	65	4	2	–
truffles	1 piece (0.4 oz)	59	4	3	–
3 Musketeers					
Bar	1 (2.1 oz)	260	8	5	0
Fun Size	3 bars (1.6 oz)	190	6	4	0
Miniatures	7 (1.4 oz)	170	5	4	0
5th Avenue					
Bar	1 (0.56 oz)	80	4	2	–
Almond Joy					
Bar	1 (0.68 oz)	90	5	4	–
Altoids					
All Flavors	3 pieces	10	0	0	0
Anastasia					
Coco Rhum Bites	2 pieces (1 oz)	110	5	3	–
Andes					
Dark Chocolate Covered Cherries	2 (1 oz)	110	5	3	0
Thins Cherry Jubilee	8 pieces (1.3 oz)	200	13	11	0
Thins Creme De Menthe	8 pieces (1.3 oz)	200	13	11	0
At Last!					
Chocolate Almond	1 bar	120	10	6	–
Chocolate Crisp	1 bar	110	9	6	–
Chocolate Mint	1 bar	110	10	6	–
Chocolate Peanut Butter	1 bar	120	11	7	–
Atkins					
Endulge Caramel Nut Chew	1 bar (1.23 oz)	140	9	4	–
Endulge Chocolate Bar	1 bar (1.1 oz)	150	12	7	–
Endulge Chocolate Crunch	1 bar (1 oz)	150	12	7	–
Endulge Peanut Butter Cups	3 pieces	160	13	6	–
Baby Ruth					
Fun Size	2 bars (1.3 oz)	170	8	5	0
Snack Bars	2 (1.3 oz)	170	8	5	0
Bartons					
Cashew Toppers	1 (1 oz)	140	9	3	0
Benecol					
Smart Chews Caramel	1 piece	20	0	0	0
Blow Pop					
Regular	1 (0.6 oz)	60	0	0	0
Brach's					
Bridge Mix	16 pieces	190	8	5	–

FOOD	PORTION	CALS	FAT	SAT FAT	TRANS FAT
Candy Corn	26 pieces	140	0	0	0
Caramel Clusters	3 pieces	210	13	5	–
Circus Peanuts	6 pieces	160	0	0	0
Fruit Rippers Berry Punch	1 pkg (0.5 oz)	60	0	0	0
Fruit Slices	3 pieces	150	0	0	0
Malts	15 pieces	190	7	5	–
Mellowcreme Pumpkins	6 pieces	130	0	0	0
Milk Maid Caramels	4 pieces	160	5	1	–
Mint Patties	3 pieces	140	3	1	–
Orange Slices	2 pieces	130	0	0	0
Peanut Butter Meltaways	3 pieces	200	13	8	–
Root Beer Barrels	3 pieces	70	0	0	0
Spearmint Leaves	5 pieces	130	0	0	0
Spice Drops	12 pieces	130	0	0	0
Sprinkles	17 pieces	200	9	8	–
Star Brites Butterscotch	3 pieces	60	0	0	0
Stars	10 pieces	200	11	0	–
Wild'N Fruity Gummi Bears	14 pieces	140	0	0	0
Breath Savers					
Sugar Free Peppermint	1 piece	5	0	0	0
Butterfinger					
Bar	1 (2.1 oz)	270	11	6	0
Crisps	1 bar (1.8 oz)	250	13	6	0
Crisps Minis	4 (1.5 oz)	220	11	6	0
Minis	4 (1.4 oz)	180	7	4	0
Cadbury					
Milk Chocolate Fruit & Nut	10 blocks (1.4 oz)	200	10	5	0
Milk Chocolate Roast Almond	10 blocks (1.4 oz)	220	13	7	–
Royal Dark	10 blocks (1.4 oz)	220	13	8	–
Carbolite					
Caramel	1 bar	100	5	3	–
CarbAway	1 bar	100	5	3	–
CarboSnack	1 bar	110	6	3	–
Chocolate Truffle	1 bar (1 oz)	122	8	5	–
Chocolate Almond	1 bar (1.75 oz)	298	21	11	–
Chocolate Crisp	1 bar (1.75 oz)	256	14	11	–
Chocolate Peanut Butter	1 bar (1.75 oz)	256	21	7	–
Crisy Caramel	1 bar (1 oz)	130	9	5	–
Milk Chocolate	1 bar (1.75 oz)	263	18	11	–

FOOD	PORTION	CALS	FAT	SAT FAT	TRANS FAT
Peanut Butter Cup	1	170	14	7	–
Pecan Cluster	1 bar	120	8	3	–
CarbSlim					
Crunch Bites Chocolate Caramel	1 pkg	122	14	12	–
Crunch Bites Peanut Butter	1 pkg	171	14	12	–
Carmello					
Snack Size	1 (0.66 oz)	90	4	3	–
Cary's Of Oregon					
English Toffee Milk Chocolate Almond	1 piece (0.75 oz)	110	8	4	–
Cella's					
Milk Chocolate Covered Cherries	2 (1 oz)	120	5	2	0
Chargers					
Chocolate Covered Expresso Beans	1 pkg (0.5 oz)	60	3	2	–
Charleston Chews					
Chocolate	1 bar (1.9 oz)	230	6	5	0
Vanilla	1 bar (1.9 oz)	230	8	5	0
Charms					
Fluffy Stuff Cotton Candy	1 pkg (0.6 oz)	70	0	0	0
Sour Balls	1 (5 g)	20	0	0	0
Squares	2 pieces	20	0	0	0
Chew-ets					
Peanut Chews Original Dark	3 pieces	170	9	4	0
ChocoSoy					
Soy Milk Chocolate	1 piece (0.4 oz)	50	3	1	–
Classic Caramels					
Chocolate Creme Filled	3 pieces	80	3	2	–
Soft & Chewy	3 pieces	80	2	2	–
Cloud Nine					
Australian Orange Peel	½ bar (1.5 oz)	220	13	7	–
Butter Nut Toffee	½ bar (1.5 oz)	230	14	8	–
Cool Mint Crisp	½ bar (1.5 oz)	220	13	7	–
Espresso Bean Crunch	½ bar (1.5 oz)	220	14	8	–
Malted Milk Crunch	½ bar (1.5 oz)	230	14	8	–
Milk Chocolate	½ bar (1.5 oz)	230	15	8	–
Oregon Red Raspberry	½ bar (1.5 oz)	230	15	8	–
Peanut Butter Brittle	½ bar (1.5 oz)	230	15	8	–

FOOD	PORTION	CALS	FAT	SAT FAT	TRANS FAT
Sundried Cherry	½ bar (1.5 oz)	230	13	8	–
Toasted Coconut Crisp	½ bar (1.5 oz)	230	14	9	–
Vanilla Dark	½ bar (1.5 oz)	230	15	8	–
CocoaVia					
Dark Chocolate Blueberry & Almond Bar	1 (0.8 oz)	100	6	3	0
Dark Chocolate Covered Almonds	1 pkg (1 oz)	140	11	4	0
Dark Chocolate Crispy Bar	1 (0.7 oz)	90	5	3	0
Dark Chocolate Original Bar	1 (0.8 oz)	80	6	4	0
Milk Chocolate Almond Bar	1 (0.8 oz)	110	7	3	0
Milk Chocolate Bar	1 (0.8 oz)	110	6	4	0
Milk Chocolate Covered Raisins	1 pkg (1 oz)	150	6	3	0
Coffee Rio					
Coffee Candy All Flavors	4 pieces	60	2	1	–
Crispy Cat					
Roasted Peanut	1 bar (1 oz)	220	10	3	0
Daboga					
Organic Milk Chocolate	1 bar (2 oz)	318	20	14	–
Dare					
RealFruit Gummies All Flavors	8 pieces (1.4 oz)	120	0	0	0
Doctor's CarbRite					
Sugar Free Dark Chocolate	1 oz	124	8	–	–
Sugar Free Dark Chocolate With Almonds	4 sq (1 oz)	132	10	4	–
Sugar Free Milk Chocolate	1 oz	128	9	–	–
Sugar Free Milk Chocolate With Peanuts	4 sq (1 oz)	132	10	4	–
Sugar Free Milk Chocolate With Soy Crisps	4 sq (1 oz)	120	8	4	–
Sugar Free Mint Chocolate	1 oz	128	9	–	–
Dots					
All Flavors	12 (1.5 oz)	140	0	0	0
Dove					
Dark Chocolate	⅓ bar	170	11	6	0
Dark Chocolate Covered Almonds	13 pieces	210	15	6	0
Dark Chocolate Miniatures	5 pieces	210	13	8	0
Milk Chocolate	⅓ bar	180	11	6	0

FOOD	PORTION	CALS	FAT	SAT FAT	TRANS FAT
Milk Chocolate Covered Almonds	13 pieces	220	15	6	0
Milk Chocolate Minatures w/ Caramel	5 pieces	200	11	7	0
Milk Chocolate Miniatures	5	220	13	8	0
Milk Chocolate w/ Almonds	⅓ bar	190	12	6	0
E. Guittard					
Bar Quevedo Bittersweet 65% Cocao	1 (2 oz)	290	23	13	0
Bar Sur Del Lago Bittersweet 65% Cacao	1 (2 oz)	290	23	13	0
Eclipse					
Mints Sugarless All Flavors	3 pieces	5	0	0	0
Endangered Species					
Dark Chocolate w/ Espresso Beans	½ bar (1.5 oz)	200	15	9	0
Dark Chocolate w/ Hazelnut Toffee	½ bar (1.5 oz)	220	15	10	0
Milk Chocolate w/ Cherries	½ bar (1.5 oz)	230	14	9	0
Organic Dark Chocolate	½ bar (0.7 oz)	100	6	4	0
Organic Dark Chocolate w/ Tangerine	½ bar (0.7 oz)	100	6	4	0
Organic Milk Chocolate w/ Key Lime	½ bar (0.7 oz)	110	7	4	0
Equal Exchange					
Organic Chocolate Expresso Bean	1 bar (1.4 oz)	216	15	9	0
Organic Milk Chocolate	1 bar (1.4 oz)	230	16	9	0
Organic Very Dark Chocolate	1 bar (1.4 oz)	220	17	10	0
Estee					
Fructose Sweetened Peanut Butter Cups	5	200	12	7	–
Fructose Sweetened Dark Chocolate	½ bar (1.4 oz)	200	14	8	–
Fructose Sweetened Milk Chocolate	½ bar (1.4 oz)	230	17	10	–
Fructose Sweetened Milk Chocolate w/ Almonds	½ bar (1.4 oz)	230	17	9	–
Fructose Sweetened Milk Chocolate w/ Crisp Rice	½ bar (1.2 oz)	370	26	15	–

FOOD	PORTION	CALS	FAT	SAT FAT	TRANS FAT
Peanut Brittle	⅓ box (1.3 oz)	210	9	2	–
Sugar Free Assorted Fruit	3	15	0	0	0
Sugar Free Butterscotch	4	15	0	0	0
Sugar Free Gourmet Jelly Beans	26	70	0	0	0
Sugar Free Gum Drops Assorted Fruit	11	110	0	0	0
Sugar Free Gummy Bears Assorted Fruit	17	70	0	0	0
Sugar Free Peppermint	3	15	0	0	0
Sugar Free Sour Citrus Slices	9	60	0	0	0
Sugar Free Toffee	4	15	0	0	0
Sugar Free Tropical Fruit	3	15	0	0	0
Ethel's					
Truffles Assorted	4	200	14	6	0
Fauchon					
Assortment Truffles	3 pieces (1.3 oz)	160	11	5	–
Chocolate Assortment	3 pieces (1.1 oz)	170	11	5	–
Ferrero Rocher					
Candy	3 pieces (1.3 oz)	220	15	5	0
Figamajigs					
Fig Candy Drops Dark Chocolate Covered	1 pkg (1.4 oz)	150	4	2	0
Fig Candy Drops Orange & Yellow Chocolate Covered	1 pkg (1.4 oz)	150	3	2	0
Frooties					
Chewy Candy Fruit Flavored	12 pieces (1.3 oz)	104	3	0	1
Fruitzels					
Assorted	7 pieces	120	0	0	0
Ghirardelli					
Squares Milk Chocolate w/ Caramel Filling	3 (1.6 oz)	220	12	7	1
Squares Mint Indulgence	3 (1.6 oz)	210	11	6	1
Squares 60% Cacao Dark Chocolate	4 (1.5 oz)	220	17	10	0
Squares 60% Cacao Dark Chocolate w/ Caramel	3 (1.6 oz)	220	15	8	1
Godiva					
Chocolatier Dark Chocolate w/ Raspberry	1 bar (1.5 oz)	220	11	4	–

FOOD	PORTION	CALS	FAT	SAT FAT	TRANS FAT
Chocolatier Milk Chocolate	1 bar (1.5 oz)	230	13	5	–
Chocolatier Milk Chocolate w/ Almonds	1 bar (1.5 oz)	230	15	4	–
Sugar Free Chocolate	1 bar (1.5 oz)	190	15	9	0
Sugar Free Chocolate w/ Almonds	1 bar (1.5 oz)	200	15	8	0
Sugar Free Dark Chocolate	1 bar (1.5 oz)	190	14	8	0
Truffles Assorted	2 pieces (1.4 oz)	210	13	8	0
Goetze's					
Caramel Creams	3 pieces	130	3	1	–
Gol D Lite					
Milk Chocolate Crisp	1 bar	125	9	6	–
Seashell Truffle	1 piece	54	3	0	–
Golightly					
Sugar Free Caramels	5 pieces	150	6	3	–
Sugar Free Doublers Chews Peach & Creme	7 pieces	150	7	3	–
Sugar Free Fudgie Rolls	6 pieces	130	5	2	–
Sugar Free Hard Candy	4 pieces	45	0	0	0
Good & Plenty					
Snack Size	1 box (0.6 oz)	60	0	0	0
Green & Black's					
Organic Chocolate Fairtrade Maya Gold	1 bar (3.5 oz)	526	34	21	–
Organic Dark Chocolate	1 bar (3.5 oz)	551	41	24	–
Organic Dark Chocolate Mint	1 bar (3.5 oz)	478	27	17	–
Organic Dark Chocolate w/ Hazelnuts & Currants	1 bar (3.5 oz)	513	34	17	–
Organic Milk Chocolate	1 bar (3.5 oz)	523	30	18	–
Organic Milk Chocolate Caramel	1 bar (3.5 oz)	495	26	16	–
Organic Milk Chocolate Raisins & Hazelnuts	1 bar (3.5 oz)	556	37	19	–
Organic Milk Chocolate Whole Almonds	1 bar (3.5 oz)	578	42	17	–
Organic White Chocolate	1 bar (3.5 oz)	573	37	22	–
Guylian					
Twists Milk Chocolate Truffle	5 pieces (1.2 oz)	230	19	11	tr
Twists Original Praline	4 pieces (1.2 oz)	200	13	6	tr

FOOD	PORTION	CALS	FAT	SAT FAT	TRANS FAT
Heath					
Snack Size	1 bar (0.3 oz)	50	3	1	–
Hershey's					
Bites Almond Joy	8 pieces	100	6	4	–
Bites Cookies 'N' Creme	8 pieces	90	5	3	–
Bites Milk Chocolate w/ Almond	7 pieces	90	6	3	–
Bites Reese's	7 pieces	90	5	3	–
Bites York	9 pieces	90	2	1	–
Chocolate Miniatures Sugar Free	5 pieces (1.4 oz)	170	13	8	0
Chocolate w/ Almonds Miniatures Sugar Free	5 pieces (1.4 oz)	180	14	7	0
Cacao Reserve 65% Cacao Dark	3 blocks (1.3 oz)	180	15	9	0
Cacao Reserve 35% Cacao Milk Chocolate w/ Hazelnuts	3 sq (1.3 oz)	220	15	7	0
Dark Chocolate Miniatures Sugar Free	5 pieces (1.4 oz)	190	15	9	0
Hugs	1 piece	25	2	1	–
Kisses	1	25	2	1	–
Kisses w/ Almonds	1 piece	25	2	1	–
Milk Chocolate	1 bar (1.4 oz)	210	12	8	0
Milk Chocolate w/ Almonds	1 bar (1.4 oz)	230	14	7	0
Miniature Special Dark	1 (0.3 oz)	45	3	2	–
Nuggets Cookies 'N' Creme	4	190	10	5	–
Nuggets Dark Chocolate w/ Almonds	4	220	14	6	–
Nuggets Milk Chocolate	4	230	13	8	0
Nuggets Milk Chocolate w/ Almonds	1	60	4	2	–
Nuggets Milk Chocolate w/ Almonds & Toffee	1	50	4	2	–
Nuggets Milk Chocolate w/ Raisins & Almonds	1	50	3	2	–
Pot Of Gold	3 pieces	130	5	4	–
Sticks Special Dark	1 (0.4 oz)	60	4	2	0
Sweet Escapes Caramel & Peanut Butter Crispy	1 bar	80	3	1	–

FOOD	PORTION	CALS	FAT	SAT FAT	TRANS FAT
Sweet Escapes Crunchy Peanut Butter	1 bar (0.7 oz)	90	3	1	–
Sweet Escapes Triple Chocolate Wafer	1 bar	80	3	2	–
Take 5	2 pkg (1.5 oz)	220	11	5	–
Tastetations Butterscotch	3 pieces	60	2	1	–
Tastetations Caramel	3 pieces	60	2	1	–
Tastetations Chocolate	3 pieces	60	21	1	–
Hint Mint					
All Flavors	2 pieces	10	0	0	0
Jay's					
Cotton Candy	1 pkg (2 oz)	220	0	0	0
Jelly Belly					
Jelly Beans Sugar Free	35	80	0	0	0
Jolly Rancher					
All Flavors	4 pieces	60	0	0	0
Lollipops All Flavors	1 (0.6 oz)	60	0	0	0
Sugar Free	4 pieces (0.6 oz)	35	0	0	0
Joyva					
Halvah Chocolate Covered	1 serv (2 oz)	380	25	5	–
Halvah Marble	1 serv (2 oz)	390	25	4	–
Judy's					
Sugar Free Almond Caramel Cluster	1 piece (1.5 oz)	200	15	4	–
Sugar Free Cashew Caramel Cluster	1 piece (1.5 oz)	190	14	5	–
Sugar Free English Toffee	1 piece (1.5 oz)	220	17	5	–
Sugar Free Macadamia Caramel Cluster	1 piece (1.5 oz)	220	20	5	–
Sugar Free Peanut Brittle	¾ cup	100	6	1	–
Sugar Free Pecan Almond Cluster	1 piece (1.5 oz)	220	19	4	–
Junior					
Caramels	1 box (1.4 oz)	170	3	3	0
Mints	1 box (1.4 oz)	170	3	3	0
Kellogg's					
Fruit Flavored Snacks Hello Kitty	10 pieces	100	0	0	0
Fruit Flavored Snacks Winnie The Pooh	1 pkg	80	0	0	0

FOOD	PORTION	CALS	FAT	SAT FAT	TRANS FAT
Fruit Streamers Watermelon Madness	1 pkg (0.8 oz)	80	1	0	0
Fruit Twistables Triple Cherry Explosion	1 pkg (0.8 oz)	70	1	0	0
Gamester Rolls All Varieties	1 pkg (0.7 oz)	80	2	1	1
Yogos Crazy Berries	1 pkg (0.8 oz)	90	2	2	0
KitKat					
Bar	1 (0.5 oz)	73	4	2	0
Klein					
Sugar Free Hard Candy All Flavors	3 pieces	12	0	0	0
Krackel					
Bar	1 (0.6 oz)	90	4	3	–
Miniature	1	45	3	2	–
Lambertz					
Petits Soleils Chocolate Coated Gingerbread	1 piece (0.4 oz)	47	2	1	–
Landies Candies					
Sugar Free Almond Clusters	2 pieces (1.5 oz)	240	17	7	–
Sugar Free Bon Bons Peanut Butter	2 (1.5 oz)	240	17	7	–
Sugar Free Coconut Clusters	2 pieces (1.5 oz)	250	18	12	–
Sugar Free Cookies & Cream	2 pieces (1.5 oz)	240	15	8	–
Sugar Free Dark Almond Bark	1 piece (1.5 oz)	230	15	7	–
Sugar Free Dark Miniature Bars	7 pieces (1.5 oz)	230	14	8	–
Sugar Free Milk Miniature Bars	7 pieces (1.5 oz)	240	15	9	–
Sugar Free Mint Discs	7 pieces (1.5 oz)	240	15	9	–
Sugar Free Peanut Clusters	2 (1.5 oz)	240	17	7	–
Sugar Free White Almond Bark	1 piece (1.5 oz)	230	15	10	–
Sugar Free White Caps	6 pieces (1.5 oz)	230	15	8	–
Lean Protein Bites					
Milk Chocolate	1 pkg (1 oz)	120	6	3	–
Peanut Butter	1 pkg (1 oz)	120	5	4	–
White Chocolate	1 pkg (1 oz)	120	4	2	–
Legacy Chocolates					
Truffles Assorted	1 piece (0.5 oz)	90	6	4	–
Let's Do Organic					
Black Licorice Bars	1 (0.9 oz)	80	0	0	0
Black Licorice Chews	8 (1.4 oz)	130	0	0	0
Gummi Bears	1 pkg (0.9 oz)	80	0	0	0

FOOD	PORTION	CALS	FAT	SAT FAT	TRANS FAT
Lifesavers					
Variety	4 pieces	60	0	0	0
Lindt					
Dark Chocolate 70% Cocoa	4 blocks (1.4 oz)	220	17	10	–
Lindor Truffles 60% Extra Dark	3 pieces	210	19	13	0
Lindor Truffles Milk Chocolate	3 pieces	220	17	12	–
Love Candy					
Dark Chocolate	1 bar (1.5 oz)	190	11	6	0
Milk Chocolate	1 bar (1.5 oz)	200	11	6	0
Yogurt Supreme	1 bar (1.5 oz)	190	11	7	0
Low Carb Chef					
Gummi Bears	14 pieces	138	0	0	0
Jelly Beans	37 pieces	120	0	0	0
Sugar Free Caramel Marshmallow Treats	3 pieces	140	7	5	–
Sugar Free Cherry Cordials	3 pieces	250	8	5	–
Sugar Free Coconut Clusters	4 pieces	210	18	13	–
Sugar Free Milk Chocolate Covered Vanilla Caramels	3 pieces	160	8	5	–
Sugar Free Peanut Butter Cups	1 piece	200	16	8	–
Sugar Free Peanut Butter Truffes	2 pieces	200	16	8	–
Sugar Free Peanut Clusters	4 pieces	210	17	5	–
Sugar Free Pecan Turtles	1 piece	120	13	6	–
Sugar Free Peppermint Patties	3 pieces	150	9	5	–
M&M's					
Almond	1 pkg (1.3 oz)	200	11	4	0
Dark Chocolate	1 pkg (1.7 oz)	240	11	7	0
Milk Chocolate	1 pkg (1.7 oz)	240	10	6	0
Minis	1 pkg (1.1 oz)	150	7	5	0
Peanut	1 pkg (1.7 oz)	250	13	5	0
Peanut Butter	1 pkg (1.6 oz)	240	14	9	0
Maple Grove Farms					
Maple Sugar Candy	5 pieces (1.3 oz)	140	0	0	0
Mauna Loa					
Kona Coffee Crunch Chocolate	1 bar (1.8 oz)	270	16	9	–
Macadamia Crisp Milk Chocolate	1 bar (1.8 oz)	270	17	9	–
Macadamia Milk Chocolate	1 bar (1.8 oz)	280	18	9	–

FOOD	PORTION	CALS	FAT	SAT·FAT	TRANS FAT
Mentos					
Sugar Free Mixed Berries	1 piece	5	0	0	0
Mike & Ike					
All Flavors	1 pkg (2 oz)	200	0	0	0
Milky Way					
Bar	1 (2 oz)	260	10	7	0
Fun Size	2 bars (1.2 oz)	150	6	4	0
Midnight	1 bar (1.8 oz)	220	8	5	0
Midnight Minis	5 (1.4 oz)	180	7	4	0
Milk Chocolate Covered Caramels	5 (1.5 oz)	200	8	6	0
Minis	5 (1.5 oz)	190	7	4	0
Mon Cheri					
Hazelnut	4 pieces	260	18	9	–
Mounds					
Bar	1 (0.7 oz)	90	5	4	–
Mr. Goodbar					
Bar	1 (1.75 oz)	270	16	7	–
Miniatures	1 (0.3 oz)	45	3	2	–
Mrs. Fields					
Decadent Chocolates	3 pieces (1.8 oz)	240	12	6	–
Munch					
Nut Bar	1 (1.42 oz)	220	15	4	0
Necco					
Mint	1 piece	12	tr	–	–
Nestle					
Crunch Stix	1 (0.6 oz)	90	5	4	0
Toll House Brownie Bar	2 pieces (2 oz)	250	12	5	–
Toll House Cookie Bar	1 piece (1 oz)	130	6	3	–
Turtles Original	3 pieces	240	14	5	–
Newman's Own					
Organic Chocolate Cups Dark Chocolate Peanut Butter	1 pkg (1.2 oz)	180	12	6	–
Organic Chocolate Cups Milk Chocolate Peanut Butter	1 pkg (1.2 oz)	180	12	6	–
Organic Chocolate Cups Peppermint	1 pkg (1.2 oz)	170	11	6	0
Organic Chocolate Sweet Dark	½ bar (¼ oz)	200	13	7	–
Organic Chocolate Sweet Dark Expresso	½ bar (1.4 oz)	200	14	8	–

FOOD	PORTION	CALS	FAT	SAT FAT	TRANS FAT
Organic Chocolate Sweet Dark Orange	½ bar (1.4 oz)	200	13	8	–
Organic Milk Chocolate	½ bar (1.4 oz)	210	13	7	–
Nibs					
Licorice	9 pieces	35	0	0	0
Nutty Ducky's					
Cashew Brittle	4 pieces (1.6 oz)	240	14	3	0
Cashew Brittle Dark Chocolate	2 pieces (1.5 oz)	220	14	5	0
Peanut Brittle	4 pieces (1.6 oz)	230	12	3	0
Peanut Brittle Milk Chocolate	2 pieces (1.5 oz)	220	12	5	0
Odense					
Marzipan	2 tbsp (1.4 oz)	170	4	0	–
Payday					
Snack Size	1 (0.7 oz)	90	5	1	–
Pearson's					
Mint Patties	1	30	1	tr	–
Perlege					
Sugar Free Belgium Chocolate All Flavors	1 bar (3.5 oz)	532	42	–	–
Pez					
Candy	1 roll (0.3 oz)	35	0	0	0
Candy Sugar Free	1 roll (0.3 oz)	30	0	0	0
Pure De-Lite					
Caramel	1 bar	120	5	4	–
Caramel Crisp	1 bar	120	6	4	–
Caramel Nougat	1 bar	110	5	3	–
Caramel Peanut Butter	1 bar	120	6	3	–
Caramel Pecan	1 bar	130	7	4	–
Sugar Free Dark Chocolate	1 bar	173	14	8	–
Sugar Free Milk Chocolate	1 bar	187	14	9	–
Sugar Free Milk Chocolate w/ Almonds	1 bar	190	14	9	–
Sugar Free Milk Chocolate w/ Coconut	1 bar	190	14	9	–
Sugar Free Milk Chocolate w/ Mint	1 bar	187	14	9	–
Sugar Free Milk Chocolate w/ Orange	1 bar	187	14	9	–
Sugar Free Milk Chocolate w/ Peanuts	1 bar	190	14	9	–

FOOD	PORTION	CALS	FAT	SAT FAT	TRANS FAT
Sugar Free White Chocolate	1 bar	187	14	9	–
Truffle Bar Caramel	1 bar	140	8	5	–
Truffle Bar Dark Mint	1 bar	160	12	8	–
Truffle Bar Hazelnut	1 bar	160	12	7	–
Truffle Bar Peanut Butter	1 bar	160	11	7	–
Raisinets					
Candy	3 pkg (1.7 oz)	200	8	5	0
Reese's					
Bites	16 pieces	220	12	7	–
FastBreak	1 bar (0.7 oz)	90	5	2	0
Miniatures Peanut Butter Cups Sugar Free	5 pieces (1.4 oz)	170	12	5	0
Nutrageous	1 bar (0.6 oz)	95	6	2	–
Peanut Butter Cups Miniatures	5 (1.4 oz)	210	12	5	0
Peanut Butter Cups Snack Size	1 piece (0.5 oz)	80	5	2	0
Peanut Butter Cups Sugar Free	1 piece (1.5 oz)	180	13	6	0
Peanut Butter Eggs	1	90	5	2	–
Pieces	25	90	5	3	–
White Miniatures Peanut Butter Cups	4 pieces (1.4 oz)	210	12	5	0
White Miniatures Peanut Butter Cups Sugar Free	5 pieces (1.4 oz)	180	13	6	0
Ritter Sport					
Dark Chocolate Whole Hazelnuts	6 pieces (1.3 oz)	210	15	8	–
Robin Eggs					
Large	2 pieces	70	2	2	–
Medium	4 pieces	90	3	2	–
Mini	10 pieces	70	3	2	–
Rolo					
Caramels In Milk Chocolate	3 pieces (0.64 oz)	90	3	2	–
Russell Stover					
Assorted	3 pieces (1.4 oz)	170	7	5	0
Low Carb Pecan Delights	1 piece (1 oz)	130	9	5	–
Pecan Delights	1 pkg (2 oz)	280	18	5	–
Private Reserve Triple Chocolate Mousse	3 pieces (1.3 oz)	220	17	12	0
Private Reserve Vanilla Bean Brulee	3 pieces (1.3 oz)	180	13	8	0

FOOD	PORTION	CALS	FAT	SAT FAT	TRANS FAT
Sugar Free Peanut Butter Cups	4 pieces (1.3 oz)	200	13	6	–
Sugar Free Pecans & Caramel	2 pieces (1.2 oz)	170	12	3	–
Scharffen Berger					
Semisweet 60% Cacao	1 bar (2 oz)	320	20	13	0
Sixlets					
Sixlets	3 tubes	90	4	3	–
Skittles					
Original Fruit	1 pkg (2.2 oz)	250	3	3	0
Slim-Fast					
Protein Snack Chews Peanut Butter	1 pkg (0.9 oz)	100	4	1	0
Smucker's					
Jelly Beans	25	150	0	0	0
Snickers					
Almond	1 (1.8 oz)	230	11	4	0
Bar	1 bar (2.07 oz)	280	14	5	0
Cruncher	1 bar (1.6 oz)	220	11	6	0
Cruncher	3 fun size (1.4 oz)	230	13	5	–
Miniatures	4 (1.3 oz)	170	9	4	–
Sour Patch					
Connectors	1.5 oz	150	0	0	0
Kids	1.5 oz	140	0	0	0
Speakeasy					
Organic Mints All Flavors	4 pieces (2 g)	10	0	0	0
Starburst					
Baja California	1 pkg	240	5	5	0
Jellybeans	¼ cup	160	0	0	0
Original Fruit	1 pkg	240	0	0	0
Sour Fruit	1 pkg	240	5	1	0
Sugar Babies					
Candy	30 pieces (1.5 oz)	180	2	0	0
Chocolate	19 pieces (1.4 oz)	180	5	2	0
Sugar Daddy					
Pop	1 lg (1.7 oz)	200	3	1	0
Swedish Fish					
Aqua Life	1.5 oz	140	0	0	0
Original	20 pieces (1.5 oz)	140	0	0	0
Symphony					
Bar	1 (0.6 oz)	90	5	3	–

FOOD	PORTION	CALS	FAT	SAT FAT	TRANS FAT
Take 5					
Snack Size	2 pieces	220	11	5	0
The Chocolate Traveler					
Wedges Bittersweet	4 pieces	130	10	5	0
Wedges Dark Chocolate Coffee	4 pieces	130	8	5	0
Wedges Dark Chocolate Mint	4 pieces	130	8	5	0
Wedges Dark Chocolate Orange	4 pieces	120	8	5	0
Wedges Dark Chocolate Raspberry	4 pieces	120	8	5	0
Wedges Dark Chocolate Tiramisu	4 pieces	120	8	5	0
Wedges Milk Chocolate	4 pieces	130	8	5	0
Wedges Milk Chocolate Dulce De Leche	4 pieces	120	7	4	0
Wedges White Chocolate	4 pieces	140	9	6	0
Wedges White Chocolate Creme Brulee	4 pieces	140	9	6	0
Tobler					
Orange Dark Chocolate	5 pieces (1.5 oz)	240	13	8	–
Toblerone					
Bittersweet Chocolate w/ Honey & Almond Nougat	⅓ bar (1.2 oz)	170	9	5	–
Milk Chocolate w/ Honey & Almond Nougat	⅓ bar (1.76 oz)	170	9	5	–
Tootsie Roll					
Midgees	6	140	3	1	1
Mini Chews	30 pieces (1.4 oz)	170	7	3	1
Pops	1 (0.6 oz)	60	0	0	0
Pops Caramel Apple	1 (0.6 oz)	60	1	0	0
Torras					
Sugar Free Dark Chocolate	1 oz	136	10	6	–
Sugar Free Milk Chocolate	1 oz	140	10	6	–
Sugar Free Milk Chocolate w/ Almonds	1 oz	146	10	5	–
Sugar Free Milk Chocolate w/ Hazelnuts	1 oz	148	11	6	–
Sugar Free White Chocolate	1 oz	138	10	6	–

FOOD	PORTION	CALS	FAT	SAT FAT	TRANS FAT
Twix					
Fun Size	1 (0.6 oz)	80	4	3	0
Peanut Butter	1 bar	280	17	8	0
Twizzlers					
Cherry	1 piece	30	0	0	0
Chocolate	1	25	0	0	0
Licorice	1 piece	30	0	0	0
Pull'N'Peel Cherry	1 piece	100	0	0	0
Strawberry Snack Size	3 pkgs	130	1	–	–
Sugar Free	4 pieces (1.5 oz)	130	1	0	0
Unique Origin					
Guaranda Dark Chocolate	1 piece (0.3 oz)	54	4	3	–
Vere					
75% Chocolate Gluten Free	1 sm bar	80	6	4	0
Brownie Box Coconut Gluten Free Vegan	3 pieces (1.4 oz)	210	18	13	0
Brownie Box Peanut Butter Gluten Free	3 pieces (1.3 oz)	180	14	6	0
Brownie Box Walnut Gluten Free	3 pieces (1.3 oz)	190	15	7	0
Clusters Chocolate Coconut Gluten Free Vegan	3 pieces (1.7 oz)	280	23	18	0
Clusters Chocolate Almond Gluten Free Vegan	2 pieces (1.3 oz)	210	16	4	0
Clusters Chocolate Rice Gluten Free Vegan	3 pieces (1.3 oz)	170	8	5	0
Clusters Chocolate Seed Gluten Free Vegan	2 pieces (1.3 oz)	210	16	4	0
Wafers Cacao Nibs Gluten Free Vegan	2 (1.1 oz)	170	12	8	0
Wafers Espresso Gluten Free Vegan	3 (1.6 oz)	250	19	11	0
Wafers Pink Peppercorn Gluten Free Vegan	3 (1.6 oz)	250	19	12	0
Wafers Spicy Pepita Gluten Free	2 (1.1 oz)	170	13	8	0
Wafers Tamari Almond Gluten Free Vegan	2 (1.2 oz)	170	11	6	0
Weight Watchers					
English Toffee Squares	3 pieces	160	10	0	0

FOOD	PORTION	CALS	FAT	SAT FAT	TRANS FAT
Mint Patties	2	100	6	5	0
Peanut Butter Crunch	4 pieces	180	8	5	0
Pecan Crowns	3 pieces	150	9	5	0
Whatchamacallit					
Bar	1 (0.57 oz)	80	4	3	–
Whitman's					
Sampler	3 pieces (1.4 oz)	220	10	7	0
Whoppers					
Malted Milk Balls	18 pieces	190	7	6	0
Yamate Chocolatier					
No Sugar Almonds & Caramel	1 piece (0.6 oz)	70	6	3	–
York					
Peppermint Patty	3 (1.4 oz)	150	3	2	0
Peppermint Patty Sugar Free	3 (1.3 oz)	110	4	3	0
Yummy Earth					
Organic Lollipops All Flavors	3	70	0	0	0
Zagnut					
Snack Size	1 piece	70	3	2	–
Zero					
Bar	1	70	3	2	–
CANTALOUPE					
dried	3.5 pieces (1.4 oz)	140	0	0	0
fresh cubed	1 cup	57	tr	–	–
fresh half	½	94	1	–	–
Chiquita					
Wedge	¼ med (4.7 oz)	50	0	0	0
Del Monte					
Fresh	¼ melon (4.7 oz)	50	0	0	0
CAPERS					
capers	1 tbsp	2	tr	tr	0
CARAWAY					
seed	1 tbsp	22	1	tr	0
CARDAMOM					
ground	1 tsp	6	tr	tr	0
CARDOON					
fresh shredded	½ cup	36	tr	tr	–

FOOD	PORTION	CALS	FAT	SAT FAT	TRANS FAT
Frieda's					
Cardoon	1 cup	15	0	0	0
CARIBOU					
roasted	3 oz	142	4	1	–
CARISSA					
fresh	1	12	tr	–	–
CAROB					
carob mix	3 tsp	45	0	0	0
carob mix as prep w/ whole milk	9 oz	195	8	5	–
flour	1 cup	185	1	tr	–
flour	1 tbsp	14	tr	tr	–
Bob's Red Mill					
Powder Toasted	2 tsp	25	0	0	0
CARP					
fresh cooked	1 fillet (6 oz)	276	12	2	–
fresh cooked	3 oz	138	6	1	–
fresh raw	3 oz	108	5	1	–
roe raw	1 oz	37	tr	–	–
CARROT JUICE					
canned	6 oz	73	tr	tr	–
Bolthouse Farms					
Carrot Juice	8 oz	70	0	0	0
Hollywood					
100% Juice	1 can (12 oz)	120	1	–	–
Lakewood					
Organic	6 oz	73	0	0	0
Luvli Juices					
Zingy Carrot	1 bottle (10 oz)	145	0	0	0
Naked Juice					
Just Carrot	8 oz	80	0	0	0
Odwalla					
100% Juice	8 oz	70	0	0	0
CARROTS					
CANNED					
slices	½ cup	17	tr	tr	–
slices low sodium	½ cup	17	tr	tr	–

FOOD	PORTION	CALS	FAT	SAT FAT	TRANS FAT
Del Monte					
Savory Sides Honey Glazed	½ cup	70	0	0	0
Sliced	½ cup	35	0	0	0
Glory					
Seasoned Honey	½ cup	50	0	0	0
S&W					
Sliced	½ cup (4.3 oz)	30	0	0	0
Tillen Farms					
Crispy Carrots Pickled	5 pieces (1 oz)	30	0	0	0
FRESH					
baby raw	1 (0.5 oz)	6	tr	tr	–
raw	1 (2.5 oz)	31	tr	tr	–
raw shredded	½ cup	24	tr	tr	–
slices cooked	½ cup	35	tr	tr	–
Bolthouse Farms					
Baby	1 pkg (2.25 oz)	25	0	0	0
Matchstix	3 oz	35	0	0	0
Earthbound Farm					
Organic Tops On	1 (2.7 oz)	35	0	0	0
Organic w/ Organic Ranch Dip	1 pkg (2.2 oz)	90	8	1	0
Frieda's					
Gold	⅔ cup (3 oz)	35	0	0	0
Grimmway					
Baby	3 oz	38	0	0	0
Nature's Gold					
Fresh	1 med (2.7 oz)	40	0	0	0
River Ranch					
Shredded	¾ cup	35	0	0	0
FROZEN					
slices cooked	½ cup	26	tr	tr	–
Birds Eye					
Steam & Serve Carrots & Cranberries	1 cup	130	5	3	0
C&W					
Whole Baby	⅔ cup	35	0	0	0
Fresh Like					
Carrots Sliced	3.5 oz	42	tr	–	–
Green Giant					
Honey Glazed	1 cup	90	3	1	1

FOOD	PORTION	CALS	FAT	SAT FAT	TRANS FAT
CASABA					
cubed	1 cup	45	tr	–	–
fresh	1/10	43	tr	–	–
CASHEWS					
cashew butter w/o salt	1 tbsp	94	8	2	–
dry roasted w/ salt	18 nuts (1 oz)	160	13	3	–
oil roasted w/ salt	1 oz	163	14	3	–
oil roasted w/o salt	1 oz	163	14	3	–
Arrowhead Mills					
Organic Cashew Butter	2 tbsp	160	13	3	0
Bowlby's					
Bits	1/2 cup	200	19	3	–
Frito Lay					
Salted	3 tbsp	160	13	3	0
Good Sense					
Jumbo Honey Roasted	1/4 cup	170	11	2	–
Jumbo Roasted & Salted	1/4 cup	190	16	3	0
Kettle					
Butter Creamy Unsalted	2 tbsp	160	14	3	0
Maranatha					
Tamari Cashews	1/4 cup	160	13	3	–
Navitas Naturals					
Cashews	1 oz	160	12	2	0
Peeled Snacks					
Nut Picks Cashew Later	1 pkg (1 oz)	180	14	3	0
Planters					
Chocolate Lovers Milk Chocolate	10 pieces (1.5 oz)	230	16	7	0
Dry Roasted	19 pieces (1 oz)	160	12	2	0
Organic	23 pieces (1 oz)	170	13	2	0
Sunfood					
Organic	1 oz	164	12	2	0
Sweet Delights					
Cashew Roasters	1/3 pkg (1 oz)	170	14	–	–
CASSAVA					
fresh	3.5 oz	120	tr	tr	–

FOOD	PORTION	CALS	FAT	SAT FAT	TRANS FAT
CATFISH					
channel breaded & fried	3 oz	194	11	3	–
wolffish atlantic baked	3 oz	105	3	tr	–
Simmons					
Farm Raised	4 oz	140	6	2	0
CAULIFLOWER					
FRESH					
cooked	½ cup (2.2 oz)	14	tr	tr	–
flowerets cooked	3 (2 oz)	12	tr	tr	–
flowerets raw	3 (2 oz)	14	tr	tr	–
green cooked	1½ cups (3.2 oz)	29	tr	tr	–
green raw	1 cup (2.2 oz)	20	tr	tr	–
green raw	1 head 7 in diam (18 oz)	158	2	tr	–
green raw floweret	1 (0.9 oz)	8	tr	tr	–
raw	½ cup (1.8 oz)	13	tr	tr	–
River Ranch					
Florets	1 cup	20	0	0	0
FROZEN					
cooked	½ cup	17	tr	tr	–
Fresh Like					
Florets	3.5 oz	26	tr	–	–
Green Giant					
Cheese Sauce	½ cup	50	3	1	1
CAVIAR					
black or red	2 tbsp	81	6	1	0
CELERY					
fresh	1 lg stalk (2.2 oz)	9	tr	tr	0
pickled	½ cup	10	tr	tr	0
raw diced	½ cup	8	tr	tr	0
seed	1 tsp	1	tr	tr	0
strips	1 cup	17	tr	tr	0
Dole					
Stalks	2 med (3 oz)	20	0	0	0
Earthbound Farm					
Organic Hearts	2 stalks (3.9 oz)	20	0	0	0
Frieda's					
Celery Root	¾ cup	35	0	0	0

FOOD	PORTION	CALS	FAT	SAT FAT	TRANS FAT
River Ranch					
Sticks Fresh	4 (3 oz)	15	0	0	0
TAKE-OUT					
creamed	½ cup	87	6	1	–
stir fried	½ cup	30	2	tr	–
stuffed w/ cheese	1 (5 inch)	38	3	2	–

CELERY JUICE

juice	1 cup	42	tr	tr	0

CELTUCE

raw	3.5 oz	22	tr	–	–

CEREAL

FOOD	PORTION	CALS	FAT	SAT FAT	TRANS FAT
bran flakes	¾ cup	90	1	tr	
corn flakes	1¼ cups	110	tr	tr	–
farina as prep w/ water	¾ cup	88	tr	tr	–
granola	½ cup	285	15	3	–
oatmeal instant as prep w/ water	1 cup (8.2 oz)	138	2	tr	–
oatmeal regular & quick as prep w/ water	¾ cup (6.1 oz)	149	2	tr	–
oatmeal regular & quick not prep	⅓ cup (0.9 oz)	104	2	tr	–
puffed rice	1 cup	56	tr	tr	–
puffed wheat	1 cup	44	tr	tr	–
shredded mini wheats	1 cup	107	1	tr	–
shredded wheat rectangular	1 biscuit (0.8 oz)	85	tr	tr	–
Alpen					
Corn Flakes	1 serv (1 oz)	110	tr	–	–
Regular	1 serv (2 oz)	200	3	–	–
Alti Plano					
Hot Cereal Chai Almond	1 pkg	210	7	0	0
Hot Cereal Oaxacan Chocolate	1 pkg	170	3	0	0
Hot Cereal Orange Date	1 pkg	180	3	0	0
Hot Cereal Regular	1 pkg	190	3	0	0
Hot Cereal Spiced Apple Raisin	1 pkg	160	2	0	0
Instant Quinoa Hot Cereal Spiced Apple Raisin	1 pkg	160	2	0	–
Instant Quinoa Organic Hot Cereal Oaxacan Chocolate	1 pkg	170	3	0	–

FOOD	PORTION	CALS	FAT	SAT FAT	TRANS FAT
Alvarado Street Bakery					
Plain Granola	½ cup	220	5	1	0
Arrowhead Mills					
Organic Amaranth Flakes	1 cup	140	2	2	0
Organic Kamut Flakes	1 cup	120	1	1	0
Organic Multigrain Flakes	1 cup	170	2	0	0
Organic Nature O's	1 cup	130	2	1	0
Organic Puffed Corn	1 cup	60	1	0	0
Organic Puffed Millet	1 cup	60	1	0	0
Organic Puffed Wheat	1 cup	60	0	0	0
Organic Rice Flakes Sweetened	1 cup	180	1	0	0
Organic Shredded Wheat	1 cup	190	1	0	0
Organic Spelt Flakes	1 cup	120	1	0	0
Aunt Paula's					
Hot Flax Cereal	1 serv (1.5 oz)	100	5	5	–
Back To Nature					
Energy Start Hi Protein Crunch	½ cup	170	2	0	0
Flax & Fiber Crunch	1 cup	200	3	0	0
Granola Apple Blueberry	½ cup	200	3	0	0
Granola Classic	½ cup	180	3	0	0
Granola French Vanilla	½ cup	220	6	2	0
Heart Basics Organic Apple Cinnamon Harvest	¾ cup	180	2	0	0
Multigrain Harvest	1 cup	210	3	1	0
Oat & Soy Crisp	¾ cup	180	3	1	0
Strawberry & Seven Grains	1 cup	210	1	0	0
Barbara's Bakery					
Shredded Spoonfuls	¾ cup	120	2	0	–
Bear Naked					
Apple Cinnamon	¼ cup	140	7	2	0
Banana Nut	¼ cup	140	7	2	0
Fruit And Nut	¼ cup	140	7	2	0
Peak Protein	½ cup	200	8	1	–
Bob's Red Mill					
Farina Creamy Brown Rice not prep	¼ cup	150	1	0	0
Muesli Old Country	¼ cup	110	3	0	0
Natural Granola No Fat	½ cup	180	3	0	0
Organic Right Stuff Hot Cereal 6 Grain not prep	¼ cup	140	2	0	0

FOOD	PORTION	CALS	FAT	SAT FAT	TRANS FAT
Rolled Oats Gluten Free not prep	½ cup	160	3	1	0
Carbsense					
Hot Cereal Country Spice not prep	½ cup	130	6	1	–
Hot Cereal Roasted Hazelnut not prep	½ cup	140	9	1	–
Cascadian Farm					
Organic Clifford Crunch	1 cup	100	1	0	0
Organic Granola Oats & Honey	⅔ cup	230	6	1	0
CoCo Wheats					
Hot Cereal	⅓ cup	200	1	0	–
Country Choice Naturals					
Instant Oatmeal Apples 'N' Cinnamon	1 pkg	140	2	0	–
Instant Oatmeal Maple Syrup	1 pkg	170	2	0	–
Instant Oatmeal Organic Plus French Vanilla	1 pkg	180	3	0	–
Instant Oatmeal Organic Plus Golden Brown Sugar	1 pkg	180	3	0	–
Instant Oatmeal Regular	1 pkg	110	2	0	–
Oatmeal Steel Cut not prep	½ cup	150	3	0	–
Oats Old Fashioned not prep	½ cup	150	3	1	–
Oats Quick not prep	½ cup	150	3	1	–
Organic Multi Grain Hot Cereal not prep	½ cup	130	2	0	–
Deliciously Slim					
Granola Cranberry Cashew	¾ cup	230	13	1	–
Granola Strawberry Almond	¾ cup	230	13	1	–
Earthbound Farm					
Organic Granola Maple Almond	½ cup	260	14	2	0
Enjoy Life					
Allergen Gluten Free Granola Cinnamon	½ cup	160	3	0	0
EnviroKidz					
Organic Orangutan O's	¾ cup	120	1	0	0
Erewhon					
Apple Stroodles	¾ cup	110	1	0	–
Aztec	1 cup	110	0	0	0

FOOD	PORTION	CALS	FAT	SAT FAT	TRANS FAT
Banana O's	¾ cup	110	0	0	0
Brown Rice Cream	¼ cup	170	1	0	–
Corn Flakes	1¼ cups	210	3	0	–
Crispy Brown Rice	1 cup	110	0	0	0
Crispy Brown Rice No Salt Added	1 cup	110	0	0	0
Fruit'n Wheat	¾ cup	170	2	0	–
Kamut Flakes	⅔ cup	110	0	0	0
Raisin Bran	1 cup	170	1	0	–
Rice Twice	¾ cup	120	0	0	0
Whole Wheat Flakes	1 cup	180	1	0	–
Expert Foods					
Low Carb Hot Cereal Sub	½ cup	24	0	0	0
Fantastic					
Oatmeal Big Cup Apple Cinnamon	1 pkg	270	4	1	–
Oatmeal Big Cup Maple Raisin 3 Grain	1 pkg	270	2	0	–
General Mills					
Basic 4	1 cup (1.9 oz)	200	2	0	–
Boo Berry	1 cup (1 oz)	120	1	0	–
Cheerios	1 cup	110	2	0	0
Cheerios Apple Cinnamon	¾ cup	120	2	0	–
Cheerios Crunch Oat Cluster	¾ cups	100	1	0	0
Cheerios Frosted	1 cup (1 oz)	120	1	0	–
Cheerios Honey Nut	1 cup (1 oz)	120	2	0	–
Cheerios Yogurt Burst Strawberry	¾ cup	120	2	1	0
Cheerios Yogurt Burst Vanilla	¾ cup	120	2	1	–
Chex Corn	1 cup (1 oz)	110	0	0	0
Chex Honey Nut	¾ cup	120	1	0	–
Chex Morning Mix Cinnamon	1 pkg (1.1 oz)	130	4	1	–
Chex Morning Mix Fruit & Nut	1 pkg (1.1 oz)	180	4	1	–
Chex Multi-Bran	1 cup (2 oz)	200	2	0	–
Chex Rice	1¼ cups (1.1 oz)	120	0	0	0
Chex Whole Grain Chocolate	¾ cup	130	3	1	0
Cinnamon Grahams	¾ cup (1 oz)	120	1	0	–
Cinnamon Toast Crunch	¾ cup (1 oz)	130	4	1	–
Cocoa Puffs	1 cup (1 oz)	120	1	0	–
Cookie Crisp	1 cup (1 oz)	120	1	0	–

FOOD	PORTION	CALS	FAT	SAT FAT	TRANS FAT
Count Chocula	1 cup (1 oz)	120	1	0	–
Country Corn Flakes	1 cup (1 oz)	120	0	0	0
Curves	¾ cup	100	1	0	0
Fiber One	½ cup (1 oz)	60	1	0	0
Fiber One Honey Clusters	1¼ cups	170	1	0	0
Franken Berry	1 cup (1 oz)	120	1	0	–
French Toast Crunch	¾ cup (1 oz)	120	1	0	–
Gold Medal Raisin Bran	1⅓ cups (1.9 oz)	170	2	0	–
Golden Grahams	¾ cup (1 oz)	120	1	0	–
Honey Nut Clusters	1 cup (1.9 oz)	210	3	0	–
Kix	1⅓ cup (1 oz)	120	1	0	–
Kix Berry Berry	¾ cup (1 oz)	120	2	0	–
Lucky Charms	1 cup (1 oz)	120	1	0	–
Nature Valley Low Fat Fruit Granola	⅔ cup (1.9 oz)	210	3	0	–
Nesquik	¾ cup (1 oz)	120	2	0	–
Oatmeal Crisp Almond	1 cup (1.9 oz)	220	5	1	–
Oatmeal Crisp Apple Cinnamon	1 cup (1.9 oz)	210	2	0	–
Oatmeal Crisp Raisin	1 cup (1.9 oz)	210	2	0	–
Para Su Familia Cinnamon Stars	1 cup (1 oz)	120	1	0	–
Para Su Familia Raisin Bran	1¼ cups (2 oz)	170	2	0	–
Raisin Nut Bran	¾ cup (1.9 oz)	200	4	1	–
Reese's Puffs	¾ cup	130	3	1	–
Snack'N Dash Cinnamon Toast Crunch	1 pkg (1.2 oz)	140	4	1	–
Snack'N Dash Honey Nut Cheerios	1 pkg (1 oz)	110	1	0	–
Snack'N Dash Lucky Charms	1 pkg (1 oz)	110	1	0	–
Sunrise Organic	¾ cup (1 oz)	110	1	0	–
Total Brown Sugar & Oat	¾ cup (1 oz)	110	1	0	–
Total Honey Clusters	¾ cup	170	2	0	0
Total Protein	¾ cup	120	4	0	–
Total Raisin Bran	1 cup	170	1	0	0
Total Whole Grain	¾ cup (1 oz)	100	1	0	0
Trix	1 cup (1 oz)	120	1	0	–
Wheaties	1 cup (1 oz)	110	1	0	–
Wheaties Energy Crunch	1 cup (1.9 oz)	210	3	0	–
Wheaties Frosted	¾ cup (1 oz)	110	1	0	–

FOOD	PORTION	CALS	FAT	SAT FAT	TRANS FAT
Wheaties Raisin Bran	1 cup (1.9 oz)	180	1	0	–
Glucerna					
Crunchy Flakes 'N Raisins	1 bowl (1.6 oz)	140	1	0	0
Crunchy Flakes 'N Strawberries	1 bowl (1.5 oz)	150	1	0	0
Glutino					
Gluten Free Apple Cinnamon	½ cup	120	2	0	0
Gluten Free Honey Nut	½ cup	130	3	tr	0
Grainfield's					
Brown Rice	1 serv (1 oz)	110	1	–	–
Crisp Rice	1 serv (1 oz)	112	tr	–	–
Raisin Bran	1 serv (1 oz)	90	2	–	–
Wheat Flakes	1 serv (1 oz)	100	1	–	–
Gram's Gourmet					
Cream Of Flax not prep	½ cup	142	5	1	–
Crunch Granolas All Flavors	½ cup	349	30	6	–
Grandy Oats					
Organic Granola Classic	½ cup	252	14	2	0
Organic Granola Low Fat Cranberry Chew	½ cup	191	1	0	0
Organic Granola Mainely Maple	½ cup	204	7	tr	0
Hi-Lo					
Low Carb Cereal	½ cup	90	2	0	–
Hodgson Mill					
Hot Cereal Bulgur Wheat w/ Soy not prep	¼ cup	115	1	0	–
Hot Cereal Oat Bran not prep	¼ cup	120	3	1	–
Honest Foods					
Granola Planks Maple Almond Crunch	½ bar (2 oz)	250	10	1	0
Kashi					
7 Whole Grain Flakes	1 cup	180	1	0	0
7 Whole Grain Honey Puffs	1 cup	120	1	0	0
7 Whole Grain Nuggets	½ cup	210	2	0	0
7 Whole Grain Pilaf as prep	½ cup	170	3	0	0
7 Whole Grain Puffs	1 cup	70	1	0	0
GoLean	1 cup	140	1	0	0
GoLean Crunch	1 cup	190	3	0	0
GoLean Crunch Honey Almond Flax	1 cup	200	5	0	0

FOOD	PORTION	CALS	FAT	SAT FAT	TRANS FAT
GoLean Instant Hot Cereal Creamy Truly Vanilla	1 pkg	150	2	0	0
GoLean Instant Hot Cereal Hearty Honey & Cinnamon	1 pkg	150	2	0	0
Good Friends	1 cup	170	2	0	0
Granola Mountain Medley	½ cup	220	7	1	0
Heart To Heart Instant Oatmeal Golden Brown Maple	1 pkg	160	2	0	0
Heart To Heart Instant Oatmeal Raisin Spice	1 pkg	150	2	0	0
Heart To Heart Oat Flakes & Blueberry Clusters	1¼ cups	200	3	1	0
Heart To Heart Toasted Oat	¾ cup	110	2	0	0
Mighty Bites All Flavors	1 cup	110	2	0	0
Organic Promise Autumn Wheat	1 cup	190	1	0	0
Organic Promise Cinnamon Harvest	1 cup	190	1	0	0
Organic Promise Strawberry Fields	1 cup	120	0	0	0
Vive Probiotic Digestive Wellness	1¼ cups	170	3	1	0
Kellogg's					
All-Bran	½ cup	80	1	0	0
All-Bran Extra Fiber	½ cup	50	1	0	0
Apple Jacks	1 cup	130	1	0	0
Caramel Nut Crunch	1 cup	210	4	2	0
Cocoa Krispies	¾ cup	120	1	1	0
Complete Oat Bran Flakes	¾ cup	110	1	0	0
Corn Flakes	1 cup	100	0	0	0
Corn Pops	1 cup	120	0	0	0
Cracklin' Oat Bran	¾ cup	200	7	3	0
Crispix	1 cup	110	0	0	0
Frosted Flakes	¾ cup	120	0	0	0
Frosted Flakes ⅓ Less Sugar	1 cup	120	0	0	0
Fruit Harvest	¾ cup	120	2	2	0
Fruit Loops	1 cup	120	1	1	0
Fruit Loops ⅓ Less Sugar	1¼ cups	120	1	1	0
Granola Low Fat w/ Raisins	⅔ cup	230	3	1	0
Honey Smacks	¾ cup	100	1	0	0

FOOD	PORTION	CALS	FAT	SAT FAT	TRANS FAT
Mini-Wheat Frosted	5 (1.8 oz)	180	1	0	0
Mueslix Raisins Dates & Almonds	⅔ cup	200	3	0	0
Organic Mini Wheats Frosted	24 pieces	190	1	0	0
Organic Raisin Bran	1 cup	190	1	0	0
Organic Rice Krispies	1¼ cups	120	0	0	0
Product 19	1 cup	100	0	0	0
Raisin Bran	1 cup	190	2	0	0
Rice Krispies	1¼ cups	120	0	0	0
Smart Start Antioxidants	1 cup	190	1	0	0
Smart Start Healthy Heart	1¼ cups	230	2	0	0
Smorz	1 cup	120	2	1	0
Special K	1 cup	110	0	0	0
Special K Fruit & Yogurt	¾ cup	120	1	1	0
Special K Low Carb Lifestyle Protein Plus	¾ cup	100	3	1	0
Special K Red Berries	1 cup	110	0	0	0
Special K Vanilla Almond	¾ cup	110	2	0	0
Keto					
Cocoa Crisp	½ cup	110	2	0	–
Frosted Flakes All Flavors	¾ cup	110	1	0	–
Hot Cereal Apple Cinnamon	2 scoops	150	4	1	–
Hot Cereal Strawberry & Creme	2 scoops	150	4	1	–
Low Carb Crispy Soy	¾ cup	110	2	–	–
Oatmeal Old Fashioned	2 scoops	150	4	1	–
Liquid Cereal					
Apple & Cinnamon	1 can (11 oz)	160	1	0	–
Chocolate	1 can (11 oz)	170	1	0	–
Fruit	1 can (11 oz)	150	0	0	0
Peanut Butter	1 can (11 oz)	170	2	0	–
Lundberg					
Purely Organic Hot'n Creamy Rice	⅓ cup	190	2	0	0
Malt-O-Meal					
Balance	¾ cup	120	1	0	0
Cinnamon Toasters	¾ cup	130	4	1	0
Colossal Crunch	¾ cup	120	2	0	0
Creamy Hot Wheat not prep	3 tbsp	130	0	0	0
Crispy Rice	1¼ cups	130	0	0	0

FOOD	PORTION	CALS	FAT	SAT FAT	TRANS FAT
Frosted Flakes	¾ cup	120	0	0	0
Frosted Mini Spooners	1 cup	190	1	0	0
Honey & Oat Blenders	¾ cup	120	2	0	0
Honey Buzzers	1⅓ cup	110	1	0	0
Instant Oatmeal Apple & Cinnamon	1 pkg	130	2	0	0
Instant Oatmeal Cinnamon & Spice	1 pkg	170	2	0	0
Instant Oatmeal Maple & Brown Sugar	1 pkg	160	2	0	0
Original Hot Wheat not prep	3 tbsp	130	1	0	0
Puffed Rice	1 cup	60	0	0	0
Raisin Bran	1 cup	220	1	0	0
McCann's					
Irish Oatmeal Instant Apples & Cinnamon	1 pkg (1 oz)	130	2	0	–
Irish Oatmeal Instant Maple & Brown Sugar	1 pkg (1 oz)	160	2	0	–
Irish Oatmeal Instant Regular	1 pkg (1 oz)	100	2	0	–
MiniCarb					
Milk Chocolate Hot Cereal not prep	½ cup	140	6	1	–
Mom's Best Naturals					
Oatmeal Instant	1 pkg	160	2	0	0
Raisin Bran	1 cup	230	2	0	0
Toasted Wheat-fuls	1 cup	200	1	0	0
Toasty O's	1 cup	120	2	0	0
Mother's					
Cinnamon Oat Crunch	1 cup	230	3	1	–
Cocoa Bumpers	1 cup	120	1	0	–
Groovy Grahams	¾ cup	100	1	0	–
Honey Round-Ups	¾ cup	110	1	0	–
Multigrain Hot Cereal	½ cup	130	1	0	–
Oat Bran Hot Cereal	½ cup	150	3	1	–
Oatmeal Instant	½ cup	150	3	1	–
Peanut Butter Bumpers	1 cup	130	3	1	–
Rolled Oats	½ cup	150	3	1	–
Toasted Oat Bran	¾ cup	120	2	0	–
Whole Wheat Hot Cereal	½ cup	130	1	0	–

FOOD	PORTION	CALS	FAT	SAT FAT	TRANS FAT
Natural Ovens					
Great Granola	¼ cup	110	4	1	–
Paul's Oatmeal not prep	⅓ cup	120	3	0	–
Nature's Path					
Optimum Organic ReBound	¾ cup	190	6	1	0
Organic Flax Plus Pumpkin Raisin Crunch	¾ cup	200	4	1	0
Organic Smart Bran	⅔ cup	90	1	0	0
Organic Granola Pomegran Plus	½ cup	140	5	2	0
Organic Zen Instant Oatmeal Cranberry Ginger	1 pkg	150	3	1	0
Organic Oatmeal Hemp Plus	1 pkg	160	3	0	0
Perky's					
Nutty Flax	¾ cup	230	5	0	0
PerkyO's Original	¾ cup	120	1	0	0
Post					
100% Bran	1 (0.8 oz)	80	1	0	0
Bran Flakes	1 cup	100	1	0	0
Cocoa Pebbles	¾ cup (1 oz)	110	2	1	–
Golden Crisp	¾ cup (1 oz)	110	0	0	0
Grape-Nuts	2 oz	200	1	0	0
Grape-Nuts O's	1 cup (1 oz)	120	0	0	0
Grape-Nuts Trail Mix Crunch	1 cup (1.7 oz)	170	2	0	–
Great Grains Cruncy Pecan	1.8 oz	220	6	1	–
Honey Bunches Of Oats	¾ cup	130	2	0	0
Honey Bunches Of Oats Peaches	1 cup	120	2	0	0
Honey Bunches Of Oats Strawberry	¾ cup	120	2	0	0
Honeycomb	1⅓ cups (1 oz)	120	1	0	–
LiveActive Mixed Berry Crunch	1 cup	190	2	0	0
LiveActive Nut Harvest Crunch	1 cup	220	6	1	0
Oreo O's	1 cup	110	2	1	–
Raisin Bran	1 cup (2 oz)	190	1	0	0
Selects Banana Nut Crunch	1 cup (2 oz)	240	6	1	–
Selects Blueberry Morning	2 oz	220	3	0	–
Shredded Wheat Frosted	2 oz	180	1	0	0
Shredded Wheat 'N Bran	2 oz	200	1	0	0
Shredded Wheat Original	2 biscuits (1.6 oz)	160	1	0	0

FOOD	PORTION	CALS	FAT	SAT FAT	TRANS FAT
Shredded Wheat Spoon Size	1 cup	170	1	0	0
Toasties Corn Flakes	1 cup (1 oz)	100	0	0	0
Quaker					
Instant Oatmeal Cinnamon & Spice	1 pkg	170	2	1	0
Instant Oatmeal Cinnamon Roll	1 pkg	160	2	1	0
Instant Oatmeal Crunch Mixed Berry	1 pkg	190	3	1	0
Instant Oatmeal Express Baked Apple	1 pkg	200	3	1	0
Instant Oatmeal For Kids Dinosaur Eggs	1 pkg	190	4	2	0
Instant Oatmeal Lower Sugar Maple & Brown Sugar	1 pkg	120	2	0	0
Instant Oatmeal Maple Brown Sugar w/ Pecans	1 pkg	160	4	1	0
Instant Oatmeal Nutrition For Women Golden Brown Sugar	1 pkg	170	2	1	0
Instant Oatmeal Organic Regular	1 pkg	100	2	1	0
Instant Oatmeal Regular	1 pkg	100	2	0	0
Instant Oatmeal Simple Harvest Apples w/ Cinnamon	1 pkg	150	2	1	0
Instant Oatmeal Strawberries & Cream	1 pkg	130	3	1	0
Instant Oatmeal Supreme Apple Raisin	1 pkg	150	2	0	0
Instant Oatmeal Supreme Cinnamon Pecan	1 pkg	180	4	1	0
Instant Oatmeal Take Heart Golden Maple	1 pkg	160	3	1	0
Instant Oatmeal Weight Control Banana Bread	1 pkg	160	3	1	0
Instant Oatmeat Crunch Maple & Brown Sugar	1 pkg	190	3	1	0
Life	¾ cup	120	2	0	0
Life Cinnamon	¾ cup	120	2	0	0
Life Honey Graham	¾ cup	120	2	0	0
Life Vanilla Yogurt Crunch	1¼ cups	210	3	1	0
Oat Bran Hot Cereal not prep	½ cup	150	3	1	0

FOOD	PORTION	CALS	FAT	SAT FAT	TRANS FAT
Old Fashioned Oats not prep	½ cup	150	3	1	0
Quick Oats Sun Country Iron Fortified	1 pkg	150	3	1	0
Ralston					
100% Hot Wheat	⅓ cup	150	1	0	–
Apple Dapples	1 cup	120	1	0	–
Cocoa Crumbles	1 cup	120	1	0	–
Confruity Crisp	¾ cup	110	1	0	–
Corn Biscuits	1 cup	110	0	0	0
Corn Flakes	1 cup	100	0	0	0
Crisp Crunch	¾ cup	120	1	0	–
Crisp Crunch Berry Treats	1 cup	120	1	0	–
Crisp Rice	1¼ cups	120	0	0	0
Enriched Bran Flakes	¾ cup	90	1	0	–
Farina	3 tbsp	120	0	0	0
Freaky Fruits	1 cup	120	1	0	–
Frosted Flakes	¾ cup	120	0	0	0
Fruit Rings	1 cup	120	1	0	–
Grits	¼ cup	140	1	0	–
Instant Oats Bananas & Cream	1 pkg	130	4	3	–
Magic Stars	¾ cup	120	1	0	–
Oats & More W/ Almonds	¾ cup	130	2	0	–
Oats Instant	1 pkg	100	2	0	–
Oats Instant Apples & Cinnamon	1 pkg	130	2	0	–
Oats Instant Blueberries & Cream	1 pkg	130	3	1	–
Oats Instant Cinnamon & Spice	1 pkg	170	2	1	–
Oats Instant For Kids Cinnawow	1 pkg	140	2	0	–
Oats Instant For Kids Maplicious & Brown Sugar	1 pkg	150	2	0	–
Oats Instant For Kids Roarin' Raspberry	1 pkg	150	3	1	–
Oats Instant For Kids Strawberries & Stars	1 pkg	140	2	0	–
Oats Instant Maple Brown Sugar	1 pkg	160	2	0	–
Oats Instant Peaches & Cream	1 pkg	130	3	1	–
Oats Instant Raisins & Spice	1 pkg	150	2	1	–

FOOD	PORTION	CALS	FAT	SAT FAT	TRANS FAT
Oats Instant Strawberries & Cream	1 pkg	140	3	1	–
Oats Old Fashioned	½ cup	150	3	1	–
Oats Quick	½ cup	140	3	1	–
Raisin Bran	1 cup	200	2	0	0
Rice Biscuits	1¼ cups	120	0	0	0
Shredded Wheat Frosted Bite Size	1¼ cups	200	1	0	0
Silly Spheres	1½ cups	110	1	0	–
Tasteeos	1 cup	110	2	0	–
Tasteeos Apple Cinnamon	¾ cup	120	2	0	–
Tasteeos Honey Nut	1 cup	120	2	0	–
South Beach					
Crunch Strawberry Harvest	1 cup	170	2	0	0
Crunch Vanilla Almond	1 cup	180	4	0	0
Granola Clusters Cherry Almond	1 pkg (1 oz)	130	4	1	0
Granola Clusters Mixed Berry	1 pkg (1 oz)	130	4	1	0
Stark Sisters					
Granola Lo-Fat Raspberry Blueberry	½ cup	230	7	1	–
Granola Nutty Maple	½ cup	250	11	3	–
Granola Original Maple Almond	½ cup	240	10	1	–
Sunbelt					
Granola Low Fat Cinnamon & Raisins	½ cup	250	3	1	0
Uncle Sam					
Cereal	1 cup (1.9 oz)	190	1	0	–
Zoe's					
Granola Cinnamon Raisin	½ cup	190	5	0	0
Granola Cranberries Currants	½ cup	190	5	0	0
Granola Honey Almond	½ cup	190	5	0	0
O's Cinnamon	¾ cup	120	2	0	0
O's Honey	¾ cup	120	2	0	0
O's Natural	¾ cup	120	2	0	0

CEREAL BARS (see also ENERGY BARS)
Attune

FOOD	PORTION	CALS	FAT	SAT FAT	TRANS FAT
Wellness Yogurt & Granola Lemon Creme	1 (1.4 oz)	180	7	3	0

FOOD	PORTION	CALS	FAT	SAT FAT	TRANS FAT
Wellness Yogurt & Granola Strawberry Bliss	1 (1.4 oz)	180	7	3	0
Back To Nature					
Bakery Squares Banana Walnut	1 (1.1 oz)	130	5	1	0
Chewy Trail Mix Cherry Pecan	1 (1 oz)	120	5	1	0
Fruit & Grain Apple	1 (1.1 oz)	110	2	0	0
Cascadian Farm					
Organic Chewy Granola Fruit & Nut	1 (1.2 oz)	140	4	1	0
CocoaVia					
Dark Chocolate Almond	1 (0.8 oz)	90	2	1	0
Enjoy Life					
Allergen Gluten Free Caramel Apple	1 (1 oz)	110	3	0	0
Entenmann's					
Multi-Grain Chocolate Chip	1	140	3	1	–
Multi-Grain Rainbow Chip	1	180	8	3	–
Multi-Grain Real Strawberry	1 (1.3 oz)	140	3	0	0
EnviroKidz					
Crispy Rice Panda Peanut Butter	1 (1 oz)	110	3	0	0
Estee					
Rice Crunchy Chocolate	1	60	1	0	–
Rice Crunchy Chocolate Chip	1	70	1	0	–
Rice Crunchy Vanilla	1	70	0	0	0
General Mills					
Milk 'N Cereal Bars Chex	1 (1.6 oz)	160	4	2	–
Milk 'N Cereal Bars Cinnamon Toast Crunch	1 (1.6 oz)	180	4	2	–
Team Cheerios Strawberry	1	160	4	0	0
Trix	1	160	4	0	0
Glenny's					
Organic Muesli Raisins & Dates	1 (1.6 oz)	170	3	1	0
Organic Museli Chocolate Chip	1 (1.6 oz)	170	3	1	0
Slim Carb Bars Brownie Cheesecake	1 (1.3 oz)	130	3	2	0
Slim-1 w/ Acai Very Berry Blast	1 (1.1 oz)	100	3	2	0
Slim-1 w/ GreenTea Double Fudge	1 (1.1 oz)	100	3	2	0

FOOD	PORTION	CALS	FAT	SAT FAT	TRANS FAT
Slim-1 w/ Hoodia Peanut Butter Caramel	1 (1.1 oz)	100	4	2	0
Glutino					
Gluten Free Breakfast Bar Apple	1 (1.4 oz)	120	1	0	0
Gluten Free Breakfast Bar Chocolate	1 (1.4 oz)	110	1	1	0
Gluten Free Organic Chocolate & Peanut	1 (1 oz)	110	3	1	0
Gluten Free Organic Wildberry	1 (1 oz)	100	1	0	0
Hershey's					
Crispy Rice Peanut Butter	1 (0.5 oz)	60	2	1	–
Honest Foods					
Cran Lemon Zest	1 (2.2 oz)	240	9	1	0
Farmer's Trail Mix	1 (2.2 oz)	240	9	1	0
Kashi					
TLC Chewy Granola Honey Almond Flax	1 (1.2 oz)	140	5	1	0
TLC Chewy Granola Peanut Peanut Butter	1 (1.2 oz)	140	5	1	0
TLC Chewy Trail Mix	1 (1.2 oz)	140	5	1	0
Kellogg's					
All-Bran Brown Sugar Cinnamon	1	130	3	1	0
All-Bran Honey Oat	1	130	3	1	0
All-Bran Oatmeal Raisin	1	120	3	1	0
Crunchy Nut Sweet & Salty Chocolatey Almond	1 (1.1 oz)	160	8	3	0
Nutri-Grain Apple Cinnamon	1	140	3	1	0
Nutri-Grain Banana Muffin	1	170	4	1	0
Nutri-Grain Chewy Granola Chocolatey Chunk	1	110	4	2	0
Nutri-Grain Cinnamon Raisin Muffin	1	170	4	1	0
Nutri-Grain Yogurt Vanilla	1	140	3	1	0
Smart Start Healthy Heart Cinnamon	1 (1.4 oz)	150	3	0	0
Snack Bites	1 pkg (0.8 oz)	90	2	1	0
Special K Chocolatey Drizzle	1 (0.8 oz)	90	2	1	0

FOOD	PORTION	CALS	FAT	SAT FAT	TRANS FAT
Special K Meal Bar Chocolate Peanut Butter	1 (1.6 oz)	190	6	4	0
Special K Snack Bar Chocolate Peanut	1 (0.9 oz)	110	4	2	0
Special K Strawberry	1 (0.8 oz)	90	2	1	0
Special K Vanilla Crisp	1 (0.8 oz)	90	2	1	0
Kind					
Almond & Coconut	1	193	14	5	–
Almonds & Apricot In Yogurt	1	208	13	6	–
Banana & Oatbran	1	160	7	6	–
Nut Delight	1	203	15	2	–
Walnut & Date	1	150	7	4	–
Kudos					
Granola Chocolate Chip	1	120	4	2	0
Granola Peanut Butter	1	130	6	3	0
Granola w/ M&M's	1	100	3	2	0
Granola w/ Snickers	1	100	3	2	0
Natural Ovens					
Great Granola Chocolate Almond	1	150	6	1	–
Great Granola Fruit & Lemon	1	130	3	0	–
Great Granola Mixed Fruit	1	130	3	0	–
Nature Valley					
Chewy Granola Blueberry Yogurt	1	140	4	2	0
Chewy Granola Lemon Yogurt	1	140	4	2	0
Chewy Granola Vanilla Yogurt	1	140	4	2	0
Chewy Trail Mix Granola Apple Cinnamon	1	140	4	1	0
Chewy Trail Mix Granola Fruit & Nut	1	140	4	1	0
Chewy Trail Mix Granola Mixed Berry	1	140	4	0	0
Crunchy Granola Apple Crisp	1	140	4	2	0
Crunchy Granola Banana Nut	2	190	7	1	0
Crunchy Granola Maple Brown Sugar	2	180	6	1	0
Crunchy Granola Peanut Butter	2	160	7	1	0

FOOD	PORTION	CALS	FAT	SAT FAT	TRANS FAT
Crunchy Granola Roasted Almond	2	190	7	1	0
Healthy Heart Granola Oatmeal Raisin	1	150	2	1	0
Heart Healthy Chewy Granola Honey Nut	1	160	4	1	0
Sweet & Salty Granola Almond	1	160	7	2	0
Sweet & Salty Granola Peanut	1	170	9	3	0
Nutri-Grain					
Nutri-Grain Blueberry	1	140	3	1	0
Nutri-Grain Mixed Berry	1	140	3	1	0
Post					
Honey Bunches Of Oats Banana Nut	1 (1.2 oz)	140	4	2	–
Honey Bunches Of Oats Oatmeal Raisin	1 (1.2 oz)	130	3	0	–
Quaker					
Breakfast Graham Strawberry	1 (1 oz)	120	4	1	0
Breakfast Bar Apple Crisp	1 (1.3 oz)	130	3	1	0
Breakfast Bar Iced Raspberry	1 (1.3 oz)	130	3	1	0
Breakfast Bites Iced Raspberry	1 pkg (1.3 oz)	130	3	1	0
Breakfast Bites Strawberry	1 pkg (1.3 oz)	130	3	1	0
Chewy Chocolate Chip	1 (0.8 oz)	100	3	2	0
Chewy Cookies & Cream	1 (0.8 oz)	90	3	1	0
Chewy 90 Calorie Cinnamon Sugar	1 (1 oz)	90	2	0	0
Chewy 90 Calorie Honey Nut	1 (0.8 oz)	90	2	0	0
Chewy Dipps Peanut Butter	1 (1 oz)	150	7	4	–
Chewy Low Fat S'mores	1 (1 oz)	110	2	1	0
Crunchy Granola Oats & Berries	1 (1 oz)	130	4	1	0
Oatmeal To Go Oatmeal Raisin	1 (2.1 oz)	220	4	1	0
Oatmeal To Go Raspberry Streusel	1 (2.1 oz)	220	4	1	0
Q-Smart Cranberry Vanilla Almond	1 (1 oz)	120	6	2	0
Trail Mix Cranberry Raisin & Almond	1 (1.2 oz)	150	5	1	0
Rice Krispies					
Split Stix Chocolatey	1 (1 oz)	130	5	3	–

FOOD	PORTION	CALS	FAT	SAT FAT	TRANS FAT
Split Stix Original	1 (1 oz)	120	5	3	–
Treats Original	1 (0.8 oz)	90	3	1	0
Skippy					
Peanut Butter	1	180	11	3	–
Peanut Butter & Fudge	1	190	12	3	–
Peanut Butter & Marshmallow	1	140	12	3	–
Peanut Butter & Strawberry	1	170	12	3	–
South Beach					
100 Calorie Chocolate Delight	1 (1 oz)	100	3	2	0
100 Calorie Peanut Butter Chocolate Chip	1 (1 oz)	100	3	2	0
100 Calorie Snack Bar Mixed Berry	1 (1 oz)	100	3	2	0
High Protein Chocolate	1 (1.2 oz)	140	5	3	0
High Protein Cranberry Almond	1 (1.2 oz)	140	5	2	0
High Protein Maple Nut	1 (1.2 oz)	140	5	2	0
High Protein Peanut Butter	1 (1.2 oz)	140	5	2	0
Wings Of Nature					
Organic Apple Cinnamon	1 (1.2 oz)	119	4	tr	0
Organic Cafe Mocha Coffee	1 (1.2 oz)	153	9	3	0
Organic Cappuccino Coffee	1 (1.2 oz)	153	9	2	0

CHAMPAGNE

FOOD	PORTION	CALS	FAT	SAT FAT	TRANS FAT
mimosa	1 serv	117	tr	tr	–
punch	1 serv	113	0	0	0
sekt german champagne	3.5 oz	84	0	0	0

CHAYOTE

FOOD	PORTION	CALS	FAT	SAT FAT	TRANS FAT
fresh cooked	1 cup	38	1	–	–
raw	1 (7 oz)	49	1	–	–
raw cut up	1 cup	32	tr	–	–

CHEESE (see also CHEESE DISHES, CHEESE SUBSTITUTES, COTTAGE CHEESE, CREAM CHEESE, NEUFCHATEL)

FOOD	PORTION	CALS	FAT	SAT FAT	TRANS FAT
american	1 oz	93	7	4	–
american cheese spread	1 oz	82	6	4	–
beaufort	1 oz	115	9	6	–
bel paese	1 oz	112	9	–	–
blue	1 oz	100	8	6	–
blue crumbled	1 cup (4.7 oz)	477	39	25	–

FOOD	PORTION	CALS	FAT	SAT FAT	TRANS FAT
bocconcini smoked	1 oz	90	6	4	0
brick	1 oz	105	8	5	–
brie	1 oz	95	8	–	–
cacio di roma sheep's milk cheese	1 oz	130	10	6	–
caerphilly	1.4 oz	150	13	–	–
camembert	1 oz	85	7	4	–
cantal	1 oz	105	9	6	–
caraway	1 oz	107	8	–	–
chabichou	1 oz	95	8	5	–
chaource	1 oz	83	7	4	–
cheddar	1 oz	114	9	6	–
cheddar low fat	1 oz	49	2	1	–
cheddar low sodium	1 oz	113	9	6	–
cheddar reduced fat	1.4 oz	104	6	–	–
cheddar shredded	1 cup	455	37	24	–
cheshire	1 oz	110	9	–	–
cheshire reduced fat	1.4 oz	108	6	–	–
colby	1 oz	112	9	6	–
colby low fat	1 oz	49	2	1	–
colby low sodium	1 oz	113	9	6	–
comte	1 oz	114	9	5	–
coulommiers	1 oz	88	7	5	–
crottin	1 oz	105	9	6	–
derby	1.4 oz	161	14	–	–
edam	1 oz	101	8	5	–
edam reduced fat	1.4 oz	92	4	–	–
emmentaler	1 oz	115	9	–	–
feta	1 oz	75	6	4	–
fontina	1 oz	110	9	5	–
frais	1.6 oz	51	3	–	–
gjetost	1 oz	132	8	5	–
gloucester double	1.4 oz	162	14	–	–
goat fresh	1 oz	23	2	1	–
goat hard	1 oz	128	10	7	–
gorgonzola	1 oz	107	9	–	–
gouda	1 oz	101	8	5	–
grana padano parmesan shaved	1 tbsp	20	2	1	0
gruyere	1 oz	117	9	5	–

FOOD	PORTION	CALS	FAT	SAT FAT	TRANS FAT
lancashire	1.4 oz	149	12	–	–
leicester	1.4 oz	160	14	–	–
limburger	1 oz	93	8	5	–
lymeswold	1.4 oz	170	16	–	–
maroilles	1 oz	97	8	5	–
monterey	1 oz	106	9	–	–
morbier	1 oz	99	8	5	–
mozzarella	1 oz	80	6	4	–
mozzarella fresh	1 oz	80	6	4	–
mozzarella part skim	1 oz	72	5	3	–
muenster	1 oz	104	9	5	–
parmesan grated	1 tbsp	23	2	1	–
parmesan hard	1 oz	111	7	5	–
picodon	1 oz	99	8	5	–
pimento	1 oz	106	9	6	–
pont l'eveque	1 oz	86	7	4	–
port du salut	1 oz	100	8	5	–
provolone	1 oz	100	8	5	–
pyrenees	1 oz	101	8	5	–
quark 20% fat	1 oz	33	1	–	–
quark 40% fat	1 oz	48	3	–	–
quark made w/ skim milk	1 oz	22	tr	–	–
queso anego	1 oz	106	9	5	–
queso asadero	1 oz	101	8	5	–
queso chichuahua	1 oz	106	8	5	–
queso fresco	1 oz	41	2	–	–
queso manchego	1 oz	107	8	–	–
queso panela	1 oz	74	5	–	–
raclette	1 oz	102	8	5	–
reblochon	1 oz	88	7	5	–
ricotta part skim	½ cup (4.4 oz)	171	10	6	–
ricotta whole milk	½ cup (4.4 oz)	216	16	10	–
romadur 40% fat	1 oz	83	6	–	–
romano	1 oz	110	8	–	–
roquefort	1 oz	105	9	5	–
rouy	1 oz	95	8	5	–
saint marcellin	1 oz	94	8	5	–
saint nectaire	1 oz	97	8	5	–
saint paulin	1 oz	85	6	4	–
sainte maure	1 oz	99	8	5	–

FOOD	PORTION	CALS	FAT	SAT FAT	TRANS FAT
selles sur cher	1 oz	93	8	5	–
stilton blue	1.4 oz	164	14	–	–
stilton white	1.4 oz	145	13	–	–
swiss	1 oz	107	8	5	–
swiss processed	1 oz	95	7	5	–
tilsit	1 oz	96	7	5	–
tome	1 oz	92	7	5	–
triple creme	1 oz	113	11	7	–
vacherin	1 oz	92	8	5	–
wensleydale	1.4 oz	151	13	–	–
whey cheese	1 oz	126	8	5	–
yogurt cheese	1 oz	80	7	3	–
Alouette					
Garlic & Herbs	2 tbsp (0.8 oz)	70	7	5	–
Athenos					
Blue	1 oz	100	8	5	0
Feta	1 oz (1 in cube)	80	6	4	0
Feta Crumbled	¼ cup	90	7	4	0
Feta Reduced Fat	1 in cube (1 oz)	60	4	3	0
Gorgonzola Crumbled	3 tbsp	110	9	6	0
Back To Nature					
Organic American Slices	1 slice (0.7 oz)	80	7	4	–
Organic Cheddar Cubes	8 pieces (1.1 oz)	130	11	7	–
Organic Cheddar Shredded	¼ cup	110	10	6	–
Organic Mozzarella Shredded	¼ cup	80	5	4	–
Organic White Cheddar Slices Reduced Fat	1 slice (0.7 oz)	60	4	3	–
Bel Gioioso					
Mozzarella Fresh	1 in cube (1 oz)	80	6	4	0
Boar's Head					
American	1 oz	100	9	6	0
American 25% Lower Sodium 25% Lower Fat	1 oz	90	6	5	0
ButterKase	1 oz	100	9	6	0
Cheddar Sharp	1 oz	110	9	5	0
Colby Jack	1 oz	110	9	6	0
Cream Havarti	1 oz	110	10	7	0
Creamy Blue	1 oz	90	8	5	0
Double Glouster Yellow	1 oz	110	10	6	0
Edam	1 oz	90	7	5	0

FOOD	PORTION	CALS	FAT	SAT FAT	TRANS FAT
Feta	1 oz	60	4	3	0
Gouda	1 oz	110	9	5	0
Lacey Swiss	1 oz	90	6	4	0
Longhorn Colby	1 oz	110	9	5	0
Monterey Jack	1 oz	100	9	6	0
Mozzarella	1 oz	90	7	5	–
Muenster	1 oz	100	8	5	0
Muenster Low Sodium	1 oz	100	8	5	0
Provolone 42% Lower Sodium	1 oz	100	8	5	0
Provolone Picante Sharp	1 oz	100	8	5	0
Swiss No Salt Added	1 oz	110	8	5	0
Boursin					
Garlic & Fine Herbs	2 tbsp	120	13	9	–
Cabot					
American	1 slice (0.7 oz)	80	7	4	–
Cheddar	1 oz	110	9	5	–
Cheddar Smoked	1 oz	110	9	5	–
Cheddar Light 50% Reduced Fat	1 oz	70	5	3	–
Cheddar Light 50% Reduced Fat Jalapeno	1 oz	70	5	3	–
Cheddar Light 75% Reduced Fat	1 oz	60	3	2	–
Cheddar Shake	2 tsp	25	2	1	–
Colby Jack	1 oz	110	9	5	–
Fancy Blend Shredded	¼ cup	100	7	4	–
Monterey Jack	1 oz	110	9	5	–
Mozzarella Shredded	¼ cup	80	6	4	–
Pepper Jack	1 oz	110	9	5	–
Swiss Slices	1 slice (1 oz)	110	8	5	–
Cantare					
Baked Brie En Croute	1 oz	100	7	5	0
Chavrie					
Goat's Milk	2 tbsp	50	4	3	–
Connoisseur					
Asiago Spread	1 tbsp	90	7	4	–
Brie Spread	2 tbsp	90	7	4	–
Gorgonzola Spread	1 tbsp	90	7	5	0
Wheel Asiago Pesto	2 tbsp	90	6	4	–
Wheel Swiss Bacon	2 tbsp	90	7	4	–

FOOD	PORTION	CALS	FAT	SAT FAT	TRANS FAT
Cracker Barrel					
Fontina	1 slice (0.7 oz)	80	7	4	0
Sharp Cheddar 2% Milk	1 oz	90	6	4	0
Crystal Farms					
American Singles	1 slice (0.7 oz)	70	5	2	0
American Singles 2%	1 slice (0.7 oz)	50	3	2	0
American Singles Fat Free	1 slice (0.7 oz)	30	0	0	0
Blue Crumbled	2 tbsp	100	8	5	0
Cheese Curds	8 pieces (1 oz)	110	9	6	0
Cheezoids Sticks	1 piece (0.8 oz)	70	5	3	0
Danish Havarti	1 oz	110	10	7	0
Deli Slices Muenster	1 slice (0.8 oz)	80	7	4	0
Deli Slices Swiss	1 slice (0.7 oz)	80	6	4	0
Feta Crumbled	¼ cup	90	7	5	0
Gorgonzola Crumbled	2 tbsp	100	8	5	0
It's So Cheesy Cheddar Aerosol	2 tbsp	90	7	3	0
Little Chunks To Go	1 pkg (0.7 oz)	80	7	4	0
Marble Jack	1 oz	110	9	6	0
Parmesan Grated	2 tsp	25	2	1	0
Pepper Jack	1 oz	110	9	6	0
Ricotta	¼ cup	90	6	4	0
Shredded Mexican 4 Cheese	¼ cup	100	8	5	0
Shredded Mozzarella	¼ cup	80	6	4	0
Shredded Pizza Blend	¼ cup	100	8	5	0
Shredded Sharp Cheddar	¼ cup	110	9	6	0
Smoked Gouda	1 oz	100	8	5	0
String	1 piece (1 oz)	80	5	3	0
Dragone					
Mozzarella Whole Milk	1 oz	90	7	5	–
Parmesan Wedge	1 oz	100	7	4	–
Ricotta Part Skim	¼ cup (2.2 oz)	90	6	4	–
Easy Cheese					
American	2 tbsp (1.1 oz)	90	6	3	0
Cheddar	2 tbsp (1.1 oz)	90	6	3	0
Fage					
Feta	1 oz	80	7	4	0
Finlandia					
Muenster	1 slice (1.1 oz)	120	10	7	0

FOOD	PORTION	CALS	FAT	SAT FAT	TRANS FAT
Formaggio					
Fresh Mozzarella	1 oz	90	6	4	–
Friendship					
Farmer	2 tbsp (1 oz)	50	3	2	0
Frigo					
Mozzarella Part Skim	1 oz	80	6	4	–
Parmesan Shredded	¼ cup (1 oz)	100	7	4	–
Ricotta Whole Milk	¼ cup (2.2 oz)	110	8	5	–
Romano Shredded	¼ cup (1 oz)	100	7	5	–
Heluva Good Cheese					
Cheddar Extra Sharp	1 oz	110	9	5	0
Horizon Organic					
American	1 slice (0.7 oz)	60	5	4	0
Cheddar	1 oz	110	9	5	0
Montery Jack	1 oz	100	8	5	0
Shred Mexican	¼ cup	110	9	5	0
Shred Parmesan	1 tbsp	20	2	1	0
Slice Provolone	1 slice (0.7 oz)	70	6	4	0
Sticks Colby	1 (1 oz)	110	9	5	0
String Mozzarella	1 stick (1 oz)	80	5	3	0
J.L. Kraft					
Spreadable Feta & Spinach	2 tbsp	80	7	4	0
Jordan's					
Provolone	1 slice (1 oz)	100	8	4	0
Kraft					
Cheddar Extra Sharp	1 oz	120	10	6	0
Cheddar Sharp Shredded 2% Milk	¼ cup	80	6	4	0
LiveActive 2% Milk Marbled Colby & Monterey Jack	1 stick (1 oz)	90	6	4	0
LiveActive Cheddar Cheese Sticks	1 (1 oz)	120	10	6	0
LiveActive Colby & Monterey Jack Cubes	7 (1 oz)	110	9	6	0
LiveActive Mozzarella Sticks	1 (1 oz)	80	5	3	0
Shredded Mexican Style Cheddar & Monterey Jack	¼ cup	110	9	5	0
Singles American 2%	1 (0.7 oz)	50	3	2	0
Land O Lakes					
Cheddar Mild	1 slice (1 oz)	110	9	6	0

FOOD	PORTION	CALS	FAT	SAT FAT	TRANS FAT
Co-Jack	1 slice (1 oz)	110	9	6	0
Swiss	1 slice (1 oz)	110	8	5	0
Laughing Cow					
Cheese Bites Light	6 pieces (0.8 oz)	35	2	1	–
Creamy French Onion Light	1 wedge	35	2	1	–
Creamy Garlic & Herb Light	1 wedge (0.7 oz)	35	2	1	–
Creamy Swiss Light Original	1 wedge (0.7 oz)	35	2	1	–
Creamy Swiss Original	1 wedge (0.7 oz)	50	4	3	–
Mini Babybel Bonbel	1 piece (0.7 oz)	70	6	4	–
Mini Babybel Gouda	1 piece (0.7 oz)	80	6	4	–
Mini Babybel Light Original	1 piece (0.7 oz)	50	3	2	–
Mini Babybel Mild Cheddar	1 piece (0.7 oz)	70	5	3	–
Mini Babybel Original	1 piece (0.7 oz)	70	6	4	–
Lifeway					
Farmer's Kefir	2 tbsp	25	2	1	–
Farmer's Kefir Lite	2 tbsp	25	1	1	–
Sweet Kiss Peach	1 oz	45	1	1	–
Meza					
Baked Brie In Pastry w/ Cranberries & Spiced Almonds	1 oz	110	7	4	0
Miller's					
Mozzarella	1 slice (1 oz)	81	5	3	–
Mont Chevre					
Assorted Crottins	1 oz	70	6	4	0
Mt Vikos					
Feta Sheep & Goat Milk	1 oz	80	7	4	0
Organic Valley					
Blue Crumbles	1 oz	100	8	5	0
Cheddar Mild	1 oz	110	9	6	0
Feta	1 oz	60	4	3	0
Monterey Jack Shredded	¼ cup	80	5	4	0
Muenster	1 slice (0.7 oz)	80	6	4	0
Provolone	1 slice (0.7 oz)	70	6	4	0
Swiss	1 oz	110	9	6	0
Polly-O					
Mozzarella Part Skim	1 oz	70	5	3	0
Mozzarella Shredded	¼ cup	90	7	4	0
Ricotta Part Skim	¼ cup	90	6	4	0
Ricotta Lite	¼ cup	70	3	2	–

FOOD	PORTION	CALS	FAT	SAT FAT	TRANS FAT
String-Ums	1 stick (1 oz)	80	6	4	–
President					
Feta	1 oz	90	7	5	–
Sargento					
4 Cheese Italian Shredded	¼ cup	80	5	3	–
4 Cheese Mexican Reduced Fat Shredded	¼ cup (1 oz)	80	6	3	–
American Burger	1 slice (0.7 oz)	70	6	4	–
Bistro Blends Shredded Mozzarella w/ Sun Dried Tomato & Basil	¼ cup	90	6	5	–
Blue Crumbled	¼ cup (1 oz)	100	8	5	–
Cheddar Chipotle Shredded	¼ cup	100	8	5	0
Cheddar Chipotle Sticks	1 (0.7 oz)	80	6	4	0
Cheddar Mild Cubes	7 (1 oz)	120	10	8	–
Cheddar Mild Shredded Reduced Fat	¼ cup (1 oz)	80	6	4	–
Cheddar White Vermont Sharp	1 slice (0.7 oz)	80	7	4	0
Cheddar White Vermont Sharp Shredded	¼ cup (1 oz)	110	9	5	0
Cheese Dips Cheddar & Buttery Pretzels	1 pkg (3.8 oz)	360	16	5	–
Cheese Dips Cheddar & Tortilla Chips	1 pkg (3 oz)	320	21	6	–
Colby-Jack Shredded	¼ cup (1 oz)	110	9	6	–
Fancy 6 Cheese Italian Shredded	¼ cup	90	7	4	–
Jarlsberg	1 slice (0.8 oz)	80	6	4	–
Monterey Jack Shredded	¼ cup (1 oz)	110	9	5	–
Mozzarella Reduced Fat Shredded	¼ cup (1 oz)	80	5	2	–
Mozzarella Shredded	¼ cup (1 oz)	80	6	4	–
Muenster	1 slice (0.7 oz)	80	6	4	–
Nacho & Taco Shredded	¼ cup (1 oz)	110	9	5	–
Parmesan Grated	2 tsp (5 g)	25	2	1	–
Parmesan Shredded	2 tsp	20	2	1	–
Pepper Jack	1 slice (0.7 oz)	80	6	4	–
Provolone	1 slice (0.7 oz)	70	5	4	–
Provolone Reduced Fat	1 slice (0.7 oz)	50	4	2	–
Ricotta Fat Free	¼ cup	50	0	0	0

FOOD	PORTION	CALS	FAT	SAT FAT	TRANS FAT
Ricotta Light	¼ cup	60	3	2	–
Ricotta Whole Milk	¼ cup	90	8	4	–
String	1 piece (1 oz)	80	6	4	–
String Light	1 piece (0.7 oz)	50	3	2	–
Swiss Reduced Fat	1 slice (0.7 oz)	80	4	2	–
Swiss Shredded	¼ cup (1 oz)	110	8	5	–
Swiss Thick Slice	1 slice (1 oz)	110	8	5	–
Swiss Thin Sliced	1 slice (0.6 oz)	70	5	3	–
Smart Balance					
Cheddar Shredded	1 oz	80	5	2	0
Mozzarella Shredded	1 oz	80	5	2	0
Sorrento					
Mozzarella Fresh	1 oz	90	6	4	0
Mozzarella w/ Tomato & Basil Shredded	¼ cup	80	5	3	–
Pizza Cheese Shredded	¼ cup	90	7	5	–
Stringsters	1 stick (1 oz)	80	5	3	–
Stella					
3 Cheese Italian Shredded	¼ cup	100	7	4	–
Asiago Wedge	1 oz	110	9	6	–
Gorgonzola Wedge	1 oz	100	9	6	–
Kasseri Wedge	1 oz	110	9	6	–
Suisse Delicat					
Healthy Swiss	1 oz	90	6	5	–
Treasure Cave					
Blue Cheese Crumbled	¼ cup (1 oz)	100	8	5	–
Feta Crumbled	¼ cup (1 oz)	60	5	4	–
Gorgonzola Crumbled	¼ cup (1 oz)	100	8	5	–

CHEESE DISHES
Alexia

FOOD	PORTION	CALS	FAT	SAT FAT	TRANS FAT
Mozzarella Stix	2 pieces	120	7	1	0

Farm Rich

FOOD	PORTION	CALS	FAT	SAT FAT	TRANS FAT
Cheese Sticks Breaded	2 (2.1 oz)	210	12	4	0
Mozzarella Bites Breaded	4 (2.2 oz)	150	7	4	0
Original Cheese Bites Breaded	7 (2.1 oz)	180	11	4	0

Fillo Factory

FOOD	PORTION	CALS	FAT	SAT FAT	TRANS FAT
Tyropita Cheese Fillo Appetizers	3 (3 oz)	230	14	8	0

FOOD	PORTION	CALS	FAT	SAT FAT	TRANS FAT
Stouffer's					
Welsh Rarebit	¼ pkg (2.5 oz)	140	10	6	0
TAKE-OUT					
fondue	½ cup (3.8 oz)	247	15	9	–
fried mozzarella sticks	3 (4.6 oz)	503	32	16	–
souffle	1 serv (7 oz)	504	38	17	–
welsh rarebit	1 slice	228	16	–	–

CHEESE SUBSTITUTES

mozzarella	1 oz	70	3	1	–
Playfood					
Cheesey Cheese	1 oz	60	5	1	0
Sheese					
Blue Style	1 oz	100	8	5	0
Cheddar Style Medium	1 oz	100	8	5	0
Creamy Mexican	2 tbsp	80	7	3	0
Creamy Original	2 tbsp	80	7	3	0

CHERIMOYA

fresh	1	515	2	–	–

CHERRIES

CANNED					
maraschino	1 (4 g)	7	tr	tr	0
maraschino	¼ cup (1.4 oz)	66	tr	tr	0
sour in light syrup	½ cup	94	tr	tr	0
sour water packed	½ cup	44	tr	tr	0
sour in heavy syrup	½ cup	116	tr	tr	0
sweet juice pack	½ cup	68	tr	tr	0
sweet pitted in heavy syrup	½ cup	105	tr	tr	0
sweet water pack	½ cup	57	tr	tr	0
Del Monte					
Sweet Dark Pitted In Heavy Syrup	½ cup	100	0	0	0
DRIED					
bing unsulfured	¼ cup	130	0	0	0
montmorency tart pitted	⅓ cup	160	1	0	–
rainier unsulfured	⅓ cup	140	1	0	–
tart	½ cup	200	1	0	0
yogurt covered	¼ cup	170	6	6	–

FOOD	PORTION	CALS	FAT	SAT FAT	TRANS FAT
Bob's Red Mill					
Tart	⅓ cup	140	0	0	0
De-Lite					
Tart	1 oz	95	tr	0	0
Eden					
Montmorency	¼ cup	140	0	0	0
Frieda's					
Bing	¼ cup (1.4 oz)	120	0	0	0
Tart	⅓ cup (1.4 oz)	150	0	0	0
Good Sense					
Cherries	⅓ cup	145	0	0	0
Peeled Snacks					
Fruit Picks Cherry-Go-Round	1 pkg (1.5 oz)	130	0	0	0
Sunsweet					
Tart & Sweet	¼ cup (1.4 oz)	100	0	0	0
FRESH					
sour	1 cup	52	tr	tr	0
sour pitted	1 cup	78	tr	tr	0
sweet	20	86	1	tr	0
Chiquita					
Cherries	21	90	1	0	–
Rainier					
Sweet Premium Northwest	1 cup	90	1	0	0
Super Cherry					
Rainier	21	90	0	0	0
FROZEN					
sour unsweetened	½ cup	36	tr	tr	0
sweet sweetened	½ cup	115	tr	tr	0
CHERRY JUICE					
tart cherry concentrate	1 cup	140	0	0	0
Eden					
Organic Montmorency	8 oz	140	1	0	0
Froose					
Cheerful Cherry	1 box (4.2 oz)	80	0	0	0
HP					
Tart Montmorency Concentrate	1 oz	80	0	0	0
L&A					
Black Cherry 100% Juice	8 oz	180	0	0	0

FOOD	PORTION	CALS	FAT	SAT FAT	TRANS FAT
Ocean Spray					
Black Cherry	8 oz	140	0	0	0
Old Orchard					
100% Pure Tart Cherry	8 oz	140	0	0	0

CHERVIL
seed	1 tsp	1	tr	–	–

CHESTNUTS
chinese steamed	3 (1 oz)	43	tr	tr	–
creme de marrons	1 oz	73	tr	tr	–
japanese roasted	1 oz	57	tr	tr	–
ready-to-eat vacuum packed	5 (1 oz)	40	0	0	0
roasted	3 (1 oz)	70	1	tr	–

CHEWING GUM
bubble gum	1 block	20	tr	tr	0
stick	1 piece	7	tr	tr	0
sugarless	1 piece	5	tr	tr	0
Bazooka					
Bubble Gum	1 piece (4 g)	15	0	0	0
Big Red					
Gum	1 piece	10	0	0	0
Brach's					
Abra Cabubble	1 piece	45	0	0	0
CareFree					
Koolerz Lemonaide	1 piece	5	0	0	0
Doublemint					
Gum	1 piece	10	0	0	0
Dubble Bubble					
Gumball	1 piece	10	0	0	0
Eclipse					
Flash All Flavors	1 piece	0	0	0	0
Sugarless All Flavors	2 pieces	5	0	0	0
Extra					
Sugar Free All Flavors	1 piece	5	0	0	0
Sugar Free Bubble Gum	1 piece	5	0	0	0
Flare					
Warming Cinnamon	1 piece	5	0	0	0
Glee Gum					
Peppermint	2 pieces (2.5 g)	5	0	0	0

FOOD	PORTION	CALS	FAT	SAT FAT	TRANS FAT
Juicy Fruit					
Gum	2 pieces	10	0	0	0
Orbit					
Sugarless All Flavors	2 pieces	5	0	0	0
White Melon Breeze	2 pieces	5	0	0	0
Skittles					
Bubble Gum	2 pieces	10	0	0	0
Speakeasy					
Natural Rainforest All Flavors	2 pieces	10	0	0	0
SteviaDent					
Gum	2 pieces	3	0	0	0
Stride					
All Flavors	1 piece	<5	0	0	0
Winterfresh					
Gum	1 stick	10	0	0	0
Thin Ice Mountain Rush	1 piece	0	0	0	0
Wrigley's					
Spearmint	1 stick	10	0	0	0
Xylichew					
Licorice	2 pieces	4	0	0	0
CHIA SEEDS					
dried	1 oz	134	7	3	–

CHICKEN (see also CHICKEN DISHES, CHICKEN SUBSTITUTES, DINNER, HOT DOG)

FOOD	PORTION	CALS	FAT	SAT FAT	TRANS FAT
CANNED					
breast meat in water	2 oz	70	1	0	0
w/ broth	½ can (2.5 oz)	117	6	2	–
Swanson					
Chunk Breast In Water	2 oz	50	1	0	0
Tyson					
Preium Chunk Breast	½ can (2 oz)	60	1	0	–
Premium Chunk	½ can (2 oz)	60	3	1	–
Valley Fresh					
Chunk White	2 oz	70	1	0	–
White & Dark Chunk	2 oz	80	2	1	–
FRESH					
broiler/fryer breast w/ skin batter dipped & fried	½ breast (4.9 oz)	364	18	5	–
broiler/fryer breast w/ skin roasted	½ breast (3.4 oz)	193	8	2	–

FOOD	PORTION	CALS	FAT	SAT FAT	TRANS FAT
broiler/fryer breast w/ skin stewed	½ breast (3.9 oz)	202	8	2	–
broiler/fryer breast w/o skin fried	½ breast (3 oz)	161	4	1	–
broiler/fryer breast w/o skin roasted	½ breast (3 oz)	142	3	1	–
broiler/fryer drumstick w/ skin batter dipped & fried	1 (2.6 oz)	193	11	3	–
broiler/fryer drumstick w/ skin floured & fried	1 (1.7 oz)	120	7	2	–
broiler/fryer drumstick w/ skin roasted	1 (1.8 oz)	112	6	2	–
broiler/fryer drumstick w/ skin stewed	1 (2 oz)	116	6	2	–
broiler/fryer drumstick w/o skin fried	1 (1.5 oz)	82	3	1	–
broiler/fryer drumstick w/o skin roasted	1 (1.5 oz)	76	2	1	–
broiler/fryer drumstick w/o skin stewed	1 (1.6 oz)	78	3	1	–
broiler/fryer leg w/ skin batter dipped & fried	1 (5.5 oz)	431	26	7	–
broiler/fryer leg w/ skin floured & fried	1 (3.9 oz)	285	16	4	–
broiler/fryer leg w/ skin roasted	1 (4 oz)	265	15	4	–
broiler/fryer leg w/ skin stewed	1 (4.4 oz)	275	16	4	–
broiler/fryer leg w/o skin fried	1 (3.3 oz)	195	9	2	–
broiler/fryer leg w/o skin roasted	1 (3.3 oz)	182	8	2	–
broiler/fryer leg w/o skin stewed	1 (3.5 oz)	187	8	2	–
broiler/fryer neck w/ skin stewed	1 (1.3 oz)	94	7	2	–
broiler/fryer neck w/o skin stewed	1 (.6 oz)	32	1	tr	–
broiler/fryer skin floured & fried	from ½ chicken (2 oz)	281	24	7	–

FOOD	PORTION	CALS	FAT	SAT FAT	TRANS FAT
broiler/fryer skin roasted	from ½ chicken (2 oz)	254	23	6	–
broiler/fryer skin stewed	from ½ chicken (2.5 oz)	261	24	7	–
broiler/fryer thigh w/ skin batter dipped & fried	1 (3 oz)	238	14	4	–
broiler/fryer thigh w/ skin floured & fried	1 (2.2 oz)	162	9	3	–
broiler/fryer thigh w/ skin roasted	1 (2.2 oz)	153	10	3	–
broiler/fryer thigh w/ skin stewed	1 (2.4 oz)	158	10	3	–
broiler/fryer thigh w/o skin fried	1 (1.8 oz)	113	5	1	–
broiler/fryer thigh w/o skin roasted	1 (1.8 oz)	109	6	2	–
broiler/fryer thigh w/o skin stewed	1 (1.9 oz)	107	5	1	–
broiler/fryer w/ skin floured & fried	½ chicken (11 oz)	844	47	13	–
broiler/fryer w/ skin fried	½ chicken (16.4 oz)	1347	81	22	–
broiler/fryer w/ skin roasted	½ chicken (10.5 oz)	715	41	11	–
broiler/fryer w/ skin stewed	½ chicken (11.7 oz)	730	42	12	–
broiler/fryer w/ skin neck & giblets batter dipped & fried	1 chicken (2.3 lbs)	2987	180	48	–
broiler/fryer w/ skin neck & giblets roasted	1 chicken (1.5 lbs)	1598	90	25	–
broiler/fryer w/ skin neck & giblets stewed	1 chicken (1.6 lbs)	1625	93	26	–
broiler/fryer w/o skin fried	1 cup	307	13	3	–
broiler/fryer w/o skin roasted	1 cup (5 oz)	266	10	3	–
broiler/fryer w/o skin stewed	1 cup (5 oz)	248	9	3	–
broiler/fryer wing w/ skin batter dipped & fried	1 (1.7 oz)	159	11	3	–
broiler/fryer wing w/ skin floured & fried	1 (1.1 oz)	103	7	2	–

FOOD	PORTION	CALS	FAT	SAT FAT	TRANS FAT
broiler/fryer wing w/ skin roasted	1 (1.2 oz)	99	7	2	–
broiler/fryer wing w/ skin stewed	1 (1.4 oz)	100	7	2	–
capon w/ skin neck & giblets roasted	1 chicken (3.1 lbs)	3211	165	46	–
cornish hen w/skin roasted	½ hen (4 oz)	296	21	6	–
cornish hen w/ skin roasted	1 hen (8 oz)	595	42	12	–
cornish hen w/o skin & bone roasted	1 hen (3.8 oz)	144	4	1	–
cornish hen w/o skin & bone roasted	½ hen (2 oz)	72	2	1	–
roaster dark meat w/o skin roasted	1 cup (5 oz)	250	12	3	–
roaster light meat w/o skin roasted	1 cup (5 oz)	214	6	2	–
roaster w/ skin neck & giblets roasted	1 chicken (2.4 lbs)	2363	140	39	–
roaster w/ skin roasted	½ chicken (1.1 lbs)	1071	64	18	–
roaster w/o skin roasted	1 cup (5 oz)	469	28	3	–
stewing dark meat w/o skin stewed	1 cup (5 oz)	361	21	6	–
stewing w/ skin neck & giblets stewed	1 chicken (1.3 lbs)	1636	107	29	–
stewing w/ skin stewed	½ chicken (9.2 oz)	744	49	13	–
Amish Select					
Boneless Skinless Breast w/ Honey Dijon Mustard	1 serv (4 oz)	130	2	0	–
Murray's					
Breast Boneless & Skinless	4 oz	110	1	0	–
Ground	3 oz	130	7	2	–
Whole Lean	4 oz	170	9	3	–
Perdue					
Boneless Skinless Breasts Cooked	3 oz	110	2	tr	–
Burger Cooked	1 (3 oz)	160	10	3	–
Chicken Breast Seasoned Italian Cooked	1 piece (3 oz)	90	1	tr	–

FOOD	PORTION	CALS	FAT	SAT FAT	TRANS FAT
Ground Cooked	3 oz	170	11	4	–
Ovenables Breast Lemon Pepper Cooked	1 piece (3 oz)	90	1	–	–
Seasoned Roasting Chicken Toasted Garlic Dark Meat	3 oz	190	14	4	–
Seasoned Roasting Chicken Toasted Garlic White Meat	3 oz	160	9	3	–
Tyson					
Breasts Boneless Skinless	4 oz	110	3	1	0
Cornish Hen	1 serv (4 oz)	200	14	4	–
Drumsticks	4 oz	150	9	3	0
Thigh Cutlets Boneless Skinless	4 oz	130	7	2	0
Whole Cut Up	4 oz	220	16	5	–
Wings	4 oz	220	17	5	0
FROZEN					
Barber					
Buffalo Fingers	1 (3.3 oz)	160	4	1	0
Nuggets 4 Cheese Stuffed	3 (3 oz)	230	16	3	0
Nuggets Cheddar & Bacon Stuffed	3 (3 oz)	240	17	4	0
Potato Chip Sticks	2 pieces (4.5 oz)	350	24	4	0
Bell & Evans					
Breaded Breast Nuggets	1 serv (4 oz)	190	6	1	–
Breaded Whole Breast Tenders	1 (4 oz)	190	6	1	–
Burgers	1 (3 oz)	120	6	2	–
Chicken Sandwich Steaks	1 serv (2 oz)	60	1	tr	–
Country Skillet					
Bites	5	270	16	3	–
Breast Tenders	3	240	14	4	–
Chunks	5	270	18	3	–
Fried	3 oz	270	18	5	–
Nuggets	10	280	17	4	–
Patties	1	190	12	3	–
Southern Fried Chunks	5	270	18	4	–
Southern Fried Patties	1	190	12	3	–
Ian's					
Fingers	3 pieces	190	8	2	–
Nuggets	5 pieces	190	8	2	0
Nuggets Allergy Free	5 pieces	190	8	2	0
Patties	1 (3.4 oz)	220	9	2	–

FOOD	PORTION	CALS	FAT	SAT FAT	TRANS FAT
Organic Prairie					
Ground	4 oz	200	12	3	–
Whole Young Small	4 oz	260	17	5	–
Tyson					
Any'tizers Barbeque Style Wings	3 pieces (3.2 oz)	200	13	4	0
Any'tizers Homestyle Chicken Fries	7 (3.2 oz)	230	11	3	0
Any'tizers Popcorn Chicken	6 (2.8 oz)	220	10	2	0
Breast Pattie	1 (2.6 oz)	180	11	3	0
Cordon Bleu	1 piece (5.9 oz)	380	24	8	0
Diced Strips	1 serv (3 oz)	90	1	0	0
Kiev	1 piece (5.9 oz)	480	37	17	1
Weaver					
Breast Strips	3 pieces	230	14	4	–
Breast Tenders	5 pieces	240	15	3	–
Buffalo Popcorn Chicken	7 pieces	230	14	2	–
Crispy Breast Strips	2 pieces	220	14	4	–
Crispy Mini Drums	5 pieces	250	16	4	–
Croquettes	2 + gravy	230	14	4	–
Honey Batter Breast Tenders	5 pieces	220	13	3	–
Hot Wings Buffalo Style	3 pieces	190	13	4	–
Nuggets	4 pieces	210	15	4	–
Patties Italian	1	210	14	3	–
Patties Breast	1	170	10	3	–
Patties Original	1	180	11	3	–
Wings Honey BBQ	3	200	11	3	–
Wellshire					
Chicken Bites Dinosaur Shaped Gluten Free	5 pieces	160	10	2	–
READY-TO-EAT					
chicken salad sandwich spread	¼ cup	104	7	2	–
Boar's Head					
Breast Hickory Smoked	2 oz	60	1	0	–
Breast Oven Roasted	2 oz	60	1	0	–
Healthy Ones					
Oven Roasted 97% Fat Free	4 slices (2 oz)	60	2	1	0
Hillshire Farm					
Smoked Breast	6 slices (2 oz)	60	1	0	–

FOOD	PORTION	CALS	FAT	SAT FAT	TRANS FAT
Oscar Mayer					
Breast Oven Roasted Thin Sliced	⅓ pkg (2 oz)	60	2	1	0
Breast Strips Breaded	½ pkg (3 oz)	170	6	1	1
Breast Strips Grilled	½ pkg (3 oz)	110	3	1	0
Perdue					
Cutlets Cooked	1 (3.5 oz)	220	11	3	–
Nuggets	5 (3.4 oz)	210	11	3	–
Nuggets Chicken & Cheese	5 (3.4 oz)	230	13	5	–
Short Cuts Chicken Breast Honey Roasted	½ cup (2.5 oz)	90	3	1	0
Short Cuts Chicken Strips Fajita Style	½ cup	90	3	1	0
Short Cuts Grilled Chicken Breast	½ cup (2.5 oz)	90	2	1	0
Short Cuts Grilled Italian	½ cup	90	3	1	0
Short Cuts Grilled Lemon Pepper	½ cup (2.5 oz)	80	1	0	0
Sara Lee					
Breast Oven Roasted	2 slices (1.6 oz)	45	1	0	–
Tyson					
Chicken Strips Fajita	1 serv (3 oz)	110	2	1	–
Honey Roasted Breast	2 slices (1.6 oz)	50	1	0	–
Hot Wings Buffalo Style	4	220	15	4	–
Roasted Whole Chicken Lemon Pepper	1 serv (3 oz)	120	6	2	–
Salad Kit Chunk Chicken	1 pkg (3.4 oz)	210	9	2	–
TAKE-OUT					
oven roasted breast of chicken	2 oz	60	1	0	–

CHICKEN DISHES
FROZEN

FOOD	PORTION	CALS	FAT	SAT FAT	TRANS FAT
Barber					
Broccoli & Cheese Reduced Fat	1 piece (5.5 oz)	250	13	3	0
Cordon Bleu	1 piece (6 oz)	370	23	7	0
Cordon Bleu Reduced Fat	1 piece (5.5 oz)	260	13	4	0
Creme Brie & Apple	1 piece (6 oz)	350	21	5	0
Kiev	1 piece (6 oz)	430	29	11	1
Mashed Potato Stuffed	1 piece (6 oz)	340	18	8	–
Skinless Breast Stuffed	1 piece (6 oz)	280	11	3	0

FOOD	PORTION	CALS	FAT	SAT FAT	TRANS FAT
Maple Leaf Farms					
Chicken Breast Stuffed Broccoli & Cheese	1 serv (6 oz)	340	19	6	–
REFRIGERATED					
Lloyd's					
Barbecue Shredded Chicken	¼ cup (2 oz)	90	2	1	–
Lunchables					
Chicken Shake-Up	1 pkg	220	6	2	0
Old El Paso					
For Tacos Shredded Chicken	¼ cup	60	2	1	–
Tyson					
Chicken Breast Medallions In White Wine & Garlic Sauce	1 serv (5 oz)	140	6	2	0
Ventera					
Rollatini w/ Rice Stuffing & Marsala Wine Sauce	1 serv + sauce (6 oz)	230	10	5	0
Wellshire					
Shredded Chicken In BBQ Sauce	¼ cup	70	3	1	–
TAKE-OUT					
arroz con pollo	1 serv (16 oz)	579	14	7	–
barbecued pulled chicken	1 serv (9 oz)	312	2	1	–
boneless breast w/ apple stuffing	1 serv (5 oz)	260	9	2	–
breast & wing breaded & fried	2 pieces (5.7 oz)	494	30	8	–
chicken & dumplings	¾ cup	256	12	4	–
chicken & noodles	1 cup	365	18	5	–
chicken a la king	1 cup	470	34	13	–
chicken cacciatore	¾ cup	394	24	6	–
chicken paprikash	1½ cups	296	10	–	–
chicken pie w/ top crust	1 slice (5.6 oz)	472	31	–	–
chicken cordon bleu	1 serv (5 oz)	280	13	4	–
chicken meatloaf	1 lg slice (5 oz)	243	9	3	–
chicken satay + peanut sauce	2 skewers	239	12	6	0
drumstick breaded & fried	2 pieces (5.2 oz)	430	27	7	–
grilled breast strips	4 strips (3 oz)	100	2	1	–
groundnut stew hkatenkwan	1 serv (15.7 oz)	576	40	10	–
jamaican jerk wings	4 wings (9.9 oz)	709	51	14	–
kobete turkish chicken w/ pastry	1 serv	513	13	4	–

FOOD	PORTION	CALS	FAT	SAT FAT	TRANS FAT
sancocho de pollo dominican chicken stew	1 serv	702	30	8	–
sukiyaki	1 serv (18 oz)	436	8	2	–
tandoori chicken breast	1 serv	260	13	–	–
tandoori chicken leg & thigh	1 serv	300	17	–	–
thigh breaded & fried	2 pieces (5.2 oz)	430	27	7	–

CHICKEN SUBSTITUTES
Boca
Chik'n Nuggets	1 serv (3 oz)	180	7	1	0
Chik'n Patties	1 (2.5 oz)	160	6	1	0

Gardenburger
Chik'n Grill	1 patty (2.5 oz)	100	3	0	0

Lightlife
Smart Cutlet Seasoned Chicken	1 (4 oz)	180	4	1	–
Smart Menu Chick'n Nuggets	4 pieces	220	11	2	–
Smart Menu Chick'n Patties	1 patty	160	7	1	–
Smart Menu Chick'n Strips	1 serv (3 oz)	80	0	0	0

Loma Linda
Fried Chik'n w/ Gravy	2 pieces (2.8 oz)	150	10	2	0

Morningstar Farms
Chik'n Roasted Herb	1 patty (2.2 oz)	110	3	1	0
Meal Starters Chik'n Strips	12 pieces (3 oz)	140	4	1	0

Quorn
Cutlets	1 (3.5 oz)	200	8	1	–
Gruyere Cutlet	1 (4 oz)	260	15	4	0
Naked Cutlet	1 (2.4 oz)	80	3	1	–
Nuggets	3-4 pieces (3 oz)	180	8	1	–
Patties	1 patty (2.6 oz)	160	7	1	–
Tenders	1 cup (3 oz)	90	2	1	–

Viana
Veggie Chickin Fillets	1 (3.7 oz)	260	14	3	1
Veggie Chickin Nuggets	3 pieces (2.6 oz)	200	12	2	1

Worthington
FriChik Original	2 pieces (3.2 oz)	140	8	1	0
Meatless Chicken Style	1 slice (2 oz)	90	5	1	0

Yves
Meatless Chicken Burger	1 (2.6 oz)	100	3	0	0

FOOD	PORTION	CALS	FAT	SAT FAT	TRANS FAT
Meatless Smoked Chicken Slices	4 (2.2 oz)	100	2	0	0

CHICKPEAS
CANNED
chickpeas	1 cup	285	3	tr	–
Eden					
Organic Garbanzo	½ cup	130	1	0	0
Green Giant					
Garbanzo Beans	½ cup	100	2	0	–
Progresso					
ChickPeas	½ cup	100	2	0	0
DRIED					
cooked	1 cup	269	4	tr	–
Arrowhead Mills					
Organic Dried Chickpeas not prep	¼ cup	160	3	0	0
REFRIGERATED					
Sabra					
Balela Vinaigrette	2 oz	100	5	1	–
Spicy Armenian Salad	2 oz	50	3	0	–

CHICORY
endive fresh chopped	½ cup	4	tr	tr	–
greens raw chopped	½ cup	21	tr	tr	–
root raw	1 (2.1 oz)	44	tr	tr	–
roots raw cut up	½ cup (1.6 oz)	33	tr	tr	–
witloof head raw	1 (1.9 oz)	9	tr	tr	–
witloof raw	½ cup (1.6 oz)	8	tr	tr	–
Frieda's					
Belgian Endive	2 cups	115	0	0	0

CHILI
powder	1 tbsp	24	1	tr	0
Amy's					
Chili & Cornbread	1 pkg (10.5 oz)	320	6	2	–
Organic Black Bean	1 cup	200	2	0	–
Organic Medium	1 cup	190	6	1	–
Organic Medium w/ Vegetables	1 cup	190	6	1	–

FOOD	PORTION	CALS	FAT	SAT FAT	TRANS FAT
Boca					
Chili w/ Ground Burger	1 pkg (9.4 oz)	150	1	0	0
Bush's					
ChiliMagic Chili Starter as prep	1 cup	250	11	4	–
Original No Beans	1 cup	240	14	5	–
Carroll Shelby's					
Original Texas Chili Kit	2 tbsp	60	1	0	–
Del Monte					
Sauce	1 tbsp	20	0	0	0
Fantastic					
3 Bean	1 pkg (8 oz)	180	4	0	0
Vegetarian Mix not prep	¼ cup	100	1	0	–
Gringo Billy's					
Chili Mix	1 tbsp	24	1	0	–
Hunt's					
Family Favorites Chili	¼ cup (2.2 oz)	25	0	0	0
Lean Cuisine					
Cafe Classics Three Bean Chili	1 pkg (10 oz)	260	7	2	0
Lightlife					
Smart Chili	1 pkg	200	0	0	0
McCormick					
Mexican Style Chili Powder	¼ tsp	0	0	0	0
McIhenny					
Original Recipe	½ cup	50	1	0	0
Mimi's Gourmet					
Organic Vegan Gluten Free 3 Bean w/ Rice	1 pkg (11.5 oz)	270	6	1	0
Organic Vegan Gluten Free Black Bean & Corn	1 pkg (10.5 oz)	250	6	1	0
Organic Vegan Gluten Free White Bean	1 pkg (10.5 oz)	230	6	1	0
Nature's Entree					
Texas Chili	1 pkg (12 oz)	320	7	2	–
Pacific Foods					
Beef Steak w/ Beans	1 cup	250	7	2	0
Ro-Tel					
Chili Fixin's	½ cup	35	1	0	–
Soy7					
Chili Mix as prep	1 cup	150	2	0	–

FOOD	PORTION	CALS	FAT	SAT FAT	TRANS FAT
Spice Hunter					
Powder Blend Salt Free	¼ tsp	0	0	0	0
Stagg					
Chunkero w/ Beans	1 cup	300	15	7	–
Classic w/ Beans	1 cup	330	17	8	–
Country Blend	1 cup	330	17	7	1
Country Blend w/ Beans	1 cup	33	17	7	1
Ranch House Chicken w/ Beans	1 cup	290	9	3	–
Silverado Beef w/ Beans	1 cup	230	3	1	–
Turkey Ranchero w/ Beans	1 cup	240	3	1	–
Vegetable Garden Four Bean	1 cup	200	1	0	–
Wick Fowler's					
2 Alarm Chili Kit	3 tbsp	60	2	0	–
False Alarm Chili Kit	2 tbsp	50	2	0	–
Worthington					
Vegetarian	1 cup	280	10	2	0
TAKE-OUT					
chiles rellenos cheese filled	1 (5 oz)	365	30	13	0
chili con carne w/ beans	1 cup	264	11	4	–
con carne w/ beans & rice	1 cup	298	9	4	–
vegetarian con carne	1 cup	272	7	1	–

CHILI PEPPER (see PEPPERS)

CHINESE PRESERVING MELON

FOOD	PORTION	CALS	FAT	SAT FAT	TRANS FAT
cooked	½ cup	11	tr	tr	

CHINESE FOOD (see ASIAN FOOD)

CHIPS (see also SNACKS)

FOOD	PORTION	CALS	FAT	SAT FAT	TRANS FAT
apple chips	10	101	5	tr	–
corn	1 oz	153	10	1	–
corn barbecue	1 oz	148	9	1	–
corn cones	1 oz	145	8	6	–
corn cones nacho	1 oz	152	9	8	–
corn onion	1 oz	142	6	1	–
potato	1 oz	152	10	3	–
potato cheese	1 bag (6 oz)	842	46	15	–
potato cheese	1 oz	140	8	2	–
potato light	1 oz	134	6	1	–
potato sour cream & onion	1 oz	150	10	3	–

FOOD	PORTION	CALS	FAT	SAT FAT	TRANS FAT
potato sticks	1 pkg (1 oz)	148	10	3	–
potato sticks	½ cup (0.6 oz)	94	6	2	–
taco	1 bag (8 oz)	1089	55	11	–
taco	1 oz	136	7	1	–
taro	1 oz	141	7	2	–
taro	10 (0.8 oz)	115	6	1	–
tortilla	1 oz	142	7	1	–
tortilla nacho	1 oz	141	7	1	–
tortilla nacho light	1 oz	126	4	1	–
tortilla ranch	1 oz	139	7	1	–
Bachman					
Potato Golden Crisps	1 pkg (1 oz)	150	9	3	–
Bravos!					
Tortilla Nacho Cheese	1 oz	150	8	2	0
Cape Cod					
Potato 40% Reduced Fat	19	130	6	2	0
Potato Beachside BBQ	19	150	8	2	0
Potato Classic	19	150	8	3	0
Potato Fresh Garden Herb Reduced Fat	19	130	6	1	0
Potato Jalapeno & Cheddar	19	140	8	2	0
Potato No Salt	19	150	10	3	0
Potato Robust Russet	19	150	8	2	0
Potato Salt & Vinegar	19	150	8	2	0
Potato Sea Salt & Cracked Pepper	19	140	7	2	0
Tortilla Reduced Carb	10	140	6	1	0
Tortilla Veggie	12	140	6	1	0
Corazonas					
Tortilla Jalapeno Jack	1 oz	140	7	1	0
Tortilla Original	1 oz	140	7	1	0
Tortilla Salsa Picante	1 oz	140	7	1	0
Deliciously Slim					
Tortilla Black Bean & Sour Cream	1 oz	140	9	2	–
Tortilla Lightly Salted	1 oz	140	8	2	–
Tortilla Ranch	1 oz	140	9	2	–
Doritos					
Baked Cooler Ranch	15 (1 oz)	120	4	1	0
Baked Nacho Cheesier	15	120	4	1	0

FOOD	PORTION	CALS	FAT	SAT FAT	TRANS FAT
Cooler Ranch	12	140	7	1	0
Four Cheese	12	140	8	1	0
Guacamole	12	150	8	2	0
Light Nacho Cheesier	11	90	1	0	0
Natural White Nacho Cheese	11	150	8	1	0
Ranchero	12	150	1	1	0
Rollitos Cooler Ranch	17	140	8	2	0
Rollitos Zesty Taco	17	150	8	2	0
Toasted Corn	13	140	7	1	0
Eatsmart					
Cafe Fries Malt Vinegar & Sea Salt	1 oz	150	7	1	0
Cafe Fries Tangy Tomato & Spices	1 oz	150	7	1	0
CheddAirs	1 oz	135	5	1	0
Soy Crisps Parmesan Garlic & Olive Oil	1 oz	160	9	1	0
Soy Crisps Tomato Romano & Olive Oil	1 oz	160	9	1	0
Veggie Crisps	1 oz	140	7	1	0
Veggie Crisps Cheddar & Jalapeno	1 oz	130	7	1	0
Veggie Crisps Sundried Tomato & Pesto	1 oz	140	7	1	0
Eden					
Brown Rice Chips	25	150	7	2	0
Sea Vegetable Chips	25	140	5	2	0
Vegetable	25	130	4	2	0
Wasabi	25	130	4	2	0
Flat Earth					
Baked Fruit Crisps Apple Cinnamon Grove	14 (1 oz)	130	5	1	0
Baked Fruit Crisps Peach Mango Paradise	14 (1 oz)	130	5	1	0
Baked Fruit Crisps Wild Berry Patch	14 (1 oz)	130	5	1	0
Baked Veggie Crisps Farmland Cheddar	14 (1 oz)	130	5	1	0
Baked Veggie Crisps Garlic & Herb Field	14 (1 oz)	130	5	1	0

FOOD	PORTION	CALS	FAT	SAT FAT	TRANS FAT
Baked Veggie Crisps Tangy Tomato Ranch	14 (1 oz)	130	5	1	0
French's					
Potato Sticks Barbecue	¾ cup	160	10	5	0
Potato Sticks Cheddar	¾ cup	170	12	5	0
Potato Sticks Original	¾ cup	190	12	5	0
Fritos					
Corn Chips King Size	12	160	10	2	0
Original	32	160	10	2	0
Scoops	10	160	10	2	0
Twists	23	150	9	2	0
Garden Of Eatin'					
Organic Pita Baked Brown Sugar & Cinnamon	8	120	3	0	0
Organic Tortilla Blue Corn	7	140	7	1	0
Organic Tortilla Blue No Salt Added	16	140	7	1	0
Organic Tortilla White Corn	7	140	6	1	0
Glenny's					
Organic Soy Barbeque	1 oz	110	3	0	0
Organic Soy Creamy Ranch	1 oz	110	3	0	0
Soy Crisps Apple Cinnamon	½ pkg (0.6 oz)	70	2	0	–
Soy Crisps Caramel	½ pkg (1.3 oz)	70	2	0	0
Soy Crisps Low Fat Lightly Salted	½ pkg (0.6 oz)	70	1	0	–
Soy Crisps No Salt	½ pkg (0.6 oz)	70	1	0	0
Soy Crisps Salt & Pepper	½ pkg (0.6 oz)	70	1	0	–
Soy Crisps White Cheddar	½ pkg (0.6 oz)	70	2	0	–
Spud Delites Sea Salt	1 pkg (1.1 oz)	100	1	0	–
Veggie Fries	½ pkg (0.6 oz)	70	1	0	0
Zen Health Tortilla Crisps Original	1 oz	110	3	0	0
Guiltless Gourmet					
Potato Au Gratin	1 oz	100	3	0	0
Potato Pico De Gallo	1 oz	100	3	0	0
Potato Sea Salt	1 oz	90	2	0	0
Tortilla Chili Lime	18 (1 oz)	110	2	0	–
Tortilla Chili Verde	18 (1 oz)	120	2	0	0
Tortilla Chipotle	18 (1 oz)	120	2	0	0
Tortilla Red Corn	18 (1 oz)	110	2	0	–

FOOD	PORTION	CALS	FAT	SAT FAT	TRANS FAT
Tortilla Spicy Black Bean	18 (1 oz)	110	2	0	–
Tortilla Sweet White Corn	18 (1 oz)	110	2	0	0
Tortilla Yellow Corn Unsalted	18 (1 oz)	110	1	0	–
Herr's					
Potato	1 oz	140	8	3	–
Husman's					
Potato Sour Cream & Onion	18 (1 oz)	150	9	3	–
Jay's					
Potato	1 oz	150	10	2	–
Keto					
Low Carb Tortilla All Flavors	1 oz	150	8	1	–
Kettle					
Bakes Potato Aged White Cheddar	1 oz	120	3	1	0
Bakes Potato Hickory Honey Barbeque	1 oz	120	3	0	0
Bakes Potato Lightly Salted	1 oz	120	3	0	0
Krinkle Cut Potato Barbeque	1 oz	150	9	1	0
Krinkle Cut Potato Dill & Sour Cream	1 oz	150	9	1	0
Krinkle Cut Potato Lightly Salted	1 oz	150	9	1	0
Krinkle Cut Potato Salt & Fresh Ground Pepper	1 oz	150	9	1	0
Organic Tortilla Blue Corn	1 oz	140	6	1	0
Organic Tortilla Brown Rice & Black Bean w/ Garlic & Onions	1 oz	120	6	1	0
Organic Tortilla Fire Roasted Chili	1 oz	140	7	1	0
Organic Tortilla Five Grain Yellow Corn	1 oz	140	6	1	0
Organic Tortilla Lightly Salted Yellow Corn	1 oz	140	6	1	0
Organic Tortilla Little Dippers	1 oz	140	6	1	0
Organic Tortilla Sesame Blue Moons	1 oz	150	8	1	0
Potato Cheddar Beer	1 oz	150	9	1	0
Potato Honey Dijon	1 oz	150	9	1	0
Potato Sea Salt & Vinegar	1 oz	150	9	1	0

FOOD	PORTION	CALS	FAT	SAT FAT	TRANS FAT
Potato Spicy Thai	1 oz	150	9	1	0
Potato Unsalted	1 oz	150	9	1	0
Potato Yogurt & Green Onion	1 oz	150	9	1	0
Lay's					
Baked KC Masterpiece	11 (1 oz)	120	3	0	0
Baked Sour Cream & Onion	12 (1 oz)	120	3	0	0
Chile Limon	1 oz	150	10	3	0
Classic	1 pkg (1 oz)	150	10	3	0
Deli Style Original	17 (1 oz)	150	10	3	0
Dill Pickle	20 (1 oz)	160	10	3	0
Flamin' Hot	17 (1 oz)	160	10	3	0
KC Masterpiece BBQ	15 (1 oz)	150	10	3	0
Kettle Cooked Jalapeno	15 (1 oz)	140	8	2	0
Kettle Cooked Mesquite BBQ	18 (1 oz)	140	8	3	0
Kettle Cooked Original	22 (1 oz)	150	8	3	0
Kettle Cooked Sea Salt & Vinegar	18 (1 oz)	140	7	2	0
Light Fat Free KC Masterpiece	20 (1 oz)	75	0	0	0
Light Fat Free Original	20 (1 oz)	75	0	0	0
Limon	17 (1 oz)	150	10	3	0
Natural Country BBQ	14 (1 oz)	150	9	1	0
Natural Sea Salt & Vinegar	16 (1 oz)	150	9	1	0
Natural Sea Salted	16 (1 oz)	150	9	1	0
Original Baked	11 (1 oz)	110	2	0	0
Salt & Vinegar	17 (1 oz)	150	10	3	0
Sour Cream & Onion	17 (1 oz)	160	11	3	0
Stax	13 (1 oz)	160	10	3	0
Wavy	11 (1 oz)	150	10	3	0
Wavy Au Gratin	13 (1 oz)	150	10	3	0
Wavy Hickory Barbecue	13 (1 oz)	150	9	2	0
Wavy Ranch	12 (1 oz)	150	10	3	0
Lundberg					
Rice Chips Original Sea Salt	1 oz	140	7	1	0
Rice Chips Sesame Seaweed	1 oz	140	7	1	0
Rice Chips Wasabi	1 oz	140	6	1	0
Madhouse Munchies					
Potato Sea Salt	16	150	9	1	0
Potato Sea Salt & Vinegar	16	150	9	1	0
Tortilla White	9	140	6	0	0

FOOD	PORTION	CALS	FAT	SAT FAT	TRANS FAT
Manny's					
Organic Tortilla Blues	1 oz	150	7	0	–
Tortilla No Salt Added	1 oz	150	7	3	–
Maui					
Shrimp Chips	17	140	8	2	0
Met-Rx					
Pro Chips Bar-B-Que	1 pkg (2 oz)	260	9	1	–
Pro Chips Nacho	1 pkg (2 oz)	260	10	2	–
Moore's					
Corn Chips	1 oz	160	10	3	0
New York Deli					
Potato Kettle Cooked	1 oz	150	9	3	0
Pita-Snax					
Cheddar Cheese	34 (1 oz)	110	2	0	–
Chili & Lime	34 (1 oz)	120	2	0	–
Cinnamon	34 (1 oz)	120	2	0	–
Dill Ranch	34 (1 oz)	120	2	0	–
Garlic	34 (1 oz)	120	2	0	–
Lightly Salted	34 (1 oz)	110	1	0	–
Popchips					
Corn Hint Of Butter	23 (1 oz)	120	5	0	0
Potato Barbeque	19 (1 oz)	120	5	0	0
Potato Original	22 (1 oz)	120	5	0	0
Rice Sea Salt	19 (1 oz)	120	5	0	0
Rice Wasabi	20 (1 oz)	120	5	0	0
Pringles					
Jalapeno	15 (1 oz)	150	10	3	0
Loaded Baked Potato	15 (1 oz)	150	10	3	0
Minis Cheddar Cheese	1 pkg	120	7	2	0
Minis Original	1 pkg	120	7	2	0
Original	14 (1 oz)	160	11	3	0
Pizza	15 (1 oz)	150	10	3	0
Select Cinnnamon Sweet Potato	28 (1 oz)	150	9	2	0
Select Parmesan Garlic	28 (1 oz)	140	9	2	0
Snack Stacks Original	1 pkg	140	10	3	0
Racquet					
Wheat Chips All Flavors	6 chips	30	1	0	–
Revival					
Baked Soy Pasta Chips Lightly Salted Sunshine	1 bag (0.9 oz)	100	2	0	–

FOOD	PORTION	CALS	FAT	SAT FAT	TRANS FAT
Baked Soy Pasta Chips Naturally Nice	1 bag (0.9 oz)	80	1	0	–
Baked Soy Pasta Chips Rev It Up Ranch	1 bag (0.9 oz)	105	3	0	–
Ruffles					
Baked Original	10	120	3	0	0
Cheddar & Sour Cream	11	160	10	3	0
KC Masterpiece Mesquite BBQ	11	150	10	3	0
Light Cheddar & Sour Cream	15	75	0	0	0
Light Original	17	70	0	0	0
Original	12	160	10	3	0
Potato Crisps	16	160	10	2	0
Reduced Fat Sea Salted	15	140	7	1	0
Sour Cream & Onion	11	160	10	3	0
Santitas					
White Corn	9	130	6	1	0
Yellow Corn	9	130	6	1	0
Snyder's Of Hanover					
Kosher Dill	1 oz	140	6	2	0
MultiGrain Sunflower	1 oz	140	6	1	0
MultiGrain Sunflower Southwestern Cheddar	1 oz	140	6	1	0
MultiGrain Tortilla Lightly Salted	1 oz	130	5	0	0
MultiGrain Tortilla Strips Flaxseed Gold	1 oz	140	6	1	0
Organic Veggie Crisps	1 oz	140	7	1	0
Potato Original	1 oz	150	7	2	0
Sweet Potato Baked	1 oz	110	2	0	0
Tortilla White Corn	1 oz	140	5	0	0
Tortilla Pounder Multi-Grain	1 oz	130	5	0	0
Solea					
Polenta Corn	1 oz	120	4	0	0
Potato Olive Oil Sea Salt	1 oz	120	6	1	0
Stacy's					
Pita Chips Multigrain	1 pkg	140	6	1	0
Pita Chips Parmesan Garlic & Herb	1 oz	140	5	1	0
Pita Chips Texarkana Hot	1 oz	130	5	1	0

FOOD	PORTION	CALS	FAT	SAT FAT	TRANS FAT
Soy Thin Chips Sticky Bun	18 (1 oz)	130	5	1	0
Soy Thin Crisps Simply Cheese	18 (1 oz)	130	6	1	0
SunChips					
French Onion	10	140	6	1	0
Original	1 pkg (1 oz)	140	6	1	0
Tastee					
Potato Yukon Gold	1 oz	130	5	1	–
Terra					
Exotic Vegetable Original	14 (1 oz)	150	9	1	0
Exotic Vegetable Zesty Tomato	14 (1 oz)	150	9	1	0
Kettles Potato Sea Salt & Pepper	15 (1 oz)	140	6	1	0
Parsnip Chips	12 (1 oz)	150	10	1	0
Potato Au Natural	18 (1 oz)	150	9	1	0
Potato Blues	1 oz	130	6	1	0
Potato Golds Original	1 oz	130	5	1	0
Potato Potpourri	1 oz	140	7	1	0
Potato Red Bliss	1 oz	140	7	1	0
Potato Frites Sea Salt & Vinegar	1 oz	150	8	1	0
Stix Original Exotic Vegetable	1 oz	150	9	1	0
Sweet Potato	17 (1 oz)	160	11	1	0
Sweets & Beets	16 (1 oz)	150	9	1	0
Taro	1 oz	140	6	1	0
Tostitos					
Blue Corn	6	140	6	1	0
Crispy Rounds	13	140	7	1	0
Gold	6	140	7	1	0
Light Restaurant Style	6	90	1	0	0
Original Bite Size	20	110	1	0	0
Restaurant Style	6	130	6	1	0
Santa Fe	7	140	6	1	0
Scoops	13	140	7	1	0
Yellow Corn	6	140	6	1	0
Utz					
Pita Natural w/ Sea Salt	1 oz	120	5	1	0
Potato	20 (1 oz)	150	9	2	0
Potato Baked	1 oz	110	2	0	0
Potato BBQ	20 (1 oz)	150	10	3	0
Potato Grandma Kettle	1 oz	140	8	3	0

FOOD	PORTION	CALS	FAT	SAT FAT	TRANS FAT
Potato Homestyle Kettle	1 oz	140	8	2	4
Potato Kettle Classics	20 (1 oz)	150	9	2	0
Potato Mystic Kettle	1 oz	150	9	2	0
Potato Mystic Kettle Reduced Fat	1 oz	130	6	2	0
Potato Natural Lightly Salted Kettle	1 oz	140	8	1	0
Potato No Salt Added	20 (1 oz)	150	9	2	0
Potato Onion & Garlic	1 oz	150	9	2	0
Potato Ripple	20 (1 oz)	150	10	3	0
Sweet Potato Kettle Classics	20 (1 oz)	150	9	2	0
Tortilla Baked	10	120	2	1	0
Tortilla Organic Yellow Corn	1 oz	140	6	1	0
Vegetable Natural Exotic Medley	1 oz	160	10	1	0
Wise					
Dipsy Doodles Corn Chips	1 oz	160	10	3	0
Potato	1 pkg (1 oz)	150	10	3	0
Potato Lightly Salted	1 oz	150	10	3	0
Potato Ridgies	1 oz	150	10	3	0
Potato Unsalted	1 oz	150	10	3	0

CHITTERLINGS

pork cooked	3 oz	258	24	9	–

CHIVES

freeze-dried	1 tbsp	1	tr	tr	–
fresh chopped	1 tbsp	1	tr	tr	–
fresh chopped	1 tsp	0	tr	tr	–

CHOCOLATE (see also CANDY, CHOCOLATE SPREAD, CHOCOLATE SYRUP, COCOA, HOT COCOA, ICE CREAM TOPPINGS, MILK DRINKS)

baking	1 oz	145	15	9	–
baking grated unsweetened	¼ cup	165	17	11	–
baking liquid unsweetened	1 oz	134	14	7	–
baking squares unsweetened	1 square (1 oz)	145	15	9	–
chips milk chocolate	1 cup (6 oz)	862	52	31	–
chips semisweet	1 cup (6 oz)	804	50	30	–
chips semisweet	60 pieces (1 oz)	136	9	5	–
drink mix powder	2-3 heaping tsp	75	1	tr	–
mexican baking	1 sq (0.7 oz)	85	3	2	–

FOOD	PORTION	CALS	FAT	SAT FAT	TRANS FAT
Baker's					
Chips Chocolate Chunks	13 pieces (0.5 oz)	70	5	3	–
E. Guittard					
Chips Cappuccino	30 (0.5 oz)	80	5	5	0
Chips Milk Chocolate	12 (0.5 oz)	80	5	3	0
Chips Semisweet	30 (0.5 oz)	70	4	3	0
Ghirardelli					
Chips Semi-Sweet	33 (0.5 oz)	70	4	3	–
Hershey's					
Chips Milk Chocolate	1 tbsp	80	5	3	–
Chips Mini Milk Chocolate	1 tbsp	80	4	3	–
Chips Raspberry	1 tbsp	80	4	3	–
Chips Semi-Sweet	1 tbsp	80	4	3	–
Chips Semi-Sweet Mini	1 tbsp	80	4	3	–
Holiday Baking Bits	1 tbsp	70	3	2	–
Mini Kisses For Baking	11 pieces	80	5	3	–
Premier White Milk Chips	1 tbsp	80	4	3	–
Skor English Toffee Baking Bits	1 tbsp	70	5	3	–
Love'n Bake					
Chocolate Schmear	2 tbsp	140	8	0	–
M&M's					
Baking Bits Milk Chocolate	1 tbsp	70	4	2	0
Baking Bits Semi-Sweet Chocolate	1 tbsp	70	4	2	0
Sunfood					
Organic Cacao Beans	1 oz	171	13	8	0
Organic Cacao Nibs	1 oz	171	13	8	0
Organic Powder	2 tbsp (1 oz)	120	4	2	0
MIX					
drink mix powder as prep w/ whole milk	9 oz	226	9	5	–

CHOCOLATE MILK (see MILK DRINKS)

CHOCOLATE SPREAD
Twist

FOOD	PORTION	CALS	FAT	SAT FAT	TRANS FAT
Sugar Free Chocolate Spread	2 tbsp	170	12	2	–

CHOCOLATE SYRUP

FOOD	PORTION	CALS	FAT	SAT FAT	TRANS FAT
chocolate fudge	1 cup (11.9 oz)	1176	46	19	–
chocolate fudge	1 tbsp (0.7 oz)	73	3	1	–

FOOD	PORTION	CALS	FAT	SAT FAT	TRANS FAT
syrup	1 cup	653	3	2	–
syrup	2 tbsp	82	tr	tr	–
syrup as prep w/ whole milk	9 oz	232	9	5	–
Colac					
Chocolate Topping	1 tbsp	37	1	tr	–
DaVinci Gourmet					
Sugar Free	2 tbsp	15	0	0	0
Hershey's					
Chocolate Fudge	1 tbsp	70	3	2	–
Double Chocolate	1 tbsp	50	0	0	0
Lite	2 tbsp	50	0	0	0
Syrup	2 tbsp	100	0	0	0
Nesquik					
Calcium Fortified	2 tbsp	100	0	0	0
Smucker's					
Sundae Syrup Chocolate	2 tbsp	110	0	0	0
Walden Farms					
Sugar Free	2 tbsp	0	0	0	0
Whoppers					
Chocolate Malt	2 tbsp	100	0	0	0
CHUTNEY					
apple	1.2 oz	68	0	–	0
coconut	2 oz	87	9	7	–
fresh mint	2 oz	18	0	0	–
mango	1 tbsp	54	2	–	–
tomato	1 oz	90	7	1	–
Patak's					
Major Grey	1 tbsp	60	0	0	0
Mango Hot	1 tbsp	60	0	0	0
Mango Sweet	1 tbsp	60	1	0	–
Robert Rothchild Farm					
Hot Peach & Apple	2 tbsp	45	0	0	0
School House Kitchen					
Bardshar	1 oz	80	0	0	0
CILANTRO					
fresh	¼ cup	1	tr	tr	0
fresh sprigs	5 (5 g)	1	tr	tr	0
Dorot					
Chopped Cube frzn	1 (4 g)	5	tr	tr	0

FOOD	PORTION	CALS	FAT	SAT FAT	TRANS FAT
CINNAMON					
cinnamon sugar	1 tsp	16	tr	tr	–
ground	1 tsp	6	tr	tr	0
sticks	0.5 oz	39	tr	tr	–
Gringo Billy's					
Cinnamon Sweetener	½ tsp	0	0	0	0
CISCO					
raw	3 oz	84	2	tr	–
smoked	1 oz	50	3	tr	–
CLAMS					
CANNED					
liquid only	1 cup	6	tr	–	–
liquid only	3 oz	2	tr	–	–
meat only	1 cup	236	3	tr	–
meat only	3 oz	126	2	tr	–
Brunswick					
Baby	2 oz	50	1	0	–
Bumble Bee					
Baby	¼ cup	50	1	1	0
Chopped Or Minced	¼ cup	25	0	0	0
Smoked	¼ cup	130	9	2	–
Chicken Of The Sea					
Chopped	¼ cup	30	0	0	0
Minced	¼ cup	30	0	0	0
Whole Baby	¼ cup	30	0	0	0
Orleans					
Clam Juice	1 tbsp	0	0	0	0
FRESH					
cooked	20 sm	133	2	tr	–
cooked	3 oz	126	2	tr	–
raw	20 sm (6.3 oz)	133	2	tr	–
raw	9 lg (6.3 oz)	133	2	tr	–
raw	3 oz	63	1	tr	–
FROZEN					
Mrs. Paul's					
Fried	18 (3 oz)	270	13	3	0
TAKE-OUT					
breaded & fried	20 sm	379	21	5	–

FOOD	PORTION	CALS	FAT	SAT FAT	TRANS FAT
CLEMENTINE JUICE					
Izze					
Sparkling Clementine	8 oz	100	0	0	0
CLEMENTINES					
Haddon House					
In Light Syrup	½ cup	80	0	0	0
Sunkist					
Fresh	2	80	0	0	0
Tina					
Fresh	1	50	1	0	–
CLOVES					
ground	1 tsp	7	tr	tr	0
COCOA (see also HOT COCOA)					
powder unsweetened	1 cup (3 oz)	197	12	7	–
powder unsweetened	1 tbsp (5 g)	11	1	tr	–
Hershey's					
Cocoa	1 tbsp	20	1	0	–
European Cocoa	1 tbsp	20	1	0	–
COCONUT					
dried sweetened shredded	¼ cup	116	8	7	0
dried toasted	1 oz	168	13	12	0
dried unsweetened	1 oz	187	18	16	0
fresh from 1 coconut	14 oz	1405	133	118	0
fresh shredded	¼ cup	71	7	6	0
Bob's Red Mill					
Shredded	3 tbsp	120	11	10	0
Frieda's					
White	¼ cup (1.4 oz)	140	13	12	–
Let's Do Organic					
Organic Reduced Fat Shredded	1 can (0.5 oz)	70	6	5	0
Shredded	3 tbsp (0.5 oz)	110	10	9	0
Prosperity					
Organic Coconut Flax Butter Garlic & Onion	1 tbsp	140	15	9	0
COCONUT JUICE					
coconut water fresh	½ cup	23	tr	tr	0
creamed sweetened canned	½ cup	264	12	11	0
milk canned	½ cup	276	29	25	0

FOOD	PORTION	CALS	FAT	SAT FAT	TRANS FAT
A Taste Of Thai					
Coconut Milk	⅓ cup	140	15	14	–
Lite Coconut Milk	⅓ cup	45	4	4	–
Amy & Brian					
Juice	8 oz	76	0	0	0
Goya					
Coconut Water	1 can (11.8 oz)	120	1	0	0
Let's Do Organic					
Creamed	1 oz	220	19	17	0
Milk	¼ cup	100	11	10	0
O.N.E.					
Natural Coconut Water	1 box (11 oz)	60	0	0	0
Thai Kitchen					
Milk	2 oz	124	12	7	–
Vita Coco					
Coconut Water	1 box (11 oz)	65	0	0	0
Coconut Water w/ Fruit Juice All Flavors	1 box (11 oz)	110	0	0	0
Zico					
Coconut Water Mango	11 oz	60	0	0	0
Coconut Water Natural	11 oz	60	0	0	0
Coconut Water Passion Fruit + Orange Peel	11 oz	60	0	0	0
COD					
atlantic canned	1 can (11 oz)	327	3	1	–
atlantic canned	3 oz	89	1	tr	–
atlantic dried	3 oz	246	2	tr	–
atlantic fresh cooked	1 fillet (6.3 oz)	189	2	tr	–
atlantic fresh cooked	3 oz	89	1	tr	–
atlantic fresh raw	3 oz	70	1	tr	–
pacific fresh baked	3 oz	95	1	tr	–
roe canned	1 oz	34	1	–	–
roe tarama	3.5 oz	547	55	–	–
Mrs. Paul's					
Filets Lightly Breaded	1 (4 oz)	220	11	5	0
TAKE-OUT					
roe baked w/ butter & lemon juice	1 oz	36	1	–	–

FOOD	PORTION	CALS	FAT	SAT FAT	TRANS FAT
COFFEE (see also COFFEE BEVERAGES, COFFEE SUBSTITUTES)					
INSTANT					
decaffeinated as prep	8 oz	2	0	0	0
decaffeinated powder	1 rounded tsp	4	0	0	0
powder	1 rounded tsp	4	tr	tr	0
REGULAR					
brewed	8 oz	2	tr	tr	0
roasted beans	1 oz	64	4	–	–
Flavia					
English Breakfast	1 bag	0	0	0	0
Espresso Roast	1 bag	0	0	0	0
French Roast	1 bag	0	0	0	0
French Vanilla	1 bag	0	0	0	0
Revival					
Soy Caramal Corn	1 cup (8 oz)	0	0	0	0
Soy Hazelnut	1 cup (8 oz)	0	0	0	0
Soy Original Roast	1 cup (8 oz)	0	0	0	0
Soy Java					
All Flavors	1 tbsp	20	0	0	0
Spava					
Calm Decaffeinated	1 cup	0	0	0	0
COFFEE BEVERAGES					
AchievONE					
All Flavors	1 bottle (9.5 oz)	120	0	–	0
America's Best Brew					
Iced Coffee All Flavors	8 oz	110	2	0	–
Big Train					
Low Carb Blended Ice Mocha as prep	1 serv (16 oz)	90	5	1	–
Cafe Sepia					
House Blend	1 bottle (6.2 oz)	80	0	0	0
Mocha	1 bottle (6.2 oz)	70	0	0	0
Cinnabon					
Latte Caramel Nut	1 can (8 oz)	170	6	3	–
Latte Cinnamon Vanilla	1 can (8 oz)	170	6	3	–
Lattes All Flavors	1 can (9.5 oz)	190	5	–	–
Cool Java					
Cappuccino Dark Roast	1 bottle (11 oz)	190	3	–	–

FOOD	PORTION	CALS	FAT	SAT FAT	TRANS FAT
Cappuccino French Vanilla	1 bottle (11 oz)	190	3	–	0
Cappuccino Mocha	1 bottle (11 oz)	190	3	–	–
Double Bean Elixir					
Coffee Soda All Flavors	8 oz	90	0	0	0
Double Hit					
Maximum Energy Coffee Drink	1 can (12 oz)	80	0	0	0
Flavour Creations					
Coffee Flavoring Tablets All Flavors	1 tablet	0	0	0	0
Frappio					
Iced Coffee Energy Drink	1 can (15 oz)	260	4	4	0
Froid					
Original or French Vanilla	1 bottle (11 oz)	180	3	–	–
General Foods					
International Coffees Cafe Francais	1 serv	60	3	3	0
International Coffees Cafe Vienna	1 serv	70	2	2	0
International Coffees Cafe Vienna Sugar Free	1 serv	30	2	2	0
International Coffees Creme Caramel	1 serv	60	2	2	0
International Coffees French Vanilla Cafe	1 serv	60	3	1	0
International Coffees French Vanilla Sugar & Fat Free Decaffeinated	1 serv	30	3	2	0
International Coffees French Vanilla Sugar Free	1 serv	30	3	2	0
International Coffees Italian Cappuccino	1 serv	50	2	2	0
International Coffees Orange Cappuccino	1 serv	70	2	2	0
International Coffees Suisse Mocha	1 serv	60	2	2	0
International Coffees Suisse Mocha Decaffeinated Sugar Free	1 serv	30	5	2	0
International Coffees Suisse Mocha Sugar Free	1 serv	30	2	2	0

FOOD	PORTION	CALS	FAT	SAT FAT	TRANS FAT
International Coffees Swiss White Chocolate	1 serv	70	3	3	0
International Coffees Vanilla Creme Decaffeinated Sugar Free	1 serv	35	3	2	0
International Coffees Vanilla Creme Decaffeinated	1 serv	60	3	2	0
International Coffees Viennese Chocolate Cafe	1 serv	50	2	2	0
Godiva					
Latte French Vanilla	1 bottle (12 oz)	200	4	3	0
Mocha Dark Chocolate	1 bottle (16 oz)	200	4	3	–
Iced 'Spresso					
Ultra Light American Vanilla	1 bottle (9.5 oz)	90	3	–	–
Ultra Light Espresso Latte	1 bottle (9.5 oz)	70	0	0	0
Jakada					
Latte Mocha	1 bottle (10.5 oz)	180	3.5	0	–
Latte Vanilla	1 bottle (10.5 oz)	180	4	2	–
Loco-Joe					
Iced Coffee	1 box (8.25 oz)	160	4	–	–
Low Carb Creations					
Cappuccino	1 cup	30	2	0	–
Shock					
Latte	8 oz	150	3	2	–
Triple Latte	1 can (8 oz)	125	2	–	–
Triple Mocha	1 can (8 oz)	125	2	–	–
Silk					
Coffee Soylatte	1 bottle (11 oz)	220	5	1	–
Sipper Sweets					
Sugar Free Low Carb Cappuccino	1 serv	50	3	0	–
Starbucks					
DoubleShot	1 (6.5 oz)	140	6	–	–
Frappuccino	1 bottle (9.5 oz)	190	3	2	–
Frappuccino Mocha	1 bottle (9.5 oz)	190	3	2	–
Frappuccino Vanilla	1 bottle (9.5 oz)	190	3	2	–
Stomping Grounds					
Latte Caramel not prep	⅓ cup	70	0	0	0
Latte Espresso not prep	⅓ cup	35	0	0	0

FOOD	PORTION	CALS	FAT	SAT FAT	TRANS FAT
Latte Mocha not prep	⅓ cup	60	0	0	0
Latte Vanilla not prep	⅓ cup	60	0	0	0
Tully's Coffee					
Bellaccino All Flavors	1 bottle (9.5 oz)	210	4	3	0
Wolfgang Puck					
Gourmet Heated Lattes All Flavors	1 can (10 oz)	100	5	3	–
TAKE-OUT					
cafe amaretto w/ alcohol	1 serv	192	9	6	–
cafe au lait	1 cup (8 oz)	77	4	3	–
cafe brulot	1 cup	48	0	0	0
cafe brulot w/ alcohol	1 serv	130	tr	tr	–
cappuccino	1 cup (8 oz)	77	4	3	0
coffee con leche	1 cup (6 oz)	104	4	2	0
espresso	1 cup (4 oz)	2	tr	tr	0
irish coffee	1 serv (8 oz)	209	11	6	0
latte w/ skim milk	1 serv (13 oz)	88	tr	tr	–
latte w/ whole milk	1 serv (14 oz)	143	6	3	0
mocha	1 serv (17 oz)	403	9	5	0
turkish	1 cup (4 oz)	50	1	0	0

COFFEE SUBSTITUTES
Pixie

FOOD	PORTION	CALS	FAT	SAT FAT	TRANS FAT
Mate Latte Chai	½ cup (4 oz)	80	0	0	0
Mate Latte Dark Roast	½ cup (4 oz)	70	0	0	0
Mate Latte Mocha	½ cup (4 oz)	70	0	0	0
Mate Latte Original	½ cup (4 oz)	70	0	0	0
Teeccino					
Herbal Coffee All Flavors	1 cup	15	0	0	0

COFFEE WHITENERS
Coffee-Mate

FOOD	PORTION	CALS	FAT	SAT FAT	TRANS FAT
Half & Half Original	2 tbsp	40	4	3	–
Half & Half Vanilla	2 tbsp	60	4	3	–
Latte Classic	2 tbsp	100	6	5	–
Latte Mocha	2 tbsp	90	4	4	–
Latte Vanilla	2 tbsp	90	4	4	–
Liquid All Flavors	1 tbsp	40	2	0	–
Liquid French Vanilla Fat Free	1 tbsp	10	0	0	0
Liquid Original	1 tbsp	20	1	0	–
Liquid Original Fat Free	1 tbsp	10	0	0	0

FOOD	PORTION	CALS	FAT	SAT FAT	TRANS FAT
Liquid Original Low Fat	1 tbsp	10	1	0	–
Original Powder	1 tsp	10	0	0	0
Original Lite Powder	1 tsp	10	0	0	0
Sugar Free All Flavors	1 tbsp	15	1	0	0
Farmland					
Nondairy Creamer	2 tbsp	40	3	2	–
Hood					
Country Creamer Non Dairy	1 tbsp	20	2	0	0
International Delight					
Amaretto	1 tbsp	40	2	1	0
Fat Free Amaretto	1 tbsp	30	0	0	0
Fat Free French Vanilla	1 tbsp	30	0	0	0
Fat Free Irish Creme	1 tbsp	30	0	0	0
French Vanilla	1 tbsp	45	2	1	0
Sugar Free French Vanilla	1 tbsp	20	2	1	0
Silk					
Creamer	1 tbsp	15	1	0	–
Creamer French Vanilla	1 tbsp	20	1	0	–
Creamer Hazelnut	1 tbsp	15	1	0	–
WildWood					
Soymilk Creamer Plain	1 tbsp	15	2	0	0

COLESLAW
Dole

FOOD	PORTION	CALS	FAT	SAT FAT	TRANS FAT
Classic Cole Slaw	1½ cups (3 oz)	25	0	0	0
Fresh Express					
3 Color Deli	1½ cups	20	0	0	0
Cole Slaw Kit as prep	2 cups	120	8	1	–
River Ranch					
Country Homestyle Kit	1 cup	140	9	2	–
Honey Dijon Peppercorn Kit	1 cup	120	8	1	–
Mix	1¼ cups	25	0	0	0
TAKE-OUT					
coleslaw w/ dressing	¾ cup	147	11	2	–
vinegar & oil coleslaw	3.5 oz	150	9	1	–

COLLARDS

FOOD	PORTION	CALS	FAT	SAT FAT	TRANS FAT
fresh cooked	½ cup	17	tr	–	–
frzn chopped cooked	½ cup	31	tr	–	–
raw chopped	½ cup	6	tr	–	–

FOOD	PORTION	CALS	FAT	SAT FAT	TRANS FAT
Allens					
Seasoned Southern Style	½ cup	35	1	0	–
Glory					
Green Fresh	2 cups	25	0	0	0
Seasoned canned	½ cup	35	0	0	0
Sensibly Seasoned canned	½ cup	20	0	0	0

COOKIES
MIX

FOOD	PORTION	CALS	FAT	SAT FAT	TRANS FAT
chocolate chip	1 (0.56 oz)	79	4	1	–
oatmeal	1 (0.6 oz)	74	3	1	–
oatmeal raisin	1 (0.6 oz)	74	3	1	–
Aunt Paula's					
Low Carb Chef Chocolate Chip as prep	1	66	4	1	–
Low Carb Chef Peanut Butter as prep	1	66	4	1	–
Betty Crocker					
Chocolate Peanut Butter as prep	1 bar	180	9	2	–
Date Bar as prep	1 bar	150	6	2	–
Oatmeal as prep	2	150	6	1	–
Big Train					
Low Carb Chocolate Chip as prep	2	140	9	4	–
Low Carb Peanut Butter as prep	2	140	9	4	–
Bob's Red Mill					
Gluten Free Chocolate Chip as prep	2	260	10	6	0
Keto					
Chocolate Chip as prep	1	47	2	–	–
Oatmeal Raisin as prep	2	59	3	–	–
King Arthur					
Chocolate Chip Whole Grain not prep	2 tbsp	90	3	2	0
MiniCarb					
All Flavors as prep	1	110	2	0	–
Nature's Path					
Organic Chocolate Chip	⅒ pkg	150	2	2	0

FOOD	PORTION	CALS	FAT	SAT FAT	TRANS FAT
Pillsbury					
Ready To Bake Chocolate Chip Sugar Free	1	90	4	1	–
READY-TO-EAT					
animal crackers	1 (2.5 g)	11	tr	tr	–
animal crackers	11 (1 oz)	126	4	1	–
animal crackers	1 box (2.4 oz)	299	9	4	–
australian anzac biscuit	1	98	3	1	–
butter	1 (5 g)	23	1	1	–
chocolate chip	1 (0.4 oz)	48	2	1	–
chocolate chip	1 box (1.9 oz)	233	12	5	–
chocolate chip low fat	1 (0.25 oz)	45	2	tr	–
chocolate chip low sugar low sodium	1 (0.24 oz)	31	1	1	–
chocolate chip soft-type	1 (0.5 oz)	69	4	1	–
chocolate w/ creme filling	1 (0.35 oz)	47	2	tr	–
chocolate w/ creme filling chocolate coated	1 (0.60 oz)	82	5	1	–
chocolate w/ creme filling sugar free low sodium	1 (0.35 oz)	46	2	1	–
chocolate w/ extra creme filling	1 (0.46 oz)	65	3	1	–
chocolate wafer	1 (0.2 oz)	26	1	tr	–
cream cheese	1 (1.1 oz)	141	9	6	–
digestive biscuits plain	2	141	7	–	–
fig bars	1 (0.56 oz)	56	1	tr	–
fortune	1 (0.28 oz)	30	tr	tr	–
fudge	1 (0.73 oz)	73	1	tr	–
gingersnaps	1 (0.24 oz)	29	1	tr	–
graham	1 squares (0.24 oz)	30	1	tr	–
graham chocolate covered	1 (0.49 oz)	68	3	2	–
graham honey	1 (0.24 oz)	30	1	tr	–
hermits	1 (1 oz)	117	5	2	–
jumbles coconut	1 (1 oz)	121	7	5	–
ladyfingers	1 (0.38 oz)	40	1	tr	–
macaroons	1 (0.8 oz)	97	3	3	–
madeleines	1 (0.8 oz)	86	5	3	–
marshmallow chocolate coated	1 (0.46 oz)	55	2	1	–

FOOD	PORTION	CALS	FAT	SAT FAT	TRANS FAT
marshmallow pie chocolate coated	1 (1.4 oz)	165	7	2	–
molasses	1 (0.5 oz)	65	2	tr	–
oatmeal	1 (0.6 oz)	81	3	1	–
oatmeal soft-type	1 (0.5 oz)	61	2	tr	–
oatmeal raisin	1 (0.6 oz)	81	3	1	–
oatmeal raisin low sugar no sodium	1 (0.24 oz)	31	1	1	–
oatmeal raisin soft-type	1 (0.5 oz)	61	2	tr	–
peanut butter sandwich	1 (0.5 oz)	67	3	1	–
peanut butter sandwich sugar free low sodium	1 (0.35 oz)	54	3	1	–
peanut butter soft-type	1 (0.5 oz)	69	4	1	–
pinenut cookies	1 (1.1 oz)	134	9	1	–
raisin soft-type	1 (0.5 oz)	60	2	1	–
reginette queen's biscuit	1 (0.8 oz)	86	3	1	–
shortbread	1 (0.28 oz)	40	2	tr	–
shortbread pecan	1 (0.49 oz)	79	5	1	–
spritz	1 (0.4 oz)	42	2	1	–
sugar	1 (0.52 oz)	72	3	1	–
sugar low sugar sodium free	1 (0.24 oz)	30	1	tr	–
sugar wafers w/ creme filling	1 (0.12 oz)	18	1	tr	–
sugar wafers w/ creme filling sugar free sodium free	1 (0.14 oz)	20	1	tr	–
toll house original	1 (0.8 oz)	105	6	2	–
vanilla sandwich	1 (0.35 oz)	48	2	tr	–
vanilla wafers	1 (0.21 oz)	28	1	tr	–
zeppole	1 (0.8 oz)	78	6	2	–
ABC					
Vegan Colossal Chocolate Chip	1 (2.1 oz)	240	7	3	–
Vegan Double Chocolate Decadence	1 (2.1 oz)	240	8	3	–
Vegan Luscious Lemon Poppyseed	1 (2.1 oz)	240	7	2	–
Vegan Mac The Chip	1 (2.1 oz)	250	10	4	–
Vegan Peanut Butter Chocolate Chip	1 (2.1 oz)	240	8	3	0
Vegan Phenomenal Pumpkin Spice	1 (2.1 oz)	220	7	2	–
Alex & Dani's					
Original Hazelnut	3 (1 oz)	130	6	2	–

FOOD	PORTION	CALS	FAT	SAT FAT	TRANS FAT
Annie's Homegrown					
Bunny Grahams All Flavors	26	130	4	0	0
Archway					
Fruit Filled Apricot	1 (0.8 oz)	90	3	1	–
Fruit Filled Raspberry	1 (0.8 oz)	90	3	1	–
Oatmeal Raisin	1	120	4	1	–
Windmill	1	90	4	1	–
Arico					
Gluten Free Casein Free Almond Cranberry	1 bar (1.4 oz)	140	6	2	0
Gluten Free Casein Free Double Chocolate	1 (0.9 oz)	100	5	2	0
Gluten Free Casein Free Lemon Ginger	1 (0.9 oz)	90	4	1	0
Gluten Free Casein Free Peanut Butter	1 bar (1.4 oz)	160	7	2	0
Arrowroot					
Biscuit	1 (5 g)	20	1	0	–
Back To Nature					
Chocolate Chunk	2	130	6	2	0
Crispy Oatmeal	2	120	5	0	0
Sandwich Chocolate & Mint Creme	2	130	6	2	0
Sandwich Classic Creme	2	130	6	2	0
Bahlsen					
Butter Leaves	7 (1 oz)	140	7	4	–
Delice	6 (1 oz)	140	6	2	–
Hanover Waffelin	5 (1 oz)	160	10	9	–
Nuss Dessert	3 (1.1 oz)	170	11	6	0
Baker's Breakfast Cookie					
Apple Pie	1 (3 oz)	204	2	tr	–
Banana Walnut	1 (3 oz)	274	8	1	–
Chocolate Chunk Raisin	1 (3 oz)	260	5	1	–
Double Chocolate Chunk	1 (3 oz)	250	5	1	–
Fruit & Nut	1 (3 oz)	270	5	1	–
Lemon Poppy Seed	1 (3 oz)	230	3	1	–
Mocha Chocolate Chunk	1 (3 oz)	250	5	1	–
Oatmeal Raisin	1 (3 oz)	250	4	1	–
Peanut Butter	1 (3 oz)	290	8	2	–
Peanut Butter & Jelly	1 (3 oz)	320	9	1	–

FOOD	PORTION	CALS	FAT	SAT FAT	TRANS FAT
Pumpkin Spice	1 (3 oz)	230	3	1	–
Vegan Chocolate Chunk	1 (3 oz)	260	6	2	–
Vegan Peanut Butter Chocolate Chunk	1 (3 oz)	310	10	2	–
Barnum's					
Animal Crackers	10 (1 oz)	120	4	1	0
Bolands					
Custard Creams	1	62	3	2	–
Cameo					
Sandwich Creme	2 (1 oz)	130	5	1	–
Carbolite					
Chocolate Chip	1 (1 oz)	120	9	2	–
Peanut Butter	1 (1 oz)	120	9	2	–
Shortbread	1 (1 oz)	180	9	2	–
Chips Ahoy!					
Chocolate Chip	1 pkg (1.4 oz)	190	9	3	–
Reduced Fat	1 pkg (1.1 oz)	140	5	2	–
Country Choice Naturals					
Chocolate Chip Walnut	1	100	4	1	–
Double Fudge Brownie	1 (0.8 oz)	90	3	1	–
Ginger	1	90	2	0	–
Ginger Snaps	5	120	5	0	–
Lemon	1	90	3	0	–
Oatmeal Chocolate Chip	1 (0.8 oz)	100	4	1	–
Oatmeal Raisin	1 (0.8 oz)	100	3	1	–
Old Fashioned Oatmeal	1 (0.8 oz)	100	3	0	–
Peanut Butter	1	100	5	1	–
Sandwich Cremes Chocolate	1	130	5	1	–
Sandwich Cremes Duplex	2	130	5	1	–
Sandwich Cremes Ginger Lemon	2	130	5	1	–
Sandwich Cremes Mint Creme	2	130	5	1	–
Sandwich Cremes Vanilla	2	130	5	1	–
Vanilla Wafers	7	120	5	0	–
Crummy					
Organic Chocolate Chip	1 (2 oz)	240	10	6	0
Organic Lavender Chocolate Chip	1 (2 oz)	240	10	6	0
Dare					
Breaktime Coconut	4	140	5	3	0

FOOD	PORTION	CALS	FAT	SAT FAT	TRANS FAT
Breaktime Ginger	4	130	4	1	0
Creme Chocolate Fudge	1	100	5	3	0
Maple Leaf Creme	1	80	4	1	0
Whipper	2	130	5	3	0
David's					
Hamantash Raspberry	1 (0.7 oz)	85	6	3	–
De Beukelaer					
Pirouline	8 (1 oz)	130	4	3	–
DiCamillo					
Biscotti DiPrato	5 (1 oz)	130	4	0	0
Doritos					
Barras De Coco	5	120	4	1	1
Dove					
Beyond Chocolate Chunk	1 (0.7 oz)	110	5	3	0
Chocolate Walnut Rendezvous	1 (0.7 oz)	110	6	3	0
Milk Chocolate Moment	3 (1.1 oz)	160	9	5	0
Mint Chocolate Serenade	3 (1.1 oz)	160	8	5	0
Dunkaroos					
Chocolate Graham	1 pkg	120	5	1	–
Cinnamon Graham	1 pkg	130	5	2	–
Honey Graham	1 pkg	120	5	1	–
Earthbound Farm					
Organic Ginger Snaps	2	120	6	4	0
Elite					
Tea Biscuits Chocolate	4	80	2	1	–
English Bay					
Strawberry Fruit Bar	1 (1.2 oz)	120	3	1	–
Enjoy Life					
Allergen Gluten Free Gingerbread Spice	2 (1 oz)	100	4	0	0
Allergen Gluten Free No Oats Oatmeal	2 (1 oz)	120	4	0	0
Allergen Gluten Free Snickerdoodle	2 (1 oz)	130	5	0	0
Snack Bar Sunbutter Crunch	1 (1 oz)	140	5	1	0
Entenmann's					
Original Chocolate Chip	3	140	7	3	0
Soft Baked Chocolate Chunk	1 (1.3 oz)	190	9	5	0
Estee					
Fructose Sweetened Chocolate Chip	4	160	8	2	–

FOOD	PORTION	CALS	FAT	SAT FAT	TRANS FAT
Fructose Sweetened Lemon	4	160	6	2	–
Fructose Sweetened Sandwich Chocolate	3	170	6	2	–
Fructose Sweetened Sandwich Original	3	170	6	2	–
Fructose Sweetened Sandwich Peanut Butter	3	190	8	2	–
Fructose Sweetened Vanilla	4	160	7	2	–
Fructose Sweetened Vanilla Sandwich	3	170	6	2	–
Sugar Free Chocolate Chip	3	110	4	1	–
Sugar Free Lemon	3	110	3	0	–
Sugar Free Wafer Chocolate Creme	4	150	8	2	–
Sugar Free Wafer Lemon Creme	4	150	9	2	–
Sugar Free Wafer Peanut Butter Creme	4	150	9	3	–
Sugar Free Wafer Strawberry Creme	4	150	9	2	–
Sugar Free Wafer Vanilla Creme	4	150	9	2	–
Fauchon					
Assorted Chocolate	4 (2 oz)	330	15	10	0
Fox's					
Golden Crunch Creams	1	75	4	2	–
French Meadow Bakery					
Gluten Free Chocolate Chip	1 (1.3 oz)	190	10	2	0
Frieda's					
Asian Almond	2 (1 oz)	170	10	3	–
Gak's Snacks					
Organic Brownie Chip	1 (1 oz)	130	5	1	0
Organic Chocolate Chip	1 (1 oz)	140	6	1	0
Organic Oatmeal	1 (1 oz)	120	4	0	0
Gamesa					
Animalitos	14	110	1	0	0
Arcoiris Marshmallow	2	120	5	4	0
Arcoiris Merengue	6	200	3	3	1
Emperador Chocolate	2	120	4	1	1
Emperador Fresa	2	120	4	1	1

FOOD	PORTION	CALS	FAT	SAT FAT	TRANS FAT
Emperador Limon	6	270	8	2	3
Emperador Vanilla	2	120	4	1	1
Hawaianas	3	130	4	1	–
Marias	8	120	2	0	0
Ricanelas	8	140	4	1	1
Roscas	3	130	4	1	1
Sugar Wafers Chocolate	3	160	7	2	2
Sugar Wafers Strawberry	3	160	6	1	2
Sugar Wafers Vanilla	3	160	7	2	2
Ginger Snaps					
Cookies	4 (1 oz)	120	3	0	–
Girl Scout					
Cafe Cookies	5	150	7	2	2
Lemon Cooler Reduced Fat	5	130	4	2	0
Samoas	2	150	8	5	1
Tagalongs	2	130	9	5	0
Thin Mints	4	140	7	4	1
Trefoils	4	130	6	2	2
Gluten-Free Pantry					
Gluten Free Buckwheat Raisin	1 (1 oz)	140	6	3	0
Gluten Free Chocolate Chunk	1 (1 oz)	140	8	4	0
Glutino					
Gluten Free Wafers Chocolate	4	160	8	5	0
Gluten Free Wafers Lemon	3	150	6	4	0
Godiva					
Biscotti Dipped In Milk Chocolate	1 (0.9 oz)	120	6	3	–
Gol D Lite					
Low Carb Pizzelle	1 (0.3 oz)	46	2	0	–
Golightly					
Fabulous Tastes Caramel Dulce De Leche	4	100	6	4	–
Goody Man					
Marshmallow Crispy Squares	1 (1.17 oz)	130	3	1	–
Gottena					
Exquisit	5	170	10	9	0
Gourmet Pastries					
Kourabiethes Butter Almond	1 (1.1 oz)	150	9	5	0
Phoenicia Honey & Spice	1 (1.3 oz)	140	5	2	0

FOOD	PORTION	CALS	FAT	SAT FAT	TRANS FAT
Grandma's					
Homestyle Big Chocolate Chip	1 (1.4 oz)	190	9	3	2
Homestyle Big Fudge Chocolate Chip	1 (1.4 oz)	170	7	2	1
Homestyle Big Oatmeal Raisin	1 (1.4 oz)	180	6	2	–
Homestyle Big Peanut Butter	1 (1.4 oz)	200	10	3	–
Mini Vanilla Creme	9	150	7	2	–
Peanut Butter Sandwich	5	210	10	3	2
Rich N'Chewy Chocolate Chip	1 pkg	270	12	4	2
Vanilla Creme Sandwich	5	210	10	3	0
Granny Oats					
Low Carb Oatmeal	4	98	6	4	–
Healthy Handfuls					
Organic Crocodile Cookies	1 pkg (1 oz)	130	5	0	0
Organic Koala Krackers	1 pkg (1 oz)	120	4	2	0
Heavenly					
Meringues All Flavors Sugar Free Fat Free	1	0	0	0	0
Honey Maid					
Grahams Honey	1 (1.1 oz)	130	4	1	0
Grahams Honey Low Fat	1 (1.1 oz)	120	2	0	0
Jacob's					
Oat Crumbles Chocolate & Pecan	1	107	6	3	–
Jacques Gourmet					
Palmier Cinnamon	3 (1 oz)	140	9	4	–
Palmier Vanilla	3 (1 oz)	140	9	4	–
Joseph's					
Almond Sugar Free	4	100	5	1	0
Chocolate Chip Sugar Free	4	95	5	1	0
Lemon Sugar Free	4	95	4	1	0
Oatmeal Chocolate Chip w/ Pecans Sugar Free	4	100	6	1	0
Peanut Butter Sugar Free	4	95	5	1	0
Karen's					
Fabulous Tastes Heavenly Chocolate Chip	4	90	5	4	–
Fabulous Tastes Luscious Raspberry Almond	4	110	6	2	–

FOOD	PORTION	CALS	FAT	SAT FAT	TRANS FAT
Fabulous Tastes Pecan Vanilla Pralines	4	120	8	3	–
Kashi					
TLC Happy Trail Mix	1 (1 oz)	130	5	1	0
TLC Oatmeal Raisin Flax	1 (1 oz)	130	5	1	0
TLC Oatmeal Dark Chocolate	1 (1 oz)	130	5	2	0
Kedem					
Tea Biscuits Chocolate	2	32	1	tr	–
Tea Biscuits Orange	2	32	1	tr	–
Keebler					
100 Calorie Pack Sandies Shortbread	1 pkg	100	3	1	0
Chips Deluxe	1 (0.5 oz)	80	5	2	–
Chocolate Dip & Cookie Sticks	1 pkg (1 oz)	130	6	2	–
Graham Honey	8 (1.1 oz)	140	4	1	–
Sandies Fruit Delights Lemon	1 (0.6 oz)	80	4	1	–
Sandies Fudge Drops	4 (1 oz)	140	7	4	0
S'mores Snack	1 pkg (0.8 oz)	110	6	3	–
Soft Batch Chocolate Chip	1 (0.6 oz)	80	4	1	–
Keto					
Low Carb Biscotti Chocolate	1 (1.2 oz)	157	9	9	–
Low Carb Biscotti Lemon Nut	1 (1.2 oz)	157	9	4	–
Low Carb Biscotti Vanilla Almond	1 (1.2 oz)	157	9	9	–
La Dolce Vita					
Biscotti Chocolate Passion	1 (1.2 oz)	130	8	5	–
Landies Candies					
Sugar Free Dark Royal Pecan Shortbread	2	167	9	4	–
Sugar Free Milk Chocolate Chip	2	173	11	5	–
Sugar Free Milk Chocolate Peanut Butter	2	171	8	5	–
Sugar Free White Chocolate Lemon	2	177	11	8	–
Laura's Wholesome Junk Food					
Anna Banana Split	1	105	5	2	–
Gluten Free Charlotte's Chocolate Chip	2	120	6	2	0
Gluten Free Sally's Raisin	2	110	5	1	0

FOOD	PORTION	CALS	FAT	SAT FAT	TRANS FAT
Lemon Vanilla	2	120	6	1	0
Oatmeal Chocolate Chip	2	110	5	2	–
Oatmeal Raisin	2	100	4	1	–
Wheat Free X-Treme Chocolate Fudge	2	110	5	2	–
Lee's					
Dreamy Mallows	2	150	5	4	0
Leibniz					
Butter Biscuits	6	130	3	2	0
Little Debbie					
Apple Flips	1 (1.2 oz)	150	5	2	–
Marshmallow Crispy Bar	1 (1.3 oz)	140	4	1	–
Liz Lovely					
Vegan Cowboy	½ cookie (1.3 oz)	190	9	2	0
Vegan Cowgirl	½ cookie (1.5 oz)	210	9	2	0
Vegan Ginger Snapdragons	½ cookie (1.5 oz)	190	7	0	0
Lorna Doone					
Shortbread	4 (1 oz)	140	7	2	0
Low Carb Creations					
Chocolate Chip	1 (1 oz)	140	10	4	–
Coconut	1 (1 oz)	140	10	5	–
Lemon	1 (1 oz)	140	11	5	–
Snickerdoodle	1 (1 oz)	140	11	4	–
LU					
Le Bastogne	2 (0.8 oz)	120	5	3	–
Le Chocolatier	3 (1 oz)	150	9	7	0
Le Fondant	4 (1.1 oz)	170	10	9	–
Le Petit Beurre	4 (1.2 oz)	140	4	3	0
Le Petit Ecolier Dark Chocolate	2 (0.9 oz)	130	6	4	–
Le Petit Ecolier Extra Dark Chocolate	2	120	7	4	–
Le Petit Ecolier Milk Chocolate	2 (0.9 oz)	130	6	4	0
Le Petit Fruit Strawberry	5 (1.2 oz)	110	1	0	–
Pim's Orange	2 (0.9 oz)	90	3	2	–
Pim's Sensation Bar Chocolate	1	110	6	3	–
Pim's Sensation Bar Hazelnut	1	110	6	3	–
Shortbread	2	140	8	5	1
Mallomars					
Cookies	2	120	5	3	0

FOOD	PORTION	CALS	FAT	SAT FAT	TRANS FAT
Mamma Says'					
Biscotti Almond Pistachio	1 (0.5 oz)	50	3	1	–
Biscotti Chocolate Macadamia	1 (0.5 oz)	45	3	1	–
Biscotti Orange Citrine	1 (0.5 oz)	60	2	1	–
Mauna Loa					
Macadamia Nut Chocolate Chip	2	130	6	1	–
Macadamia Nut Hawaiian Crunch	2	150	8	2	–
Macadamia Nut White Chocolate Chip	2	130	6	1	–
Miss Meringue					
Chocolettes Crunchy Chocolate	4	110	10	0	–
Chocolettes Strawberry Vanilla	4	130	4	2	–
Classiques Cappuccino	4	110	0	0	0
Classiques Chocolate Chip	4	120	2	1	–
Classiques Dulce De Leche Artisan	4	110	0	0	0
Macaroons Traditional	1 (1.3 oz)	180	10	9	–
Madeleines Traditional	2 (1.2 oz)	160	9	5	–
Minis Vanilla	13 (1.1 oz)	110	0	0	0
Minis Vanilla Sugar Free	13	35	0	0	0
MoonPie					
Chocolate	1 (2.75 oz)	330	10	6	–
Murray's					
Sugar Free Chocolate Chip	3 (1.1 oz)	160	9	4	0
Sugar Free Chocolate Sandwich	3 (1 oz)	130	7	3	0
Sugar Free Fudge Dipped Grahams	4 (1 oz)	150	8	6	0
Sugar Free Ginger Snap	7 (1.1 oz)	130	5	2	0
Sugar Free Oatmeal	3 (1.1 oz)	140	7	3	0
Sugar Free Shortbread	8 (1 oz)	130	5	2	0
Nabisco					
100 Calorie Barnmus's Animal Choco	1 pkg	100	3	0	0
100 Calorie Pack Alpha-Bits Mini	1 pkg	100	3	2	0

FOOD	PORTION	CALS	FAT	SAT FAT	TRANS FAT
100 Calorie Pack Lorna Doone	1 pkg	100	3	2	0
100 Calorie Pack Teddy Grahams Mini Cinnamon	1 pkg	100	3	0	0
Biscos Sugar Wafers	8 (1 oz)	140	6	3	0
Chips Ahoy! Mini	1 pkg (1.2 oz)	170	8	3	0
Nutter Butter Bites	1 pkg (1.2 oz)	170	7	2	0
Oreo Mini	1 pkg (1.2 oz)	160	7	2	0
Social Tea	6	140	4	1	0
Nana's					
No Gluten Berry Vanilla	1 bar (1.2 oz)	130	4	0	0
No Gluten Chocolate	1 (3.5 oz)	360	12	0	0
No Gluten Ginger	1 (3.5 oz)	360	10	0	0
No Gluten Nana Banana	1 bar (1.2 oz)	130	5	0	0
No Wheat Oatmeal Raisin	1 (3.5 oz)	280	10	0	0
Vegan Chocolate Chip	1 (4 oz)	320	14	2	0
Vegan Peanut Butter	1 (4 oz)	360	16	1	0
Vegan Sunflower	1 (3.5 oz)	380	14	2	0
Natural Ovens					
Carob Chip	1	90	4	0	–
Chocolate Raspberry	1	120	5	2	–
Oatmeal Raisin	1	90	3	0	–
Nature's Path					
Organic Animal Vanilla	9	120	4	2	0
Organic Signature Lemon Poppyseed	4	130	4	2	0
New York Style					
Biscotti Almond	3 (1 oz)	130	5	1	0
Newman's Own					
Organic Champion Chip Chocolate Chip	4	160	7	3	–
Organic Champion Chip Chocolate Chocolate Chip	4	160	8	4	–
Organic Champion Chip Double Chocolate Mint Chip	4	160	8	4	–
Organic Champion Chip Espresso Chocolate Chip	4	150	7	3	–
Organic Champion Chip Orange Chocolate Chip	4	160	7	3	–
Organic Champion Chip Wheat Free Dairy Free	4	160	8	4	–

FOOD	PORTION	CALS	FAT	SAT FAT	TRANS FAT
Organic Fig Newmans Fat Free	2	120	0	0	0
Organic Fig Newmans Low Fat	2	140	2	1	–
Organic Fig Newmans Wheat Free Dairy Free	2	120	2	0	–
Organic Newman-O's Chocolate Creme	2	130	5	2	–
Organic Newman-O's Ginger-O's	2	120	5	2	–
Organic Newman-O's Mint Creme	2	130	5	2	–
Organic Newman-O's Original	2	130	5	2	–
Organic Newman-O's Tops & Bottoms	6	120	3	0	–
Organic Newman-O's Wheat Free Dairy Free	2	130	5	2	–
Newtons					
Fig	2 (1.1 oz)	110	2	0	0
Fig 100% Whole Grain	2 (1.3 oz)	130	3	1	0
Fig Fat Free	2 (1 oz)	90	0	0	0
Raspberry	2 (1 oz)	100	2	0	0
Nilla Wafers					
Cookies	1 oz	140	6	2	0
Reduced Fat	1 oz	110	2	0	–
Nonni's					
Biscotti Decadence	1 (1.1 oz)	130	5	3	–
Biscotti Original	1 (1 oz)	100	4	2	–
NutraBalance					
High Fibre	1 (0.7 oz)	90	4	1	–
Nutter Butter					
Sandwich Cookie	1 (1 oz)	130	6	1	–
Oreo					
Cakesters	2 (2 oz)	250	12	3	0
Oreo Double Stuff	1 (1 oz)	140	7	3	0
Sandwich Cookie	2 (1.2 oz)	160	7	2	0
Pepperidge Farm					
Chantilly Raspberry	2	120	3	2	0
Chessmen	3 (0.9 oz)	120	5	3	0
Dark Chocolate Mint Chocolate Chunk	1	140	7	4	0
Gingerman	4	130	4	2	0

FOOD	PORTION	CALS	FAT	SAT FAT	TRANS FAT
Medallion Milk Chocolate	5	160	8	5	0
Milano	3	180	10	5	0
Milano French Vanilla	2	130	5	5	0
Milano Mint Chocolate Covered	4	130	6	3	0
Milano Sugar Free	3	170	9	4	0
Nantucket Chocolate Dipped	1	150	8	4	0
Nantucket Dark Chocolate Chunk	1	140	7	4	0
Pirouettes Cappuccino	2	120	5	3	0
Pirouettes Chocolate Mint	2	120	5	3	0
Sausalito Milk Chocolate Macadamia Nut	1	140	8	4	0
Shortbread	2	140	7	4	0
Soft Baked Milk Chocolate	1	150	7	3	0
Soft Baked Oatmeal Cranberry	1	130	4	2	0
Soft Baked Sugar	1	140	5	3	0
Tahiti	2	170	10	6	0
Verona Apricot Raspberry	3	140	5	3	0
Pure De-Lite					
High Protein Chocolate Fudge	1 (2.2 oz)	210	8	2	–
High Protein Peanut Butter Crunch	1 (2.2 oz)	210	8	2	–
Quaker					
Breakfast Cookie Oatmeal Raisin	1	180	5	2	0
Right Direction					
Chocolate Chip	1	60	6	3	0
SnackWell's					
Cookie Cakes Chocolate Mint	1 (0.6 oz)	50	1	0	–
Creme Sandwich	1 pkg (1.7 oz)	210	5	2	0
Devil's Food Fat Free	1 (0.5 oz)	50	0	0	0
Sugar Free Lemon Creme	2 (1.1 oz)	130	6	2	0
Sugar Free Shortbread	2 (1 oz)	130	6	2	0
South Beach					
Wafer Sticke Dark Chocolate Hazelnut Creme	1 pkg	100	6	3	0
Wafer Sticke Dark Chocolate Peanut Butter	1 pkg	100	6	3	0

FOOD	PORTION	CALS	FAT	SAT FAT	TRANS FAT
Soybite					
All Flavors	1	79	5	1	–
Stella D'Oro					
Almond Delight	1 (1 oz)	150	8	4	0
Angelica Goodies	1 (0.7 oz)	90	3	1	0
Anginetti	4 (1.1 oz)	130	3	1	0
Biscotti Almond	1 (0.7 oz)	90	4	2	0
Biscotti French Vanilla	1 (0.7 oz)	90	3	2	0
Breakfast Treats Chocolate	1 (0.9 oz)	110	4	2	0
Breakfast Treats Original	1 (0.7 oz)	90	3	2	0
Coffee Treats Almond Toast	2 (0.9)	100	2	0	0
Coffee Treats Angel Wings	3 (1 oz)	160	10	5	0
Coffee Treats Anisette Sponge	2 (0.9 oz)	90	1	0	0
Coffee Treats Anisette Toast	3 (1.2 oz)	130	1	0	0
Coffee Treats Roman Egg Biscuits	1 (1.1 oz)	130	5	2	0
Egg Jumbo	3 (1.2 oz)	120	2	0	0
Lady Stella	3 (1 oz)	130	5	3	0
Margherite	2 (1 oz)	130	5	2	0
Swiss Fudge	3 (1.2 oz)	170	9	5	0
Super Chip					
Chocolate Chip	2 (0.9 oz)	100	7	–	–
Teddy Grahams					
Chocolate	24 (1.1 oz)	130	5	1	0
Honey	24 (1 oz)	130	4	1	0
Temptations					
Chocolate Alps	1 bar (1.6 oz)	170	7	0	0
Chocolate Mocha	1 bar (1.6 oz)	170	6	5	0
No Gluten Chocolate Rush	1 bar (1.6 oz)	170	9	7	0
Tree Of Life					
Wheat Free Carob	1 (0.8 oz)	100	5	0	–
Zwieback					
Toast	1 (8 g)	35	1	0	–
REFRIGERATED					
chocolate chip	1 (0.42 oz)	59	3	1	–
chocolate chip unbaked	1 oz	126	6	2	–
oatmeal	1 (0.4 oz)	56	3	1	–
oatmeal raisin	1 (0.4 oz)	56	3	1	–
peanut butter	1 (0.4 oz)	60	3	1	–
peanut butter dough	1 oz	130	7	2	–

FOOD	PORTION	CALS	FAT	SAT FAT	TRANS FAT
sugar	1 (0.42 oz)	58	3	1	–
sugar dough	1 oz	124	6	2	–
TAKE-OUT					
biscotti w/ nuts chocolate dipped	1 (1.3 oz)	117	6	3	–
black & white	1 lg (3 oz)	302	9	5	–
finikia	1 (1.2 oz)	171	5	5	–
koulourakia butter cookie twist	1 (0.9 oz)	113	6	3	–
linzer tart	1 (2.4 oz)	280	14	4	–

CORIANDER

FOOD	PORTION	CALS	FAT	SAT FAT	TRANS FAT
cilantro fresh	1 tsp (2 g)	tr	tr	0	–
leaf dried	1 tsp	2	tr	tr	0
leaf fresh	¼ cup	1	tr	–	–
seed	1 tsp	5	tr	tr	0

CORN
CANNED

FOOD	PORTION	CALS	FAT	SAT FAT	TRANS FAT
cream style	½ cup	93	1	tr	–
w/ red & green peppers	½ cup	86	1	tr	–
white	½ cup	66	1	tr	–
yellow	½ cup	66	1	tr	–
Del Monte					
Cream Style	½ cup	60	1	0	–
Cream Style No Salt Added	½ cup	60	1	0	0
Fiesta	½ cup	50	1	0	–
Gold & White	½ cup	80	1	0	0
Savory Sides In Butter Sauce	½ cup	90	3	1	0
Savory Sides Santa Fe	½ cup	70	1	0	0
Summer Crisp	½ cup	70	1	0	–
White	½ cup	60	1	0	–
Green Giant					
Mexicorn	⅓ cup	70	1	0	0
Super Sweet Yellow & White	⅓ cup	60	1	0	0
S&W					
Cream Style	½ cup (4.4 oz)	60	1	0	–
Whole Kernel	⅓ cup (3 oz)	70	2	0	–
FRESH					
white cooked	½ cup	89	1	tr	–
white raw	½ cup	66	1	tr	–
yellow cooked	1 ear (2.7 oz)	83	1	tr	–

FOOD	PORTION	CALS	FAT	SAT FAT	TRANS FAT
yellow cooked	½ cup	89	1	tr	–
yellow raw	1 ear (3 oz)	77	1	tr	–
yellow raw	½ cup	66	1	tr	–
FROZEN					
cooked	½ cup	67	tr	tr	–
on the cob cooked	1 ear (2.2 oz)	59	tr	tr	–
Birds Eye					
Steamfresh Southwestern	⅔ cup	90	2	0	0
Steamfresh Super Sweet	⅔ cup	70	1	0	0
Steamfresh Sweet Mini Corn On The Cob	1	90	1	0	0
C&W					
Cheddar Bacon	½ cup	130	5	2	0
Early Harvest Supersweet Petite	⅔ cup	70	1	0	0
Salsa Corn	1 cup	90	1	0	0
Europe's Best					
Baby Sweet	⅔ cup	50	1	0	0
Fresh Like					
Cut	3.5 oz	85	1	–	–
On The Cob	1 ear (3 in)	96	1	–	–
Glory					
Savory Accents Fried Corn	½ cup	110	2	1	0
Green Giant					
Cream Style	½ cup	110	1	0	0
Nibblers On-The-Cob	1 (2.1 oz)	70	1	0	0
Niblets & Butter Sauce Low Fat	⅔ cup	110	2	1	0
Pictsweet					
Cut Corn	⅔ cup	100	1	0	–
Roast Works					
Flame Roasted Cob Corn	1 cob (3 oz)	130	1	0	0
Stouffer's					
Souffle	½ pkg (6 oz)	150	5	1	0
TAKE-OUT					
fritters	1 (1 oz)	62	2	tr	–
on the cob w/ butter cooked	1 ear	155	3	2	–
scalloped	1 cup	257	11	3	0

CORN CHIPS (see CHIPS)

CORNISH HEN (see CHICKEN)

FOOD	PORTION	CALS	FAT	SAT FAT	TRANS FAT
CORNMEAL					
cornmeal mush as prep w/ water	1 cup	223	1	tr	0
cornmeal yellow	1 cup	505	2	tr	0
harina de maize con leche	1 cup	295	7	4	0
Expert Foods					
Low Carb Grits Mix	1½ tsp	15	0	0	0
Indian Head					
Stone Ground	¼ cup	100	1	–	0
McKenzie's					
Hush Puppies	1 serv (1.9 oz)	190	10	3	–
Quaker					
Old Fashioned Grits not prep	¼ cup	140	1	–	–
Quick Grits not prep	¼ cup	130	1	–	0
Yellow	3 tbsp (1 oz)	90	1	–	–
TAKE-OUT					
corn pone	1 piece (2.1 oz)	128	3	1	0
fritter puerto rican style	1 (1.4 oz)	109	7	2	0
harina de maiz con coco	½ cup	383	27	24	0
hush puppies	1 (0.8 oz)	74	3	tr	0
johnnycake	1 piece (1.7 oz)	134	4	1	0
CORNSTARCH					
cornstarch	1 cup (4.5 oz)	488	tr	tr	–
Argo					
Cornstarch	1 tbsp	30	0	0	0
Bob's Red Mill					
Cornstarch	1 tbsp	30	0	0	0
Kingsford's					
Cornstarch	1 tbsp	30	0	0	0
COTTAGE CHEESE					
creamed	1 cup (7.4 oz)	217	9	6	–
creamed	4 oz	117	5	3	–
creamed w/ fruit	4 oz	140	4	2	–
dry curd	1 cup (5.1 oz)	123	1	tr	–
dry curd	4 oz	96	tr	tr	–
lowfat 1%	1 cup (7.9 oz)	164	2	1	–
lowfat 1%	4 oz	82	1	1	–
lowfat 2%	1 cup (7.9 oz)	203	4	3	–
lowfat 2%	4 oz	101	2	1	–

FOOD	PORTION	CALS	FAT	SAT FAT	TRANS FAT
Breakstone's					
Fat Free	½ cup	80	0	0	0
LiveActive	1 pkg (4 oz)	90	2	2	0
LiveActive Mixed Berries	1 pkg (4 oz)	120	2	1	0
Cabot					
Cottage Cheese	½ cup	100	5	3	–
No Fat	½ cup	70	0	0	0
Hood					
4% Fat w/ Pineapple	½ cup	130	4	2	0
Fat Free	½ cup	80	0	0	0
Low Fat	½ cup	90	1	1	0
Low Fat No Salt Added	½ cup	90	1	1	0
Low Fat w/ Peaches	½ cup	110	1	1	0
Horizon Organic					
Lowfat	½ cup	100	3	2	0
Regular	½ cup	120	5	3	0
Knudsen					
LiveActive Pineapple	1 pkg (4 oz)	110	2	1	0
Kraft					
LiveActive 1% Milk Cheddar Cubes	7 (1 oz)	90	6	4	0
Light N'Lively					
Lowfat	½ cup	80	2	1	0
Organic Valley					
Low Fat	½ cup	100	2	2	0
COTTONSEED					
kernels roasted	1 tbsp	51	4	1	–
COUSCOUS					
cooked	1 cup (5.5 oz)	176	tr	tr	–
dry	1 cup (6.1 oz)	650	1	tr	–
Hodgson Mill					
Whole Wheat not prep	⅓ cup	210	1	0	–
Marrakesh Express					
Mango Salsa as prep	1 cup	190	0	0	0
Mushroom as prep	1 cup	190	1	0	–
Plain as prep	1 cup	270	0	0	0
Near East					
Broccoli & Cheese as prep	1 cup	230	3	2	–
Curry as prep	1 cup	220	4	tr	–

FOOD	PORTION	CALS	FAT	SAT FAT	TRANS FAT
Herbed Chicken as prep	1 cup	220	3	tr	–
Original as prep	1 cup	230	5	0	–
Parmesan as prep	1 cup	220	5	2	–
Roasted Garlic Olive Oil as prep	1 cup	230	5	1	–
Toasted Pine Nut as prep	1 cup	230	6	1	–
Tomato Lentil as prep	1 cup	220	3	tr	–
Wild Mushroom Herb as prep	1 cup	230	4	2	–
Rice Select					
All Varieties not prep	¼ cup	150	0	0	0

CRAB
CANNED
blue	½ cup	67	1	tr	–
blue drained	1 can (6.5 oz)	124	2	tr	–
Ace Of Diamonds					
Fancy w/ Leg Meat	¼ cup (2 oz)	40	0	0	0
Brunswick					
Crabmeat 15% Leg	2 oz	40	1	0	–
Fancy Lump	2 oz	45	1	0	–
Bumble Bee					
Lump	¼ cup	40	1	0	–
Pink	¼ cup	35	1	0	–
White	¼ cup	40	1	0	0
Chicken Of The Sea					
Fancy	½ can (2 oz)	40	0	0	0
Lump	½ can (2 oz)	35	1	–	–
Madam					
Crab Meat	½ cup	40	1	0	–
Terry's					
Crabmeat	¼ cup	40	0	0	0
FRESH					
alaska king meat only steamed	3 oz	82	1	tr	–
blue cooked flaked	1 cup (4 oz)	120	2	tr	–
dungeness steamed	3 oz	94	1	tr	–
queen steamed	3 oz	98	1	tr	–
FROZEN					
Margaritaville					
Coral Reef Cakes + Sauce	1	200	10	2	–

FOOD	PORTION	CALS	FAT	SAT FAT	TRANS FAT
Mrs. Paul's					
Deviled Crab Cakes	1 (3 oz)	220	12	2	0
Phillips Seafood					
Carb Cakes	1 (3 oz)	160	10	2	0
Crab Meat Stuffing	1 serv (3.5 oz)	170	4	2	0
Mini Cakes	4	160	10	2	0
Slammers	2	150	9	4	0
TAKE-OUT					
alaska king leg steamed	1 leg (4.7 oz)	130	2	tr	–
baked	1 (3.8 oz)	160	2	tr	–
cakes	2 (4.2 oz)	186	9	2	–
crab imperial	1 crab (6.8 oz)	289	15	3	–
crab salad	1 serv (5.5 oz)	285	21	3	–
crab thermidor	1 serv (6.4 oz)	456	37	22	–
deviled	1 serv (4.5 oz)	254	13	3	–
dungeness steamed	1 crab (4.5 oz)	140	2	tr	–
empanada de jueyes	1 (4.4 oz)	341	16	4	–
fried crab puffs	4 (3.2 oz)	323	18	10	–
kenagi korean crab cooked	1 serv (3 oz)	71	tr	–	–
salmorejo de jueyes (in tomato sauce)	1 serv (4.5 oz)	215	14	2	–
soft-shell breaded & fried	1 med (2.3 oz)	216	13	3	–
taco de jueyes	1 (4.2 oz)	266	14	5	–
CRACKER CRUMBS					
cracker meal	1 cup	440	2	tr	0
graham cracker crumbs	1 cup	355	8	1	0
Kellogg's					
Corn Flake Crumbs	6 tbsp (1.2 oz)	120	0	0	0
CRACKERS					
melba toast round	1	12	tr	tr	0
oyster cracker	¼ cup	48	1	tr	0
saltines	1	13	tr	tr	0
water biscuits	3	92	3	–	–
zwieback	1 oz	107	1	–	–
American Vintage					
Wine Biscuits All Flavors	5	140	7	1	–
Andre's					
CarboSave Crackerbread All Flavors	1 oz	140	8	1	–

FOOD	PORTION	CALS	FAT	SAT FAT	TRANS FAT
Annie's Homegrown					
Cheddar Bunnies BBQ	50	130	6	1	0
Cheddar Bunnies Original	50	150	7	1	–
Cheddar Bunnies Ranch	50	130	6	1	0
Cheddar Bunnies Whole Wheat	50	130	6	1	0
Back To Nature					
Classic Rounds	5	70	2	0	0
Crispy Wheats	17	130	4	0	0
Rice Thin Sesame Ginger	16	120	3	0	0
Rice Thin White Cheddar	16	120	3	0	0
Better Cheddars					
Original	1.1 oz	160	8	2	0
Blue Diamond					
Nut-Thins Almond	16	130	3	0	0
Nut-Thins Hazelnut	16	130	3	0	0
Nut-Thins Pecan	16	130	4	0	0
Bran-A-Crisp					
Low Carb Wheat Bran	1	20	0	0	0
Bremner Wafers					
Cracked Wheat	7	70	2	0	0
Low Sodium	7	70	2	0	0
Original	7	70	2	0	0
Brown Rice Snaps					
Cheddar	6	60	1	0	0
Original Tamari Seaweed	9	60	0	0	0
Unsalted Plain	8	60	0	0	0
Cheese Nips					
Cheddar	1 pkg (1.2 oz)	170	7	2	–
Cheeters					
Low Carb All Flavors	1 pkg (1 oz)	104	8	1	–
Cheetos					
Cheddar	1 pkg	240	14	4	–
Chicken Biskit					
Original	1.1 oz	160	8	2	0
Dare					
Breton Minis	13	80	4	2	0
Breton Multigrain	3 (0.5 oz)	80	4	2	0
Breton Original	3	60	3	2	0
Breton Reduced Fat & Sodium	7	120	2	1	0

FOOD	PORTION	CALS	FAT	SAT FAT	TRANS FAT
Cabaret	3	70	4	2	0
Crispy Baguettes Original	9	110	2	1	0
Crispy Baguettes Three Cheese	8	130	5	1	0
Grainsfirst	4	90	3	1	0
Vinta	2 (0.5 oz)	70	3	2	0
Vivant	3	60	3	2	–
Water Crackers Original	5	60	2	1	–
Doritos					
Jalapeno Cheese	1 pkg	230	13	4	–
Nacho Cheesier	1 pkg	240	14	3	–
Dr. Kracker					
Flatbread Klassic Seed	1 (1 oz)	120	5	1	0
Flatbread Pumpkin Seed Cheddar	1 (1 oz)	120	5	2	0
Flatbread Seeded Spelt	1 (1 oz)	120	6	1	0
Flatbread Seedlander	1 (1 oz)	120	5	2	0
Flatbread Spelt Sunflower Cheddar	1 (1 oz)	120	6	2	0
Krispy Grahams	5 (1 oz)	110	3	1	0
Eden					
Brown Rice	8 (1.1 oz)	120	2	0	0
Nori Nori Rice	15 (1 oz)	110	0	0	0
Foods Alive					
Golden Flax Maple & Cinnamon	5	150	8	1	0
Golden Flax Mexican Harvest	5	150	8	1	0
Golden Flax Onion Garlic	5	140	7	1	0
Golden Flax Organic Hemp	5	130	6	1	0
Golden Flax Regular	5	150	9	1	0
Gamesa					
Sabrisas	11	150	2	2	2
Glutino					
Gluten Free	4 (0.5 oz)	70	2	1	0
Gluten Free Rusks	2 (0.7 oz)	80	2	1	0
Gold'n Krackle					
Cheese	½ oz	65	2	1	–
Healthy Handfuls					
Lucky Duckies Cheddar Cheese	1 pkg (1 oz)	100	4	1	0

FOOD	PORTION	CALS	FAT	SAT FAT	TRANS FAT
Heavenly					
All Flavors Cholesterol Free Sugar Free	1	16	4	1	–
Jacob's					
Table Cracker Bran	1	33	1	1	–
Kashi					
TLC Country Cheddar	18 (1 oz)	130	5	1	0
TLC Honey Sesame	15 (1 oz)	130	3	0	0
TLC Natural Ranch	15 (1 oz)	130	3	0	0
TLC Original 7 Grain	15 (1 oz)	130	3	0	0
TLC Party Mediterranean Bruschetta	4	120	4	1	0
TLC Snack Fire Roasted Vegetable	5	130	4	0	0
Keebler					
Sandwich Cracker Wheat & Cheddar	1 pkg	200	10	2	–
Toasteds Buttercrisp	5 (0.6 oz)	80	4	1	–
Toasteds Sesame	5 (0.6 oz)	80	4	1	–
Toasteds Wheat	5 (0.6 oz)	80	4	1	–
Kitchen Table Bakers					
Aged Parmesan	3	80	6	4	0
Everything	3	80	6	4	0
Garlic	3	80	6	4	0
Jalapeno	3	80	6	4	0
Lance					
Cheese On Wheat	1 pkg (1.4 oz)	190	9	2	0
Mary's Gone Crackers					
Wheat Free Gluten Free Black Pepper	13 (1 oz)	140	5	1	0
Wheat Free Gluten Free Onion	13 (1 oz)	140	5	1	0
Wheat Free Gluten Free Original Seed	13 (1 oz)	140	5	1	0
Milton's					
Multi-Grain	2	70	4	0	0
Nabisco					
Garden Harvest Apple Cinnamon	16 (1 oz)	120	3	0	0
Garden Harvest Banana	16 (1 oz)	120	3	0	0
Garden Harvest Tomato Basil	16 (1 oz)	120	4	0	0

FOOD	PORTION	CALS	FAT	SAT FAT	TRANS FAT
Garden Harvest Vegetable Medley	16 (1 oz)	120	4	0	0
Vegetable Thins	21 (1 oz)	150	7	2	0
Water Original	4	60	1	0	0
Wheat	4	90	4	0	0
Nature's Path					
Signature Tamari Flax	15	110	3	1	0
New York Style					
Crispini Seeds & Spice	6	120	4	1	0
Panatini Three Cheese	2	80	5	2	0
Panetini Original	2	80	4	2	0
Pita Chips Garlic	7	130	5	3	0
Pita Chips Natural Whole Wheat	7	120	5	3	0
No-Carb Kitchen					
Cheese	1	25	3	1	–
Old London					
Mediterranean Toast	3	60	2	1	–
Pepperidge Farm					
100 Calorie Pack Goldfish Cheddar	1 pkg	100	4	1	0
100 Calorie Pack Goldfish Pretzel	1 pkg	100	2	0	0
Goldfish Cinnamon Graham	1 pkg	210	8	6	0
Goldfish Pizza	55	140	5	1	0
Goldfish w/ Whole Grain	55	140	5	1	0
Reduced Sodium Goldfish Cheddar	60	140	5	1	0
Snack Sticks Pumpernickel	15	120	2	0	0
Water Crackers	4	60	1	0	0
Wheat Crisps Spicy Salsa	16	140	6	1	0
Peter Pan					
Peanut Butter Cheese	1 pkg	210	10	3	–
Peanut Butter Toast	1 pkg	210	11	3	–
Premium					
Saltine Fat Free	5 (0.5 oz)	60	0	0	0
Saltine Multigrain	5 (0.5 oz)	60	2	0	0
Saltine Unsalted Tops	5	60	2	0	0
Saltines Low Sodium	0.5 oz	80	2	0	–
Saltines Original	0.5 oz	60	2	0	0

FOOD	PORTION	CALS	FAT	SAT FAT	TRANS FAT
Ritz					
Crackers	0.5 oz	80	5	1	0
Low Sodium	0.5 oz	80	4	1	0
Reduced Fat	5 (0.5 oz)	70	2	0	0
Whole Wheat	0.5 oz	70	3	1	–
Rykrisp					
Seasoned	2	60	2	0	–
San-J					
Brown Rice Black Sesame	5	140	6	–	–
Brown Rice Sesame	5	130	5	–	–
Brown Rice Tamari	6	170	1	–	–
Sara Lee					
Cracked Pepper Trio	7	130	4	1	–
English Water	7	130	4	1	–
Harvest Vegetable	6	140	6	1	–
Sociables					
Original	0.5 oz	70	4	1	0
South Beach					
Whole Wheat	1 pkg	100	4	0	0
Tree Of Life					
Saltine Cracked Pepper Fat Free	4 (0.5 oz)	60	0	0	–
Saltine Fat Free	4 (0.5 oz)	50	0	0	–
Triscuit					
Deli-Style Rye	1 oz	120	5	1	0
Original	1 oz	120	5	1	0
Reduced Fat	1 oz	120	3	0	0
Utz					
Cheese Peanut Butter	6	200	10	2	0
Vegetable Thins					
Original	1 oz	150	7	2	0
Wasa					
Crisp'N Light 7 Grain	3	60	0	0	0
Fiber Rye	1	30	1	0	0
Hearty Rye	1	45	0	0	0
Oats	1	60	1	0	0
Sourdough Rye	1	35	0	0	0
Westminster					
Oyster	1 pkg (0.5 oz)	66	2	tr	0

FOOD	PORTION	CALS	FAT	SAT FAT	TRANS FAT
Wheat Thins					
100% Whole Grain	1 oz	140	6	1	0
Low Sodium	1.1 oz	150	6	1	0
Original	1.1 oz	150	6	1	0
Reduced Fat	1 oz	130	4	1	0
Wheatsworth					
Crackers	5 (0.5 oz)	80	4	1	0
Wisecrackers					
Low Fat Roasted Garlic	10	110	2	0	–
CRANBERRIES					
cranberry orange relish	¼ cup	118	tr	tr	0
cranberry sauce	¼ cup	109	tr	tr	0
dried	½ cup	85	tr	tr	0
dried organic	⅓ cup	120	1	0	–
fresh chopped	1 cup	13	tr	tr	0
fresh whole	1 cup	11	tr	tr	0
sauce	1 slice (2 oz)	86	tr	tr	0
De-Lite					
Dried Sweetened	1 oz	92	tr	tr	0
Earthbound Farm					
Organic Dried	⅓ cup	130	0	0	0
Eden					
Organic Dried	⅓ cup	140	1	0	0
Fool					
Cranberry Spread	1 tbsp	30	0	0	0
Frieda's					
Dried	⅓ cup (1.4 oz)	110	1	0	–
Good Sense					
Cranberries 'N More	¼ cup	170	10	2	–
Dried Sweetened	½ cup	130	0	0	0
Jok'n'Al					
Cranberry Sauce	1 tbsp	8	0	0	0
Lollipop Tree					
Cranberry Curd	1 tbsp	50	1	1	–
Mariani					
Dried Sweetened	⅓ cup	130	0	0	0
Newman's Own					
Organic Dried	¼ cup	130	0	0	0

FOOD	PORTION	CALS	FAT	SAT FAT	TRANS FAT
Ocean Spray					
Craisins	⅓ cup	130	0	0	0
Cranberry Sauce Jellied	¼ cup	110	0	0	0
Cranorange	¼ cup	120	0	0	0
Whole Berry Sauce	¼ cup	110	0	0	0
Steel's					
Spiced Cranberry Sauce	⅓ cup	20	0	0	0
Sunsweet					
Dried	⅓ cup (1.5 oz)	140	0	0	0
CRANBERRY BEANS					
canned	½ cup	108	tr	tr	–
dried cooked w/o salt	½ cup	120	tr	tr	–
CRANBERRY JUICE					
cranberry juice cocktail low calorie w/ vitamin C	8 oz	46	tr	0	0
cranberry juice cocktail w/ vitamin C	8 oz	137	tr	tr	0
unsweetened	8 oz	116	tr	tr	0
Apple & Eve					
100% Juice	8 oz	130	0	0	0
Keto					
Kooler	½ tsp	0	0	0	0
Lakewood					
Organic	6 oz	50	0	0	0
Organic Light	6 oz	45	0	0	0
Langers					
Cranberry 100	8 oz	140	0	0	0
Nantucket Nectars					
Big Cran	8 oz	140	0	0	0
Northland					
100% Juice	8 oz	130	0	0	0
Ocean Spray					
Cocktail	8 oz	140	0	0	0
Cocktail Light Low Calorie	8 oz	40	0	0	0
Cocktail Reduced Calorie	8 oz	50	0	0	0
Cranberry Drink	8 oz	130	0	0	0
Cranberry Spritzer	8 oz	160	0	0	0
Crantastic	8 oz	100	0	0	0
White Cran Peach	8 oz	120	0	0	0

FOOD	PORTION	CALS	FAT	SAT FAT	TRANS FAT
White Cranberry	8 oz	120	0	0	0
White Cranberry Strawberry	8 oz	120	0	0	0
Old Orchard					
Cocktail	8 oz	140	0	0	0
SSips					
Cocktail	1 box (7 oz)	110	0	0	0
CRAYFISH					
cooked	3 oz	97	1	tr	–
raw	3 oz	76	1	tr	–
raw	8	24	tr	tr	–
CREAM (see also WHIPPED TOPPINGS)					
clotted cream	2 tbsp (1 oz)	164	18	–	–
creme fraiche	2 tbsp (1 oz)	100	11	–	–
half & half	1 cup (8.5 oz)	315	28	17	–
half & half	1 tbsp (0.5 oz)	20	2	1	–
heavy whipping	1 tbsp (0.5 oz)	52	6	3	–
heavy whipping whipped	1 cup (4.1 oz)	411	44	27	–
light coffee	1 cup (8.4 oz)	496	46	29	–
light coffee	1 tbsp (0.5 oz)	29	3	2	–
light whipping	1 tbsp (0.5 oz)	44	5	3	–
light whipping whipped	1 cup (4.2 oz)	345	37	23	–
Cabot					
Whipped	2 tbsp	30	2	2	–
Coffee-Mate					
Half & Half Fat Free	2 tbsp	20	0	0	0
Hood					
Half & Half	2 tbsp	40	4	2	0
Light	1 tbsp	30	3	2	0
Simply Smart Fat Free Half & Half	2 tbsp	15	0	0	0
Whipping Cream	1 tbsp	45	5	3	0
Horizon Organic					
Half & Half	2 tbsp	35	3	2	0
Heavy Whipping	1 tbsp	50	5	4	0
Organic Valley					
Half & Half	2 tbsp (1 oz)	40	4	2	0
CREAM CHEESE					
cream cheese	1 oz	99	10	6	–
cream cheese	1 pkg (3 oz)	297	30	19	–

FOOD	PORTION	CALS	FAT	SAT FAT	TRANS FAT
Back To Nature					
Organic Cream Cheese	⅛ pkg (1 oz)	100	10	6	–
Boar's Head					
Cream Cheese	2 tbsp (1 oz)	100	10	7	0
Connoisseur					
Wheel Mango Peach	2 tbsp	110	7	5	–
Wheel Wild Blueberry	2 tbsp	100	7	5	–
Crystal Farms					
Regular	1 oz	90	9	6	1
Tub	2 tbsp	100	9	7	0
Whipped	2 tbsp	70	7	5	0
Horizon Organic					
Reduced Fat	2 tbsp	70	7	4	0
Spreadable	2 tbsp	110	10	6	0
Lifeway					
Lox & Onion	2 tbsp	80	8	5	–
Vegetable	2 tbsp	80	7	5	–
Whipped	2 tbsp	80	8	5	–
Organic Valley					
Cream Cheese	1 oz	100	10	6	0
Soft	2 tbsp	90	9	6	0
Philadelphia					
⅓ Less Fat	1 oz	70	6	4	0
Fat Free	1 oz	30	0	0	0
Original	1 oz	100	9	6	0
Whipped	2 tbsp	60	6	4	0

CREAM CHEESE SUBSTITUTE
WholeSoy & Co.

Soy Cream Cheese Organic Original & Flavored	2 tbsp	70	6	1	0

CREAM OF TARTAR

cream of tartar	1 tsp	8	0	0	0

CREAM SUBSTITUTES
ExpertExtras

RealCream	1 tsp	14	1	1	–

CREPES

basic crepe unfilled	1 (7 in)	112	6	2	0

FOOD	PORTION	CALS	FAT	SAT FAT	TRANS FAT
Frieda's					
Ready-To-Use	1 (0.5 oz)	30	1	0	–
CROAKER					
atlantic breaded & fried	3 oz	188	11	3	–
atlantic raw	3 oz	89	3	1	–
CROCODILE					
cooked	3 oz	78	1	–	–
CROISSANT					
apple	1 (2 oz)	145	5	3	–
cheese	1 (2 oz)	236	12	5	–
plain	1 (2 oz)	232	12	7	–
plain	1 mini (1 oz)	115	6	3	–
Sara Lee					
Croissant	1 (1.5 oz)	170	8	3	–
Petite	2 (2 oz)	230	11	4	–
TAKE-OUT					
w/ egg & cheese	1 (4.5 oz)	368	25	14	–
w/ egg cheese & bacon	1 (4.5 oz)	413	28	15	–
w/ egg cheese & ham	1 (5.3 oz)	474	34	17	–
w/ egg cheese & sausage	1 (5.6 oz)	523	38	18	–
CROUTONS					
plain	1 cup (1 oz)	122	2	tr	–
seasoned	1 cup (1.4 oz)	186	7	2	–
Cardini's					
Italian	2 tbsp	30	2	0	0
Edward & Sons					
Organic Lightly Salted	2 tbsp	30	1	0	0
Fresh Gourmet					
Butter & Garlic	7 (7 g)	35	2	0	0
Cornbread Sweet Butter	½ cup (1 oz)	110	1	0	0
Country Ranch	6 (7 g)	35	2	0	0
Fat Free Garlic Caesar	12 (7 g)	30	0	0	0
Italian Seasoned	6 (7 g)	35	2	0	0
Organic Seasoned	5 (7 g)	30	2	0	0
Pepperidge Farm					
Whole Grain Seasoned	6	30	1	0	0
Zesty Italian	6	30	1	0	0

FOOD	PORTION	CALS	FAT	SAT FAT	TRANS FAT
Rothbury Farms					
Seasoned	2 tbsp	30	1	–	0
CUCUMBER					
fresh peeled	1 med (7 oz)	24	tr	tr	0
fresh sliced	1 cup	14	tr	tr	0
fresh w/ peel sliced	½ cup	34	tr	tr	0
Chiquita					
Cucumber	⅓ med (3.5 oz)	15	0	0	0
Frieda's					
Japanese	⅔ cup	10	0	0	0
Seedless Hothouse	⅔ cup	110	0	0	0
TAKE-OUT					
cucumber & onion salad w/ vinegar	1 cup	52	tr	tr	0
cucumber salad w/ oil & vinegar	1 cup	183	15	2	0
cucumber salad w/ sour cream dressing	1 cup	68	6	3	0
kimchee	½ cup (1.8 oz)	36	2	tr	–
tzatziki	½ cup (3.4 oz)	72	6	1	–
CUMIN					
seed	1 tsp	8	tr	tr	0
CURRANT JUICE					
black currant nectar	7 oz	110	0	–	0
red currant nectar	7 oz	108	tr	–	–
CurrantC					
Black Currant Juice	8 oz	130	0	0	0
CURRANTS					
black fresh	½ cup	36	tr	tr	–
zante dried	½ cup	204	tr	tr	–
Sun-Maid					
Zante	¼ cup	130	0	0	0
CURRY					
curry powder	1 tsp	7	tr	tr	–
paste	1 tube (6 oz)	465	36	12	tr
A Taste Of Thai					
Curry Paste Green	1 tsp	15	2	0	–

FOOD	PORTION	CALS	FAT	SAT FAT	TRANS FAT
Curry Paste Panang	1 tsp	25	2	1	–
Curry Paste Red	1 tsp	20	2	1	0
Curry Paste Yellow	1 tsp	30	3	0	–
Patak's					
Curry Paste Biryani	2 tbsp	180	16	2	–
Garam Masala Paste	2 tsp	130	12	1	–
Tandoori Paste	2 tbsp	30	1	0	–
Vandaloo Paste	2 tbsp	160	16	1	–
Spice Hunter					
Curry Seasoning Salt Free	¼ tsp	0	0	0	0
TAKE-OUT					
beef curry	1 cup	432	31	7	–
chicken curry ½ breast	1 serv	160	9	2	–
chicken curry boneless	1 serv (6.2 oz)	219	12	2	–
chicken curry leg & thigh	1 serv	180	10	2	–
chickpea curry	1 serv (8.3 oz)	305	15	8	–
lamb curry	1 cup	257	14	4	–
mixed vegetable curry	1 serv (7.7 oz)	398	33	–	–
pea & potato curry	1 serv (7 oz)	284	22	–	–
pork vandaloo curry	1 serv	620	47	–	–
potato	1 serv (6 oz)	292	16	–	–
sambhar dhal curry	1 serv (10 oz)	177	7	4	–

CUSK
fillet baked	3 oz	106	1	–	–

CUSTARD
MIX

as prep w/ 2% milk	½ cup (4.7 oz)	148	4	2	–
as prep w/ whole milk	½ cup (4.7 oz)	163	5	3	–
flan as prep w/ 2% milk	½ cup (4.7 oz)	135	2	1	–
flan as prep w/ whole milk	½ cup (4.7 oz)	150	4	3	–
Betty Crocker					
Flan w/ Caramel Sauce as prep	1 serv	330	7	4	–
READY-TO-EAT					
Kozy Shack					
Flan	1 pkg (4 oz)	145	4	2	–
TAKE-OUT					
baked	½ cup (5 oz)	148	7	3	–
flan	½ cup (5.4 oz)	220	6	3	–
flan de calabaza	1 piece (3.5 oz)	225	10	2	0

FOOD	PORTION	CALS	FAT	SAT FAT	TRANS FAT
flan de coco	1 piece (4.2 oz)	340	13	8	–
tocino del cielo heaven's delight	1 cup	856	21	7	–
zabaione	½ cup (57.2 g)	135	5	2	–

CUTTLEFISH
steamed	3 oz	134	1	tr	–

DANDELION GREENS
fresh cooked	½ cup	17	tr	–	–
raw chopped	½ cup	13	tr	–	–

Frieda's
Dandelion Greens	2 cups	40	0	0	0

DANISH PASTRY
FROZEN
Morton
Honey Buns	1 (2.28 oz)	270	13	3	–
Honey Buns Mini	1 (1.3 oz)	160	8	2	–

READY-TO-EAT
Entenmann's
Danish Ring Walnut	⅙ ring (2 oz)	260	16	5	0

TAKE-OUT
cheese	1 (2.5 oz)	266	16	5	–
cinnamon	1 (5 oz)	572	32	8	–
fruit	1 (5 oz)	527	27	7	–
lemon	1 (2.5 oz)	263	13	2	–
raisin nut	1 (2.3 oz)	280	16	4	–

DATES
deglet noor dried	10	240	0	–	0
dried chopped	1 cup	489	1	–	–
dried whole	10	228	tr	–	–
jujube dried	1 oz	75	tr	–	–
jujube fresh	1 oz	30	tr	–	–
jujube preserved in sugar	1 oz	91	tr	–	–
medjool	2–3 (1.4 oz)	120	0	0	0

Bob's Red Mill
Dried Crumbles	⅓ cup	130	0	0	0

Earthbound Farm
Organic Dried	6 (1.4 oz)	120	0	0	0

FOOD	PORTION	CALS	FAT	SAT FAT	TRANS FAT
Frieda's					
Medjool	2–3 (1.4 oz)	120	0	0	0
SunDate					
Fancy Medjool	3 (1.4 oz)	120	0	0	0
Sunsweet					
California Pitted	5–6 (1.4 oz)	120	0	0	0

DEER (see VENISON)

DELI MEATS/COLD CUTS (see also BEEF, CHICKEN, HAM, MEAT SUBSTITUTES, TURKEY)

FOOD	PORTION	CALS	FAT	SAT FAT	TRANS FAT
barbecue loaf pork & beef	1 slice (0.8 oz)	40	2	1	–
beerwurst beef	1 slice (4 in x ⅛ in)	75	7	3	–
beerwurst beef	2 oz	155	13	5	–
berliner pork & beef	1 slice (0.8 oz)	53	4	1	–
blood sausage	1 slice (0.9 oz)	95	9	3	–
bologna beef	1 slice (1 oz)	88	8	3	–
bologna beef low fat	1 slice (1 oz)	57	4	2	–
bologna beef reduced sodium	1 slice (1 oz)	88	8	3	–
bologna beef & pork	1 slice (1 oz)	87	7	3	–
bologna beef & pork low fat	1 slice (1 oz)	64	5	2	–
braunschweiger pork	1 slice (1 oz)	92	8	3	–
dutch brand loaf pork & beef	1 slice (1.3 oz)	104	9	3	–
headcheese pork	1 slice (1.6 oz)	71	5	2	–
honey loaf pork & beef	1 slice (1 oz)	35	1	tr	–
lebanon bologna beef	2 slices (1 oz)	105	6	2	–
mortadella beef & pork	1 slice (0.5 oz)	47	4	1	–
olive loaf pork	2 slices (2 oz)	134	9	3	–
pastrami beef	1 slice (1 oz)	41	2	1	–
peppered loaf pork & beef	1 slice (1 oz)	41	2	1	–
pepperoni pork & beef	15 slices (1 oz)	135	12	5	–
picnic loaf pork & beef	1 slice (1 oz)	65	5	2	–
salami cooked beef & pork	1 slice (0.8 oz)	58	5	2	–
salami hard pork	3 slices (0.9 oz)	14	8	3	–
salami hard pork & beef less sodium	1 slice (1 oz)	113	9	3	–
sandwich spread pork & beef	¼ cup	141	10	4	–
summer sausage thuringer cervelat	2 oz	203	17	6	–
Boar's Head					
Abruzzese Hot & Sweet	1 oz	100	8	3	–
Bologna 25% Lowered Sodium	2 oz	150	13	5	–

FOOD	PORTION	CALS	FAT	SAT FAT	TRANS FAT
Bologna Beef	2 oz	150	13	4	–
Bologna Garlic	2 oz	150	13	5	–
Bologna Lebanon	2 oz	100	5	3	–
Bologna Pork & Beef	2 oz	150	13	5	–
Braunschweiger Lite	2 oz	120	8	5	–
Capocollo Hot & Sweet	1 oz	80	5	2	–
Dutch Loaf	2 oz	150	12	5	–
Liverwurst Smoked	2 oz	170	15	6	–
Mortadella	2 oz	160	14	5	–
Olive Loaf	2 oz	130	12	5	–
Pastrami	2 oz	70	3	1	–
Pickle & Pepper Loaf	2 oz	150	13	7	–
Prosciutto	1 oz	60	3	1	–
Salami Beef	2 oz	120	9	3	–
Salami Cooked	2 oz	130	11	5	–
Salami Hard	1 oz	110	9	4	–
Sopressata Hot & Sweet	1 oz	100	7	3	–
Spiced Ham	2 oz	120	10	5	–
Healthy Ones					
Pastrami 97% Fat Free	4 slices (2 oz)	60	2	1	0
Hebrew National					
Bologna Beef	1 slice (1 oz)	80	8	4	–
Bologna Lean Beef	4 slices (2 oz)	90	5	3	–
Salami Beef	3 slices (2 oz)	150	13	6	–
Salami Lean Beef	4 slices (2 oz)	90	5	3	–
Hormel					
Pepperoni Sliced	16 slices (1 oz)	140	13	5	–
Oscar Mayer					
Salami Beef	3 slices (1.8 oz)	150	13	6	1
Russer					
Turkey Breast Honey Roasted	1 slice (1 oz)	25	1	0	0
Sara Lee					
Corned Beef	1 slice (2 oz)	50	2	1	–
Pastrami	2 slices (1.6 oz)	60	3	1	–
Salami Genoa	4 slices (1 oz)	110	10	4	–
Salami Hard	4 slices (1 oz)	120	11	4	–
Wellshire					
Salami Genoa	1 oz	100	8	2	–
Salami Hard	1 oz	100	8	2	–
Sopressata Sliced	1 oz	100	8	2	–

FOOD	PORTION	CALS	FAT	SAT FAT	TRANS FAT
TAKE-OUT					
corned beef brisket	2 oz	90	5	2	–
DILL					
seed	1 tsp	6	tr	tr	0
sprigs fresh	5 (0.3 oz)	0	tr	tr	0
weed dry	1 tbsp	8	tr	tr	0

DINNER (see also ASIAN FOOD, PASTA DINNERS, POT PIES, SPANISH FOOD)

Amy's

FOOD	PORTION	CALS	FAT	SAT FAT	TRANS FAT
Country Dinner Vegetable Salisbury Steak	1 pkg (11 oz)	380	12	4	–
Banquet					
Beef Patty w/ Country Style Vegetables	1 meal (9.5 oz)	310	20	8	–
Boneless White Fried Chicken	1 meal (8.25 oz)	540	34	9	–
Chicken Parmigiana	1 meal (9.5 oz)	320	18	7	–
Chicken Fried Beef Steak	1 pkg (10 oz)	420	23	12	–
Extra Helping Boneless Pork Riblet	1 meal (15.25 oz)	720	40	15	–
Extra Helping Fried Beef Steak	1 meal (16 oz)	820	50	23	–
Extra Helping Fried Chicken	1 meal (14.7 oz)	910	55	13	–
Extra Helping Meatloaf	1 meal (16 oz)	610	40	15	–
Extra Helping Salisbury Steak	1 meal (16.5 oz)	740	54	21	–
Extra Helping Turkey & Gravy w/ Dressing	1 meal (17 oz)	620	32	8	–
Extra Helping White Fried Chicken	1 meal (13 oz)	690	48	12	–
Extra Helping Yankee Pot Roast	1 meal (14.5 oz)	410	20	7	–
Family Size Brown Gravy & Salisbury Steak	1 serv	240	20	10	–
Family Size Brown Gravy & Sliced Beef	1 serv	140	8	4	–
Family Size Chicken & Broccoli Alfredo	1 serv	270	12	7	–
Family Size Country Style Chicken & Dumplings	1 serv	290	14	5	–
Family Size Hearty Beef Stew	1 cup	170	7	3	–
Honey Roast Turkey Breast	1 meal (9 oz)	270	12	3	–
Our Original Fried Chicken	1 meal (9 oz)	470	27	9	–

FOOD	PORTION	CALS	FAT	SAT FAT	TRANS FAT
Pork Cutlet Meal	1 meal (10.25 oz)	420	25	7	–
Sliced Beef	1 meal (9 oz)	270	10	5	–
Turkey Meal	1 meal (9.25 oz)	290	13	3	–
Veal Parmagiana	1 meal (8.75 oz)	330	14	5	–
Western Style Beef Patty	1 meal (9.5 oz)	360	21	10	–
White Meat Fried Chicken	1 meal (8.75 oz)	460	28	11	–
Yankee Pot Roast	1 meal (9.4 oz)	230	10	4	–
Birds Eye					
Voila! Pasta Primavera w/ Chicken	1⅔ cups	250	3	0	0
Voila! Shrimp Scampi	1¾ cups	190	3	1	0
Voila! Southwestern Chicken	2 cups	250	6	3	0
Boston Market					
Glazed Rotisserie Chicken w/ Mashed Potatoes Gravy Vegetables	1 pkg (16 oz)	390	15	3	0
Meatloaf w/ Mashed Potatoes & Gravy	1 pkg (16 oz)	880	55	23	–
C&W					
Stir Fry Feast Pot Sticker + Sauce	2 cups	200	4	1	–
Stir Fry Feast Ultimate + Sauce	1½ cups	190	5	1	0
Campbell's					
Supper Bakes Cheesy Chicken w/ Pasta	⅙ pkg	170	4	2	1
Supper Bakes Garlic Chicken w/ Pasta	⅙ pkg	220	2	1	0
Supper Bakes Savory Pork Chops w/ Herb Stuffing	⅙ box	160	2	1	0
Supper Bakes Traditional Roast Chicken w/ Stuffing	⅙ pkg	160	3	1	0
Contessa					
Beef Goulash not prep	1¾ cups	210	5	2	0
Chicken Cacciatore not prep	1¾ cups	230	7	2	0
Chicken Alfredo not prep	1¾ cups	330	18	10	0
Fantastic					
Ginger Shitake w/ Rice Noodles	1 pkg (7.4 oz)	340	10	2	–
Fillo Factory					
Organic Fillo Pie Eggplant & Red Pepper	1 serv (5 oz)	230	9	2	0

FOOD	PORTION	CALS	FAT	SAT FAT	TRANS FAT
Glory					
Savory Singles Chicken & Dumplings	1 pkg	290	8	3	0
Savory Singles Chicken Smoked Sausage & Rice Casserole	1 pkg	440	18	5	0
Savory Singles Ham & Sausage Jambalaya	1 pkg	400	18	6	0
Savory Singles Turkey & Gravy w/ Cornbread Stuffing	1 pkg	440	18	4	0
Glutino					
Gluten Free Chicken Pomodoro w/ Brown Rice & Vegetables	1 pkg (9.1 oz)	190	3	0	0
Gluten Free Chicken Ranchero w/ Brown Rice	1 pkg (9.1 oz)	180	2	0	0
Golden Cuisine					
Beef Stew	1 pkg	350	10	4	tr
Boneless Pork Patty	1 pkg	504	25	9	tr
Breaded Baked Fish w/ Rice Pilaf	1 pkg	300	5	1	tr
Chicken Cacciatore	1 pkg	417	10	4	0
Chicken & Noodles	1 pkg	331	8	2	3
Chicken Parmesan	1 pkg	430	19	4	1
Chicken w/ Marinara Sauce	1 pkg	329	8	2	0
Meatloaf Patty & Gravy	1 pkg	340	14	6	tr
Mesquite Chicken	1 pkg	320	5	1	0
Pot Roast w/ Gravy	1 pkg	343	11	4	tr
Salisbury Steak & Mushroom Sauce	1 pkg	350	10	4	tr
Swedish Meatballs	1 pkg	440	26	12	tr
Turkey Tetrazzini	1 pkg	304	6	2	0
Green Giant					
Create A Meal Stir Fry Sweet & Sour as prep	1 cup	280	7	1	0
Skillet Meal Chicken Teriyaki as prep	1½ cups	240	1	0	0
Healthy Choice					
Beef Merlot	1 pkg	240	8	2	–
Beef Pot Roast	1 pkg	320	9	3	–
Beef Stroganoff	1 pkg	320	9	3	–

FOOD	PORTION	CALS	FAT	SAT FAT	TRANS FAT
Beef Teriyaki	1 pkg	310	7	3	–
Beef Tips Portabello	1 pkg	300	8	3	0
Blackened Chicken	1 pkg	300	6	2	–
Boneless Beef Ribs w/ Classic BBQ Sauce	1 pkg	360	9	3	–
Charbroiled Beef Patty	1 pkg	310	9	3	–
Cheesy Rice & Chicken	1 pkg	250	5	3	–
Chicken Breast & Vegetables	1 pkg	260	7	2	–
Chicken Broccoli Alfredo	1 pkg	300	7	3	–
Chicken Carbonara	1 pkg	290	7	3	–
Chicken Margherita	1 pkg	340	8	2	–
Chicken Parmigiana	1 pkg	320	9	3	–
Chicken Piccata	1 pkg	260	5	3	–
Chicken Teriyaki	1 pkg	270	6	2	–
Chicken Tuscany	1 pkg	340	9	3	–
Country Breaded Chicken	1 pkg	370	9	3	–
Country Glazed Chicken	1 pkg	230	5	2	–
Country Herb Chicken	1 pkg	280	6	3	0
Creamy Herb Roasted Chicken	1 pkg	240	5	2	–
Grilled Basil Chicken	1 pkg	330	9	3	–
Grilled Chicken Breast & Pasta	1 pkg	250	7	3	–
Grilled Chicken Breast w/ Mashed Potatoes	1 pkg	190	5	2	–
Grilled Chicken Caesar	1 pkg	300	8	3	–
Grilled Chicken Marinara	1 pkg	270	5	2	–
Grilled Steak w/ Roasted Garlic Sauce	1 pkg	220	7	3	–
Grilled Turkey Breast	1 pkg	250	5	2	–
Grilled Whiskey Steak	1 pkg	280	6	2	–
Herb Baked Fish	1 pkg	360	9	3	–
Homestyle Chicken & Pasta	1 pkg	250	6	3	–
Honey Glazed Chicken	1 pkg	320	6	2	–
Lemon Pepper Fish	1 pkg	280	5	2	0
Mandarin Chicken	1 pkg	250	4	1	–
Mesquite Chicken BBQ	1 pkg	300	5	2	–
Mixed Grills Chicken Honey BBQ w/ Dipping Sauce	1 pkg	380	7	2	–
Mixed Grills Chicken Honey Mustard w/ Dipping Sauce	1 pkg	360	7	2	–

FOOD	PORTION	CALS	FAT	SAT FAT	TRANS FAT
Mixed Grills Chicken Teriyaki w/ Dipping Sauce	1 pkg	340	7	2	–
Mixed Grills Chicken Tomato Garlic w/ Dipping Sauce	1 pkg	370	7	2	–
Mixed Grills Steak w/ BBQ Sauce	1 pkg	420	8	3	–
Mixed Grills Steak Teriyaki w/ Dipping Sauce	1 pkg	350	9	3	–
Mixed Grills Steak w/ Zesty Steak Sauce	1 pkg	350	8	3	–
Oriental Style Beef	1 pkg	310	9	3	–
Oriental Style Chicken	1 pkg	240	5	2	–
Oven Roasted Beef	1 pkg	280	7	3	–
Princess Chicken	1 pkg	310	7	2	–
Roast Turkey Breast	1 pkg	220	6	2	–
Roasted Chicken Breast	1 pkg	280	8	3	–
Roasted Chicken Chardonnay	1 pkg	290	8	3	–
Salisbury Steak	1 pkg	360	9	4	–
Salisbury Steak w/ Red Skin Mashed Potatoes	1 pkg	200	6	3	–
Sesame Chicken	1 pkg	260	6	2	–
Slow Roasted Turkey Breast w/ Mashed Potatoes	1 pkg	210	7	2	–
Sweet & Sour Chicken	1 pkg	340	7	2	–
Traditional Meatloaf	1 pkg	300	9	3	–
Traditional Turkey Breast	1 pkg	300	4	1	0
Tuna Casserole	1 pkg	270	7	2	–
Helen's Kitchen					
Indian Curry w/ Tofu Steaks & Rice	1 pkg (9 oz)	300	8	1	0
Ian's					
Chicken Finger Meal Allergen Free	1 pkg (7 oz)	368	9	2	0
Chicken Nugget Meal	1 pkg (8 oz)	440	14	2	–
Fish Stick Meal	1 pkg (8.4 oz)	480	11	2	–
Hamburger Meal	1 pkg (7 oz)	296	9	2	0
Pizza Meal	1 pkg (6.7 oz)	340	7	3	–
Popcorn Turkey Dog Meal Allergen Free	1 pkg (7 oz)	442	17	2	0
Kashi					
Black Bean Mango	1 pkg (10 oz)	340	8	1	0

FOOD	PORTION	CALS	FAT	SAT FAT	TRANS FAT
Lemon Rosemary Chicken	1 pkg (10 oz)	330	9	2	0
Lime Cilantro Shrimp	1 pkg (10 oz)	250	8	2	0
Southwest Style Chicken	1 pkg (10 oz)	240	5	0	0
Sweet & Sour Chicken	1 pkg (10 oz)	320	4	1	0
Kid Cuisine					
All American Fried Chicken	1 meal	500	21	5	2
All Star Chicken Breast Nuggets	1 meal	460	19	5	0
Bug Safari Chicken Breast Nuggets	1 meal	450	16	4	0
Carnival Corn Dog	1 meal	430	12	3	0
Deep Sea Adventure Fish Sticks	1 meal	400	12	2	0
Fiesta Beef Taco Dippers	1 meal	370	16	6	0
Pop Star Popcorn Chicken	1 meal	410	10	3	0
Laura's Lifestyle					
Carb Conscious Chicken Puttanesca	1 pkg (9 oz)	270	10	2	–
Carb Conscious Chicken Chow Mein	1 pkg (9 oz)	260	8	4	–
Carb Conscious Chicken Santa Fe	1 pkg (9 oz)	280	9	2	–
Carb Conscious Thai Chicken	1 pkg (9 oz)	280	8	2	–
Lean Cuisine					
Cafe Classics Baked Chicken Florentine	1 pkg (8 oz)	200	8	2	0
Cafe Classics Baked Lemon Pepper Fish	1 pkg (9 oz)	220	6	2	0
Cafe Classics Beef Peppercorn	1 pkg (8.75 oz)	220	7	3	0
Cafe Classics Beef Portabello	1 pkg (9 oz)	200	5	3	0
Cafe Classics Beef Pot Roast	1 pkg (9 oz)	190	6	2	0
Cafe Classics Bowl Creamy Basil Chicken	1 pkg (10.5 oz)	310	9	3	0
Cafe Classics Bowl Grilled Chicken Caesar	1 pkg (9 oz)	270	7	3	0
Cafe Classics Chicken Carbonara	1 pkg (9 oz)	280	7	2	0
Cafe Classics Chicken & Vegetables	1 pkg (10.5 oz)	240	5	2	0
Cafe Classics Chicken L'Orange	1 pkg (9 oz)	230	2	1	0
Cafe Classics Chicken Marsala	1 pkg (8.1 oz)	140	4	2	0

FOOD	PORTION	CALS	FAT	SAT FAT	TRANS FAT
Cafe Classics Chicken Parmesan	1 pkg (10.9 oz)	280	5	2	0
Cafe Classics Chicken Tuscan	1 pkg (12 oz)	300	7	3	0
Cafe Classics Chicken w/ Almonds	1 pkg (8.5 oz)	260	4	1	0
Cafe Classics Chicken w/ Basil Cream Sauce	1 pkg (8.5 oz)	270	7	3	0
Cafe Classics Fiesta Grilled Chicken	1 pkg (9.5 oz)	250	6	3	0
Cafe Classics Garlic Beef & Broccoli	1 pkg (9 oz)	170	6	2	0
Cafe Classics Glazed Chicken	1 pkg (8.5 oz)	220	4	1	0
Cafe Classics Glazed Turkey Tenderloins	1 pkg (9 oz)	260	5	2	0
Cafe Classics Grilled Chicken	1 pkg (9.4 oz)	160	5	1	0
Cafe Classics Grilled Chicken w/ Teriyaki Glaze	1 pkg (10 oz)	270	3	1	0
Cafe Classics Herb Roasted Chicken	1 pkg (8 oz)	190	4	1	0
Cafe Classics Honey Dijon Grilled Chicken	1 pkg (8 oz)	220	4	3	0
Cafe Classics Honey Mustard Chicken	1 pkg (8 oz)	250	4	1	0
Cafe Classics Honey Roasted Pork	1 serv (9.5 oz)	230	9	4	0
Cafe Classics Mandarin Chicken	1 pkg (9 oz)	270	4	1	0
Cafe Classics Meatloaf w/ Gravy & Whipped Potatoes	1 pkg (9.4 oz)	280	9	4	0
Cafe Classics Orange Peel Chicken	1 pkg (12 oz)	390	9	2	0
Cafe Classics Oven Roasted Beef	1 pkg (9.25 oz)	210	8	4	0
Cafe Classics Roasted Garlic Chicken	1 pkg (8.8 oz)	200	8	3	0
Cafe Classics Roasted Turkey & Vegetables	1 pkg (8 oz)	150	5	1	0
Cafe Classics Roasted Turkey Breast	1 pkg (12 oz)	280	6	1	0

FOOD	PORTION	CALS	FAT	SAT FAT	TRANS FAT
Cafe Classics Roasted Turkey Breast w/ Dressing	1 pkg (9.75 oz)	270	2	1	0
Cafe Classics Salisbury Steak	1 pkg (12.5 oz)	310	8	4	0
Cafe Classics Salisbury Steak w/ Mac & Cheese	1 pkg (9.5 oz)	280	8	5	0
Cafe Classics Sesame Chicken	1 pkg (9 oz)	330	8	2	0
Cafe Classics Southern Beef Tips	1 pkg (8.75 oz)	250	5	2	0
Cafe Classics Steak Tips Portabello	1 pkg (7.5 oz)	180	7	2	0
Cafe Classics Steak Tips Dijon	1 pkg (12 oz)	320	8	3	0
Cafe Classics Stuffed Cabbage	1 pkg (9.5 oz)	200	6	2	0
Cafe Classics Swedish Meatballs	1 pkg (9.1 oz)	290	8	3	0
Cafe Classics Sweet & Sour Chicken	1 pkg (10 oz)	290	3	1	0
Cafe Classics Three Cheese Chicken	1 pkg (8 oz)	230	10	3	0
Comfort Classics Baked Chicken	1 pkg (8.6 oz)	230	5	1	0
Dinnertime Selects Balsamic Glazed Chicken	1 pkg (12 oz)	400	8	3	0
Dinnertime Selects Chicken Florentine	1 pkg (13.25 oz)	420	8	4	0
Dinnertime Selects Chicken Portabello	1 pkg (12 oz)	370	6	2	0
Dinnertime Selects Lemon Garlic Shrimp	1 pkg (12 oz)	350	7	4	0
Skillet Beef Teriyaki & Rice	1 serv	190	3	1	0
Spa Cuisine Chicken Mediterranean	1 pkg (10.5 oz)	240	4	1	0
Spa Cuisine Chicken In Peanut Sauce	1 pkg (9 oz)	280	7	2	0
Spa Cuisine Chicken Pecan	1 pkg (9 oz)	260	6	2	0
Spa Cuisine Lemon Chicken	1 pkg (9 oz)	290	7	2	0
Spa Cuisine Lemongrass Chicken	1 pkg (9.4 oz)	240	6	4	0
Spa Cuisine Pork w/ Cherry Sauce	1 pkg (8.25 oz)	260	5	2	0
Spa Cuisine Rosemary Chicken	1 pkg (8.25 oz)	230	5	3	0

FOOD	PORTION	CALS	FAT	SAT FAT	TRANS FAT
Spa Cuisine Salmon w/ Beef	1 pkg (9.5 oz)	360	8	3	0
Luzianne					
Cajun Creole Dirty Rice	1 serv	160	1	0	–
Cajun Creole Etouffee	1 serv	200	1	0	–
Cajun Creole Gumbo	1 serv	160	1	0	–
Cajun Creole Jambalaya	1 serv	200	1	0	–
Marie Callender's					
Beef Stroganoff w/ Noodles	1 meal (13 oz)	600	27	11	–
Beef Tips In Mushroom Sauce	1 meal (13 oz)	430	19	7	–
Breaded Chicken Parmigiana	1 meal (16 oz)	860	32	8	–
Breaded Fish w/ Mac & Cheese	1 meal (12 oz)	550	28	9	–
Cheesy Rice w/ Chicken & Broccoli	1 meal (12 oz)	390	13	9	–
Chicken & Dumplings	1 meal (14 oz)	390	20	10	–
Chicken Teriyaki	1 meal (13 oz)	510	12	3	–
Grilled Southwestern Style Chicken	1 meal (14 oz)	410	11	6	–
Honey Smoked Ham Steak w/ Macaroni & Cheese	1 meal (14 oz)	490	13	7	–
Meatloaf & Gravy w/ Mashed Potatoes	1 meal (14 oz)	540	30	12	–
Old Fashioned Beef Pot Roast & Gravy	1 meal (15 oz)	500	17	6	–
Roast Beef	1 meal (14.5 oz)	390	19	8	–
Sirloin Salisbury Steak & Gravy	1 meal (14 oz)	550	25	11	–
Skillet Meal Au Gratin Potatoes	⅔ cup (5 oz)	190	10	7	–
Skillet Meal Beef Pot Roast	½ pkg	290	9	4	–
Skillet Meal Beef Stroganoff	½ pkg	310	11	7	–
Skillet Meal Chicken & Rice w/ Broccoli & Cheese	½ pkg	440	14	10	–
Skillet Meal Chicken Teriyaki	½ pkg	340	1	1	–
Skillet Meal Herb Chicken	½ pkg	290	4	2	–
Skillet Meal Roasted Chicken & Vegetables	½ pkg	260	6	2	–
Skillet Meal White & Wild Rice In Cheese Sauce	1 cup	300	13	8	–
Swedish Meatballs	1 meal (12.5 oz)	520	26	12	–
Sweet & Sour Chicken	1 meal (14 oz)	570	15	3	–
Turkey w/ Gravy & Dressing	1 meal (14 oz)	500	19	9	–

FOOD	PORTION	CALS	FAT	SAT FAT	TRANS FAT
Mon Cuisine					
Vegan Moroccan Couscous	1 pkg (10 oz)	280	4	1	–
Vegan Veal Schnitzel In Sauce	1 pkg (10 oz)	300	8	1	–
Vegetarian Stuffed Cabbage In Tomato Sauce	1 pkg (10 oz)	220	5	0	–
Morton					
Breaded Chicken Pattie	1 meal (6.75 oz)	290	17	4	–
Chicken Nuggets	1 meal (7 oz)	340	19	5	–
Chili Gravy w/ Beef Enchilada & Tamale	1 meal (10 oz)	270	9	4	–
Fried Chicken	1 meal (9 oz)	470	30	10	–
Gravy & Charbroiled Beef Patty	1 meal (9 oz)	310	18	9	–
Gravy & Salisbury Steak	1 meal (9 oz)	310	20	8	–
Gravy & Turkey w/ Stuffing	1 meal (9 oz)	240	10	4	–
Tomato Sauce w/ Meat Loaf	1 meal (9 oz)	250	13	5	–
Veal Parmagiana w/ Tomato Sauce	1 meal (8.75 oz)	290	15	5	–
Nature's Choice					
Broccoli Parmesan Alfredo	1 pkg (12 oz)	270	9	3	–
Nature's Entree					
Hearty Stew	1 pkg (12 oz)	290	9	3	–
Tuscany White Bean	1 pkg (12 oz)	330	8	2	–
Organic Classics					
Chicken Marsala w/ Mashed Potatoes	1 pkg (9.5 oz)	330	16	8	0
Jamaican Style Jerk Chicken w/ Wehani Rice	1 pkg (9.5 oz)	270	7	1	0
Lemon Chicken w/ Wehani Rice	1 pkg (9.5 oz)	320	8	2	0
Pacific Foods					
Beef Steak Stew	1 cup	250	7	2	–
Chicken Stew	1 cup	200	5	3	0
Patak's					
Vegetable Curry w/ Rice Creamy Coconut	1 pkg	400	18	10	–
Vegetable Curry w/ Rice Rich Tomato & Onion	1 pkg (10.5 oz)	290	6	1	–
Vegetable Curry w/ Rice Tangy Lemon & Cilantro	1 pkg	300	7	2	–

FOOD	PORTION	CALS	FAT	SAT FAT	TRANS FAT
Patio					
Ranchera	1 pkg (13 oz)	470	22	10	–
Quorn					
Meat Free Simply Saute Indian	½ pkg	240	4	2	–
Meat Free Simply Saute Mexican	½ pkg	340	7	3	–
Meat Free Simply Saute Thai	½ pkg	240	9	3	–
Savvy Faire					
Baja Jack Scramble	1 pkg (8.2 oz)	370	25	11	–
Braised Beef	1 pkg (9.4 oz)	320	18	4	–
Herb Crusted Chicken	1 pkg (9.7 oz)	430	21	5	–
Seeds Of Change					
Chicken Teriyaki	1 pkg (10 oz)	300	4	1	0
Mushroom Wild Pilaf	1 pkg (11 oz)	350	16	9	0
Seven Grain Pilaf	1 pkg (11 oz)	390	14	8	0
Shady Brook					
Roasted Carved Turkey	1 pkg (18.6 oz)	550	18	4	–
South Beach					
Beef & Broccoli & Asian Style Noodles	1 pkg	320	13	4	0
Caprese Style Chicken w/ Cauliflower & Broccoli	1 pkg	250	8	3	0
Cashew Chicken w/ Sugar Snap Peas	1 pkg	360	13	3	0
Chicken Alfredo A La Roma	1 pkg	270	8	4	0
Chicken Basilico w/ Rotini	1 pkg	280	10	2	0
Chicken Santa Fe Style Rice & Beans	1 pkg (8.9 oz)	340	12	4	0
Garlic Herb Chicken w/ Green Beans Almondine	1 pkg	250	12	2	0
Garlic Parmesan Chicken w/ Penne	1 pkg	290	11	3	0
Garlic Sesame Beef w/ Cauliflower Sugar Snap Peas & Peppers	1 pkg	250	11	3	0
Kung Pao Chicken Breast Strips w/ Peppers & Broccoli	1 pkg	300	11	2	0
Meatloaf w/ Gravy	1 pkg (8.9 oz)	210	9	3	0

FOOD	PORTION	CALS	FAT	SAT FAT	TRANS FAT
Orange Beef Slices & Brown Rice In Sauce w/ Broccoli & Carrots	1 pkg	260	8	2	0
Roasted Turkey	1 pkg (9.4 oz)	240	9	2	0
Savory Beef w/ Cheesy Broccoli	1 pkg	240	8	4	0
Savory Pork w/ Pecans & Green Beans	1 pkg	260	13	4	–
Szechwan Pork & Asian Noodles In Sauce	1 pkg	270	8	2	0
Stouffer's					
Beef Stew	1 pkg (11 oz)	280	9	3	0
Beef Stroganoff	1 pkg (9.75 oz)	380	17	5	0
Chicken A La King	1 pkg (11.5 oz)	360	12	4	0
Corner Bistro Burbon Steak Tips	1 pkg (12 oz)	520	22	6	1
Corner Bistro Sesame Chicken	1 pkg (12.63 oz)	510	15	3	0
Country Fried Beef Steak	1 pkg (16 oz)	610	33	10	2
Creamed Chipped Beef	½ pkg (5.5 oz)	140	7	4	0
Fish Filet	1 pkg (9 oz)	400	16	5	1
Fried Chicken Breast	1 pkg (8.88 oz)	360	18	5	0
Green Pepper Steak	1 pkg (10.5 oz)	240	4	2	0
Grilled Chicken Teriyaki	1 pkg (9.38 oz)	300	4	1	0
Grilled Lemon Pepper Chicken	1 pkg (9 oz)	240	8	2	0
Meatloaf	1 pkg (6 oz)	560	29	12	2
Pork Cutlet	1 pkg (10 oz)	370	21	4	1
Roast Pork	1 pkg (9.5 oz)	320	11	3	0
Roast Turkey Breast	1 pkg (16 oz)	390	13	4	0
Salisbury Steak	1 pkg (16 oz)	470	24	8	1
Stuffed Pepper	1 pkg (10 oz)	220	10	4	0
Swedish Meatballs	1 pkg (11.5 oz)	560	27	12	1
Swanson					
Chicken & Dumplings	1 cup	230	10	5	0
Chicken A La King	1 can	270	18	4	0
Tamarind Tree					
Alu Chole	1 pkg (9.25 oz)	320	7	0	–
Channa Dal Masala	1 pkg (9.25 oz)	290	3	0	–
Dal Makhani	1 pkg (9.25 oz)	350	6	2	–
Navratan Korma	1 pkg (9.25 oz)	370	15	4	–
Palak Paneer	1 pkg (9.25 oz)	350	17	7	–
Saag Chole	1 pkg (9.25 oz)	330	9	1	–
Vegetable Jalfrazi	1 pkg (9.25 oz)	280	7	1	–

FOOD	PORTION	CALS	FAT	SAT FAT	TRANS FAT
Taste Above					
Meatless Zesty BBQ w/ Veggie Beef & Rice	1 pkg (10 oz)	280	6	1	0
TastyBite					
Beans Masala & Basmati Rice	1 pkg (12 oz)	426	8	2	0
Green Curry Vegetables & Jasmine Rice	1 pkg (12 oz)	320	10	6	0
Spinach Dal & Basmati Rice	1 pkg (12 oz)	372	9	1	0
Stir Fry Vegetables & Jasmine Rice	1 pkg (12 oz)	450	16	2	0
Vegetable Supreme & Basmati Rice	1 pkg (12 oz)	317	6	1	0
Yellow Curry Vegetables & Jasmine Rice	1 pkg (12 oz)	380	13	8	0
Yves					
Meatless Santa Fe Beef	1 pkg (10.5 oz)	360	9	1	0
DIP					
spinach sour cream	¼ cup	155	15	4	–
Blue Bunny					
Incrediples	2 tbsp	30	1	1	–
Incrediples Taco Fiesta	2 tbsp	30	1	1	–
Spicy Buffalo	2 tbsp	30	1	1	–
Bravos!					
Salsa	2 tbsp	15	0	0	0
Salsa Con Queso	1 tbsp	25	2	0	0
Cabot					
Bac'n Horseradish	2 tbsp	50	5	3	–
Clam	2 tbsp	50	5	3	–
French Onion	2 tbsp	50	5	–	–
Ranch	1 tbsp	50	5	3	–
Salsa Grande	2 tbsp	50	5	3	–
Veggie	2 tbsp	50	5	3	–
Cedarlane					
Organic Five Layer Mexican	2 tbsp	60	3	2	0
Eatsmart					
Flame Roasted Salsa Con Queso	2 tbsp	35	2	0	0
Garden Style Sweet Salsa	2 tbsp	20	0	0	0
Jalapeno & Lime Tres Bean	2 tbsp	25	0	0	0

FOOD	PORTION	CALS	FAT	SAT FAT	TRANS FAT
Fritos					
Bean	2 tbsp	40	1	0	–
Chili Cheese	2 tbsp	45	3	1	–
Hot Bean	2 tbsp	40	1	1	–
Jalapeno Cheddar Cheese	2 tbsp	50	4	1	–
Mild Cheddar	2 tbsp	60	4	2	–
Gringo Billy's					
Guacamole Mix	1 tsp	10	0	0	0
Guiltless Gourmet					
Black Bean Mild	2 tbsp	30	0	0	0
Roasted Red Pepper Salsa	2 tbsp	15	0	0	0
Southwestern Grill Salsa	2 tbsp	15	0	0	0
Marie's					
French Onion Roasted	2 tbsp	100	10	3	0
Guacamole	2 tbsp	40	3	2	0
Honey Vanilla Cream Fruit Dip	2 tbsp	60	5	3	0
Spinach Parmesan	2 tbsp	90	9	3	0
Marzetti					
Veggie Fat Free Ranch	2 tbsp	35	7	0	–
Veggie Dip Light Veggie	1 pkg (3.25 oz)	170	17	3	0
Phillips Seafood					
Crab & Spinach	2 tbsp	50	5	3	0
Maryland Crab	2 tbsp	70	6	4	0
Racquet					
Hot Cheddar Jalapeno	2 tbsp	30	3	1	–
Road's End Organics					
Nacho Cheese Gluten Free	2 tbsp	20	0	0	0
Robert Rothchild Farm					
Artichoke	2 tbsp	60	5	1	0
Ruffles					
French Onion	¼ cup	200	15	3	–
Ranch	2 tbsp	60	5	3	–
Snyder's Of Hanover					
Three Bean	2 tbsp	25	0	0	0
Utz					
Jalapeno Cheddar	2 tbsp	260	4	1	1
Sour Cream & Onion	2 tbsp	60	5	3	0
Walden Farms					
Low Carb Bruschetta	2 tbsp	35	3	–	–
Low Carb Pesto Bruschetta	1 tsp	10	1	–	–

FOOD	PORTION	CALS	FAT	SAT FAT	TRANS FAT
Wise					
French Onion	2 tbsp	60	5	0	0
Nacho Cheese	2 tbsp	50	5	1	2
DOCK					
fresh cooked	3½ oz	20	1	–	
raw chopped	½ cup	15	tr	–	
DOUGHNUTS					
cake type unsugared	1 (1.6 oz)	198	11	2	–
chocolate glazed	1 (1.5 oz)	175	8	3	–
chocolate sugared	1 (1.5 oz)	175	8	3	–
chocolate coated	1 (1.5 oz)	204	13	4	–
creme filled	1 (3 oz)	307	21	6	–
french cruller glazed	1 (1.4 oz)	169	8	2	–
frosted	1 (1.5 oz)	204	13	4	–
honey bun	1 (2.1 oz)	242	14	3	–
jelly	1 (3 oz)	289	16	4	–
old fashioned	1 (1.6 oz)	198	11	2	–
sugared	1 (1.6 oz)	192	10	3	–
wheat glazed	1 (1.6 oz)	162	9	1	–
wheat sugared	1 (1.6 oz)	162	9	1	–
yeast glazed	1 (2.1 oz)	242	14	3	–
Entenmann's					
Crumb	1	260	12	6	0
Frosted Devil's Food	1	310	19	12	0
Glazed	1	260	13	7	0
Glazed Popems	4	220	10	5	0
Mini Frosted	1 (1 oz)	150	11	7	0
Plain Old Fashion	1	230	14	7	0
Rich Chocolate Frosted	1	280	18	12	0
Snack & Smile					
Mini Donuts Chocolate	6	370	19	10	–
Mini Donuts Glazed	6	340	16	40	–
Mini Donuts Powdered Sugar	6	320	13	4	–
Super Bakery					
Daily Donut	1 (2.2 oz)	250	14	3	0
Proballs Slam	1 (1.3 oz)	130	6	3	–
Powdered Baseballs					

FOOD	PORTION	CALS	FAT	SAT FAT	TRANS FAT
DRINK MIXERS					
whiskey sour mix not prep	1 pkg (0.6 oz)	64	0	0	0
whiskey sour mix	2 oz	55	0	0	0
Baja Bob's					
Bloody Mary Mix Lean & Mean	4 oz	20	0	0	0
Pina Colada	4 oz	30	1	0	–
Sugar Free Margarita Mix	4 oz	10	0	0	0
Sugar Free Margarita Mix Desert Lime	4 oz	10	0	0	0
Sugar Free Margarita Mix Wild Strawberry	4 oz	10	0	0	0
Sweet-n-Sour Mix	4 oz	10	0	0	0
McIlhenny					
Bloody Mary Mix as prep	1 cup	70	0	0	0
Ocean Spray					
Bloody Mary Mix	4 oz	40	0	0	0
Margarita Mix	4 oz	160	0	0	0
Sour Mix	4 oz	140	0	0	0
DRUM					
freshwater fillet baked	5.4 oz	236	10	2	–
freshwater baked	3 oz	130	5	1	–
DUCK					
w/ skin roasted	1 cup (4.9 oz)	472	40	14	–
w/ skin w/ bone leg roasted	3 oz	184	10	3	–
w/ skin w/o bone breast roasted	3 oz	172	9	2	–
w/o skin roasted	1 cup (4.9 oz)	281	16	6	–
w/o skin w/ bone leg braised	1 cup (6.1 oz)	310	10	2	–
w/o skin w/o bone breast broiled	1 cup (6.1 oz)	244	4	1	–
wild w/ skin raw	½ duck (9.5 oz)	571	41	14	–
wild w/o skin breast raw	½ breast (2.9 oz)	102	4	1	–
Maple Leaf Farms					
Breast Filet	4 oz	360	33	9	–
Leg Quarters	4 oz	420	33	11	–
Orange Breast Filet	4 oz	320	28	8	–
DUMPLING					
Kahiki					
Potstickers Chicken	5 (3.3 oz)	230	11	2	0

FOOD	PORTION	CALS	FAT	SAT FAT	TRANS FAT
Samosas Coconut Curry Chicken	4 (2.8 oz)	170	3	1	0
Pepperidge Farm					
Apple	1	250	11	3	4
Peach	1	320	11	3	4
Traveling Chef					
Potstickers Chicken + Dipping Sauce	5 pieces + 1 tbsp sauce	285	7	1	0
TAKE-OUT					
bread dumpling	1 lg	330	10	–	–
gyoza potstickers vegetable	8 (4.9 oz)	210	4	1	–
DURIAN					
fresh	3.5 oz	141	2	–	–
EEL					
fresh cooked	1 fillet (5.6 oz)	375	24	5	–
fresh cooked	3 oz	200	13	3	–
raw	3 oz	156	10	2	–
smoked	3.5 oz	330	28	7	–
EGG (*see also* EGG DISHES, EGG SUBSTITUTES)					
CHICKEN					
hard or soft cooked	1	77	5	2	–
pickled	1	72	5	2	–
poached	1	73	5	2	–
scrambled plain	2	199	15	6	–
sunny side up	2	155	12	3	–
white cooked	1	17	tr	0	–
yolk cooked	1	55	4	2	–
Crystal Farms					
In Shell Pasteurized	1	70	5	2	0
Peeled Hard Cooked	1	70	5	2	0
Davidson's					
Pasteurized Shell Eggs	1 lg	75	5	2	0
Egg-Land's Best					
Extra Large	1 (2 oz)	80	5	2	0
Large	1	70	4	1	0
Organic Brown	1	70	4	1	0
Eggology					
100% Organic Egg Whites	¼ cup	30	0	0	0

FOOD	PORTION	CALS	FAT	SAT FAT	TRANS FAT
Gold Circle Farms					
Cage Free	1 large	70	5	2	0
Horizon Organic					
Jumbo	1 (2.2 oz)	90	5	2	0
Land O Lakes					
Farm Fresh Brown Extra Large	1 (1.8 oz)	70	5	2	0
Organic Valley					
Egg Whites Pasteurized	¼ cup	25	0	0	0
Large Omega-3	1	70	5	2	0
Pete And Gerry's					
Organic	1	70	5	1	0
Sunny Fresh					
Eggs ASAP!	2	140	10	3	0
OTHER POULTRY					
duck 100 year old	1 (1 oz)	49	3	–	–
duck cooked	1 (2.5 oz)	129	10	3	–
duck preserved hard core	1 (1.8 oz)	80	6	2	–
duck preserved soft core	1 (1.8 oz)	80	6	2	–
duck salted	1 (1 oz)	54	4	–	–
goose cooked	1 (5 oz)	265	19	5	–
quail canned	1 (0.3 oz)	14	1	tr	–
quail cooked	1 (0.5 oz)	24	2	1	–
turkey raw	1 (2.8 oz)	135	9	3	–
EGG DISHES					
Aunt Jemima					
Eggs & Sausage	1 pkg (6.2 oz)	370	27	9	–
Omelet Ham & Cheese	1 pkg (5.2 oz)	250	15	6	0
Cedarlane					
Zone Omelette Cheese	1 pkg (10.4 oz)	350	14	8	0
TAKE-OUT					
deviled	1 half	62	5	1	–
eggs benedict	2	825	64	30	–
omelet cheese	3 eggs	387	29	11	–
omelet mushroom	3 eggs	251	17	5	–
omelet mushroom & onion	3 eggs	294	20	6	–
omelet plain	3 eggs	338	25	7	–
omelet spanish	3 eggs	496	38	9	–
omelet spinach	3 eggs	279	19	6	–
omelet western	3 eggs	355	23	7	–

FOOD	PORTION	CALS	FAT	SAT FAT	TRANS FAT
salad	½ cup	353	34	6	–
scotch egg	1 (4.2 oz)	301	21	–	–
tortilla de amarillo omelet w/ plantain	3 eggs	536	35	7	–
EGG ROLLS					
egg roll wrapper fresh	1	83	tr	tr	–
Chun King					
Chicken Mini	6	210	9	3	–
Chicken Restaurant Style	1 (3 oz)	190	9	5	–
Pork & Shrimp Mini	6	210	9	3	–
Shrimp Mini	6	190	6	2	–
Shrimp Restaurant Style	1 (3 oz)	180	7	3	–
Frieda's					
Egg Roll Wrappers	2 (1.6 oz)	130	1	0	–
Kahiki					
Chicken	1 (3 oz)	160	6	1	0
Chipotle Lime Chicken	1 (3 oz)	170	4	2	0
Lemongrass Chicken Stix	3 (2.6 oz)	100	2	0	0
Pork & Shrimp	1 (3 oz)	140	4	1	0
Vegetable	1 (3 oz)	90	4	1	0
La Choy					
Chicken Mini	6	210	9	3	–
Chicken Restaurant Style	1 (3 oz)	210	9	5	–
Pork Restaurant Style	1 (3 oz)	220	11	3	–
Pork & Shrimp Bite Size	12	210	10	3	–
Pork & Shrimp Mini	6	210	9	3	–
Shrimp Mini	6	190	6	2	–
Shrimp Restaurant Style	1 (3 oz)	180	7	2	–
Sweet & Sour Chicken Restaurant Style	1 (3 oz)	220	9	2	–
Vegetable w/ Lobster Mini	6	190	7	2	–
Lean Cuisine					
Cafe Classics Vegetable	1 pkg (9 oz)	310	5	1	0
Loompya					
Lumpia Chicken & Vegetables	2	170	1	0	–
Nasoya					
Egg Roll Wrapper	3	170	1	0	–
Pagoda					
Sweet & Sour Chicken	1 (2.7 oz)	170	6	2	–

FOOD	PORTION	CALS	FAT	SAT FAT	TRANS FAT
Phillips					
Spring Rolls Crab & Shrimp w/ Sauce	3 (3.75 oz)	220	7	2	0
TAKE-OUT					
chicken	1 (3 oz)	140	4	2	–
lobster	1 (4.8 oz)	270	7	2	–
lumpia vegetable & shrimp	2 (3 oz)	120	0	0	–
meat & shrimp	1 (4.8 oz)	320	12	3	–
pork & shrimp	1 (5 oz)	300	10	4	–
shrimp	1 (3 oz)	170	5	1	–
spicy pork	1 (3 oz)	200	9	2	–
vegetable	1 (3 oz)	170	4	1	–

EGG SUBSTITUTES

FOOD	PORTION	CALS	FAT	SAT FAT	TRANS FAT
Better'n Eggs					
All Whites	¼ cup	30	0	0	0
Ham & Cheese	¼ cup	45	2	1	0
Original	¼ cup (2 oz)	30	0	0	0
Plus	¼ cup	35	0	0	0
Three Cheese	¼ cup	45	1	1	0
Bob's Red Mill					
Egg White Dried	2 tsp	15	0	0	0
Vegetarian Egg Replacer	1 tbsp	30	1	0	0
Deb-El					
Just Whites	2 tsp	12	0	0	0
Egg Beaters					
Original	¼ cup	30	0	0	0
EggPro					
Powder	1 tbsp	15	0	0	0
Fantastic					
Tofu Scrambler not prep	1 tbsp	35	0	0	0
Horizon Organic					
Liquid Egg	¼ cup	35	0	0	0
Land O Lakes					
Liquid Egg	¼ cup	30	0	0	0
Quick Eggs					
Fat Free Cholesterol Free	¼ cup	30	0	0	0

EGGNOG

FOOD	PORTION	CALS	FAT	SAT FAT	TRANS FAT
eggnog	1 cup	342	19	11	–
eggnog	1 qt	1368	76	45	–

FOOD	PORTION	CALS	FAT	SAT FAT	TRANS FAT
eggnog flavor mix as prep w/ milk	9 oz	260	8	5	–
Farmland					
Egg Nog	½ cup	180	8	5	–
Hood					
Fat Free Sugar Free	1 cup	110	0	0	0
Golden	½ cup	180	9	5	0
Light	½ cup	140	4	3	0
Horizon Organic					
Lowfat	½ cup	140	3	2	0
Organic Valley					
Ultra Pasteurized	½ cup	180	10	6	0
TAKE-OUT					
eggnog	1 cup	306	22	14	–

EGGNOG SUBSTITUTES
Silk

FOOD	PORTION	CALS	FAT	SAT FAT	TRANS FAT
Nog	½ cup	90	2	0	–

EGGPLANT

FOOD	PORTION	CALS	FAT	SAT FAT	TRANS FAT
cubed cooked w/ oil	1 cup	133	8	1	–
pickled	½ cup	33	tr	tr	–
slices grilled	1 (2 oz)	36	2	tr	–
Cedarlane					
Eggplant Mediterranean	1 pkg (10 oz)	230	10	4	0
Celentano					
Eggplant Parmigiana	1 serv (7 oz)	330	22	5	0
Frieda's					
Chinese	⅔ cup (3 oz)	20	0	0	0
Japanese Nasu	⅔ cup (3 oz)	20	0	0	0
Peloponnese					
Baba Ghanoush	2 tbsp	40	3	0	–
Sabra					
Baba Ghanoush	2 oz	50	6	0	–
Stonewall Kitchen					
Eggplant Spread	1 tbsp	25	1	–	–
TastyBite					
Punjab Eggplant	½ pkg (5 oz)	144	9	1	0
TAKE-OUT					
baba ghannouj	¼ cup	55	4	–	–
caponata	2 tbsp (1 oz)	30	2	–	–

FOOD	PORTION	CALS	FAT	SAT FAT	TRANS FAT
iman bayildi eggplant w/ onion & tomato	1 serv (15.6 oz)	345	28	4	–
indian eggplant runi	1 serv	180	14	4	–
moussaka	1 serv (9 oz)	372	24	6	–
papoutsaki little shoes	1 serv (15.5 oz)	245	16	7	–

ELDERBERRIES

fresh	1 cup	105	1	–	–

ELDERBERRY JUICE

elderberry	7 oz	76	0	0	0

ELK

eye of round roasted	3.5 oz	151	3	1	tr
ground cooked	3.5 oz	143	3	1	tr

ENERGY BARS (see also CEREAL BARS, NUTRITION SUPPLEMENTS)
Activex

Organic All Flavors	1 (1.6 oz)	200	12	3	0

All In One

All Flavors	1 (1.8 oz)	180	5	4	–

Amino Vital

Fit Apple Pie	1 (1.76 oz)	150	2	2	0
Fit Chocolate Peanut	1 (1.76 oz)	190	8	4	0
Fit Toasted Nut Cranberry	1 (1.76 oz)	180	8	5	0

Atkins

Advantage Almond Brownie	1 (1.6 oz)	220	8	4	–
Advantage Chocolate Coconut	1 (1.6 oz)	230	11	8	–
Advantage Chocolate Decadence	1 (1.6 oz)	220	11	7	–
Advantage Chocolate Mocha Crunch	1 (1.6 oz)	220	10	6	–
Advantage Chocolate Peanut Butter	1 (1.6 oz)	240	12	6	–
Advantage Cookies 'N Creme	1 (1.6 oz)	220	11	7	–
Advantage S'mores	1 (1.6 oz)	220	10	5	–
Morning Start Apple Crisp	1 bar	170	9	4	–
Morning Start Blueberry Muffin	1 bar	160	7	4	–
Morning Start Chocolate Chip Crisp	1 bar	160	7	3	–

FOOD	PORTION	CALS	FAT	SAT FAT	TRANS FAT
Attune					
Wellness Chocolate Crisp	1 (0.7 oz)	100	6	4	0
Wellness Cool Mint Chocolate	1 (0.7 oz)	100	6	4	0
Balance					
Big Bar Honey Peanut	1 bar	310	10	4	–
Chocolate Banana + Antioxidants	1 bar	200	6	4	–
Chocolate Mint + Antioxidants	1 bar	200	6	4	–
Gold Caramel Nut Blast	1 bar	210	7	4	–
Gold Chocolate Peanut Butter	1 bar	210	7	4	–
Gold Crunch Chocolate Chocolate	1 bar	210	6	4	–
Gold Crunch Chocolate Mint Cookie	1 bar	210	6	4	–
Gold Crunch S'mores	1 bar	210	7	4	–
Gold Rocky Road	1 bar	210	7	4	–
Gold Triple Chocolate Chaos	1 bar	200	6	4	–
Honey Peanut + Ginseng	1 bar	200	6	3	–
Lemon Meringue + Calcium	1 bar	190	6	3	–
Original Almond Brownie	1 bar	200	6	2	–
Original Chocolate	1 bar	200	6	4	–
Original Chocolate Raspberry Fudge	1 bar	200	6	3	–
Original Honey Peanut	1 bar	200	6	3	–
Original Mocha Chip	1 bar	200	6	4	–
Original Peanut Butter	1 bar	200	6	3	–
Original Yogurt Honey Peanut	1 bar	200	6	3	–
Outdoor Chocolate Crisp	1 bar	200	6	2	–
Outdoor Crunchy Peanut	1 bar	200	6	1	–
Outdoor Honey Almond	1 bar	200	6	1	–
Outdoor Nut Berry	1 bar	200	6	1	–
Satisfaction Apple Cinnamon Oatmeal	1 bar	280	5	4	–
Satisfaction Chocolate Crisp	1 bar	280	6	4	–
Satisfaction Chocolate Peanut	1 bar	280	6	4	–
Satisfaction Peanut Butter Crisp	1 bar	280	6	4	–
Yogurt Berry + Antioxidants	1 bar	200	6	3	–
Be Natural					
Almond & Apricot	1 bar	218	14	7	–

FOOD	PORTION	CALS	FAT	SAT FAT	TRANS FAT
Almond & Coconut	1 bar	248	18	6	–
Banana & Wheat Bran	1 bar	201	9	8	–
Fruit & Nut Delight	1 bar	225	14	2	–
Macadamia & Apricot	1 bar	224	15	8	–
Nut Delight	1 bar	266	20	3	–
Sesame Nut Split	1 bar	256	17	2	–
Walnut & Date	1 bar	147	9	1	–
Yogurt Coated Almond & Apricot	1 bar	233	14	3	–
Yogurt Coated Fruit & Nut	1 bar	190	12	1	–
Belly-bar					
Baby Needs Chocolate	1 bar	170	6	3	0
Berry Nutty Cravings	1 bar	170	4	1	0
Mellow Oat	1 bar	180	5	2	0
Boomi Bar					
Almond Protein Plus	1	270	18	1	–
Cashew Almond Delicacy	1	260	17	2	–
Cranberry Apple	1	210	9	1	–
Merry Macadamia	1	220	14	2	–
Pistachio Pineapple	1	200	9	2	–
Boost					
Chocolate Crunch	1 (1.5 oz)	190	7	4	–
Bora Bora					
Organic Cranberry Crunch	1 (1.4 oz)	170	10	2	0
Organic Peanut Peanut	1 (1.4 oz)	230	17	3	0
Organic Sesame Raisin	1 (1.4 oz)	170	11	2	0
Carb Options					
Chocolate Chip	1 bar	200	8	4	–
Chocolate Peanut	1 bar	200	8	4	–
Cinnamon Delight	1 bar	200	8	4	–
CarbWise					
Chocolate S'Mores Crunch	1 bar	240	9	6	–
Choice					
Berry Almond Crispy	1 bar	50	1	0	–
Fudge Brownie	1 bar	140	5	3	–
Peanut Butter Crispy	1 bar	60	2	2	–
Peanutty Chocolate	1 bar	140	5	3	–
Clif					
Banana Nut Bread	1 (2.4 oz)	250	6	1	0
Builders Chocolate Mint	1 (2.4 oz)	270	8	5	0

FOOD	PORTION	CALS	FAT	SAT FAT	TRANS FAT
Builders Peanut Butter	1 (2.4 oz)	270	8	5	0
Carrot Cake	1 (2.4 oz)	240	4	2	0
Chocolate Brownie	1 (2.4 oz)	240	5	2	0
Chocolate Chip	1 (2.4 oz)	250	5	2	0
Cool Mint Chocolate	1 (2.4 oz)	250	5	2	0
Crunchy Peanut Butter	1 (2.4 oz)	250	6	2	0
Mojo Mixed Nuts	1 (1.6 oz)	220	9	2	0
Mojo Mountain Mix	1 (1.6 oz)	200	8	2	0
Nectar Cinnamon Pecan	1 (1.6 oz)	170	9	1	0
Nectar Lemon Vanilla Cashew	1 (1.6 oz)	180	6	1	0
Oatmeal Raisin Walnut	1 (2.4 oz)	240	5	1	0
ZBar Peanut Butter	1 (1.3 oz)	140	5	1	0
Deliciously Slim					
Chocolate Fudge Cake	1 (2.1 oz)	200	6	3	–
Ensure					
All Flavors	1 (2.1 oz)	230	6	4	–
Fast Fuel Up					
Natural Chocolate Crunch	1 (2.3 oz)	300	19	7	–
Natural Chocolate Espresso	1 (2.3 oz)	300	19	7	–
Organic Chocolate Crunch	1 (1.8 oz)	230	15	6	–
Organic Chocolate Espresso	1 (1.8 oz)	230	15	5	–
Gatorade					
All Flavors	1 (2.3 oz)	260	5	1	–
GeniSoy					
Soy Protein Southern Style Chunky Peanut Butter Fudge	1 (2.2 oz)	240	6	3	–
Soy Protein Ultimate Chocolate Fudge Brownie	1 (2.2 oz)	230	5	3	–
Glucerna					
All Flavors	1 (0.7 oz)	80	3	1	0
Gnu					
Flavor & Fiber Banana Walnut	1 (1.4 oz)	130	3	1	0
Flavor & Fiber Orange Cranberry	1 (1.4 oz)	130	3	0	0
Hi-Lo					
Chocolate Caramel	1 (1.76 oz)	200	8	5	–
Chocolate Mint	1 (2.1 oz)	200	6	4	–
Chocolate Peanut Butter	1 (2.1 oz)	210	7	4	–
Chocolate Raspberry	1 (2.1 oz)	200	6	3	–

FOOD	PORTION	CALS	FAT	SAT FAT	TRANS FAT
Hooah!					
Chocolate Crisp	1 (2.29 oz)	280	9	5	0
Ideal					
Mixed Berry Tart	1 (1.7 oz)	200	7	3	–
JojoBar					
Chocolate Cashew	1 (1.8 oz)	220	14	5	0
Peanut Butter & Jelly	1 (1.8 oz)	220	13	4	0
Kashi					
GoLean Chocolate Almond Toffee	1 (2.7 oz)	290	6	5	0
GoLean Cookies 'N Cream	1 (2.7 oz)	290	6	4	0
GoLean Malted Chocolate Chip	1 (2.7 oz)	290	6	4	0
GoLean Oatmeal Raisin Cookie	1 (2.7 oz)	280	5	3	0
GoLean Peanut Butter & Chocolate	1 (2.7 oz)	290	6	5	0
GoLean Crunchy Chocolate Peanut	1 (1.8 oz)	180	5	2	0
GoLean Roll Caramel Peanut	1 (1.9 oz)	200	5	2	0
GoLean Roll Fudge Sundae	1 (1.9 oz)	190	5	2	0
TLC Chewy Granola Cherry Dark Chocolate	1 (1.2 oz)	120	2	1	0
TLC Crunchy Granola Honey Toasted 7 Grain	1 (1.4 oz)	180	6	1	0
TLC Crunchy Granola Pumpkin Spice	1 (1.4 oz)	180	6	1	0
TLC Crunchy Granola Roasted Almond	1 (1.4 oz)	180	6	1	0
LaraBar					
Apple Pie	1	190	9	1	0
Banana Cookie	1	210	10	0	0
Cashew Cookie	1	230	13	3	0
Cherry Pie	1	190	9	0	0
Chocolate Coconut Chew	1	220	12	2	0
Ginger Snap	1	220	13	1	0
Jocolat	1 (1 oz)	110	6	1	0
Living Harvest					
Organic Hemp Protein Forbidden Fruit	1 (1.6 oz)	170	6	1	0
Luna					
Caramel Nut Brownie	1 (1.7 oz)	190	6	3	0

FOOD	PORTION	CALS	FAT	SAT FAT	TRANS FAT
Chai Tea	1 (1.7 oz)	180	4	3	0
Dulce De Leche	1 (1.7 oz)	180	3	1	0
Iced Oatmeal Raisin	1 (1.7 oz)	180	4	3	0
Key Lime Pie	1 (1.7 oz)	180	4	3	–
LemonZest	1 (1.7 oz)	180	4	3	0
Nutz Over Chocolate	1 (1.7 oz)	180	5	3	0
Met-Rx					
Big 100 Gram Bar Peanut Butter	1 (3.5 oz)	340	4	2	–
Source/One Chocolate Cheesecake	1 (2.1 oz)	160	5	4	–
Momentum					
Chocolate Caramel Nut	1 bar	150	6	3	–
Chocolate Peanut Butter	1 bar	150	6	4	–
Double Chocolate	1 bar	150	6	4	–
Mommy Munchies					
Chocolate Mint	1 (1.8 oz)	180	7	2	0
Cinnamon Bun	1 (1.8 oz)	180	6	3	0
Moto Bar					
Bodacious Banana Split	1 bar	300	6	2	–
Charming Cherry Almond	1 (2.9 oz)	300	6	1	–
Cozy Pumpkin Pie	1 bar	300	6	1	–
Jazzy Peanut Butter & Jelly	1 bar	300	3	1	–
Kooky Cappuccino	1 bar	300	6	1	–
Luscious Lemon Blueberry	1 bar	300	5	1	–
Saucy Apple Cinnamon	1 bar	280	4	1	–
Zany Cranberry Orange	1 bar	300	5	1	–
Mrs. May's					
Trio Blueberry	1 (1.2 oz)	170	12	2	0
Trio Tropical	1 (1.2 oz)	170	12	9	0
Nature's Path					
Optimum Blueberry Flax & Soy	1 (2 oz)	200	3	0	0
Optimum Cranberry Ginger & Soy	1 (2 oz)	200	3	0	0
Optimum Peanut Butter	1 (2 oz)	230	8	1	0
Optimum Pomegran Cherry	1 (2 oz)	230	5	1	0
Optimum ReBound	1 (2 oz)	190	4	1	0
New You					
Chocolate Crisp	1 (1.65 oz)	180	4	3	–

FOOD	PORTION	CALS	FAT	SAT FAT	TRANS FAT
NuGo					
Banana Chocolate Protein	1 bar	190	3	1	–
Blue Berry Boom	1 bar	180	3	2	–
Chocolate Blast	1 bar	180	3	2	–
Coffee Break	1 bar	180	3	2	–
Orange Smoothie Protein	1 bar	190	3	2	–
Peanut Butter Pleaser	1 bar	180	3	2	–
Nutiva					
Organic Flax & Raisin	1 (1.4 oz)	200	15	2	–
Organic Flaxseed Flax Chocolate	1 (1.4 oz)	200	12	2	–
Original Organic Hempseed	1 (1.4 oz)	210	14	2	–
Nutribar					
Chocolate Covered Belgian Chocolate	1 (2.3 oz)	252	8	3	–
Chocolate Covered Caramel	1 (2.3 oz)	261	8	3	–
Chocolate Covered Chocolate Fudge	1 (2.3 oz)	267	8	3	–
Chocolate Covered Hazelnut	1 (2.3 oz)	261	8	3	–
Chocolate Covered Mocha Almond	1 (2.3 oz)	261	8	3	–
Chocolate Covered Peanut	1 (2.3 oz)	262	9	3	–
Yogurt Covered Peach Apricot	1 (2.3 oz)	261	8	3	–
Yogurt Covered Raspberry	1 (2.3 oz)	261	8	3	–
Yogurt Covered Wildberry	1 (2.3 oz)	261	8	3	–
Odwalla					
Berries GoMega	1 bar	220	5	1	0
Carrot	1 bar	220	4	2	0
Choco-walla	1 bar	240	6	2	0
Cranberry C Monster	1 bar	220	3	1	0
Super Protein	1 bar	230	5	2	0
Superfood	1 bar	230	4	2	0
Oh Mama!					
Chocolate Peanut Butter	1 (1.8 oz)	190	6	3	–
Frosted White Lemon	1 (1.8 oz)	180	5	4	–
Frosted White Raspberry	1 (1.8 oz)	180	5	4	–
Peacekeeper					
Nuts About Peace All Flavors	1 (1.4 oz)	180	10	1	–
Perfect 10					
Bliss Apricot	1 (1.8 oz)	215	9	2	0

FOOD	PORTION	CALS	FAT	SAT FAT	TRANS FAT
Bliss Cranberry	1 (1.8 oz)	215	12	3	0
Natural Apricot	1 (1.8 oz)	205	10	1	0
Natural Cranberry	1 (1.8 oz)	164	10	1	0
Natural Lemon	1 (1.8 oz)	210	12	1	0
PermaLean					
Protein Crunch Chocoholic Chocolate	1 (1.8 oz)	170	3	2	–
Protein Crunch Chocolate Raspberry	1 (1.8 oz)	180	2	2	–
Protein Crunch Stark Raving Peanutz	1 (1.8 oz)	180	4	2	–
PowerBar					
Harvest Apple Cinnamon Crisp	1 (2.3 oz)	240	4	1	0
Harvest Chunky Cherry Crunch	1 (2.3 oz)	240	4	1	0
Harvest Peanut Butter Chocolate Chip	1 (2.3 oz)	240	4	1	0
Harvest Strawberry Crunch	1 (2.3 oz)	230	4	1	0
Harvest Dipped Double Chocolate Crisp	1 (2.3 oz)	250	5	3	0
Harvest Dipped Oatmeal Raisin Cookie	1 (2.3 oz)	250	5	2	0
Harvest Dipped Toffee Chocolate Chip	1 (2.3 oz)	250	5	3	0
Performance Apple Cinnamon	1 (2.3 oz)	230	3	1	0
Performance Banana	1 (2.3 oz)	230	3	1	0
Performance Cappuccino	1 (2.3 oz)	230	2	1	0
Performance Chocolate	1 (2.3 oz)	230	2	1	0
Performance Chocolate Peanut Butter	1 (2.3 oz)	240	3	1	0
Performance Cookies & Cream	1 (2.3 oz)	240	4	1	0
Performance Malt Nut	1 (2.3 oz)	230	3	1	0
Performance Oatmeal Raisin	1 (2.3 oz)	230	3	1	0
Performance Peanut Butter	1 (2.3 oz)	230	4	1	0
Performance Strawberry Cream	1 (2.3 oz)	230	2	1	0
Performance Vanilla Crisp	1 (2.3 oz)	230	3	1	0
Performance Wild Berry	1 (2.3 oz)	230	3	1	0
Protein Plus Carb Select Chocolate	1 (2.5 oz)	260	7	4	0

FOOD	PORTION	CALS	FAT	SAT FAT	TRANS FAT
Protein Plus Carb Select Chocolate Caramel Crunch	1 (2.6 oz)	270	11	7	0
Protein Plus Carb Select Chocolate Peanut Butter	1 (2.5 oz)	270	9	4	0
Protein Plus Carb Select Peanut Caramel	1 (2.6 oz)	270	11	7	0
Protein Plus Chocolate Fudge Brownie	1 (2.7 oz)	270	5	3	0
Protein Plus Chocolate Peanut Butter	1 (2.7 oz)	290	5	3	0
Protein Plus Cookies & Cream	1 (2.7 oz)	290	5	4	0
Protein Plus Vanilla Yogurt	1 (2.7 oz)	290	5	4	0
Triple Treat Caramel Peanut Crisp	1 (1.9 oz)	220	5	2	0
Triple Treat Caramel Peanut Fusion	1 (1.9 oz)	230	8	5	0
Triple Treat Chocolate Caramel Fusion	1 (1.9 oz)	230	8	5	0
Triple Treat Chocolate Peanut Butter Crisp	1 (1.9 oz)	220	5	2	0
Prana Bar					
Apricot Goji	1 (1.7 oz)	220	13	2	–
Coconut Acai	1 (1.7 oz)	220	13	2	–
Pear Ginseng	1 (1.7 oz)	220	15	2	–
Pria					
Carb Select Caramel Nut Brownie	1 (1.7 oz)	170	8	5	0
Carb Select Chocolate Mocha Crisp	1 (1.7 oz)	130	6	4	0
Carb Select Chocolate Peanut Butter Crisp	1 (1.7 oz)	130	6	4	0
Carb Select Cookies N' Caramel	1 (1.7 oz)	170	7	4	0
Carb Select Peanut Butter Caramel Nut	1 (1.7 oz)	170	8	5	0
Chocolate Peanut Crunch	1 (1 oz)	110	4	2	0
Complete Nutrition Chocolate Mint Crisp	1 (1.6 oz)	170	6	4	0
Complete Nutrition Chocolate Peanut Butter Crisp	1 (1.6 oz)	170	6	4	0

FOOD	PORTION	CALS	FAT	SAT FAT	TRANS FAT
Complete Nutrition French Vanilla Crisp	1 (1.6 oz)	170	5	4	0
Creme Carmel Crisp	1 (1 oz)	110	3	3	0
Double Chocolate Cookie	1 (1 oz)	110	3	3	0
French Vanilla Crisp	1 (1 oz)	110	3	3	0
Mint Chocolate Cookie	1 (1 oz)	110	4	3	0
Strawberry Shortcake	1 (1 oz)	110	3	3	0
Pure Protein					
Blueberry Cheesecake	1 bar	190	3	2	–
PureFit					
Almond Crunch	1 (2 oz)	230	6	1	0
Peanut Butter Crunch	1 (2 oz)	240	7	2	0
Resource					
Mini Nutrition Bar	1 bar	90	3		–
Revival					
Soy Apple Cinnamon Celebration	1 bar	200	5	4	–
Soy Autumn Frost Low Carb	1 bar	200	5	4	–
Soy Chocolate Raspberry Zing Low Carb	1 bar	200	5	3	–
Soy Chocolate Temptation	1 bar	220	3	1	–
Soy Marshmallow Krunch	1 bar	220	3	1	–
Soy Peanut Butter Chocolate Pal	1 bar	240	5	1	–
Soy Peanut Butter Pal	1 bar	240	5	1	–
Simply Nutrilite					
Sweet & Salty	1 (1.6 oz)	170	6	2	0
Slim-Fast					
Classic Meal Bar Chocolate Cookie Dough	1 bar	220	5	4	0
Classic Meal Bar Milk Chocolate Peanut	1 bar	220	5	3	0
High Protein Granola Bar Chocolate Chip	1 bar	190	6	3	0
High Protein Granola Bar Peanut	1 bar	200	7	3	0
Low Carb Breakfast Bar Apple Cobbler	1 bar	180	6	4	0
Low Carb Breakfast Bar Peanut Butter	1 bar	190	8	4	0

FOOD	PORTION	CALS	FAT	SAT FAT	TRANS FAT
Low Carb Snack Bar Caramel Nut	1 bar	120	5	3	0
Low Carb Snack Bar Coconut Almond	1 bar	120	5	3	0
Low Carb Snack Bar Peanut Butter Crunch	1 bar	120	5	2	0
Optima Meal Bar Apple Crisp	1 bar	180	3	2	0
Optima Meal Bar Caramel Crispy Peanut	1 bar	220	6	4	0
Optima Meal Bar Chewy Granola Trail Mix	1 bar	210	5	1	0
Optima Snack Bar Banana Nut Muffin	1 bar	150	8	1	0
Optima Snack Bar Blueberry Muffin	1 bar	140	57	1	0
Optima Snack Bar Chocolate Peanut Nougat	1 bar	120	4	3	0
Optima Snack Bar Oatmeal Raisin Cookie	1 bar	120	4	2	0
Snickers Marathon					
Chewy Chocolate Peanut	1 (1.9 oz)	210	8	3	0
SoBe					
Milk Chocolate	1 (1.75 oz)	240	14	9	–
Solo GI					
Berry Bliss	1 (1.6 oz)	190	5	3	0
Chocolate Charger	1 (1.6 oz)	190	6	3	0
Mint Mania	1 (1.6 oz)	190	6	3	0
Peanut Power	1 (1.6 oz)	200	7	3	0
South Beach					
Energy Mix	1 pkg (1 oz)	160	13	3	0
SoyJoy					
Fruit & Soy Bar Berry	1 (1.1. oz)	130	5	2	0
Fruit & Soy Bar Mango Coconut	1 (1.1 oz)	140	6	4	0
Fruit & Soy Bar Raisin Almond	1 (1.1 oz)	130	6	2	0
Strive					
Crunchy Chocolate Smores	1 (2.1 oz)	200	9	5	–
T.H.E. Bar					
Granola Raisin	1 (1.8 oz)	200	6	3	0

FOOD	PORTION	CALS	FAT	SAT FAT	TRANS FAT
Think5					
Red Berry	1 (2.5)	240	4	1	0
Red Berry Chocolate Covered	1 (2.8 oz)	290	8	4	0
ThinkPink					
Blueberry Dark Chocolate	1 (2.1 oz)	240	8	4	0
Lemon Burst	1 (2.1 oz)	230	7	4	0
Peanut Butter Caramel	1 (2.1 oz)	230	8	4	0
White Chocolate Raspberry	1 (2.1 oz)	240	8	4	0
Zoe's					
Chocolate Delight	1 (1.7 oz)	190	7	3	0
Chocolate Peanut Butter Bliss	1 (1.7 oz)	200	8	3	0
Heavenly Apple	1 bar	180	5	1	0
Peanut Butter Paradise	1 (1.7 oz)	190	6	1	0

ENERGY DRINKS

FOOD	PORTION	CALS	FAT	SAT FAT	TRANS FAT
1In3Trinity					
Energy Drink	1 can (8.4 oz)	10	0	0	0
Accelerade					
All Flavors	8 oz	80	0	0	0
Amino Vital					
Amino Acid Supplement All Flavors	8 oz	35	0	0	0
Pro Fruit Punch	8 oz	35	0	0	0
Pro Tropic Fruit	8 oz	40	0	0	0
Puredge All Flavors	8 oz	50	0	0	0
AMP					
Energy Drink	1 can (8.4 oz)	120	0	0	0
Arizona					
Diet Green Tea Energy Drinks	8 oz	10	0	0	0
Extreme Energy Shot	1 bottle (8.3 oz)	130	0	0	0
Green Tea Energy Drink	8 oz	100	0	0	0
Pomegranate Lite	8 oz	70	0	0	0
B52					
Zero Sugar Citrus Berry	8 oz	10	0	0	0
Balance					
Chocolate as prep w/ 2% milk	1 serv	310	11	4	–
Vanilla as prep w/ 2% milk	1 serv	310	11	4	–
Bally Blast					
Energy Drink	1 can (8.3 oz)	120	0	0	0
Sugar Free	1 can (8.3 oz)	10	0	0	0

FOOD	PORTION	CALS	FAT	SAT FAT	TRANS FAT
Banzai					
Energy Drink	8 oz	120	0	0	0
Bawls					
Guarana	8 oz	90	0	0	0
Guaranexx Sugar Free	1 bottle (10 oz)	0	0	0	0
Beaver Buzz					
Citrus	1 can	140	0	0	0
Black Hole					
Blueberry	8 oz	100	0	0	0
Citrus	8 oz	110	0	0	0
Bliss					
Energy Drink	1 can (8.4 oz)	110	0	0	0
Low Carb	1 can (8.4 oz)	26	0	0	0
Bloom					
All Flavors	1 can (10.5 oz)	100	0	0	0
Blox					
Black Cherry	8 oz	86	0	0	0
Orange Rush	8 oz	103	0	0	0
Original	8 oz	105	0	0	0
Blu Fuel					
Energy Drink	1 can (10 oz)	133	0	0	0
BooKoo					
Energy Drink	8 oz	110	0	0	0
Shot All Flavors	1 can (5.57 oz)	80	0	0	0
Zero Carb	8 oz	0	0	0	0
Boost					
High Protein Vanilla	8 oz	240	6	–	–
Bossa Nova					
Acai Juice Mango	1 bottle (10 oz)	132	0	0	0
Acai Juice Original	1 bottle (10 oz)	138	1	–	0
Acai Juice Passion Fruit	1 bottle (10 oz)	132	1	–	0
Brain Toniq					
Functional Drink	1 can (8.4 oz)	80	0	0	0
Brain Twist					
Flu & Cold Defense All Flavors	8 oz	70	0	0	0
C1.5					
Extreme	1 can (8.4 oz)	120	0	0	0
Caballo Negro					
Double Kick	8 oz	120	0	0	0
Energy Drink	1 can (8.4 oz)	120	0	0	0

FOOD	PORTION	CALS	FAT	SAT FAT	TRANS FAT
Cascabel					
Energy Drink	1 can (8.4 oz)	110	0	0	0
Sugar Free	1 can (8.4 oz)	10	0	0	0
Cheetah					
Energy Drink	1 can (12 oz)	80	0	0	0
Choice					
Chocolate	1 can (8 oz)	220	10	2	–
Chocolate Fudge Sugar Free	1 pkg (11 oz)	125	3	1	–
French Vanilla Sugar Free	1 pkg (11 oz)	100	3	0	–
Strawberries'n Cream Sugar Free	1 pkg (11 oz)	100	3	0	–
Vanilla	1 can (8 oz)	220	10	2	–
Cintron					
Citrus Mango	8 oz	110	0	0	0
Citrus Mango Sugar Free	8 oz	0	0	0	0
Coca-Cola					
Zero	8 oz	1	0	0	0
Coolah					
Original	8 oz	120	0	0	0
Crunk					
Energy Drink	1 can	120	0	0	0
Cytomax					
Sport Drinks All Flavors	1 bottle (20 oz)	130	0	0	0
Defcon3					
Healthy Energy Soda	1 can (12 oz)	45	0	0	0
Defense					
Effervescent Supplement	1 can	150	0	0	0
Diablo					
Energy Drink	1 can (8.7 oz)	151	0	0	0
DNA Energy					
Low Carb Citrus	8 oz	0	0	0	0
Double Hit					
Maximum Energy Coffee Drink Sugar Free	1 can (12 oz)	0	0	0	0
Emu					
Energy Drink	1 bottle (8.4 oz)	170	0	0	0
EQ Thrist Equalizer					
All Flavors	8 oz	60	0	0	0
Everlast					
High Energy Citrus Blast	1 can (8.3 oz)	140	0	0	0

FOOD	PORTION	CALS	FAT	SAT FAT	TRANS FAT
Freedom					
Energy Drink	1 can (12 oz)	160	0	0	0
Full Throttle					
Energy Drink	8 oz	100	0	0	0
Fury	8 oz	110	0	0	0
Function					
Alternative Energy	8 oz	60	0	0	0
Brainac Carambola Punch	8 oz	60	0	0	0
Urban Detox Citrus Prickly Pear	8 oz	60	0	0	0
Youth Trip Acai Grape	8 oz	60	0	0	0
Fuze					
Energize Blackberry Grape	8 oz	100	0	0	0
Energize Exotic Punch	8 oz	100	0	0	0
Energize Mojo Mango	8 oz	100	0	0	0
Essential Cranberry Grapefruit	8 oz	90	0	0	0
Focus Orange Carrot	8 oz	90	0	0	0
Refresh Banana Colada	8 oz	90	0	0	0
Refresh Mixed Berry	8 oz	90	0	0	0
Refresh Peach Mango	8 oz	90	0	0	0
Replenish Agave Cactus	8 oz	90	0	0	0
Stamina Grape & Aronia Punch	8 oz	80	0	0	0
Vitaboost Citrus Starfruit Punch	8 oz	90	0	0	0
Gatorade					
All Flavors	8 oz	50	0	0	0
Lemonade All Flavors	8 oz	50	0	0	0
Nutrition Shake All Flavors	1 can (11 oz)	370	6	1	–
Rain All Flavors	8 oz	50	0	0	0
X-Factor All Flavors	8 oz	50	0	0	0
GeniSoy					
Soy Protein Shake Chocolate	1 scoop (1.2 oz)	120	0	0	0
Soy Protein Shake Strawberry Banana	1 scoop	130	0	0	0
Soy Protein Shake Vanilla	1 scoop (1.2 oz)	130	0	0	0
Gleukos					
Preformance All Flavors	8 oz	70	0	0	0
Go Fast					
Energy Drink	1 can (8.4 oz)	90	0	0	0
Light	1 can (8.4 oz)	20	0	0	0
Sportsman's	1 can (8.4 oz)	90	0	0	0

FOOD	PORTION	CALS	FAT	SAT FAT	TRANS FAT
Guaraviton					
Energy Drink	8 oz	98	0	0	0
Guayaki					
Organic Empower Mint	8 oz	38	0	0	0
Organic Raspberry Revolution	8 oz	50	0	0	0
Organic Unsweetened	8 oz	15	0	0	0
Guru					
Energy Drink	1 can (8.3 oz)	100	0	0	0
Lite	1 can (8.3 oz)	5	0	0	0
Hansen's					
Energy Peach	8 oz	130	0	0	0
Energy Punch	8 oz	120	0	0	0
Happy Bunny					
Spaz Juice	1 can (8.4 oz)	110	0	0	0
Her Energy					
Pink Lemonade	1 can (8.4 oz)	130	0	0	0
Pink Lemonade Sugar Free	1 can (8.4 oz)	0	0	0	0
Hiball					
All Flavors	1 bottle (10 oz)	10	0	0	0
High Voltage					
Sugar Free	8 oz	5	0	0	0
Hooah!					
Soldier Fuel All Flavors	1 can (12 oz)	160	0	0	0
Hydrive					
All Flavors	1 bottle (11.2 oz)	25	0	0	0
Hype					
Classic Energy	1 can (8.3 oz)	110	0	0	0
Invigor8					
Energy Boost	1 can	110	0	0	0
Nutrition Boost	1 can	110	0	0	0
Iron Energy					
All Flavors	8 oz	90	0	0	0
Jet Set					
Club Soda	1 can (12 oz)	0	0	0	0
Ginger Ale	1 can (12 oz)	150	0	0	0
Original	1 can (12 oz)	105	0	0	0
Tonic Water	1 can (12 oz)	150	0	0	0
KaBoom					
All Flavors	8 oz	105	0	0	0
Krank'd					
All Flavors	1 bottle (16 oz)	80	0	0	0

FOOD	PORTION	CALS	FAT	SAT FAT	TRANS FAT
Liv Naturals					
All Flavors	8 oz	70	0	0	0
Lolli's Pop					
Cheery Energy Drink	1 bottle	170	0	0	0
Passion Stimulating Elixir	1 bottle	140	0	0	0
Marquis Platinum					
Vitality Drink	1 can	30	0	0	0
Mix1					
All Flavors	1 bottle (11 oz)	200	3	0	0
Mr. Re					
Restorative	1 can (11 oz)	80	0	0	0
Natural Ovens					
Ultra Omega Balance	1 tbsp	75	5	0	–
Zesty Flax Energy Mix	1 tbsp	40	2	1	–
New York Minute					
Energy Drink	1 can (8.4 oz)	130	0	0	0
Nexcite					
Herbal Fizz	1 bottle	72	0	0	0
Nitro2Go					
High Energy	1 can	110	0	0	0
High Energy Lite	1 can	20	0	0	0
NOS					
High Performance	8 oz	110	0	0	0
Odwalla					
Berries GoMega	8 oz	160	2	0	0
Mo' Beta	8 oz	150	0	0	0
Super Protein Original	8 oz	190	1	0	0
Superfood	8 oz	130	1	0	0
Wellness	8 oz	150	1	0	0
Peep One					
Erotic Drink	1 can (8.3 oz)	109	tr	–	–
Pickle Juice					
Dill	8 oz	0	0	0	0
Sport	8 oz	7	0	0	0
Pimpjuice					
Energy Drink	1 can (8 oz)	140	0	0	0
PJ Tight	1 can (8 oz)	20	0	0	0
Pink					
Diet	1 can	10	0	0	0

FOOD	PORTION	CALS	FAT	SAT FAT	TRANS FAT
Piranha					
Phunky Fruit Punch	1 can (8.4 oz)	140	0	0	0
Pit Bull					
Energy Drink	1 can (8.4 oz)	110	0	0	0
Sugar Free	1 can (8.4 oz)	0	0	0	0
Power Trip					
Xtreme	1 can (10.5 oz)	140	0	0	0
Powerade					
Arctic Shatter	8 oz	64	0	0	0
Fruit Punch	8 oz	65	0	0	0
Green Squall	8 oz	64	0	0	0
Jagged Ice	8 oz	65	0	0	0
NASCAR Grape	8 oz	64	0	0	0
Olympic Citrus	8 oz	63	0	0	0
Option All Flavors	8 oz	10	0	0	0
PowerBar					
Endurance Sport Drink	1 pkg (0.6 oz)	70	0	0	0
Performance Recovery Drink	1 pkg (0.8 oz)	90	0	0	0
Pure Power					
Energy Drink	1 can (8.4 oz)	110	0	0	0
Shotz	1 can (5.75 oz)	80	0	0	0
Purity Organic					
Acerola Cherry	1 bottle	60	0	0	0
Pomegranate Blueberry	1 bottle	60	0	0	0
Pomegranate Raspberry	1 bottle	60	0	0	0
Rawlings EX2					
Sustained Energy	1 can (8.4 oz)	132	0	0	0
Red Bull					
Energy Drink	1 can (8.3 oz)	110	0	0	0
Sugar Free	1 can	10	0	0	0
Red Eye					
Classic	1 bottle (12 oz)	208	0	0	0
Extreme	1 bottle (12 oz)	140	0	0	0
Gold	1 bottle (12 oz)	208	0	0	0
Passion	1 bottle (12 oz)	149	0	0	0
Platinum	1 bottle (12 oz)	149	0	0	0
Rehab					
Recovery Supplement	1 can (12 oz)	150	0	0	0
RESQ					
Energy Drink	1 can (8 oz)	126	0	0	0

FOOD	PORTION	CALS	FAT	SAT FAT	TRANS FAT
Resurrect					
Daily Detox & Anti-Hangover Elixir	1 can (12 oz)	5	0	0	0
Rip It					
Citrus X	8 oz	130	0	0	0
Citrus X Sugar Free	8 oz	0	0	0	0
Energy Fuel	8 oz	130	0	0	0
Energy Lite	8 oz	0	0	0	0
Rockstar					
Energy Cola	8 oz	120	0	0	0
Energy Drink	8 oz	140	0	0	0
Juiced	8 oz	90	0	0	0
Ronin					
Diet	1 can (16 oz)	15	0	0	0
Original	1 can (16 oz)	180	0	0	0
Rox					
Energy Drink	1 can	110	0	0	0
Zero	1 can	10	0	0	0
Rumba					
Energy Juice	8 oz	120	0	0	0
Simply Nutrilite					
Berry Antioxidant	1 can (8.4 oz)	120	0	0	0
Slim-Fast					
Classic Ready-To-Drink Creamy Milk Chocolate	1 can	220	3	1	0
Classic Ready-To-Drink French Vanilla	1 can	220	3	1	0
High Protein Ready-To-Drink All Flavors	1 can	190	5	2	0
Low Carb Diet Ready-To-Drink All Flavors	1 can	190	9	2	0
Snapple A Day					
Meal Replacement All Flavors	1 bottle (11.5 oz)	210	0	0	0
SoBe					
Adrenaline Rush	1 can (8.3 oz)	140	0	0	0
Black & Blue Berry Brew	8 oz	120	0	0	0
Courage Cherry Citrus	8 oz	110	0	0	0
Drive	8 oz	120	0	0	0
Elixir Cranberry Grapefruit	8 oz	110	0	0	0
Elixir Orange Carrot 3C	8 oz	90	0	0	0

FOOD	PORTION	CALS	FAT	SAT FAT	TRANS FAT
Elixir Pomegranate Cranberry	8 oz	100	0	0	0
Energy	8 oz	120	0	0	0
Fuerte	8 oz	130	0	0	0
Karma	8 oz	120	0	0	0
Lean Diet Citrus	8 oz	5	0	0	0
Long John Lizard's Grape Grog	8 oz	120	0	0	0
Power	8 oz	120	0	0	0
Synergy All Flavors	1 can (11.5 oz)	120	0	0	0
Tsunami	8 oz	110	0	0	0
Wisdom	8.5 oz	110	0	0	0
Zen Blend	8.5 oz	90	0	0	0
Sol Mate					
All Flavors	1 bottle	90	0	0	0
Source Burn					
2	8 oz	130	0	0	0
Energy Drink	8 oz	140	0	0	0
Sugar Free	8 oz	10	0	0	0
Speed Zone					
Energy Drink	1 can (8.4 oz)	110	0	0	0
Steaz					
Organic Fuel	8 oz	90	0	0	0
Stevita					
All Flavors	2 tsp	0	0	0	0
Stewie's					
Domination Serum	1 can (8.45 oz)	110	0	0	0
Mind Erase Elixir	1 can (8.45 oz)	100	0	0	0
Stinger					
All Flavors	1 can (8.4 oz)	130	0	0	0
Sugar Free All Flavors	1 can (8.4 oz)	0	0	0	0
Sum Poosie					
Energy Drink	1 bottle (12 oz)	170	0	0	0
Swing Juice					
Energy Drink	8 oz	60	0	0	0
Tantra					
Erotic	1 can (8.4 oz)	130	0	0	0
The Beast					
Energy Drink	1 can (8.3 oz)	120	0	0	0
Tornado					
Energy Drink	8 oz	110	0	0	0

FOOD	PORTION	CALS	FAT	SAT FAT	TRANS FAT
Vault					
Enegry Drink	8 oz	120	0	0	0
Vipa					
Energy Drink	1 can (12 oz)	0	0	0	0
Who's Your Daddy					
Original	8 oz	110	0	0	0
Sugar Free	8 oz	0	0	0	0
Wide Open Performance					
Energy Drink	1 can (8.3 oz)	120	0	0	0
Wired					
Energy Drink	8 oz	110	0	0	0
Sugar Free	8 oz	5	0	0	0
X 3000 Taurine	8 oz	110	0	0	0
Xcyto					
Sugar Free	1 can (12.5 oz)	10	0	0	0
XL					
Diet	1 can (8.8 oz)	10	0	0	0
Energy Drink	1 can (8.8 oz)	113	0	0	0
XO					
Balance	8 oz	50	0	0	0
Berry	1 bottle	90	0	0	0
Citrus	1 bottle	90	0	0	0
Defense	8 oz	40	0	0	0
Diet	1 bottle	15	0	0	0
Endurance	8 oz	50	0	0	0
Energy	8 oz	40	0	0	0
Essential	8 oz	40	0	0	0
Focus	8 oz	40	0	0	0
Grape	1 bottle	90	0	0	0
Multi-V	8 oz	40	0	0	0
Original	1 bottle	110	0	0	0
Peach	1 bottle	90	0	0	0
Power-C	8 oz	40	0	0	0
Rescue	8 oz	40	0	0	0
Revive	8 oz	50	0	0	0
Stress-B	8 oz	40	0	0	0
Vanilla	1 bottle	90	0	0	0
XS Energy					
Citrus Blast	1 can (8.4 oz)	8	0	0	0
Cranberry Grape	1 can (8.4 oz)	8	0	0	0

FOOD	PORTION	CALS	FAT	SAT FAT	TRANS FAT
Electric Lemon Blast	1 can (8.4 oz)	16	0	0	0
Tropical Blast	1 can (8.4 oz)	8	0	0	0
Xtazy					
All Flavors	1 can	160	0	0	0
YET					
Your Energy Drink	1 can	8	0	0	0
Youth Juice					
Drink	2 oz	10	0	0	0

ENGLISH MUFFIN
READY-TO-EAT

FOOD	PORTION	CALS	FAT	SAT FAT	TRANS FAT
apple cinnamon	1	138	2	tr	–
crumpets	1 (1.5 oz)	80	0	0	0
granola	1	155	1	tr	–
mixed grain	1	155	1	tr	–
plain	1	134	1	tr	–
plain toasted	1	133	1	tr	–
raisin cinnamon	1	138	2	tr	–
sourdough	1	134	1	tr	–
wheat	1	127	1	tr	–
whole wheat	1	134	1	tr	–
Crystal Farms					
English Muffin	1	130	1	0	0
Food For Life					
7 Sprouted Grains	1	160	2	–	–
Ezekiel 4:9 Cinnamon Raisin	1	160	0	0	0
Ezekiel 4:9 Sprouted Grain	1	160	1	–	–
Genesis 1:29 Original	1	180	4	–	–
Pepperidge Farm					
100% Whole Wheat	1	140	2	1	0
Original	1	130	2	1	0
Rudi's Organic Bakery					
MultiGrain w/ Flax	1 (2 oz)	130	1	0	–
Whole Grain Wheat	1 (2 oz)	120	1	0	–
Sara Lee					
Heart Healthy Wheat w/ Honey	1	140	1	1	0
Original w/ Whole Grain	1	140	1	0	0
Thomas'					
100 Calories	1	100	1	0	0
Carb Consider	1	100	2	0	–

FOOD	PORTION	CALS	FAT	SAT FAT	TRANS FAT
Corn	1	150	1	1	0
Hearty Grains 100% Whole Wheat	1	120	1	0	0
Hearty Grains Honey Wheat	1	130	1	0	0
Light Multi-Grain	1	100	2	0	0
Oatmeal & Honey	1	130	1	0	0
Original	1	120	1	0	0
Original Whole Grain	1	130	1	0	0
Raisin Cinnamon	1	140	1	0	0
Sandwich Size Original	1	190	2	0	0
Super Size Multi Grain	1	240	3	0	0
TAKE-OUT					
w/ butter	1 (2.2 oz)	189	6	2	–
w/ cheese & sausage	1 (4 oz)	393	24	10	–
w/ egg cheese & canadian bacon	1 (4.8 oz)	289	13	5	–
w/ egg cheese & sausage	1 (5.8 oz)	487	31	12	–
EPAZOTE					
fresh	1 tbsp (1 g)	tr	0	–	0
fresh sprig	1 (2 g)	1	tr	–	–
EPPAW					
raw	½ cup	75	1	–	–
FALAFEL					
Near East					
Falafel as prep	2½ patties	230	16	2	–
Sabra					
Burger	1 (1.8 oz)	90	3	1	–
VeggieLand					
FalafelBurger	1 (4 oz)	190	6	1	–
TAKE-OUT					
falafel	1 (1.2 oz)	57	3	tr	–
FAT (see also BUTTER, BUTTER SUBSTITUTES, MARGARINE, OIL)					
bacon grease	1 tbsp	116	13	5	–
beef shortening	1 tbsp	115	13	6	–
beef suet	1 oz	242	27	15	–
chicken	1 cup	1846	205	61	–
chicken	1 tbsp	115	13	4	–
cocoa butter	1 tbsp	120	14	8	–

FOOD	PORTION	CALS	FAT	SAT FAT	TRANS FAT
duck	1 tbsp (13 g)	115	13	4	–
goose	1 oz	257	29	2	–
goose	1 tbsp	115	13	4	–
lamb new zealand	1 oz	182	19	10	–
lard	1 cup (205 g)	1849	205	80	–
lard	1 tbsp (13 g)	115	13	5	–
meat pan drippings	½ tbsp	124	14	6	–
nutmeg butter	1 tbsp	120	14	12	–
pork raw	1 oz	230	25	9	0
salt pork	1 cube (1 oz)	215	23	8	0
shortening	1 cup	1812	205	41	–
shortening	1 tbsp	113	13	3	–
turkey	1 tbsp	116	13	4	0
ucuhuba butter	1 tbsp	120	14	12	–
whale blubber	1 oz	244	27	–	–
Crisco					
Shortening	1 tbsp	110	12	3	0
Nebraska Land					
Pork Fatback	0.5 oz	110	11	4	–
Smart Balance					
Shortening	1 tbsp	110	12	4	0
Spectrum					
Organic Shortening	1 tbsp	110	13	6	0
FEIJOA					
fresh	1 (1.75 oz)	25	tr	–	–
puree	1 cup	119	2	–	–
FENNEL					
fresh bulb	1 (8.2 oz)	73	tr	–	0
fresh sliced	1 cup	27	tr	–	0
leaves	1 oz	7	tr	–	–
seed	1 tsp	7	tr	tr	0
stir fried	1 cup	85	6	1	–
FENUGREEK					
seed	1 tsp	12	tr	tr	0
FIBER					
apple fiber	0.5 oz	40	1	–	0
Benefiber					
Supplement	1 pkg (4 g)	20	0	0	0

FOOD	PORTION	CALS	FAT	SAT FAT	TRANS FAT
Choice					
Fiber Burst Lemon Lime	3 pieces	45	1	0	–
Fiber Burst Tropical Fruit	3 pieces	45	1	0	–
Metamucil					
Natural Fiber Regular Flavor	1 rounded tsp (7 g)	25	0	0	0
UniFiber					
Natural Fiber	1 pkg (4 g)	4	0	0	0
Wellements					
Fiber-Psyll	1 scoop (0.5 oz)	55	0	0	0
FIDDLEHEAD FERNS					
fresh	3.5 oz	34	tr	–	–
FIGS					
calimyrna	3 (5.4 oz)	120	0	0	0
canned in heavy syrup	3	75	tr	tr	–
canned in light syrup	3	58	tr	tr	–
canned water pack	3	42	tr	–	–
dried california	½ cup (3.5 oz)	200	1	–	–
dried cooked	½ cup	140	1	tr	–
dried whole	10	477	2	tr	–
fresh	1 med	50	tr	tr	–
Blue Ribbon					
California Figs	1 pkg (1.5 oz)	120	0	0	0
Figamajigs					
Chocolate Covered Bar	1 (1.4 oz)	130	3	2	0
Chocolate Covered Bar w/ Almonds	1 (1.4 oz)	150	4	2	0
Jenny					
Sundried Kalamata	4	120	0	0	0
Trucco					
Kalamata	2	100	0	0	0
FIREWEED					
leaves chopped	1 cup (0.8 oz)	24	1	–	–
FISH (see also individual names, FISH SUBSTITUTES, SUSHI)					
CANNED					
Beach Cliff					
Fish Steaks In Louisiana Hot Sauce	1 can (3.7 oz)	160	7	2	0
Fish Steaks In Mustard Sauce	1 can (3.7 oz)	160	9	2	0

FOOD	PORTION	CALS	FAT	SAT FAT	TRANS FAT
Fish Steaks In Soybean Oil	1 can (3.7 oz)	200	13	3	0
Fish Steaks w/ Hot Green Chilies	1 can (3.7 oz)	160	10	2	0
Fish Steaks w/ Jalapeno Peppers	1 can (3.7 oz)	130	14	4	0
Brunswick					
Fish Steaks In Louisiana Hot Sauce	1 can (3.7 oz)	160	7	2	0
Fish Steaks In Mustard Sauce	1 can (3.7 oz)	160	9	2	0
Fish Steaks In Soybean Oil	1 can (3.7 oz)	200	13	3	0
Fish Steaks In Spring Water	1 can (3.7 oz)	150	8	2	0
Fish Steaks w/ Hot Tabasco Peppers	1 can (3.7 oz)	220	14	4	0
Seafood Snacks Golden Smoked	1 can (3.2 oz)	170	11	2	0
Seafood Snacks In Lemon & Cracked Pepper	1 can (3.2 oz)	160	10	2	0
Seafood Snacks In Louisiana Hot Sauce	1 can (3.2 oz)	140	8	2	0
Seafood Snacks In Teriyaki Sauce	1 can (3.2 oz)	160	8	2	0
Seafood Snacks In Tomato & Basil Sauce	1 can (3.2 oz)	140	8	2	0
Seafood Snacks Kippered	1 can (3.2 oz)	160	9	2	0
Chicken Of The Sea					
Fish Steaks	½ can (2 oz)	70	3	1	–
FROZEN					
breaded fillet	1 (2 oz)	155	7	2	–
sticks	1 stick (1 oz)	76	3	1	–
Gorton's					
Grilled Garlic Butter	1 piece (3.8 oz)	100	3	1	0
Grilled Italian Herb	1 piece (3.8 oz)	100	3	1	0
Ian's					
Fillets	1 (3.4 oz)	260	8	1	–
Fish Stick Allergy Free	5 pieces	190	6	1	0
Fish Sticks	5 pieces	190	6	1	0
Van de Kamp's					
Battered Tenders	4 (4 oz)	210	10	4	0
Crisp & Healthy Breaded Fish Sticks	6 (3.6 oz)	140	1	1	0

FOOD	PORTION	CALS	FAT	SAT FAT	TRANS FAT
Crunchy Fillets	2 (3.5 oz)	230	13	5	0
Sticks	6 (4 oz)	260	13	5	0
TAKE-OUT					
fish cake	1 (4.7 oz)	166	7	2	–
jamaican brown fish stew	1 serv	426	22	5	–
kedgeree	5.6 oz	242	11	–	–
mousse	1 serv (3.5 oz)	185	14	–	–
stew	1 cup (7.9 oz)	157	4	2	–
taramasalata	2 tbsp	124	14	–	–
FISH OIL					
cod liver	1 tbsp	123	14	3	0
herring	1 tbsp	123	14	3	0
menhaden	1 tbsp	123	14	4	0
salmon	1 tbsp	123	14	3	0
sardine	1 tbsp	123	14	4	0
shark	1 oz	270	29	–	–
whale beluga	1 oz	252	28	4	–
whale bowhead	1 oz	252	28	–	–
Cormega					
Omega-E Orange	1 pkg	20	2	1	0
Spectrum					
Cod Liver Oil w/ Lemon	1 tsp	40	5	1	0
FISH PASTE					
fish paste	2 tsp	15	1	–	–
FLAXSEED					
Arrowhead Mills					
Organic	3 tbsp (1 oz)	140	9	1	0
Bob's Red Mill					
Flaxseed Meal	2 tbsp	60	5	0	0
Carringon Farms					
Organic Flax Paks	1 pkg (0.4 oz)	50	5	tr	0
Cracker Flax					
Organic Apple Raisin	1 oz	130	5	0	–
Hodgson Mill					
Milled	2 tbsp	60	5	0	–
FLOUNDER					
FRESH					
cooked	3 oz	99	1	tr	–
cooked	1 fillet (4.5 oz)	148	2	tr	–

FOOD	PORTION	CALS	FAT	SAT FAT	TRANS FAT
FROZEN					
Mrs. Paul's					
Filets Lightly Breaded	1 (2.7 oz)	150	7	4	0
TAKE-OUT					
breaded & fried	3.2 oz	211	11	3	–
stuffed w/ crab	1 piece (7.6 oz)	332	11	2	–
FLOUR					
arrowhead	1 cup	457	tr	tr	0
buckwheat whole groat	1 cup	402	4	1	–
corn masa	1 cup (4 oz)	416	4	1	–
cottonseed lowfat	1 oz	94	tr	tr	–
peanut defatted	1 cup	196	tr	tr	–
peanut lowfat	1 cup	257	13	2	–
potato	1 cup (6.3 oz)	628	1	tr	–
rice brown	1 cup (5.5 oz)	574	4	tr	–
rice white	1 cup (5.5 oz)	578	2	1	–
rye dark	1 cup (4.5 oz)	415	3	tr	–
rye light	1 cup (3.6 oz)	374	1	tr	–
rye medium	1 cup (3.6 oz)	361	2	tr	–
sesame lowfat	1 oz	95	tr	tr	–
triticale whole grain	1 cup (4.6 oz)	439	2	tr	–
white all-purpose	1 cup (4.4 oz)	455	1	tr	–
white bread	1 cup (4.8 oz)	495	2	tr	–
white cake unsifted	1 cup (4.8 oz)	496	1	tr	–
white self-rising	1 cup (4.4 oz)	443	1	tr	–
white unbleached	1 cup (4.4 oz)	455	1	tr	–
whole wheat	1 cup (4.2 oz)	407	2	tr	–
Arrowhead Mills					
Organic Barley	⅓ cup	95	1	0	–
Organic Brown Rice	⅓ cup	130	1	0	0
Organic Kamut	⅓ cup	130	1	0	0
Organic Oat	⅓ cup	120	3	1	0
Organic Rye	¼ cup	110	1	0	0
Organic Spelt	⅓ cup	130	1	0	0
Organic Unbleached White	¼ cup	120	1	0	0
Organic White Rice	⅓ cup	120	0	0	0
Bob's Red Mill					
Brown Rice	¼ cup	140	1	0	0
Corn	¼ cup	160	1	0	0
Graham	¼ cup	120	1	0	0

FOOD	PORTION	CALS	FAT	SAT FAT	TRANS FAT
Kamut Organic	¼ cup	94	1	0	0
Sorghum Sweet White Gluten Free	¼ cup	120	1	0	0
Spelt	¼ cup	120	1	0	0
Whole Wheat	¼ cup	110	1	0	0
Whole Wheat Hard White Organic	¼ cup	120	1	0	0
Domata Living Flour					
Gluten Free Casein Free	¼ cup	110	0	0	0
Gold Medal					
All Purpose	¼ cup (1 oz)	100	0	0	0
Better For Bread	¼ cup (1 oz)	100	0	0	0
Organic All Purpose	¼ cup (1 oz)	100	0	0	0
Self Rising	¼ cup (1 oz)	100	0	0	0
Unbleached	¼ cup (1 oz)	100	0	0	0
Wondra	¼ cup	100	0	0	0
Heckers					
All Purpose Unbleached	¼ cup	100	0	0	0
Whole Wheat	¼ cup	100	1	0	–
Hodgson Mill					
Best For Bread	¼ cup	100	0	0	0
Buckwheat	¼ cup	100	1	0	–
Oat Bran Flour	¼ cup	110	2	1	–
Kentucky Kernel					
Seasoned Flour	4 tsp	36	0	0	0
King Arthur					
All Purpose	¼ cup	110	0	0	0
All Purpose Unbleached	¼ cup	110	0	0	0
Organic White Whole Wheat	¼ cup	100	1	0	0
Organic Whole Wheat	½ cup	110	1	0	0
Organic Artisan	¼ cup	110	0	0	0
Self-Rising	¼ cup	120	0	0	0
White Whole Wheat	¼ cup	100	1	0	0
Whole Wheat	¼ cup	110	1	0	0
La Pina					
Flour	¼ cup (1 oz)	100	0	0	0
Lundberg					
Brown Rice	¼ cup	110	2	0	0
Manitoba Harvest					
Hemp Seed Flour	¼ cup	120	4	0	0

FOOD	PORTION	CALS	FAT	SAT FAT	TRANS FAT
Red Band					
All Purpose	¼ cup (1 oz)	100	0	0	0
Self-Rising	¼ cup (1 oz)	100	0	0	0
Robin Hood					
Whole Wheat	¼ cup (1 oz)	90	1	–	–

FOOD COLORS

blue	1 tsp	0	0	0	0
orange	1 tsp	0	0	0	0
red	1 tsp	tr	0	0	0
yellow	1 tsp	tr	0	0	0

FRENCH BEANS

dried cooked	1 cup	228	1	tr	–

FRENCH FRIES (see POTATOES)

FRENCH TOAST
FROZEN

french toast	1 slice (2 oz)	126	4	1	–
Aunt Jemima					
Cinnamon	2 slices (4 oz)	240	6	2	0
Whole Grain	2 slices (4 oz)	240	6	2	0
Eggo					
Toaster Sticks Original	2	220	6	2	0
Farm Rich					
Original Sticks	5 (4.2 oz)	330	15	2	0
Ian's					
Sticks	5 (3.2 oz)	250	9	2	0
TAKE-OUT					
plain	1 slice	151	7	2	–
sticks	5 (4.9 oz)	513	29	5	–
w/ butter	2 slices	356	19	8	–

FROG LEGS
TAKE-OUT

as prep w/ seasoned flour & fried	1 (0.8)	70	5	–	–

FRUCTOSE
Bob's Red Mill

Fructose	1 tsp	15	0	0	0

FOOD	PORTION	CALS	FAT	SAT FAT	TRANS FAT
Estee					
Fructose	1 tsp	15	0	0	0
Packet	1 pkg	10	0	0	0

FRUIT DRINKS (*see also individual names,* SMOOTHIES, YOGURT DRINKS)
MIX

FOOD	PORTION	CALS	FAT	SAT FAT	TRANS FAT
Bio Fruit					
Mix	1 scoop (8 g)	42	1	–	0
Crystal Light					
LiveActive On The Go	1 pkg	10	0	0	0
Sugar Free All Flavors as prep	1 serv	5	0	0	0
Luna					
Dragonfruit Kiwi	1 pkg	50	0	0	0
Pomegranate Berry	1 pkg	50	0	0	0
South Beach					
Tide Me Over Strawberry Banana	1 pkg	30	0	0	0
Tide Me Over Tropical Breeze	1 pkg	30	0	0	0
Tang					
Orange Strawberry as prep	1 serv (8 oz)	110	0	0	0
Orange Pineapple as prep	1 serv (8 oz)	100	0	0	0
READY-TO-DRINK					
fruit punch	6 oz	87	tr	0	–
After The Fall					
Banana Casablanca	8 oz	150	0	0	0
Mango Montage	8 oz	150	0	0	0
Apple & Eve					
100% Cranberry Apple Juice	8 oz	100	0	0	0
Mango Mangosteen	8 oz	120	0	0	0
Brazsoy					
Fruit Juice w/ Soy	8 oz	94	1	0	0
Capri Sun					
Fruit Punch	1 pkg (7 oz)	90	0	0	0
Ceres					
Cranberry & Kiwi	8 oz	110	0	0	0
Medley	8 oz	130	0	0	0
Youngberry	8 oz	120	0	0	0
Champion Lyte					
All Flavors	1 bottle	0	0	0	0

FOOD	PORTION	CALS	FAT	SAT FAT	TRANS FAT
Crayons					
Kiwi Strawberry	1 bottle (12 oz)	130	0	0	0
Outrageous Orange Mango	1 bottle (12 oz)	140	0	0	0
Redder Than Ever Fruitpunch	1 bottle (12 oz)	130	0	0	0
Crystal Light					
Strawberry Kiwi Sugar Free	8 oz	5	0	0	0
Essn					
Sparkling Blood Orange & Cranberry	1 can (8.4 oz)	160	0	0	0
Feel Good Drinks					
Spritz Cranberry & Lime No Sugar Added	1 bottle	159	tr	–	–
Spritz Orange & Passionfruit No Sugar Added	1 bottle	151	tr	–	–
Spritz Pink Citrus No Sugar Added	1 bottle	159	tr	–	–
Firefly					
Chill Out De-stress Drink	1 bottle (11.2 oz)	100	0	0	0
De-tox Morning After Drink	1 bottle (11.2 oz)	104	0	0	0
Five Alive					
Citrus	8 oz	120	0	0	0
Fizz Ed.					
Pomegranate Cherry	1 can (8.4 oz)	90	0	0	0
Frutzzo					
Organic 100% Juice Pomegranate Passionfruit	1 bottle (12 oz)	140	0	0	0
Organic 100% Juice Pomegranate Acai	1 bottle (12 oz)	140	0	0	0
Hansen's					
Fruit Punch 100% Juice	1 box (4.23 oz)	60	0	0	0
Hawaiian Punch					
Bodacious Berry	8 oz	110	0	0	0
Fruit Juicy Red	8 oz	80	0	0	0
Green Berry Rush	8 oz	120	0	0	0
Mazin Melon Mix	8 oz	110	0	0	0
Tropical Vibe	8 oz	110	0	0	0
Wild Purple Smash	8 oz	110	0	0	0
Hog Wash					
All Flavors	1 bottle (10 oz)	37	0	0	0

FOOD	PORTION	CALS	FAT	SAT FAT	TRANS FAT
Hood					
Fruit Punch	1 cup	120	0	0	0
Juici					
Sparkling All Flavors	1 bottle (12 oz)	105	0	0	0
Juicy Juice					
Harvest Surprise Orange Mango	8 oz	130	0	0	0
Harvest Surprise Tropical	8 oz	100	0	0	0
Kagome					
Burgundy Berry Blossom	8 oz	100	0	0	0
Golden Peach Garden	8 oz	100	0	0	0
Orange Carrot Blossom	8 oz	100	0	0	0
Purple Roots & Fruits	8 oz	130	0	0	0
L&A					
Pineapple Coconut	8 oz	140	3	3	–
Lakewood					
Lean Green	6 oz	90	0	0	0
Organic Acai Amazon Berry	6 oz	95	3	0	0
Minute Maid					
Berry Kiwi	1 can (12 oz)	160	0	0	0
Cranberry Grape	8 oz	150	0	0	0
Light Mango Tropical	8 oz	5	0	0	0
Light Orange Tangerine	8 oz	15	0	0	0
Orange Tangerine	8 oz	110	0	0	0
Pomegranate Blueberry 100% Juice	8 oz	120	1	–	0
Tropical Punch Chilled	8 oz	110	0	0	0
Naked Juice					
Berry Blast	8 oz	120	0	0	0
Blue Machine	8 oz	170	1	1	0
Green Machine	8 oz	130	0	0	0
Mango Acai	8 oz	190	3	1	0
Power C	8 oz	120	1	0	0
Protein Zone	8 oz	210	4	2	0
Red Machine	8 oz	160	3	0	0
Strawberry Banana C	8 oz	120	0	0	0
Very Berry	8 oz	130	0	0	0
Very Pro Berry	8 oz	190	1	0	0
Well Being	8 oz	140	0	0	0

FOOD	PORTION	CALS	FAT	SAT FAT	TRANS FAT
Nantucket Nectars					
Organic Banana Mango Carrot	8 oz	120	0	0	0
Organic Blueberry Banana	8 oz	120	0	0	0
Organic Cranberry Orange	8 oz	130	0	0	0
Peach Orange	8 oz	130	0	0	0
Pomegranate Pear	8 oz	110	0	0	0
Newman's Own					
Orange Mango Tango	8 oz	150	0	0	0
Noble					
Organic 100% Juice Orange Tangerine	8 oz	120	0	0	0
Northland					
Cranberry Blueberry	1 cup (8 oz)	140	0	0	0
NutraShake					
Fruit Punch Plus Fiber	1 pkg (8 oz)	120	0	0	0
Ocean Spray					
Citrus Splash Spritzer	8 oz	160	0	0	0
Cran*Grape	8 oz	170	0	0	0
Cran*Raspberry	8 oz	140	0	0	0
Cran*Strawberry	8 oz	140	0	0	0
Cranapple	8 oz	160	0	0	0
Kiwi Strawberry	8 oz	120	0	0	0
Mandarin Magic	8 oz	120	0	0	0
Orange Citrus Spritzer	8 oz	160	0	0	0
Ruby Tangerine	8 oz	120	0	0	0
White Cranberry Apple Juice	8 oz	120	0	0	0
Wildberry Spritzer	8 oz	160	0	0	0
Odwalla					
Quenchers AntioxiDance	8 oz	90	0	0	0
Quenchers B Berrier	8 oz	120	0	0	0
Old Orchard					
100% Juice Pomegranate Black Currant	8 oz	130	0	0	0
100% Juice Pomegranate Cherry	8 oz	140	0	0	0
Cocktail Apple Passion Mango	8 oz	120	0	0	0
Healthy Balance Apple Kiwi Strawberry	8 oz	30	0	0	0
Phat Phruit					
Peach Mango	8 oz	40	0	0	0
Pineapple Orange	8 oz	40	0	0	0

FOOD	PORTION	CALS	FAT	SAT FAT	TRANS FAT
Purity Organic					
Citrus Punch	8 oz	123	tr	–	–
Sabor Latino					
Guava Mango Drink	1 box (7 oz)	110	0	0	0
Nectar Strawberry Banana + Calcium	8 oz	150	0	0	0
Pina Colada	8 oz	130	0	0	0
Snapple					
Cranberry Raspberry	8 oz	120	0	0	0
Diet Carrot Apple	8 oz	10	0	0	0
Diet Plum-A-Granate	8 oz	0	0	0	0
Go Bananas	8 oz	120	0	0	0
Kiwi Strawberry	8 oz	110	0	0	0
Snapricot Orange	8 oz	120	0	0	0
Soy20					
All Flavors	1 bottle (12 oz)	90	0	0	0
SSips					
Cherry Berry	1 box (7 oz)	110	0	0	0
Sun Shower					
100% Juice Nectarine Mango	8 oz	93	0	0	0
Sundia					
Tropical Medley	½ cup	70	0	0	0
Tree Ripe					
Organic Fruit Punch	8 oz	150	0	0	0
TreeTop					
Apple Grape No Sugar Added	8 oz	130	0	0	0
Tropicana					
Fruit Punch	1 cup	130	0	0	0
Light Fruit Punch	8 oz	10	0	0	0
Orange Tangerine Juice	8 oz	110	0	0	0
Orchard Berry	8 oz	110	0	0	0
Organic Orchard Medley	8 oz	120	0	0	0
Twister Berry Blast	8 oz	120	0	0	0
Twister Citrus Spark	8 oz	120	0	0	0
Twister Fruit Fury	8 oz	120	0	0	0
Twister Light Strawberry Spiral	8 oz	40	0	0	0
V8					
Fusion Pomegranate Blueberry	8 oz	100	0	0	0
Light Peach Mango	8 oz	50	0	0	0
Splash Berry Blend	8 oz	70	0	0	0

FOOD	PORTION	CALS	FAT	SAT FAT	TRANS FAT
Splash Diet Berry Blend	8 oz	10	0	0	0
Splash Mango Peach	8 oz	80	0	0	0
Vruit					
Apple Carrot	1 box (8.45 oz)	120	0	0	0
Berry Veggie	1 box (8.45 oz)	110	0	0	0
Orange Veggie	1 box (8.45 oz)	110	1	–	–
Tropical Blend	1 box (8.45 oz)	110	0	0	0
Wadda Juice					
All Flavors	1 bottle (4 oz)	25	0	0	0
Walnut Acres					
Organic Orange Carrot	8 oz	110	0	0	0
Welch's					
White Grape Peach 100% Juice	8 oz	160	1	0	0

FRUIT MIXED (see also individual names)
CANNED

FOOD	PORTION	CALS	FAT	SAT FAT	TRANS FAT
fruit cocktail in heavy syrup	½ cup	93	tr	tr	–
fruit cocktail juice pack	½ cup	56	tr	tr	–
fruit cocktail water pack	½ cup	40	tr	tr	–
fruit salad in heavy syrup	½ cup	94	tr	tr	–
fruit salad in light syrup	½ cup	73	tr	tr	–
fruit salad juice pack	½ cup	62	tr	tr	–
fruit salad water pack	½ cup	37	tr	tr	–
mixed fruit in heavy syrup	½ cup	92	tr	tr	–
tropical fruit salad in heavy syrup	½ cup	110	tr	–	–
Del Monte					
Carb Clever Fruit Cocktail	½ cup	40	0	0	0
Fruit Cocktail In 100% Juice	½ cup	60	0	0	0
Fruit Cocktail In Extra Light Syrup	½ cup	60	0	0	0
Fruit Cocktail In Heavy Syrup	½ cup	100	0	0	0
Fruit Cup Mixed In Extra Light Syrup	1 pkg (4 oz)	50	0	0	0
Fruit Naturals Tropical Medley	½ cup	70	0	0	0
Orchard Select Premium Mixed	½ cup	80	0	0	0
Snack Cups Strawberry Banana Peaches	1 pkg	70	0	0	0
SunFresh Citrus Salad	½ cup	80	0	0	0

FOOD	PORTION	CALS	FAT	SAT FAT	TRANS FAT
Dole					
Tropical Fruit Salad	½ cup	80	0	0	0
Liberty Gold					
Fruit Cocktail In Heavy Syrup	½ cup	90	0	0	0
DRIED					
mixed	11 oz pkg	712	1	tr	–
Goodniks					
Fruit Medley	¼ cup	110	2	2	0
Mariani					
Berries 'N Cherries	¼ cup	140	0	0	0
Sun-Maid					
Mixed	¼ cup	100	0	0	0
Sunsweet					
Berry Blend	¼ cup (1.4 oz)	120	0	0	0
Orchard Mix	¼ cup (1.4 oz)	100	0	0	0
Tropical Mix	⅓ cup	150	0	0	0
FROZEN					
mixed fruit sweetened	1 cup	245	tr	tr	–
FRUIT SNACKS					
fruit leather	1 bar (0.8 oz)	81	1	1	–
fruit leather pieces	1 oz	97	2	tr	–
fruit leather pieces	1 pkg (0.9 oz)	92	2	tr	–
fruit leather rolls	1 lg (0.7 oz)	73	1	tr	–
fruit leather rolls	1 sm (0.5 oz)	49	tr	tr	–
Bare Fruit					
Bananas & Cherries	1 pkg (0.6 oz)	55	1	0	0
Betty Crocker					
Fruit By The Foot All Flavors	1 roll	80	2	–	–
Funky Monkey					
Bananamon	1 pkg (1 oz)	110	0	0	0
Carnaval Mix	1 pkg (1 oz)	110	0	0	0
Jivealime	1 pkg (1 oz)	110	0	0	0
Purple Funk	1 pkg (1 oz)	120	1	0	0
Peeled Snacks					
Fruit & Nuts FigSated	⅓ cup	150	6	1	0
Fruit & Nuts Plu-what?	⅓ cup	150	6	1	0
Sharkies					
Organic Energy Fruit Chews All Flavors	1 pkg (1.8 oz)	170	0	0	0

FOOD	PORTION	CALS	FAT	SAT FAT	TRANS FAT
Stretch Island					
Fruit Leather Bountiful Blueberry	1 pkg (0.5 oz)	45	0	0	0
Fruit Leather Harvest Grape	1 pkg (0.5 oz)	45	0	0	0
Fruit Leather Mango Sunrise	1 pkg (0.5 oz)	45	0	0	0
Fruit Leather Truly Tropical	1 pkg (0.5 oz)	45	0	0	0
Organic Smooshed Fruit Apple	1 piece (0.4 oz)	40	0	0	0
Organic Smooshed Fruit Strawberry	1 piece (0.4 oz)	40	0	0	0
Tropicana					
Fruit Wise Bars All Flavors	1 (1.4 oz)	140	0	0	0
Fruit Wise Strips All Flavors	1 strip (0.7 oz)	70	0	0	0
Welch's					
White Grape Peach	20 pieces	110	0	0	0

GARLIC

FOOD	PORTION	CALS	FAT	SAT FAT	TRANS FAT
clove	1	4	tr	tr	–
fresh chopped	1 tbsp	18	tr	tr	–
powder	1 tsp	9	tr	tr	–
Dorot					
Crushed Cubes frzn	1 cube (4 g)	7	tr	tr	0
Frieda's					
Elephant	1 tbsp	5	0	0	0
Vinegar Marinated	1 oz	30	0	0	0
McCormick					
Garlic Salt	¼ tsp	0	0	0	0

GEFILTE FISH

FOOD	PORTION	CALS	FAT	SAT FAT	TRANS FAT
sweet	1 piece (1.5 oz)	35	1	tr	–
Mrs. Adler's					
Pike'n Whitefish	1 piece (1.8 oz)	50	1	0	–

GELATIN
READY-TO-EAT
Del Monte

FOOD	PORTION	CALS	FAT	SAT FAT	TRANS FAT
Mandarin Orange In Lite Orange Gel	1 pkg (4.5 oz)	60	0	0	0
Mixed Fruit In Cherry Gel	1 pkg (4.5 oz)	90	0	0	0
Peaches In Peach Gel	1 pkg (4.5 oz)	90	0	0	0
Peaches In Raspberry Gel	1 pkg (4.5 oz)	90	0	0	0

FOOD	PORTION	CALS	FAT	SAT FAT	TRANS FAT
Peaches In Lite Strawberry Banana Gel	1 pkg (4.5 oz)	60	0	0	0
Hunt's					
Snack Pack Juicy Gels Raspberry Mixed Berry	1 serv (3.5 oz)	100	0	0	0
Snack Pack Juicy Gels Strawberry	1 serv (3.5 oz)	100	0	0	0
Snack Pack Juicy Gels Strawberry Orange	1 serv (3.5 oz)	100	0	0	0
Snack Pack Tropical Punch	1 serv (3.5 oz)	100	0	0	0
Jell-O					
Sugar Free Tropical Berry	1 serv (3.2 oz)	10	0	0	0
Kozy Shack					
Gel Treats Cherry	1 pkg (4 oz)	85	0	0	0
Gel Treats Lemon Lime	1 pkg (4 oz)	85	0	0	0
Gel Treats Orange	1 pkg (4 oz)	85	0	0	0
Gel Treats Strawberry	1 pkg (4 oz)	85	0	0	0
Gel Treats Sugar Free Orange	1 pkg (4 oz)	11	0	0	0
Gel Treats Sugar Free Strawberry	1 pkg (4 oz)	11	0	0	0
GIBLETS					
capon simmered	1 cup (5 oz)	238	8	3	–
chicken fried	1 cup (5 oz)	402	20	6	–
chicken simmered	1 cup (5 oz)	289	17	6	0
turkey simmered	1 cup (5 oz)	243	7	2	–
GINGER					
ground	1 tsp	6	tr	tr	–
pickled	0.5 oz	5	0	0	0
preserved	1.5 oz	34	0	0	–
root fresh	5 slices	9	tr	tr	–
root fresh sliced	¼ cup	19	tr	tr	–
Eden					
Pickled w/ Shiso Leaves	1 tbsp	20	0	0	0
Frieda's					
Crystallized	9 pieces (1.1 oz)	100	0	0	0
Galanga Thai Ginger	⅔ cup	60	1	0	–
McCormick					
Crystallized	¼ tsp	15	0	0	0

FOOD	PORTION	CALS	FAT	SAT FAT	TRANS FAT
GINKGO NUTS					
canned	1 oz	32	tr	tr	–
dried	1 oz	99	tr	tr	–
raw	1 oz	52	tr	tr	–
GINSENG					
dried	1 oz	90	tr	–	–
fresh	1 oz	28	tr	–	–
GIZZARDS					
chicken simmered	1 cup (5 oz)	212	4	1	tr
turkey simmered	1 (3 oz)	103	3	1	0
GNOCCHI					
Bellino					
W/ Potato	1 cup	240	1	0	–
Vantia					
Gnocchi Whole Wheat	¾ cup	210	1	0	0
GOAT					
roasted	3 oz	122	3	1	–
GOJI BERRIES					
dried	1 oz	106	3	–	0
Navitas Naturals					
Dried	1 oz	90	0	0	0
Sunfood					
Organic	1 oz	90	0	0	0
Superfood Snacks					
Organic Chocolate Goji Treats	3 pieces (1.4 oz)	150	4	1	0
GOJI JUICE					
Gojilania					
Organic	8 oz	110	0	0	0
GOOSE					
w/ skin roasted	½ goose (1.7 lbs)	2362	170	53	–
w/ skin roasted	6.6 oz	574	41	13	–
w/o skin roasted	½ goose (1.3 lbs)	1406	75	27	–
w/o skin roasted	5 oz	340	18	7	–

FOOD	PORTION	CALS	FAT	SAT FAT	TRANS FAT
GOOSEBERRIES					
canned in light syrup	½ cup	93	tr	tr	–
fresh	1 cup	67	1	tr	–
Navitas Naturals					
Cape Gooseberry Dried	1 oz	80	0	0	0
GRAPE JUICE					
bottled unsweetened	1 cup	154	tr	tr	0
Apple & Eve					
Vintage Concord	8 oz	150	0	0	0
Cascadian Farm					
Organic frzn as prep	8 oz	150	0	0	0
Ceres					
Hanepoot White Grape	8 oz	130	0	0	0
Hansen's					
White Grape 100% Juice	1 box (4.23 oz)	90	0	0	0
Juicy Juice					
Harvest Surprise	8 oz	120	0	0	0
Keto					
Kooler	½ tsp	0	0	0	0
Lakewood					
Organic Concord	6 oz	105	0	0	0
Langers					
Plus 100% Juice	8 oz	160	0	0	0
White Grape Plus 100% Juice	8 oz	160	0	0	0
Nantucket Nectars					
Organic Concord Grape	8 oz	130	0	0	0
Newman's Own					
Gorilla Grape	8 oz	140	0	0	0
Old Orchard					
100% Juice White	8 oz	160	0	0	0
Tang					
Drink Mix as prep	1 serv (8 oz)	110	0	0	0
Tree Ripe					
Organic 100% Juice	6 oz	120	0	0	0
Tropicana					
Grape	1 bottle (14 oz)	270	0	0	0
Walnut Acres					
Organic	8 oz	120	0	0	0

FOOD	PORTION	CALS	FAT	SAT FAT	TRANS FAT
Welch's					
100% Juice	8 oz	170	0	0	0
100% White	8 oz	160	0	0	0
Light White Grape	8 oz	70	0	0	0
GRAPE LEAVES					
canned	1 (4 g)	3	tr	tr	0
fresh raw	1 (3 g)	3	tr	tr	0
Sabra					
Stuffed Meatless	1	45	1	0	–
TAKE-OUT					
dolmas w/ beef & rice	1 (0.7 oz)	50	4	1	0
dolmas w/ lamb & rice	1 (0.7 oz)	56	4	1	0
dolmas w/ rice	1 (2 oz)	92	6	1	0
GRAPEFRUIT					
CANNED					
juice pack	½ cup	46	tr	tr	–
unsweetened	1 cup	93	tr	tr	–
water pack	½ cup	44	tr	tr	–
Del Monte					
Fruit Naturals Red	½ cup	60	0	0	0
SunFresh Red	½ cup	80	0	0	0
SunFresh White	½ cup	45	0	0	0
In Real Fruit Juice					
FRESH					
pink	½	37	tr	tr	–
pink sections	1 cup	69	tr	tr	–
red	½	37	tr	tr	–
red sections	1 cup	69	tr	tr	–
white	½	39	tr	tr	–
white sections	1 cup	76	tr	tr	–
Ocean Spray					
Sweet Ruby	½ med	60	0	0	0
Sunkist					
Fresh	½ med	60	0	0	0
Oroblanco	½	100	1	0	0
GRAPEFRUIT JUICE					
fresh	1 cup	96	tr	tr	–
frzn as prep	1 cup	102	tr	tr	–

FOOD	PORTION	CALS	FAT	SAT FAT	TRANS FAT
frzn not prep	6 oz	302	1	tr	–
sweetened	1 cup	116	tr	tr	–
Apple & Eve					
Ruby Red	8 oz	130	0	0	0
Crystal Light					
Sunrise Sunrise Ruby Red as prep	1 serv (8 oz)	5	0	0	0
Izze					
Sparkling Grapefruit	8 oz	160	0	0	0
Minute Maid					
Frozen + Calcium	8 oz	100	0	0	0
Ruby Red	8 oz	130	0	0	0
Ocean Spray					
100% Juice Pink	8 oz	110	0	0	0
100% White Juice	8 oz	100	0	0	0
Ruby Drink	8 oz	120	0	0	0
Ruby Red Drink	8 oz	130	0	0	0
Odwalla					
100% Juice	8 oz	90	0	0	0
Sundia					
Ruby	½ cup	70	0	0	0
Tao Tea					
Grapefruit Lemon Fusion	8 oz	72	0	0	0
Tropicana					
Sweet	8 oz	130	0	0	0
GRAPES					
seedless red or green	1 cup	110	tr	tr	0
seedless red or green	20	69	tr	tr	0
thompson seedless in heavy syrup	½ cup	93	tr	tr	0
thompson seedless water pack	½ cup	49	tr	tr	0
with seeds red or green	1 cup	106	tr	tr	0
with seeds red or green	20	80	tr	tr	0
Chiquita					
Grapes	1½ cups (4.8 oz)	90	1	0	–
Earthbound Farm					
Organic Black	1½ cups	190	1	0	0
Frieda's					
Champagne	½ cup (3 oz)	50	0	0	0

FOOD	PORTION	CALS	FAT	SAT FAT	TRANS FAT
GRAVY					
CANNED					
beef	1 can (10 oz)	155	7	3	–
beef	1 cup	124	6	3	–
chicken	1 cup	189	14	3	–
mushroom	1 cup	120	6	1	–
turkey	1 cup	122	5	1	–
Boston Market					
Roasted Chicken	¼ cup	25	2	1	–
Campbell's					
Au Jus	¼ cup	5	0	0	0
Chicken	¼ cup	40	3	1	0
Fat Free Beef	¼ cup	15	0	0	0
Fat Free Turkey	¼ cup	20	0	0	0
Mushroom	¼ cup	20	1	0	0
Franco-American					
Fat Free Slow Roast Chicken	¼ cup	20	0	0	0
Slow Roast Chicken	¼ cup	20	1	0	0
Heinz					
HomeStyle Classic Chicken	¼ cup	25	1	0	0
HomeStyle Roasted Turkey	¼ cup	25	1	0	0
Pacific Foods					
Natural Beef	1 cup	20	0	0	0
Natural Chicken	¼ cup	25	0	0	0
Natural Mushroom	¼ cup	20	0	0	0
Natural Turkey	¼ cup	25	1	0	0
FROZEN					
Tofurky					
Giblet & Mushroom	2 tbsp	30	1	0	0
MIX					
au jus as prep w/ water	1 cup	32	1	1	–
brown as prep w/ water	1 cup	75	2	1	–
chicken as prep	1 cup	83	2	1	–
mushroom as prep	1 cup	70	1	1	–
onion as prep w/ water	1 cup	77	1	tr	–
pork as prep	1 cup	76	2	1	–
turkey as prep	1 cup	87	2	1	–
Bournvita					
Extract	2 heaping tsp	34	1	–	–

FOOD	PORTION	CALS	FAT	SAT FAT	TRANS FAT
Bovril					
Extract	1 heaping tsp	9	0	–	0
Knorr					
Au Jus Instant as prep	2 oz	10	0	0	0
Beef Instant as prep	2 oz	20	1	tr	0
Brown Instant as prep	2 oz	25	0	0	0
Brown Low Sodium Instant as prep	2 oz	25	tr	0	0
Chicken Instant as prep	2 oz	25	tr	0	0
Chicken Low Sodium Instant as prep	2 oz	25	1	tr	0
Leahey Gardens					
No Beef Brown Gluten Free	¼ cup	9	tr	0	0
No Chicken Golden	¼ cup	18	2	0	0
Marmite					
Extract	1 heaping tsp	9	0	–	0
Road's End Organics					
Savory Herb Cholesterol Free Gluten Free	¼ cup	25	0	0	0
TAKE-OUT					
au jus	1 cup	62	6	2	–
giblet gravy	¼ cup	45	3	1	0
GREAT NORTHERN BEANS					
canned	1 cup	299	1	tr	–
dried cooked	1 cup	209	1	tr	–
Eden					
Organic	½ cup	110	1	0	0
GREEN BEANS					
CANNED					
drained	1 cup	27	tr	tr	–
Allens					
Italian Cut	½ cup	30	0	0	0
Del Monte					
Cut	½ cup	20	0	0	0
Cut w/ Potatoes & Ham Flavor	½ cup	30	0	0	0
French Style	½ cup	20	0	0	0
Fresh Cut Italian	½ cup	30	0	0	0
Whole	½ cup	20	0	0	0

FOOD	PORTION	CALS	FAT	SAT FAT	TRANS FAT
Gertie's Finest					
Pickled	1 oz	15	0	0	0
Green Giant					
50% Less Sodium Cut	½ cup	20	0	0	0
S&W					
Blue Lake Cut	½ cup (4.2 oz)	20	0	0	0
Tillen Farms					
Crispy Dilly Beans Pickled	¼ cup	15	0	0	0
FRESH					
cooked w/o salt	1 cup	44	tr	tr	–
raw	1 cup	34	tr	tr	0
raw whole beans	10	17	tr	tr	–
Frieda's					
Purple Wax	⅔ cup	25	0	0	0
GreenLine					
Fresh Trimmed	3 oz	25	0	0	0
FROZEN					
cooked	1 cup	38	tr	tr	0
Birds Eye					
Steamfresh Cut	½ cup	30	0	0	0
C&W					
French Cut	1 cup	30	0	0	0
Cascadian Farm					
Organic Petite Whole	1 cup	25	0	0	0
Fresh Like					
Cut	3.5 oz	29	tr	–	–
French Cut	3.5 oz	29	tr	–	–
Green Giant					
Green Bean Casserole	⅔ cup	110	8	3	1
Pictsweet					
Cut	⅔ cup	30	0	0	0
TAKE-OUT					
casserole w/ mushroom sauce	1 cup	108	6	2	–
pickled	½ cup	19	tr	tr	–

GREENS

Ready Pac

Microwave Leafy Greens as prep	½ cup	15	0	0	0

FOOD	PORTION	CALS	FAT	SAT FAT	TRANS FAT
GROUNDCHERRIES					
fresh	½ cup	37	tr	–	–
GROUPER					
cooked	1 fillet (7.1 oz)	238	3	1	–
cooked	3 oz	100	1	tr	–
raw	3 oz	78	1	tr	–
GUAR GUM					
Bob's Red Mill					
Guar Gum	1 tbsp	20	0	0	0
GUAVA					
fresh	1	45	1	tr	–
guava sauce	½ cup	43	tr	tr	–
Frieda's					
Fresh	1 (3 oz)	45	1	0	–
GUAVA JUICE					
Apple & Eve					
Nectar	5 oz	130	0	0	0
Ceres					
Guava	8 oz	120	0	0	0
Nantucket Nectars					
Guava	8 oz	130	0	0	0
Sabor Latino					
Nectar + Calcium	8 oz	160	0	0	0
GUINEA HEN					
w/ skin raw	½ hen (12.1 oz)	545	22	–	–
w/o skin raw	½ hen (9.3 oz)	292	7	–	–
HADDOCK					
fresh broiled	4 oz	127	1	tr	0
roe raw	1 oz	37	tr	–	–
smoked	1 oz	33	tr	tr	0
Van de Kamp's					
Battered Fillets	2 (3.6 oz)	210	11	4	0
TAKE-OUT					
breaded & fried	4 oz	229	10	2	0
HALIBUT					
atlantic & pacific cooked	½ fillet (5.6 oz)	223	5	1	–

FOOD	PORTION	CALS	FAT	SAT FAT	TRANS FAT
atlantic & pacific cooked	3 oz	119	2	tr	–
atlantic & pacific raw	3 oz	93	2	tr	–
greenland baked	3 oz	203	15	2	–
greenland baked	5.6 oz	380	28	5	–
FROZEN					
Van de Kamp's					
Battered Fillets	3 (4 oz)	230	11	4	0

HALVA (see SESAME)

HAM

FOOD	PORTION	CALS	FAT	SAT FAT	TRANS FAT
boneless extra lean roasted	3 oz	123	5	2	0
boneless roasted	3 oz	151	8	3	0
canned extra lean roasted	3 oz	116	4	1	0
canned lean roasted	3 oz	142	7	2	0
center slice lean & fat roasted	3 oz	173	11	4	0
deviled	¼ cup	188	17	6	0
ham salad spread	2 tbsp	65	5	2	0
patty grilled	1 (2 oz)	205	19	7	0
prosciutto	4 slices (1.3 oz)	72	3	1	0
sliced	3 slices (2.9 oz)	137	7	2	0
sliced extra lean	3 slices (2.2 oz)	69	2	1	0
westphalian smoked	1 oz	105	10	–	–
whole roasted	3 oz	207	14	5	0
Boar's Head					
Black Forest Smoked	2 oz	60	1	0	–
Deluxe	2 oz	60	1	0	–
Deluxe 42% Lowered Sodium	2 oz	60	1	0	–
Fresh Seasoned	2 oz	90	3	2	–
Maple Glazed Honey	2 oz	60	1	0	–
Pepper	2 oz	60	1	0	–
Rosemary & Sundried Tomato	2 oz	70	3	1	–
Virginia Smoked	2 oz	60	1	0	–
Healthy Ones					
Honey 97% Fat Free	7 slices (2 oz)	90	2	1	0
Hillshire					
Deli Select Honey Ham	6 slices (2 oz)	60	2	1	–
Organic Prairie					
Hardwood Smoked Bone In Spiral Sliced	3 oz	110	3	1	–

FOOD	PORTION	CALS	FAT	SAT FAT	TRANS FAT
Oscar Mayer					
Ham Brown Sugar Thin Sliced	⅓ pkg (2 oz)	70	2	0	0
Lunchables Ham Bagels	1 pkg	410	10	5	–
Virginia Shaved	2 oz	50	1	1	0
Sara Lee					
Bavarian Oven Roasted Honey	2 oz	70	4	1	–
Brown Sugar	2 oz	70	3	0	–
Homestyle Baked	2 oz	60	2	1	–
Virginia Baked	4 slices (1.8 oz)	60	2	1	0
Tyson					
Glazed Ham Maple & Brown Sugar	1 serv (5 oz)	180	5	2	–
Honey Ham	2 slices (1.6 oz)	50	2	1	–
TAKE-OUT					
croquette	1 (2.2 oz)	149	9	2	0
salad	½ cup	287	23	5	–
spam musubi	1 serv (6 oz)	253	6	2	–
thick slice fried	1 (2.2 oz)	140	9	3	0

HAMBURGER

FOOD	PORTION	CALS	FAT	SAT FAT	TRANS FAT
Ian's					
Mini	2 (4.6 oz)	360	12	4	0
Mini Cheeseburger	2 (5 oz)	420	17	6	0
Kid Cuisine					
Cheeseburger Builder	1 meal	390	11	5	0
Lean Pockets					
Cheeseburger	1 (4.5 oz)	280	7	3	–
Oscar Meyer					
Lunchables All-Star Burgers	1 pkg	420	14	9	1
Quaker Maid					
Pure Beef Patties	1 (4 oz)	240	18	7	–
Wellshire					
Beef	1 (4 oz)	260	12	7	–
Turkey Burgers	1 (4 oz)	200	2	tr	–
TAKE-OUT					
cheeseburger + condiments	1 reg (4.5 oz)	347	17	7	0
double hamburger + condiments	1 reg (5.8 oz)	384	19	7	0
single patty + condiments	1 reg (4 oz)	299	11	4	0

FOOD	PORTION	CALS	FAT	SAT FAT	TRANS FAT
HAMBURGER SUBSTITUTES (*see also* MEAT SUBSTITUTES)					
Amy's					
All American Burger	1 (2.5 oz)	120	3	0	–
California Burger	1 (2.5 oz)	130	5	1	–
Chicago Burger	1 (2.5 oz)	160	5	2	–
Boca					
American Flame Grilled	1 (2.5 oz)	90	3	1	0
Cheeseburger	1 (2.5 oz)	100	5	2	0
Grilled Vegetable	1 (2.5 oz)	70	1	0	0
Ground Burger	1 serv (2 oz)	60	1	0	0
Original	1 (2.5 oz)	70	1	0	0
Original Vegan	1 patty (2.5 oz)	70	1	0	0
Dr. Praeger's					
California Burger	1 (2.7 oz)	100	3	0	–
Fantastic					
Natures Burger Mix not prep	¼ cup	170	3	0	–
Tofu Burger Mix not prep	3 tbsp	80	3	0	–
Gardenburger					
Black Bean Chipotle	1 (2.5 oz)	80	3	0	0
Flamed Grilled	1 (2.5 oz)	90	4	0	0
GardenVegan	1 (2.5 oz)	100	1	0	0
Original	1 (2.5 oz)	100	4	1	0
Portabella	1 (2.5 oz)	90	3	1	0
Lightlife					
Light Burgers	1 (3 oz)	120	2	0	–
Smart Menu Burger	1	80	1	0	–
Morningstar Farms					
Classic Burger	1 (2.2 oz)	150	7	1	0
Garden Veggie Patties	1 patty (2.4 oz)	100	3	1	0
Harvest Burger	1	140	4	2	–
Okara Pattie	1 (2.2 oz)	120	5	1	0
Vegan Burger	1 (2.5 oz)	100	2	0	0
Tofurky					
SuperBurgers Original	1 (3.5 oz)	120	2	0	0
VeggieLand					
Veggie Burger Original	1 (3.5 oz)	132	4	0	–
Veggie Burger Peppadew	1 (5 oz)	210	5	1	0

FOOD	PORTION	CALS	FAT	SAT FAT	TRANS FAT
WildWood					
Organic Original Burgers Tofu-Veggie	1 (3.2 oz)	180	13	2	0
HAZELNUTS					
dried blanched	1 oz	191	19	1	–
dried unblanched	1 oz	179	18	1	–
dry roasted unblanched	1 oz	188	19	1	–
oil roasted unblanched	1 oz	187	18	1	–
Kettle					
Butter Creamy Unsalted	2 tbsp	180	17	1	0
Love'n Bake					
Hazelnut Praline	2 tbsp	170	12	1	–
Low Carb Creations					
Soft Hazelnut Brittle	2 pieces (1 oz)	160	12	2	–
Torras					
Hazelnut Chocolate Spread	1 tsp	27	2	2	–
Twist					
Sugar Free Chocolate Hazelnut Spread	2 tbsp	180	14	4	–
HEART					
beef simmered	3 oz	140	4	1	0
chicken cooked	1 (3 g)	5	tr	tr	0
chicken diced simmered	½ cup	134	6	2	0
lamb braised	3 oz	157	7	3	0
pork braised	1 (4.5 oz)	191	7	2	0
turkey simmered	½ cup	94	3	1	0
veal braised	3 oz	158	6	2	0
HEARTS OF PALM					
canned	1 (1.2 oz)	9	tr	tr	0
canned	½ cup	20	tr	tr	0
Del Monte					
Hearts Of Palm	2-3 pieces	20	0	0	0
Native Forest					
Organic	1 oz	15	0	0	0
HEMP					
Living Harvest					
Organic Hemp Nuts	2 tbsp (1 oz)	170	12	1	0
Organic Protein Powder	2 scoops (1 oz)	110	3	0	0

FOOD	PORTION	CALS	FAT	SAT FAT	TRANS FAT
Manitoba Harvest					
Hemp Seed Butter	2 tbsp	160	10	1	0
Protein Powder	2 scoops (1 oz)	134	6	1	0
Shelled Seed	2 tbsp	160	10	1	0
Nutiva					
Organic Protein Powder	2 scoops (1 oz)	120	3	0	–
Shelled Hempseed	2 tbsp	110	8	1	0

HERBAL TEA (see TEA/HERBAL TEA)

HERBS/SPICES (see also individual names)

FOOD	PORTION	CALS	FAT	SAT FAT	TRANS FAT
cajun seasoning	1 tbsp	19	1	–	–
chinese five spice	1 tsp	7	tr	–	–
garam masala	1 tsp	8	tr	–	–
poultry seasoning	1 tsp	5	tr	tr	0
pumpkin pie spice	1 tsp	6	tr	tr	0
A Taste Of Thai					
Chicken & Rice Seasoning	¼ pkg (6 g)	15	0	0	0
Chef Paul Prudhomme's					
Magic Blackened Redfish	¼ tsp	0	0	0	0
Magic Fajita	¼ tsp	0	0	0	0
Magic Pork & Veal	¼ tsp	0	0	0	0
Magic Poultry	¼ tsp	0	0	0	0
Cut N Clean					
Greens Seasoning	1 ½ tsp	20	0	0	0
Eden					
Shake Furikake	½ tsp	5	0	0	0
Emeril's					
Asian Essence	½ tsp	0	0	0	0
Bayou Blast!	½ tsp	0	0	0	0
Chicken Rub	½ tsp	0	0	0	0
Original Essence	½ tsp	0	0	0	0
Steak Rub	½ tsp	0	0	0	0
Gringo Billy's					
Meat Rubs Chipotle	¼ tsp	0	0	0	0
Meat Rubs Montreau	¼ tsp	0	0	0	0
Meat Rubs Ultimate	¼ tsp	0	0	0	0
Tuna Seasoning	1 tsp	5	1	0	–
McCormick					
Blends Bon Appetit	¼ tsp	0	0	0	0
Cajun Seasoning	¼ tsp	0	0	0	0

FOOD	PORTION	CALS	FAT	SAT FAT	TRANS FAT
Greek Seasoning	¼ tsp	0	0	0	0
Jamaican Jerk Seasoning	¼ tsp	0	0	0	0
Seafood Seasoning	¼ tsp	0	0	0	0
Mrs. Dash					
Grilling Blend Chicken	¼ tsp	0	0	0	0
Grilling Blend Steak	¼ tsp	0	0	0	0
Original Blend	¼ tsp	0	0	0	0
Tomato Basil Garlic	¼ tsp	0	0	0	0
Nueva Cocina					
Picadillo	2 tsp	15	0	0	0
Taco Fresco	2 tsp	15	0	0	0
Ortega					
Burrito Seasoning	1½ tsp	20	0	0	0
Fajita Seasoning	1½ tsp	20	0	0	0
Taco Seasoning	1 tbsp	20	0	0	0
Spice Hunter					
All Purpose Blend	¼ tsp	0	0	0	0
Greek Seasoning Salt Free	¼ tsp	0	0	0	0

HERRING

FOOD	PORTION	CALS	FAT	SAT FAT	TRANS FAT
atlantic baked	4 oz	230	13	3	0
dried salted	1 fillet (1.4 oz)	161	9	2	0
pickled	1 oz	74	5	1	0
pickled in cream sauce	1 oz	72	5	1	0
roe	1 tbsp	39	2	tr	0
smoked kippered	1 oz	620	4	1	0
Beach Cliff					
Kippered Snacks	1 can (4 oz)	220	16	3	0
TAKE-OUT					
breaded fried	1 serv (4 oz)	225	14	3	0

HIBISCUS

FOOD	PORTION	CALS	FAT	SAT FAT	TRANS FAT
flowers dried sweetened	⅓ cup	100	0	0	0

HICKORY NUTS

FOOD	PORTION	CALS	FAT	SAT FAT	TRANS FAT
dried	1 oz	187	18	2	–

HOMINY
CANNED

FOOD	PORTION	CALS	FAT	SAT FAT	TRANS FAT
white	1 cup (5.6 oz)	482	1	tr	–

FOOD	PORTION	CALS	FAT	SAT FAT	TRANS FAT
HONEY					
honey	1 cup (11.9 oz)	1031	0	0	0
honey	1 tbsp (0.7 oz)	64	0	0	0
orange blossom	1 tbsp	60	0	0	0
wild honey	1 tbsp	60	0	0	0
Frieda's					
Honeycomb	½ cup (3 oz)	260	0	0	0
Steel's					
Sugar Free	1 tbsp	24	0	0	0
SueBee					
Clover	1 tbsp	60	0	0	0
HONEYDEW					
balls frzn	1 cup (8 oz)	83	tr	tr	0
fresh cut up	1 cup	61	tr	tr	0
fresh wedge	⅛ melon (4.5 oz)	45	tr	tr	0
whole fresh	1 (35 oz)	360	1	tr	0
Chiquita					
Wedge Fresh	1/10 melon (4.7 oz)	50	0	0	0
HORSE					
roasted	3 oz	149	5	2	–
HORSERADISH					
sauce	1 tbsp	7	tr	tr	–
wasabi root raw	1 (5.9 oz)	184	1	–	0
wasabi root raw sliced	½ cup (2.3 oz)	71	tr	–	0
Boar's Head					
Horseradish	1 tsp (5 g)	0	0	0	0
Horseradish Sauce Pub Style	1 tsp	15	2	0	–
Horseradish & Beets	1 tsp	0	0	0	0
Eden					
Wasabi Powder	1 tsp	10	0	0	0
Robert Rothchild Farm					
Sauce	1 tsp	20	2	1	0
Sara Lee					
Horseradish Sauce	1 tbsp	20	2	0	–
HOT CHOCOLATE					
mix as prep w/ water	7 oz	103	1	1	–
mix w/ equal as prep w/ water	7 oz	48	tr	tr	–

FOOD	PORTION	CALS	FAT	SAT FAT	TRANS FAT
Carnation					
Hot Cocoa Rich Chocolate as prep w/ 2% milk	1 pkg	200	8	4	–
Country Choice Naturals					
Irish Chocolate Mint Cocoa	1 pkg	100	0	0	0
Royal Chocolate Cocoa	1 pkg	100	0	0	0
Soy Cocoa Irish Chocolate Mint	1 pkg	100	1	0	–
Soy Cocoa Royal Chocolate	1 pkg	100	1	0	–
Keto					
Hot Cocoa	1 tsp	12	0	0	0
Low Carb Creations					
Cocoa as prep	1 cup	30	2	0	–
White Hot Chocolate	1 cup	25	2	0	–
Nestle					
Hot Cocoa Carb Select Fat Free	1 pkg	25	0	0	0
Sipper Sweets					
Sugar Free Low Carb Mix	1 serv	50	3	0	–
Swiss Miss					
Caramel Cream	1 serv	110	3	0	–
Hot Cocoa Milk Chocolate Fat Free	1 pkg	50	0	0	0
Milk Chocolate	1 pkg	120	3	2	0
Milk Chocolate w/ Marshmallows	1 pkg	120	3	1	–
TAKE-OUT					
hot cocoa	1 cup	218	9	6	–
mexican hot chocolate	1 cup	173	6	4	–

HOT DOG

FOOD	PORTION	CALS	FAT	SAT FAT	TRANS FAT
beef	1 (1.5 oz)	149	13	5	–
beef & pork	1 (1.5 oz)	137	12	5	–
beef low fat	1 (2 oz)	133	11	5	–
chicken	1 (1.5 oz)	116	9	2	–
fat free	1 (2 oz)	62	1	tr	–
low fat	1 (2 oz)	88	6	2	–
low sodium	1 (2 oz)	180	16	7	–
pork and beef cheese smokie	1 (1.5 oz)	141	12	5	–
turkey	1 (1.5 oz)	102	8	3	–
Ball Park					
Franks	1 (2 oz)	180	16	6	–

FOOD	PORTION	CALS	FAT	SAT FAT	TRANS FAT
Franks Beef	1 (2 oz)	180	16	7	–
Franks Bun Size	1 (2 oz)	180	16	6	–
Franks Smoked White Turkey	1 (1.8 oz)	45	0	0	0
Franks Fat Free	1 (1.8 oz)	40	0	0	0
Franks Lite	1 (1.8 oz)	100	7	3	–
Franks Singles Cheese	1 (1.6 oz)	150	13	5	–
Grillmaster Hearty Beef	1	250	23	9	–
Grillmaster Smokehouse	1	210	24	9	–
Boar's Head					
Beef	1 (2 oz)	160	14	6	–
Beef Lite	1 (1.6 oz)	90	6	3	–
Beef Cocktail	5 (2 oz)	170	15	6	–
Pork & Beef	1 (2 oz)	150	14	5	–
Dietz & Watson					
New York Style Beef	1 (2.3 oz)	130	15	6	–
Healthy Choice					
Beef Low Fat	1 (1.8 oz)	70	3	1	–
Healthy Ones					
Beef	1 (1.8 oz)	70	3	1	0
Franks	1 (1.8 oz)	70	3	1	0
Hebrew National					
97% Fat Free Beef	1 (1.7 oz)	45	2	1	–
Beef	1 (1.7 oz)	150	14	6	–
Cocktail Franks	5 (2 oz)	180	16	7	–
Dinner Frank	1 (4 oz)	350	32	15	–
Franks In A Blanket	5 (2.8 oz)	290	24	10	–
Reduced Fat Beef	1 (1.7 oz)	120	10	5	–
Ian's					
Popcorn Turkey Corn Dog	5 pieces (3 oz)	237	13	2	0
Johnsonville					
Stadium Beef	1 (2.7 oz)	240	22	8	0
Organic Prairie					
Beef Uncured	1 (1.5 oz)	120	11	4	–
Chicken Uncured	1 (1.5 oz)	100	6	2	0
Pork Uncured	1 (1.5 oz)	130	12	4	–
Turkey Uncured	1 (1.5 oz)	80	6	1	0
Oscar Mayer					
Beef	1 (1.6 oz	140	13	6	1
Beef Light	1 (1.6 oz)	90	6	6	0

FOOD	PORTION	CALS	FAT	SAT FAT	TRANS FAT
Cheese Dogs	1 (1.6 oz)	140	13	4	0
Corn Dogs	1	210	12	4	0
Smokies	1 (1.8 oz)	150	13	5	0
State Fair					
Corn Dogs	1 (2.67 oz)	180	12	4	–
Wellshire					
Beef Premium	1 (2 oz)	110	9	4	–
Cheese Franks	1 (2 oz)	110	9	4	–
Chicken Franks	1 (1.6 oz)	70	8	2	–
Turkey Franks	1 (1.6 oz)	110	6	2	–
TAKE-OUT					
corndog	1	460	19	5	–
w/ bun chili	1	297	13	5	–
w/ bun plain	1	242	15	5	–

HOT DOG SUBSTITUTES
Lightlife

FOOD	PORTION	CALS	FAT	SAT FAT	TRANS FAT
Smart Dogs	1	45	0	0	0
Smart Franks	1 (2 oz)	110	5	0	–
Tofu Pups	1 (1.5 oz)	60	3	1	–
Loma Linda					
Big Franks	1 (1.8 oz)	110	6	1	0
Big Franks Low Fat Vegan	1 (1.8 oz)	80	3	1	0
Morningstar Farms					
Corn Dog Veggie	1 (2.5 oz)	170	6	1	0
Quorn					
Meat-Free Dogs	1 (1.5 oz)	70	4	0	–
Yves					
Meatless Hot Dog	1	50	1	0	0
Tofu Dogs	1	45	1	0	0

HUMMUS
Athenos

FOOD	PORTION	CALS	FAT	SAT FAT	TRANS FAT
Black Olive	2 tbsp	50	3	0	0
Original	2 tbsp	50	3	0	0
Travelers Hummus & Pita	1 pkg	325	13	3	–
Guiltless Gourmet					
Roasted Garlic	2 tbsp	35	2	0	0
Sabra					
Homus	2 oz	110	5	1	–
Homus Spicy	½ cup	171	4	0	–

FOOD	PORTION	CALS	FAT	SAT FAT	TRANS FAT
Tribe					
40 Spices	2 tbsp	50	4	0	0
French Onion	2 tbsp	50	4	0	0
Organic Classic	2 tbsp	50	4	0	0
Organic Roasted Red Peppers	2 tbsp	40	3	0	0
Roasted Eggplant	2 tbsp	35	3	0	0
Scallion	2 tbsp	50	4	0	0
Zesty Lemon	2 tbsp	50	3	0	0
Wild Garden					
Hummus Dip	2 tbsp	35	2	0	–
WildWood					
Organic Low Fat	2 tbsp	50	2	0	0
Organic Mid-Eastern	2 tbsp	65	4	1	0
TAKE-OUT					
hummus	⅓ cup	140	7	1	–
HYACINTH BEANS					
dried cooked	1 cup	228	1	–	–

ICE CREAM AND FROZEN DESSERTS (see also ICES AND ICE POPS, SHERBET, YOGURT FROZEN)

FOOD	PORTION	CALS	FAT	SAT FAT	TRANS FAT
chocolate	½ cup (4 oz)	143	7	4	–
dixie cup chocolate	1 (3.5 oz)	125	6	4	–
dixie cup strawberry	1 (3.5 oz)	112	5	–	–
dixie cup vanilla	1 (3.5 oz)	116	6	4	–
freeze dried ice cream chocolate strawberry & vanilla	1 pkg (0.75 oz)	158	5	2	–
strawberry	½ cup (4 oz)	127	6	–	–
vanilla	½ cup (4 oz)	132	7	4	–
vanilla soft serve	½ cup	111	2	1	–
Blue Bunny					
Bar Candy Center Crunch	1 (3.2 oz)	370	29	22	0
Bar English Toffee	1 (1.4 oz)	130	9	7	0
Bar Homemade Vanilla	1 (2.3 oz)	190	13	10	0
Bar Orange Dream	1 (2.1 oz)	80	2	1	0
Bar Strawberry Sundae Crunch	1 (2.2 oz)	170	9	4	0
Blendz Peanut Butter Cup	1 (4.4 oz)	270	11	6	0
Caramel Sundae Bite Size	4 (3.1 oz)	340	23	15	0
Chocolate	½ cup	130	7	–	0
Cone Bunny Tracks	1 (4.8 oz)	420	21	12	0

FOOD	PORTION	CALS	FAT	SAT FAT	TRANS FAT
Cone The Champ Chocolate Lovers	1 (3.5 oz)	300	15	11	0
Cone Vanilla Nutty Sundae	1 (3 oz)	250	11	7	0
Cups Vanilla & Chocolate	1 (1.7 oz)	100	5	4	0
Mint Chip	½ cup	140	7	5	0
Neapolitan	½ cup	130	6	4	0
Orange Dream	½ cup	130	5	4	0
Premium All Natural Vanilla	½ cup	160	9	6	0
Premium Bunny Tracks	½ cup	190	11	6	0
Premium Butter Pecan	½ cup	150	9	4	0
Premium Cookies & Cream	½ cup	150	8	5	0
Premium Double Strawberry	½ cup	140	6	4	0
Premium Exquisite Mint	½ cup	170	8	5	0
Premium Rocky Road	½ cup	150	7	5	0
Premium Toasted Almond Fudge	½ cup	160	9	5	0
Sandwich Big Vanilla	1 (3.7 oz)	260	10	6	–
Sandwich Chips Galore	1 (3.4 oz)	310	16	8	0
Strawberry	½ cup	120	6	4	0
Breyers					
Almond Joy	½ cup	140	5	3	–
Banana Fudge Chunk	½ cup	170	9	5	–
Bar Light Creamy Vanilla Chocolate Coated	1	160	8	5	0
Butter Almond	½ cup	160	10	5	–
Butter Pecan	½ cup	170	11	5	–
Butter Pecan Homemade	½ cup	170	11	5	–
Butter Pecan No Sugar Added	½ cup	120	7	3	–
Caramel Praline Crunch	½ cup	180	9	5	–
Caramel Toffee Crunch	½ cup	180	9	6	–
CarbSmart Chocolate	½ cup	130	10	6	–
CarbSmart Strawberry	½ cup	130	9	6	–
CarbSmart Vanilla	½ cup	130	9	6	–
Cherry Chocolate Chip	½ cup	150	8	5	–
Cherry Vanilla	½ cup	140	8	5	–
Chocolate	½ cup	150	8	5	–
Chocolate 98% Fat Free	½ cup	90	2	1	–
Chocolate Caramel No Sugar Added	½ cup	110	4	3	–
Chocolate Chip	½ cup	160	9	5	–

FOOD	PORTION	CALS	FAT	SAT FAT	TRANS FAT
Chocolate Chip Cookie Dough	½ cup	170	9	6	–
Chocolate Rainbow	½ cup	140	7	5	–
Coffee	½ cup	140	8	5	–
Cookies & Cream	½ cup	160	8	5	–
Creamsicle	½ cup	130	5	3	–
Deep Chocolate Fudge	½ cup	200	12	8	–
Dulce De Leche	½ cup	150	7	4	–
French Vanilla	½ cup	150	8	5	–
French Vanilla Light	½ cup	120	4	2	–
French Vanilla No Sugar Added	½ cup	110	5	3	–
Fresh Banana	½ cup	140	5	4	–
Heath English Toffee	½ cup	190	9	5	–
Hershey w/ Almonds	½ cup	170	8	5	–
Ice Cream Cake Oreo	1 slice	190	10	5	–
Ice Cream Cake Vanilla	1 slice	190	11	7	–
Klondike Sandwich	½ cup	160	7	4	–
Mint Chocolate Chip	½ cup	160	9	5	–
Mint Chocolate Chip Light	½ cup	130	5	3	–
Mint Oreo	½ cup	170	7	4	–
Mocha Almond Fudge	½ cup	170	9	4	–
Oreo	½ cup	160	6	5	–
Peach	½ cup	130	6	4	–
Peanut Butter & Fudge	½ cup	170	10	5	–
Reese's Peanut Butter Cups	½ cup	180	9	5	–
Rocky Road	½ cup	160	8	5	–
SpongeBob Cookie Dough	½ cup	160	7	4	–
Strawberry	½ cup	120	6	4	–
Strawberry Shortcake	½ cup	160	6	4	–
Turtle Sundae	½ cup	190	11	6	–
Vanilla	½ cup	140	8	5	–
Vanilla Calcium Rich	½ cup	130	7	4	–
Vanilla Fudge Twirl	½ cup	140	7	5	–
Vanilla Homemade	½ cup	140	8	5	–
Vanilla Lactose Free	½ cup	130	7	5	–
Vanilla Light	½ cup	110	3	2	–
Vanilla Light 2% Milk	½ cup	130	5	3	–
Vanilla No Sugar Added	½ cup	100	5	3	–
Vanilla Caramel Brownie	½ cup	170	9	5	–
Vanilla Fudge Brownie	½ cup	180	9	5	–

FOOD	PORTION	CALS	FAT	SAT FAT	TRANS FAT
Vanilla Fudge Twirl No Sugar Added	½ cup	110	4	3	–
Wild Berry Swirl	½ cup	140	8	5	–
Bubbies					
Mochi Mango	1 piece (1.3 oz)	110	4	3	0
Butterfinger					
Bar	1 (1.9 oz)	210	15	10	0
Celestial Seasonings					
Tea Dreams Cinnamon Apple Spice	½ cup	140	6	0	0
Tea Dreams Vanilla Ginger Spice Chai	½ cup	140	6	1	0
Tea Dreams Bars Chocolate Caramel Chai	1 (2.7 oz)	240	15	9	0
Dove					
Beyond Vanilla	½ cup	240	15	10	0
Give In To Mint	½ cup	300	18	12	0
Irresistibly Raspberry	½ cup	240	13	8	0
Milk Chocolate w/ Almonds	1 bar (3.3 oz)	340	23	13	0
Milk Chocolate w/ Vanilla Ice Cream	1 bar (3.3 oz)	330	21	13	0
Miniatures Milk Chocolate w/ Vanilla Ice Cream	5 pieces (3.1 oz)	300	20	13	0
Triple Chocolate	1 bar (2.8 oz)	200	18	10	0
Unconditional Chocolate	½ cup	290	17	11	0
Vanilla w/ A Chocolate Soul	½ cup	290	18	12	0
Edy's					
Carb Benefit Butter Pecan	½ cup	170	12	6	0
Carb Benefit Chocolate	½ cup	150	10	6	0
Carb Benefit Chocolate Chip	½ cup	160	11	8	0
Carb Benefit Mint Chocolate Chip	½ cup	160	11	8	0
Carb Benefit Vanilla Bean	½ cup	140	9	6	0
Dips Chocolate	26 pieces	420	32	20	0
Dips Mint	26 pieces	420	32	19	0
Dips Vanilla	26 pieces	420	32	19	0
Grand Andes Cool Mint	½ cup	170	9	6	0
Grand Butter Pecan	½ cup	170	10	5	0
Grand Chocolate	½ cup	150	8	5	0

FOOD	PORTION	CALS	FAT	SAT FAT	TRANS FAT
Grand Chocolate Caramel Swirl	½ cup	170	9	5	0
Grand Chocolate Chip	½ cup	160	8	5	0
Grand Chocolate Fudge Mousse	½ cup	160	8	5	0
Grand Chocolate Fudge Sundae	½ cup	170	9	5	0
Grand Coffee	½ cup	140	8	5	0
Grand Cookie Dough	½ cup	180	9	6	0
Grand Cookies 'N Cream	½ cup	160	8	5	1
Grand Double Fudge Brownie	½ cup	170	9	5	0
Grand Dulce De Leche	½ cup	150	7	5	0
Grand Espresso Chip	½ cup	150	8	5	0
Grand French Vanilla	½ cup	160	9	5	0
Grand Fudge Tracks	½ cup	180	11	6	0
Grand Ice Cream Sandwich	½ cup	150	7	5	0
Grand Mint Chocolate Chip	½ cup	170	9	6	0
Grand Peanut Butter Cup	½ cup	180	10	4	0
Grand Real Strawberry	½ cup	130	6	4	0
Grand Rocky Road	½ cup	170	10	5	0
Grand Spumoni	½ cup	150	8	5	–
Grand Toffee Bar Crunch	½ cup	170	9	5	0
Grand Toll House Cookie Swirl	½ cup	170	9	5	0
Grand Turtle Sundae	½ cup	160	9	5	0
Grand Ultimate Caramel Cup	½ cup	170	8	5	0
Grand Vanilla	½ cup	140	8	5	–
Neapolitan	½ cup	140	7	5	0
Slow Churned Light Butter Pecan	½ cup	120	5	2	0
Slow Churned Light Caramel Delight	½ cup	120	4	2	0
Slow Churned Light Chocolate	½ cup	110	4	2	0
Slow Churned Light Chocolate Chip	½ cup	120	5	3	0
Slow Churned Light Chocolate Fudge Chunk	½ cup	120	5	3	0
Slow Churned Light Coffee	½ cup	105	4	2	0
Slow Churned Light Cookie Dough	½ cup	130	5	3	0

FOOD	PORTION	CALS	FAT	SAT FAT	TRANS FAT
Slow Churned Light Cookies 'N Cream	½ cup	120	4	2	0
Slow Churned Light French Silk	½ cup	130	5	3	0
Slow Churned Light French Vanilla	½ cup	100	4	2	0
Slow Churned Light Fudge Tracks	½ cup	120	5	3	0
Slow Churned Light Mint Chocolate Chip	½ cup	120	5	3	0
Slow Churned Light Mocha Almond Fudge	½ cup	120	5	2	–
Slow Churned Light Neapolitan	½ cup	100	3	2	0
Slow Churned Light Rocky Road	½ cup	120	4	2	0
Slow Churned Light Strawberry	½ cup	110	3	2	0
Slow Churned Light Vanilla	½ cup	100	4	2	0
Slow Churned No Sugar Added Butter Pecan	½ cup	120	5	2	0
Slow Churned No Sugar Added Chocolate	½ cup	95	3	2	0
Slow Churned No Sugar Added Cookie Dough	½ cup	110	4	3	0
Slow Churned No Sugar Added Fat Free Chocolate Fudge	½ cup	100	0	0	0
Slow Churned No Sugar Added Fat Free Raspberry Vanilla Swirl	½ cup	90	0	0	0
Slow Churned No Sugar Added Fat Free Vanilla	½ cup	90	0	0	0
Slow Churned No Sugar Added Fat Free Vanilla Chocolate Swirl	½ cup	100	0	0	0
Slow Churned No Sugar Added Fudge Tracks	½ cup	110	4	2	0
Slow Churned No Sugar Added Mint Chocolate Chip	½ cup	110	5	3	0
Slow Churned No Sugar Added Neapolitan	½ cup	95	3	2	0

FOOD	PORTION	CALS	FAT	SAT FAT	TRANS FAT
Slow Churned No Sugar Added Triple Chocolate	½ cup	110	4	2	0
Slow Churned No Sugar Added Vanilla	½ cup	90	3	2	0
Eskimo Pie					
Milk Chocolate	1 bar (1.8 oz)	160	11	9	–
Fat Boy					
Casco Nut Sundae On A Stick	1 (3 oz)	310	24	10	0
Casco Nut Sundae On A Stick Cherry Cordial	1 (3 oz)	300	22	15	0
Sandwich Chocolate	1 (3 oz)	210	9	5	0
Sandwich Egg Nog	1 (3 oz)	220	10	5	0
Sandwich Jr. Vanilla	1 (1.6 oz)	120	5	3	0
Sandwich Vanilla	1 (3 oz)	220	10	5	0
Glace De Vino					
Chocolate Amarretto Cream Sherry	½ cup	180	7	4	0
Raspberry Merlot Cheesecake	½ cup	180	7	4	0
Good Humor					
Bar Oreo	1 (4 oz)	250	15	8	–
Bar Reese's Peanut Butter	1 (4 oz)	310	21	13	–
Bar Toasted Almond	1 (3 oz)	180	10	3	–
Bar Vanilla Dark Chocolate	1 (3 oz)	190	13	9	–
Bar Vanilla Milk Chocolate	1 (3 oz)	180	13	9	–
Bar Candy Center Crunch	1 (4 oz)	310	23	17	–
Bar Strawberry Shortcake	1 (4 oz)	230	12	4	–
Chocolate Eclair Bar	1 (4 oz)	220	11	5	–
Cone Premium Sundae	1 (4.3 oz)	270	15	8	–
Cone Strawberry Shortcake	1 (4.3 oz)	230	10	5	–
Giant Sandwich Neapolitan	1 (6 oz)	250	10	5	–
Giant Sandwich Vanilla	1 (6 oz)	250	10	5	–
King Cone	1 (4.6 oz)	250	13	6	–
Number 1 Bar	1 (4 oz)	200	11	8	–
Sandwich Chocolate Chip Cookie	1 (4.5 oz)	290	13	6	–
Sandwich Vanilla	1 (3.5 oz)	160	6	3	–
Sundae Twist Cup	1 (6 oz)	160	3	2	–
GoodBody					
Chocolate Banana	1 bar (3.5 oz)	120	1	0	0
Chocolate Double Dutch	1 bar (3.5 oz)	130	1	0	0

FOOD	PORTION	CALS	FAT	SAT FAT	TRANS FAT
Chocolate Peanut Butter	1 bar (3.5 oz)	180	7	1	0
Vanilla & Raspberry Sorbet	1 bar (3.5 oz)	120	0	0	0
Vanilla & Strawberry Sorbet	1 bar (3.5 oz)	120	0	0	0
Vanilla & Tropical Sorbet	1 bar (3.5 oz)	120	0	0	0
Green & Black's					
Organic Chocolate Covered Chocolate	1 bar (3.5 oz)	214	14	9	–
Organic Chocolate Covered Vanilla	1 bar (3.5 oz)	233	16	10	–
Haagen-Dazs					
Bars Chocolate & Almonds	1 (3.7 oz)	380	27	14	–
Bars Chocolate & Dark Chocolate	1 (3.6 oz)	350	24	15	–
Bars Chocolate Peanut Butter Swirl	1 (3 oz)	320	23	11	–
Bars Coffee & Almond Crunch	1 (3.7 oz)	370	27	15	–
Bars Cookies & Cream Crunch	1 (3.6 oz)	370	26	15	–
Bars Dulce De Leche Caramel	1 (3.7 oz)	370	24	15	–
Bars Tropical Coconut	1 (3.5 oz)	340	24	15	–
Bars Vanilla & Almonds	1 (3.7 oz)	380	28	14	–
Bars Vanilla & Dark Chocolate	1 (3.6 oz)	350	24	15	–
Bars Vanilla & Milk Chocolate	1 (3.5 oz)	340	24	14	–
Butter Pecan	½ cup	310	23	11	–
Cappuccino Commotion	½ cup	310	21	12	–
Cherry Vanilla	½ cup	240	15	9	–
Chocolate	½ cup	270	18	11	–
Chocolate Brownie w/ Walnuts	½ cup	290	19	9	–
Chocolate Chocolate Fudge	½ cup	290	18	12	–
Chocolate Chocolate Chip	½ cup	300	20	12	–
Chocolate Swiss Almond	½ cup	300	20	11	–
Cinnamon	½ cup	250	17	10	–
Coffee	½ cup	270	18	11	–
Coffee Mocha Chip	½ cup	290	19	12	–
Cookie Dough Chip	½ cup	310	20	12	–
Cookies & Cream	½ cup	270	17	10	–
Creme Caramel Pecan	½ cup	320	20	10	–
Dulce De Leche Caramel	½ cup	290	17	10	–
Low Fat Chocolate	½ cup	170	3	2	–
Low Fat Coffee Fudge	½ cup	170	3	2	–
Low Fat Strawberry	½ cup	150	2	1	–

FOOD	PORTION	CALS	FAT	SAT FAT	TRANS FAT
Low Fat Vanilla	½ cup	170	3	2	–
Macadamia Brittle	½ cup	300	20	12	–
Mango	½ cup	250	14	6	–
Mint Chip	½ cup	300	19	12	–
Pineapple Coconut	½ cup	230	12	8	–
Pistachio	½ cup	290	20	11	–
Rum Raisin	½ cup	270	17	10	–
Strawberry	½ cup	250	16	10	–
Vanilla	½ cup	270	18	11	–
Vanilla Chocolate Chip	½ cup	310	20	12	–
Vanilla Fudge	½ cup	290	18	12	–
Vanilla Swiss Almond	½ cup	300	20	11	–
Hawaiian Punch					
Cream Surfers	1 bar	90	2	1	0
Healthy Choice					
Bar Sorbet & Cream	1	100	1	1	0
Brownie Bliss	½ cup	130	2	1	–
Butter Pecan Crunch	½ cup	100	2	1	–
Cappuccino Chocolate Chunk	½ cup	120	2	1	–
Caramel Fudge Brownie	½ cup	120	2	1	–
Cherry Chocolate Mambo	½ cup	130	2	1	–
Chocolate Chocolate Chunk	½ cup	120	2	1	–
Cookies 'N Cream	½ cup	120	2	1	–
Crazy Caramel	½ cup	120	2	1	–
Double Karma	½ cup	140	2	1	–
French Silk	½ cup	120	2	1	–
Happy Together	½ cup	150	2	1	–
Jumpin' Java	½ cup	130	2	1	–
Low Fat Bar Fudge	1	90	1	1	–
Low Fat Bar Mocha Fudge	1	90	2	1	–
Low Fat Bar Strawberry & Cream	1	90	2	1	–
Mint Chocolate Chip	½ cup	120	2	1	–
No Sugar Added Chocolate Fudge Brownie	½ cup	120	2	1	–
No Sugar Added Coffee Almond Fudge	½ cup	110	2	1	–
No Sugar Added Mint Chocolate Chip	½ cup	110	2	1	–
No Sugar Added Vanilla	½ cup	100	2	1	–

FOOD	PORTION	CALS	FAT	SAT FAT	TRANS FAT
Peanut Butter Cup	½ cup	120	2	1	–
Praline & Caramel	½ cup	120	2	1	–
Rocky Road	½ cup	130	2	1	–
Sandwich Caramel	1	140	3	1	–
Sandwich Fudge Swirl	1	140	3	1	–
Sandwich Vanilla	1	130	3	1	–
Turtle Fudge Cake	½ cup	130	2	1	–
Vanilla	½ cup	110	2	1	–
Vanilla Bean	½ cup	120	2	1	–
Vanilla Caramel Fudge	½ cup	140	2	1	–
Hershey's					
Butter Pecan	½ cup	170	9	6	–
French Vanilla	½ cup	170	10	6	–
Neapolitan	½ cup	160	9	5	–
Hood					
Butterscotch Blast	½ cup	160	7	5	0
Chocolate	½ cup	140	7	5	0
Chocolate Eclair	1 bar (2.2 oz)	150	10	4	0
Cookie Dough Delight	½ cup	160	8	5	0
Creamy Coffee	½ cup	140	7	5	0
Fat Free Chocolate Passion	½ cup	100	0	0	0
Fat Free Very Vanilla	½ cup	100	0	0	0
Fudge Twister	½ cup	150	7	4	0
Grasshopper Pie	½ cup	160	7	4	0
Hoodsie Cups	1 (1.7 oz)	100	5	4	0
Light Butter Pecan	½ cup	140	6	2	0
Light Creamy Vanilla	½ cup	110	3	2	0
Low Fat No Sugar Added Vanilla Dream	½ cup	90	2	1	0
Maple Walnut	½ cup	160	9	5	0
No Sugar Added Chocolate Chip	½ cup	100	3	2	0
Nutty Royale	1 cone (2.5 oz)	220	12	7	0
Orange Cream	1 bar (2.2 oz)	90	2	1	0
Sandwich Vanilla	1	180	6	4	0
Sandwich Vanilla Light	1 (2.2 oz)	160	3	2	0
Sandwich Vanilla Lowfat	1 (2.8 oz)	80	2	1	0
Spumoni	½ cup	140	7	5	0
Klondike					
Bar Almond	1	300	21	14	–

FOOD	PORTION	CALS	FAT	SAT FAT	TRANS FAT
Bar Cappuccino	1	280	19	14	–
Bar Caramel & Peanut	1	290	19	12	–
Bar Caramel Crunch	1	270	17	13	–
Bar Chocolate	1	280	19	14	–
Bar Dark Chocolate	1	280	19	13	–
Bar Heath	1	300	20	14	–
Bar Krunch	1	280	19	14	–
Bar Oreo	1	160	10	3	–
Bar Original	1	280	19	14	–
Bar Peppermint Patty	1	280	19	13	–
Bar Reese's	1	220	15	9	–
Big Bear Sandwich Neapolitan	1	300	12	6	–
Big Bear Sandwich Vanilla	1	300	12	6	–
Big Bear Cone Vanilla	1	330	20	0	–
Big Bear Cone Vanilla Caramel	1	360	21	9	–
Big Bear Cone Vanilla Fudge	1	380	20	9	–
CarbSmart Fudge Bar	1	60	7	5	–
CarbSmart Ice Cream Bar	1	130	15	11	–
Choco Taco	1	290	16	8	–
Cone Oreo	1	250	12	6	–
Cone Reese's	1	290	15	7	–
Cookie Sandwich Chips	1	470	20	9	–
Cookie Sandwich Oreo	1	230	9	4	–
Minis	2 pieces	170	11	8	–
Sandwich Double Decker	1	370	14	7	–
Slim-A-Bear 98% Fat Free Sandwich Vanilla	1	130	2	0	0
Slim-A-Bear No Sugar Added Cone Vanilla	1	270	15	5	–
Slim-A-Bear No Sugar Added Fudge Bar	1	90	2	1	–
Slim-A-Bear No Sugar Added Reduced Fat Bar Vanilla	1	160	9	7	–
Slim-A-Bear No Sugar Added Sandwich Vanilla	1	120	3	1	–
Sundae Cup	1	280	17	10	–
M&M's					
Cone	1 (2.8 oz)	250	12	6	0
Sandwich	1 (3 oz)	260	12	7	0
Vanilla Fudge	½ cup	180	10	5	0

FOOD	PORTION	CALS	FAT	SAT FAT	TRANS FAT
Natural Choice					
Organic Double Chocolate	½ cup	230	14	8	0
Organic Strawberry	½ cup	210	13	8	0
Organic Vanilla	½ cup	220	14	9	–
No Pudge!					
Giant Chocolate Eclair Low Fat	1 bar	110	2	0	–
Giant Cone Chocolate No Sugar Added	1	110	4	3	–
Giant Cone Cookies & Cream Low Fat	1	140	3	2	–
Giant Cone Fudgy Brownie Low Fat	1	140	3	2	–
Giant Cone Vanilla No Sugar Added	1	110	4	3	–
Giant Cookie & Cream Low Fat No Sugar Added	1 bar	100	3	2	–
Giant Fudgy Fat Free No Sugar Added	1 bar	60	0	0	0
Giant Sandwich Brownie Batter Low Fat	1	140	2	0	–
Giant Sandwich Brownie Chunk Low Fat	1	140	2	0	–
Giant Sandwich Vanilla & Chocolate No Sugar Added	1	130	5	3	–
Giant Strawberry Shortcake 98% Fat Free	1 bar	90	1	1	0
Popsicle					
Bar Snoopy	1 (3.5 oz)	150	8	6	–
Bar Sprinklers	1 (2.1 oz)	130	6	3	–
Cone Crispy	1 (2.5 oz)	150	7	4	–
Creamsicle Pop	1 (1.75 oz)	70	2	1	–
Cup Cookies & Cream	1 (10 oz)	310	13	8	–
Fruit Juicee Cups	1 (4 oz)	80	0	0	0
Ice Cream Bar Vanilla	1 (3 oz)	160	11	9	–
Ice Cream Pops Minis	2 (2.8 oz)	190	13	9	–
Sandwich Cookie Rugrats	1 (2.5 oz)	140	6	4	–
Sandwiches Minis	1 (2 oz)	100	4	2	–
Scribblers Ice Cream Pops	2 (2.4 oz)	130	5	4	–
Swirl Bar Bubble Gum	1 (2.6 oz)	60	0	0	0
WWE Bar	1 (3.6 oz)	180	8	5	–
X-Men Wolverine Bar	1 (4 oz)	100	0	0	0

FOOD	PORTION	CALS	FAT	SAT FAT	TRANS FAT
Rice Dream					
Bar Vanilla Nutty	1 (3.3 oz)	320	24	11	0
Bar Vanilla w/ Chocolate Coating	1 (3 oz)	230	15	9	0
Carob Almond	½ cup	180	10	1	0
Frozen Pie Chocolate	1 (3.4 oz)	330	19	8	0
Mint Carob Chip	½ cup	170	8	1	0
Strawberry	½ cup	160	8	0	0
Silhouette					
The Skinny Cow Low Fat Ice Cream Sandwich Vanilla	1	130	2	1	–
Skinny Cow					
Bar Vanilla Strawberry Sorbet Swirl	1	110	1	1	0
Cone Chocolate w/ Fudge	1	150	3	2	0
Cone Vanilla & Caramel	1	150	3	2	0
Fudge Bar	1	100	1	1	0
Sandwich Chocolate Peanut Butter	1	150	2	1	0
Sandwich Strawberry Shortcake	1	140	2	1	0
Sandwich Vanilla	1	140	2	1	0
Sandwich Vanilla No Sugar Added	1	140	2	1	0
Slim-Fast					
Chocolate Fudge Bar	1 bar	110	2	1	–
Ice Cream Sandwich Chocolate	1	130	2	1	–
Ice Cream Sandwich Vanilla	1	130	1	1	–
Soy Dream					
Butter Pecan	½ cup	140	9	2	0
Sandwich Lil' Dreamers Chocolate	1 (1.4 oz)	100	5	1	0
Vanilla	½ cup	140	7	2	0
Starbucks					
Caramel Cappuccino Swirl	½ cup	240	12	7	–
Classic Coffee	½ cup	230	12	7	–
Coffee Almond Fudge	½ cup	250	13	7	–
Frappuccino Bar Java Fudge	1 bar	130	2	1	–
Frappuccino Bar Mocha	1 bar	120	2	1	–
Java Chip	½ cup	250	13	8	–

FOOD	PORTION	CALS	FAT	SAT FAT	TRANS FAT
Low Fat Latte	½ cup	170	3	2	–
Mud Pie	½ cup	240	11	6	–
White Chocolate Latte	½ cup	280	15	6	–
Tofutti					
Cuties Chocolate	1 (1.4 oz)	130	5	1	–
Cuties Vanilla	1 (1.4 oz)	120	5	1	0
Turkey Hill					
Black Cherry	½ cup	140	7	5	–
Black Raspberry	½ cup	140	7	–	–
Butter Pecan	½ cup	170	11	5	–
Carb IQ Vanilla Bean	½ cup	110	8	5	–
Chocolate Marshmallow	½ cup	160	7	–	–
Chocolate Mint Chip	½ cup	180	11	–	–
Chocolate Peanut Butter Cup	½ cup	180	11	–	–
Colombian Coffee	½ cup	140	8	–	–
Cookies 'N Cream	½ cup	160	9	5	–
Death By Chocolate	½ cup	160	8	–	–
Dutch Chocolate	½ cup	150	8	–	–
Egg Nog	½ cup	150	8	–	–
Fat Free No Sugar Added Caramel Fudge Decadence	½ cup	100	0	0	0
Fat Free No Sugar Added Cherry Vanilla Fudge	½ cup	90	0	0	0
Fat Free No Sugar Added Dutch Chocolate	½ cup	90	0	0	0
Fat Free No Sugar Added Vanilla Bean	½ cup	90	0	0	0
Fudge Ripple	½ cup	140	7	–	–
Light Butter Pecan	½ cup	130	6	3	–
Light Choco Mint Chip	½ cup	140	5	4	–
Light Tin Lizzie Sundae	½ cup	140	5	–	–
Light Vanilla & Chocolate	½ cup	110	3	2	–
Light Vanilla Bean	½ cup	110	3	2	–
Neapolitan	½ cup	150	8	5	–
Orange Swirl	½ cup	140	6	–	–
Original Vanilla	½ cup	140	8	–	–
Peanut Butter Ripple	½ cup	170	11	–	–
Philadelphia Style Butter Almond	½ cup	180	12	–	–

FOOD	PORTION	CALS	FAT	SAT FAT	TRANS FAT
Philadelphia Style Chocolate	½ cup	170	10	–	–
Philadelphia Style Mint Chocolate Chip	½ cup	180	11	–	–
Philadelphia Style Sweet Cherry Vanilla	½ cup	160	8	–	–
Philadelphia Style Vanilla Bean	½ cup	170	10	–	–
Rocky Road	½ cup	170	8	4	–
Rum Raisin	½ cup	150	7	–	–
Sandwich Choco Mint Chip	1	200	8	–	–
Sandwich Vanilla	1	190	8	–	–
Strawberries 'N Cream	½ cup	140	6	–	–
Sundae Cones Rocky Road	1	340	19	–	–
Sundae Cones Tin Roof Sundae	1	290	17	–	–
Tin Roof Sundae	½ cup	160	9	5	–
Vanilla & Chocolate	½ cup	150	8	5	–
Vanilla Bean	½ cup	140	8	5	–
Twix					
Ice Cream	½ cup	160	8	5	0
Ice Cream Bar	1 (1.6 oz)	170	10	7	0
Weight Watchers					
English Toffee Crunch	1 bar	110	6	5	1
Smart Ones Giant Sundae	1 serv (8 oz)	150	1	0	–
TAKE-OUT					
cone vanilla light soft serve	1 (4.6 oz)	164	6	4	–
gelato chocolate hazelnut	½ cup (5.3 oz)	370	29	4	–
gelato vanilla	½ cup (3 oz)	211	15	8	–
sundae caramel	1 (5.4 oz)	303	9	5	–
sundae hot fudge	1 (5.4 oz)	284	9	5	–
sundae strawberry	1 (5.4 oz)	269	8	4	–

ICE CREAM CONES AND CUPS

brown sugar cone	1 (10 g)	40	tr	tr	–
wafer cone	1	17	tr	tr	0
waffle cone	1 lg	121	2	tr	0

ICE CREAM TOPPINGS

butterscotch	2 tbsp (1.4 oz)	103	tr	tr	–
caramel	2 tbsp (1.4 oz)	103	tr	tr	–
marshmallow cream	1 jar (7 oz)	615	tr	–	–

FOOD	PORTION	CALS	FAT	SAT FAT	TRANS FAT
marshmallow cream	1 oz	88	tr	–	–
nuts in syrup	2 tbsp	184	9	1	0
pineapple	2 tbsp (1.5 oz)	106	0	–	0
strawberry	1 cup (11.5 oz)	863	1	–	–
strawberry	2 tbsp (1.5 oz)	107	tr	–	–
Colac					
Passion Fruit	1 tbsp	31	0	0	0
Strawberry	1 tbsp	31	0	0	0
Hershey's					
Chocolate Shoppe Caramel	2 tbsp	100	0	0	0
Chocolate Shoppe Double Chocolate	1 tbsp	60	1	1	–
Chocolate Shoppe Hot Fudge	1 tbsp	70	3	1	–
Chocolate Shoppe Hot Fudge Fat Free	2 tbsp	100	0	0	0
Sprinkles Candy Coated Milk Chocolate	1 tbsp	70	3	2	–
Lollipop Tree					
Hot Fudge Sauce	1 tbsp	80	5	3	–
Maple Walnut Cream	2 tbsp	190	12	7	0
Reese's					
Sprinkles Peanut Butter & Milk Chocolate	1 tbsp	70	4	2	–
Sanders					
Butterscotch Caramel	2 tbsp	90	4	2	–
Smucker's					
Butterscotch Caramel	2 tbsp	130	1	1	–
Dove Dark Chocolate	2 tbsp	140	5	2	–
Dove Milk Chocolate	2 tbsp	130	4	2	–
Dulce De Leche Milk Caramel Spread	2 tbsp	110	2	1	–
Hot Fudge	2 tbsp	140	4	1	–
Hot Fudge Sugar Free Fat Free	2 tbsp	90	0	0	0
Magic Shell Caramel	2 tbsp	220	18	9	–
Magic Shell Chocolate	2 tbsp	210	17	8	–
Magic Shell Chocolate Fudge	2 tbsp	120	14	8	–
Magic Shell Turtle Delight	2 tbsp	210	16	7	–
Magic Shell Twix	2 tbsp	210	15	7	–
Steel's					
Sugar Free Butterscotch	2 tbsp	60	0	0	0
Sugar Free Chocolate Fudge	2 tbsp	45	3	2	–

FOOD	PORTION	CALS	FAT	SAT FAT	TRANS FAT
Sugar Free Hot Fudge	2 tbsp	65	3	0	–
Sugar Free Peanut Butter Fudge	2 tbsp	75	6	2	–

ICED TEA
MIX
A La Source

Organic as prep	8 oz	90	0	0	0
Organic Green Tea as prep	8 oz	90	0	0	0
Organic Herbal Tea Red Rooibos	8 oz	80	0	0	0

Carb Options

Lemon as prep	1 serv	0	0	0	0

Celestial Seasonings

Blueberry Ice	1 cup	0	0	0	0

Crystal Light

On The Go All Flavors as prep	1 serv	5	0	0	0
Sugar Free All Flavors as prep	1 serv	5	0	0	0

Lipton

Chailatta Chocolate as prep	8 oz	120	2	0	–
Chailatta Hazelnut as prep	8 oz	120	2	0	–
Chailatta Original as prep	8 oz	120	2	0	–
Chailatta Vanilla as prep	8 oz	120	2	0	–
Decaffeinated Lemon Unsweetened as prep	1 serv	0	0	0	0
Decaffeinated Lemon as prep	1 serv	70	0	0	0
Diet Lemon as prep	1 serv	5	0	0	0
Diet Peach as prep	1 serv	5	0	0	0
Diet Raspberry as prep	1 serv	5	0	0	0
Green Tea as prep	1 serv	70	0	0	0
Lemon Sweetened as prep	1 serv	70	0	0	0
Sweetened All Fruit Flavors as prep	1 serv	80	0	0	0
To Go w/ Honey & Lemon	1 pkg	0	0	0	0
To Go w/ Lemon	1 pkg	0	0	0	0
To Go w/ Mandarin & Mango	1 pkg	0	0	0	0
Unsweetened as prep	1 serv	0	0	0	0

Nestea

Lemon Liquid Concentrate as prep	8 oz	80	0	0	0

FOOD	PORTION	CALS	FAT	SAT FAT	TRANS FAT
Peach Liquid Concentrate as prep	8 oz	90	0	0	0
Sugar Free w/ Lemon	2 tsp	5	0	0	0
Sweetened w/ Lemon	1⅓ tbsp	60	0	0	0
Unsweetened w/ Lemon	2 tsp	5	0	0	0
READY-TO-DRINK					
Anteadote					
All Flavors	8 oz	0	0	0	0
Arizona					
Green Tea w/ Ginseng & Honey	8 oz	70	0	0	0
Lemon	8 oz	90	0	0	0
Bina					
Lemon	8 oz	70	0	0	0
Peach	8 oz	114	0	0	0
Bolthouse Farms					
Perfectly Protein Vanilla Chai Tea w/ Soy	8 oz	160	3	1	0
Bombilla & Gourd					
Organic Eco Teas All Flavors	8 oz	40	0	0	0
Brazil Gourmet					
Nectar Tea All Flavors	8 oz	90	0	0	0
Nectar Tea Light Mango Passion	8 oz	60	0	0	0
C+Swiss					
Hemp Ice Tea	1 can (8.4 oz)	90	0	0	0
Cafe Sepia					
Matcha Latte	1 can (8.6 oz)	130	3	1	–
Crystal Light					
Sugar Free Lemon	8 oz	5	0	0	0
Delta Blues					
Spearmint Tea Punch	8 oz	90	0	0	0
Enviga					
All Flavors	1 can (12 oz)	5	0	0	0
Fuze					
LemonAID	8 oz	70	0	0	0
Slender Energy All Flavors	8 oz	20	0	0	0
Vitamin Tea Diet Peach	8 oz	5	0	0	0
Vitamin Tea Green Tea w/ Ginseng	8 oz	60	0	0	0

FOOD	PORTION	CALS	FAT	SAT FAT	TRANS FAT
Vitamin Tea Lemon	8 oz	70	0	0	0
White Tea	8 oz	60	0	0	0
White Tea No Carb Diet Pomegranate	8 oz	0	0	0	0
Glaceau Vitamin Water					
Vital-T	8 oz	50	0	0	0
Hawaiian					
Iced Tea	1 can	120	0	0	0
Honest Tea					
Assam	8 oz	17	0	0	0
Black Forest Berry	8 oz	25	0	0	0
Gold Rush	8 oz	9	0	0	0
Green Dragon	8 oz	30	0	0	0
Kashmiri Chai	8 oz	17	0	0	0
Lori's Lemon	8 oz	30	0	0	0
Moroccan Mint	8 oz	17	0	0	0
Peach Oo-La-Long	8 oz	30	0	0	0
Hood					
Iced Tea	1 cup	100	0	0	0
Inko's					
White Tea All Flavors	1 bottle (16 oz)	56	0	0	0
White Tea Honeysuckle	1 bottle	0	0	0	0
Ito En					
Apricot	8 oz	60	0	0	0
Green Tea Apple	8 oz	70	0	0	0
Mango	8 oz	50	0	0	0
Shencho Shot	1 can (6.4 oz)	0	0	0	0
White Tea Grape	8 oz	60	0	0	0
Joe Tea					
All Flavors	8 oz	100	0	0	0
Kalahari					
Rooibos Red Tea All Flavors	8 oz	50	0	0	0
Kombucha					
Wonder Drink Asian Pear Ginger	1 bottle (8.5 oz)	60	0	0	0
Wonder Drink Rooibus Red Peach	1 bottle (8.5 oz)	60	0	0	0
Lipton					
Diet Green Tea w/ Citrus	8 oz	0	0	0	0
Diet Lemon	8 oz	0	0	0	0

FOOD	PORTION	CALS	FAT	SAT FAT	TRANS FAT
Diet Sweet	8 oz	0	0	0	0
Extra Sweet	8 oz	100	0	0	0
Green Tea w/ Citrus	8 oz	80	0	0	0
Green Tea w/ Honey	8 oz	70	0	0	0
Lemon	8 oz	90	0	0	0
Original Sweetened	8 oz	70	0	0	0
Original Unsweetened	8 oz	0	0	0	0
Peach	8 oz	110	0	0	0
Raspberry	8 oz	110	0	0	0
Nestea					
Green Tea Peach	1 bottle (20 oz)	220	0	0	0
Green Tea Diet Peach	8 oz	0	0	0	0
Lemon	1 bottle (20 oz)	210	0	0	0
Lemon Diet	8 oz	0	0	0	0
Sweetened	8 oz	60	0	0	0
Sweetened Green Tea	8 oz	80	0	0	0
Sweetened Diet Green Tea	8 oz	0	0	0	0
New Leaf					
All Flavors	8 oz	75	0	0	0
Old Orchard					
Green Tea w/ Lemon & Honey	8 oz	45	0	0	0
Green Tea w/ Pomegranate	8 oz	45	0	0	0
Pacific Foods					
Organic Lemon	8 oz	70	0	0	0
Organic Peach	8 oz	70	0	0	0
Organic Raspberry	8 oz	70	0	0	0
Organic Sweetened Black Tea	8 oz	60	0	0	0
Organic Unsweetened Green Tea	8 oz	0	0	0	0
POM					
Light Tea Pomegranate Hibiscus Green	8 oz	35	0	0	0
Light Tea Pomegranate Orange Blossom	8 oz	35	0	0	0
Light Tea Pomegranate Wildberry White	8 oz	35	0	0	0
Republic Of Tea					
No Carb Unsweetened All Flavors	1 bottle (12 oz)	0	0	0	0

FOOD	PORTION	CALS	FAT	SAT FAT	TRANS FAT
Snapple					
Diet Lemonade Ice Tea	8 oz	10	0	0	0
Diet Lime Green Tea	8 oz	0	0	0	0
Just Plain Tea	8 oz	0	0	0	0
Lemonade Ice Tea	8 oz	110	0	0	0
Lime Green Tea	8 oz	100	0	0	0
Mint	8 oz	110	0	0	0
Peach	8 oz	100	0	0	0
Very Cherry	8 oz	100	0	0	0
SoBe					
Lean Diet Green Tea	8 oz	0	0	0	0
Lean Diet Peach Tea	8 oz	5	0	0	0
Lemon	8 oz	90	0	0	0
Solebury Home					
Organic All Flavors	8 oz	33	0	0	0
Soy20					
Lemon Green Tea	1 bottle (12 oz)	90	0	0	0
Sri Lankan					
Apple	8 oz	70	0	0	0
Lemon	8 oz	60	0	0	0
SSips					
Diet Green Tea w/ Honey & Ginseng	1 box (7 oz)	0	0	0	0
Green Tea w/ Honey & Ginseng	1 box (7 oz)	60	0	0	0
Lemon	8 oz	100	0	0	0
Sweet Leaf					
Diet Sweet	8 oz	0	0	0	0
Lemon & Lime	8 oz	0	0	0	0
Mint & Honey Green	8 oz	60	0	0	0
Peach	8 oz	75	0	0	0
Raspberry & Tangerine	8 oz	75	0	0	0
Sweet Tea	8 oz	75	0	0	0
T42					
A Classic Earl Grey	8 oz	60	0	0	0
Herbal All Flavors	8 oz	70	0	0	0
Jamaican Ginger Green Tea	8 oz	70	0	0	0
Lemon & Honey Green Tea	8 oz	60	0	0	0
Wake-Up Blend English Breakfast	8 oz	45	0	0	0
With Lemon	8 oz	60	0	0	0

FOOD	PORTION	CALS	FAT	SAT FAT	TRANS FAT
Tao Tea					
Grapefruit Green Tea	8 oz	71	0	0	0
Lemon Green Tea	8 oz	67	0	0	0
Tradewinds					
Diet Green Tea	8 oz	0	0	0	0
Diet Raspberry	8 oz	0	0	0	0
Mango Green Tea	8 oz	80	0	0	0
Turkey Hill					
Decaffeinated	1 cup	80	0	0	0
Decaffeinated Orange	1 cup	10	0	0	0
Diet	1 cup	0	0	0	0
Lemon	1 cup	100	0	0	0
Orange	1 cup	100	0	0	0
Peach	1 cup	110	0	0	0
Raspberry Tea	1 cup	110	0	0	0
Regular	1 cup	90	0	0	0
VidaTea					
All Flavors	1 can	90	0	0	0
VitaZest					
Green Tea Vitamin Enriched	8 oz	0	0	0	0
Weil For Tea					
Gyokuro	1 can (8.6 oz)	0	0	0	0
Turmeric	1 can (8.6 oz)	0	0	0	0
XS Energy					
Energy Tea Berry Typhoon	1 can (8.4 oz)	12	0	0	0

ICES AND ICE POPS

FOOD	PORTION	CALS	FAT	SAT FAT	TRANS FAT
Blue Bunny					
Bar Big Fudge	1 (2.7 oz)	110	2	1	0
Chill Cups Double Lemon	1 (4 oz)	100	0	0	0
FrozFruit Creamy Coconut	1 bar (3 oz)	150	10	8	0
FrozFruit Strawberries & Cream	1 bar (4 oz)	190	5	4	0
Pop Banana	1 (1.9 oz)	35	0	0	0
Pop Jolly Rancher	1 (4 oz)	120	0	0	0
Pop Root Beer	1 (1.9 oz)	40	0	0	0
The Original Bomb	1 (1.8 oz)	50	0	0	0
Breeze Freeze					
100% Fruit Juice	1 (8 oz)	54	0	0	0
Fruit Granita	1 (8 oz)	120	0	0	0

FOOD	PORTION	CALS	FAT	SAT FAT	TRANS FAT
Breyers					
Fruit Bars No Sugar Added	1 (1.75 oz)	25	0	0	0
Juice Bar Strawberry	1 (3.75 oz)	120	0	0	0
Soft Frozen Cup Lemonade	1 pkg (12 oz)	290	0	0	0
Soft Frozen Cup Strawberry	1 pkg (12 oz)	260	0	0	0
Edy's					
Sherbet Berry Rainbow	½ cup	130	2	1	0
Sherbet Key Lime	½ cup	130	2	1	0
Sherbet Orange Cream	½ cup	120	2	1	0
Sherbet Raspberry	½ cup	130	1	1	0
Sherbet Swiss Orange	½ cup	150	3	3	0
Sherbet Tropical Rainbow	½ cup	130	1	1	0
Whole Fruit Creamy Coconut	1 bar	120	3	3	0
Whole Fruit Lemonade	1 bar	80	0	0	0
Whole Fruit Lime	1 bar	80	0	0	0
Whole Fruit Orange & Cream	1 bar	80	2	1	0
Whole Fruit Peach	½ cup	90	0	0	0
Whole Fruit Strawberry	1 bar	80	0	0	0
Whole Fruit Tangerine	1 bar	80	0	0	0
Whole Fruit Tropical	1 bar	100	0	0	0
Whole Fruit Wild Berry	1 bar	80	0	0	0
Good Humor					
Great White	1 (3 oz)	70	0	0	0
Hyper Stripe	1 (2.7 oz)	80	0	0	0
Haagen-Dazs					
Sorbet Orange	½ cup	120	0	0	0
Sorbet Orchard Peach	½ cup	130	0	0	0
Sorbet Bars Orange	1 (2.5 oz)	120	5	4	–
Sorbet Bars Raspberry & Vanilla Yogurt	1 (2.5 oz)	90	0	0	0
Sorbet Bars Strawberry & Vanilla Ice Cream	1 (2.5 oz)	110	5	4	–
Hawaiian Punch					
Arctic Surfers	1 pop	50	0	0	0
Hendrie's					
Citrus N' Berry Stix	1 (1.9 oz)	15	0	0	0
Fudge Stix Fat Free	1 bar (1.8 oz)	70	0	0	0
Hood					
Hoodsie Pop	1 (3.3 oz)	60	0	0	0

FOOD	PORTION	CALS	FAT	SAT FAT	TRANS FAT
Luigi's					
Italian Ice Cherry	1 (6 oz)	130	0	0	0
Italian Ice Lemon Strawberry	1 (6 oz)	120	0	0	0
Italian Ice No Sugar Added Lemon	1 (6 oz)	60	0	0	0
Italian Ice Pina Colada	1 (6 oz)	130	0	0	0
Swirl Blue Ribbon Lemonade	1 (6 oz)	150	0	0	0
Minute Maid					
Fruit & Cream Swirl	1 tube (3 oz)	90	3	2	–
Fruit Bars	1 bar	60	0	0	0
Natural Choice					
Organic Vegan Fruit Bars Coconut	1 (2.75 oz)	90	4	3	0
Organic Vegan Fruit Bars Pink Lemonade	1 (2.75 oz)	50	0	0	0
Organic Vegan Grape	1 (2.75 oz)	50	0	0	0
Organic Vegan Sorbet Blueberry	½ cup	110	0	0	0
Organic Vegan Sorbet Lemon	½ cup	110	0	0	0
Organic Vegan Sorbet Mango	½ cup	110	0	0	0
PickleSickle					
Pop	1 (2 oz)	3	0	0	0
Popsicle					
All Natural Ice Pops	1 (1.75 oz)	50	0	0	0
Bar Bart Simpson	1 (4 oz)	110	1	–	–
Bar Dora The Explorer	1 (4 oz)	100	0	0	0
Bar Fruti Holanda Lemon Lime	1 (3 oz)	90	0	0	0
Bar Fruti Holanda Strawberry	1 (3 oz)	90	0	0	0
Bar Incredible Hulk	1 (4 oz)	100	0	0	0
Bar Jimmy Neutron	1 (4 oz)	100	0	0	0
Bar Mega Warheads	1 (4 oz)	110	1	0	–
Bar Power Ranger	1 (4 oz)	100	0	0	0
Bar Spider Man	1 (4 oz)	100	0	0	0
Bar SpongeBob	1 (4 oz)	100	0	0	0
Big Stick Pops Big Reds	1 (3.5 oz)	70	0	0	0
Big Stick Pops Cherry Pineapple	1 (3.5 oz)	50	0	0	0
Bubble Play	1 (4 oz)	100	0	0	0
Creamsicle Bar	1 (2.5 oz)	100	3	2	–
Creamsicle Sugar Free	2 (3.3 oz)	40	2	2	–

FOOD	PORTION	CALS	FAT	SAT FAT	TRANS FAT
Creamsicle Pop No Sugar Added	1 (1.75 oz)	25	0	0	0
Cup Cherry	1 (12 oz)	240	0	0	0
Cup Frostee Fudge	1 (10 oz)	280	11	7	–
Cup Lemon	1 (12 oz)	230	0	0	0
Cup Screwball	1 (3.75 oz)	110	0	0	0
Firecracker	1 (1.6 oz)	35	0	0	0
Fruita Holanda Coconut Bar	1 (3 oz)	120	3	2	–
Fudgsicle Bar	1 (2.5 oz)	90	2	1	–
Fudgsicle Bar Fat Free	1 (1.75 oz)	60	0	0	0
Fudgsicle Pop	1 (1.75 oz)	60	1	1	–
Fudgsicle Pops No Sugar Added	2 (1.75 oz)	90	1	0	–
Minis Fudge Bar	2 (2.4 oz)	80	2	2	–
Pop Great White	1 (1.75 oz)	45	0	0	0
Pop Lick-A-Color	1 (2 oz)	50	0	0	0
Pop Sherbet Cyclone	1 (1.8 oz)	50	1	0	–
Pop Towering Tornado	1 (3.5 oz)	90	0	0	0
Pop Ups Orange Burst	1 (2.75 oz)	80	1	0	–
Pop Ups Reckless Rainbow	1 (2.75 oz)	90	1	0	–
Pop Ups SpongeBob	1 (2.75 oz)	90	2	1	–
Pops Tropical Sugar Free	1 (1.75 oz)	15	0	0	0
Pops Wild Bunch	2 (2.2 oz)	60	0	0	0
Rainbow Floats	1 (1.75 oz)	60	2	1	–
Rainbow Pops	1 (1.75 oz)	45	0	0	0
Scribblers Juice Pops	2 (2.4 oz)	60	0	0	0
Shots	1 serv (1.7 oz)	40	1	–	–
Snow Cone	1 (7 oz)	30	0	0	0
Sugar Free Pops Orange Cherry Grape	1 (1.75 oz)	15	0	0	0
Super Mario Bros Bar	1 (4 oz)	100	0	0	0
Swirl Bar Cotton Candy	1 (2.6 oz)	60	0	0	0
Tingle Twister Ice Pops	1 (1.75 oz)	45	0	0	0
Torpedo Pop Cherry	1 (1.75 oz)	35	0	0	0
The Power Of Fruit					
Original Fruit Bar	1 (1.75 oz)	28	tr	tr	0
Tropicana					
Fruit Juice Bar Orange	1	45	0	0	0
Fruit Juice Bar Raspberry	1	45	0	0	0
Strawberry	1	45	0	0	0

FOOD	PORTION	CALS	FAT	SAT FAT	TRANS FAT
Wawona					
Peach	1 pop	78	tr	0	0
Strawberry	1 pop	77	tr	0	0
JACKFRUIT					
fresh	3.5 oz	70	tr	–	–
JALAPENO (see PEPPERS)					
JAM/JELLY/PRESERVE					
all flavors jam	1 pkg (0.5 oz)	34	0	0	0
all flavors jam	1 tbsp (0.7 oz)	48	0	0	0
all flavors jelly	1 pkg (0.5 oz)	38	0	0	0
all flavors jelly	1 tbsp (0.7 oz)	52	0	0	0
all flavors preserve	1 pkg (0.5 oz)	34	0	0	0
all flavors preserve	1 tbsp (0.7 oz)	48	0	0	0
apple butter	1 tbsp (0.6 oz)	33	0	0	0
orange marmalade	1 pkg (0.5 oz)	34	0	0	0
orange marmalade	1 tbsp (0.7 oz)	49	0	0	0
strawberry jam	1 tbsp (0.7 oz)	48	0	0	0
Cascadian Farm					
Organic Fruit Spread Blackberry	1 tbsp	45	0	0	0
Organic Fruit Spread Raspberry	1 tbsp	45	0	0	0
Organic Sweet Orange Marmalade	1 tbsp	45	0	0	0
Colac					
Jelly All Flavors	1 tbsp	37	0	0	0
Eden					
Organic Apple Butter	1 tbsp	20	0	0	0
Organic Apple Cherry Butter	1 tbsp	25	0	0	0
Organic Cherry Butter	1 tbsp	35	0	0	0
El Angel					
Strawberry Marmalade	1 tbsp	25	0	0	0
Jok'n'Al					
Low Carb Fruit Spreads All Flavors	1 tbsp	10	0	0	0
Lollipop Tree					
Butter Cranberry Pear	1 tbsp	25	0	0	0
Butter Pumpkin Maple Pecan	1 tbsp	30	0	0	0

FOOD	PORTION	CALS	FAT	SAT FAT	TRANS FAT
Jam Raspberry Peach	1 tbsp	50	0	0	0
Jam Triple Cherry	1 tbsp	50	0	0	0
Jelly Hot Pepper	1 tbsp	60	1	0	0
Jelly Wasabi Lime Pepper	1 tbsp	60	0	0	0
Matouk's					
Guava Jam	1 tbsp	50	0	0	0
Mango Jam	1 tbsp	50	0	0	0
Polaner					
All Fruit Apricot	1 tbsp	40	0	0	0
All Fruit Grape	1 tbsp	40	0	0	0
All Fruit Pineapple	1 tbsp	40	0	0	0
All Fruit Raspberry Seedless	1 tbsp	40	0	0	0
Robert Rothchild Farm					
Preserves Cherry Acai	1 tbsp	35	0	0	0
Sarabeth's					
Spreadable Fruit Orange Apricot	1 tbsp	30	0	0	0
Spreadable Fruit Peach Apricot	1 tbsp	40	0	0	0
Smucker's					
Cider Apple Butter	1 tbsp	45	0	0	0
Jam Concord Grape	1 tbsp	50	0	0	0
Jam Red Plum	1 tbsp	50	0	0	0
Jam Seedless Red Raspberry	1 tbsp	50	0	0	0
Jam Seedless Strawberry	1 tbsp	50	0	0	0
Jelly Apple	2 tbsp	50	0	0	0
Jelly Concord Grape	1 tbsp	50	0	0	0
Jelly Currant	1 tbsp	50	0	0	0
Jelly Elderberry	1 tbsp	50	0	0	0
Jelly Guava	1 tbsp	50	0	0	0
Jelly Mixed Fruit	2 tbsp	50	0	0	0
Low Sugar All Flavors	1 tbsp	25	0	0	0
Preserves All Flavors	1 tbsp	50	0	0	0
Simply Fruit All Flavors	1 tbsp	40	0	0	0
Sugar Free All Flavors	1 tbsp	10	0	0	0
Welch's					
Grape Jam	1 tbsp	50	0	0	0

JAPANESE FOOD (see ASIAN FOOD, SUSHI)

JELLY (see JAM/JELLY/PRESERVE)

JERKY (see MEAT STICKS)

FOOD	PORTION	CALS	FAT	SAT FAT	TRANS FAT
JICAMA					
fresh	1 sm (12.8 oz)	139	tr	tr	–
raw sliced	1 cup	46	tr	tr	0
Frieda's					
Jicama	¾ cup	35	0	0	0
JUJUBE					
dried	1 oz	82	tr	–	0
JUTE					
cooked	1 cup	32	tr	tr	–
KALE					
chopped cooked w/o salt	1 cup	36	1	tr	0
fresh cooked w/ fat	1 cup	69	4	1	–
scotch chopped cooked w/o salt	1 cup	36	1	tr	0
Glory					
Fresh Greens	1 serv (2.8 oz)	40	1	0	0
Seasoned canned	½ cup	35	1	0	0
KANGAROO					
kangaroo	3 oz	120	2	–	–
KEFIR					
kefir	8 oz	98	2	1	0
Lifeway					
Greek Style	8 oz	202	14	9	0
Nonfat All Fruit Flavors	8 oz	188	0	0	0
Nonfat Plain	8 oz	116	0	0	0
Organic Helios All Fruit Flavors	8 oz	160	4	3	0
Organic Helios Plain	8 oz	120	4	3	0
Organic Lowfat All Fruit Flavors	8 oz	160	2	2	–
Organic Lowfat Plain	8 oz	110	2	2	–
Original	8 oz	162	8	5	–
Probugs All Flavors	1 bottle	130	5	3	0
Slim6 All Flavors	8 oz	110	2	2	–
KETCHUP					
banana	1 tsp	10	0	0	0
ketchup	1 pkg (0.2 oz)	6	tr	tr	–
ketchup	1 tbsp	15	tr	tr	0
low sodium	1 tbsp	15	tr	tr	0

FOOD	PORTION	CALS	FAT	SAT FAT	TRANS FAT
Del Monte					
Ketchup	1 tbsp	15	0	0	0
Estee					
No Sugar Added	1 tbsp	15	0	0	0
Heinz					
Ketchup	1 tbsp	15	0	0	0
No Salt	1 tbsp	20	0	0	0
One Carb	1 tbsp	5	0	0	0
Organic	1 tbsp	20	0	0	0
Hunt's					
Ketchup	1 tbsp	15	0	0	0
No Salt Added	1 tbsp	20	0	0	0
Squeeze	1 tbsp	15	0	0	0
Keto					
Ketchup	1 tbsp	4	0	0	0
Muir Glen					
Organic	1 tbsp	20	0	0	0
Steel's					
Sugar Free	1 tbsp	10	0	0	0
Stokelys					
Tomato	1 tbsp	15	0	0	0
Walden Farms					
Calorie Free	1 tbsp	0	0	0	0
Wholemato					
Organic Agave	1 tbsp	15	0	0	0
KIDNEY					
beef simmered	3 oz	134	4	1	tr
lamb braised	3 oz	116	3	1	0
pork braised	3 oz	128	4	1	0
veal braised	3 oz	139	5	1	0
KIDNEY BEANS					
canned	½ cup	108	1	tr	0
dried cooked w/o salt	½ cup	112	tr	tr	0
Bush's					
Light Red	½ cup	110	0	0	0
Eden					
Chili Beans	½ cup	130	0	0	0
Organic	½ cup	100	0	0	0
Organic Cannellini	½ cup	100	1	0	0
Organic Refried	½ cup	80	1	0	0

FOOD	PORTION	CALS	FAT	SAT FAT	TRANS FAT
Goya					
Dark	½ cup	90	1	0	–
Progresso					
Red	½ cup	110	0	0	0
Rienzi					
Cannellini	½ cup	80	0	0	0
Red	½ cup	90	1	0	–
KIWI					
fresh	1 lg (3.2 oz)	56	tr	tr	0
fresh	1 med (2.6 oz)	46	tr	tr	0
Chiquita					
Fresh	2 med (5.2 oz)	100	1	0	–
Zespri					
Gold	2 med	80	1	0	0
Green	2 med	100	2	0	0
KIWI JUICE					
Auna					
Kiwifruit Juice	1 bottle (12 oz)	120	0	0	0
KNISH					
Gabila's					
Potato	1 (4.5 oz)	170	6	1	–
TAKE-OUT					
cheese	1 (2.1 oz)	205	12	3	–
meat	1 (1.8 oz)	174	11	3	–
potato	1 (2.1 oz)	212	12	3	–
potato	1 lg (7 oz)	332	12	3	–
KOHLRABI					
raw sliced	1 cup	36	tr	tr	0
sliced cooked w/o salt	1 cup	48	tr	tr	0
Frieda's					
Kohlrabi	⅔ cup	25	0	0	0
TAKE-OUT					
creamed	1 cup	150	9	2	–
KRILL					
fresh	1 oz	22	1	–	–
KUMQUATS					
canned in syrup	1	13	tr	tr	0
fresh	1	13	tr	tr	0

FOOD	PORTION	CALS	FAT	SAT FAT	TRANS FAT
KUZU					
Eden					
Root Starch	1 tbsp	30	0	0	0
LAMB					
cubed lean & fat braised	4 oz	253	10	4	0
cubed lean broiled	4 oz	211	8	3	0
ground broiled	4 oz	321	22	9	0
leg roasted	4 oz	213	15	6	0
loin chop lean & fat broiled	1 chop (4 oz)	222	16	7	0
rib chop lean & fat broiled	1 chop (1.6 oz)	165	14	6	0
rib roast baked	4 oz	386	31	13	0
shank lean & fat braised	4 oz	360	20	8	0
shoulder chop lean & fat cooked	1 chop (5.5 oz)	274	20	8	0
shoulder w/ bone braised	4 oz	231	17	7	0
LAMB DISHES					
TAKE-OUT					
moroccan pilaf w/ bulgur	1 serv	327	13	2	–
moussaka	4 in sq (16 oz)	659	43	11	–
stew w/ potatoes & vegetables	1 cup	260	6	2	–
LAMBSQUARTERS					
chopped cooked w/ salt	1 cup	58	1	tr	0
LEEKS					
chopped cooked w/o salt	¼ cup	8	tr	tr	0
cooked	1 (4.4 oz)	38	tr	tr	0
freeze dried	1 tbsp	1	0	0	0
Frieda's					
Fresh	1 cup	50	0	0	0
LEMON					
fresh	1 med (4 oz)	22	tr	tr	0
peel	1 tbsp	3	tr	tr	0
peel	1 tsp	1	0	0	0
wedge	1 (7 g)	2	tr	tr	0
Sunkist					
Fresh	1 (2 oz)	15	0	0	0
True Lemon					
Crystallized Lemon	1 pkg (1 g)	0	0	0	0

FOOD	PORTION	CALS	FAT	SAT FAT	TRANS FAT
LEMON CURD					
lemon curd made w/ egg	2 tsp	29	1	–	–
Lollipop Tree					
Lemon Curd	1 tbsp	50	2	2	0
Robert Rothchild Farm					
Lemon Curd & Tart Filling	1 tbsp	50	2	1	0
LEMON EXTRACT					
lemon extract	½ tsp	12	tr	–	–
LEMON GRASS					
fresh	1 tbsp	5	tr	tr	0
LEMON JUICE					
bottled	1 oz	6	tr	tr	0
bottled	1 tbsp	3	tr	tr	0
fresh	1 oz	8	0	0	0
from 1 lemon	1.6 oz	12	0	0	0
from wedge	6 g	1	0	0	0
Essn					
Sparkling Meyer Lemon Juice	1 can (8.4 oz)	170	0	0	0
Izze					
Sparkling Lemon	8 oz	150	0	0	0
LEMONADE					
FROZEN					
Tropicana					
Twister Light	8 oz	50	0	0	0
MIX					
A La Source					
Organic as prep	8 oz	110	0	0	0
Country Time					
Lemonade as prep	8 oz	60	0	0	0
Pink as prep	8 oz	60	0	0	0
Raspberry as prep	8 oz	80	0	0	0
Strawberry as prep	8 oz	80	0	0	0
Crystal Light					
Lemonade as prep	1 serv	5	0	0	0
On The Go as prep	1 pkg	5	0	0	0
Pink as prep	1 serv	5	0	0	0
Keto					
Kooler Pink	½ tsp	0	0	0	0

FOOD	PORTION	CALS	FAT	SAT FAT	TRANS FAT
Low Carb Creations					
Lemonade as prep	1 serv	10	0	0	0
Raspberry as prep	1 serv	10	0	0	0
Sipper Sweets					
Sugar Free Low Carb	1 serv	8	0	0	0
READY-TO-DRINK					
Adina					
Hibiscus Lemon Bissap	8 oz	80	0	0	0
Apple & Eve					
Organic	8 oz	130	0	0	0
Crystal Light					
Sugar Free	8 oz	5	0	0	0
Honest Ade					
Cranberry	8 oz	50	0	0	0
Hood					
Lemonade	1 cup	110	0	0	0
Minute Maid					
Chilled	8 oz	100	0	0	0
Lemonade	1 can (12 oz)	150	0	0	0
Light	8 oz	15	0	0	0
Naked Juice					
Just Made	8 oz	110	0	0	0
Nesbitt's					
Honey	1 bottle (12 oz)	180	0	0	0
Newman's Own					
Pink Virgin	8 oz	110	0	0	0
Roadside Virgin	8 oz	110	0	0	0
Virgin Lemon Aided	8 oz	110	0	0	0
Ocean Spray					
Spritzer	8 oz	160	0	0	0
Odwalla					
PomaGrand	8 oz	110	0	0	0
Pure Squeezed	8 oz	120	0	0	0
Purity Organic					
Lemonade	8 oz	123	tr	–	–
Santa Cruz					
Organic	1 can	160	0	0	0
Organic Raspberry	1 can	120	0	0	0
Simply					
Lemonade	8 oz	120	0	0	0

FOOD	PORTION	CALS	FAT	SAT FAT	TRANS FAT
Snapple					
Lemonade	8 oz	110	0	0	0
Super Sour	8 oz	130	0	0	0
SSips					
Lemonade	8 oz	110	0	0	0
Sweet Leaf					
Lemonade Stand All Flavors	8 oz	95	0	0	0
T42					
Lemonade	8 oz	90	0	0	0
Pink	8 oz	90	0	0	0
Three Drinks					
Sparkling	12 oz	12	0	0	0
Tropicana					
Light	1 cup	10	0	0	0
Orchard Style	8 oz	120	0	0	0
Twister Strawberry	8 oz	140	0	0	0
Turkey Hill					
Lemonade	1 cup	120	0	0	0
Uncle Matt's					
Organic	8 oz	120	0	0	0
Zeigler's					
Old Fashioned	8 oz	120	0	0	0

LENTILS

FOOD	PORTION	CALS	FAT	SAT FAT	TRANS FAT
dried cooked	1 cup	230	1	tr	0
Eden					
Organic Green w/ Onion & Bay Leaf	½ cup	90	0	0	0
Near East					
Lentil Pilaf as prep	1 cup	200	3	2	–
Sabra					
Dardara	2 oz	40	2	0	–
Shiloh Farms					
Organic Green not prep	¼ cup (1.6 oz)	150	0	0	0
TastyBite					
Jodhpur Lentils	½ pkg (5 oz)	106	4	2	0
Madras Lentils	½ pkg (5 oz)	127	5	3	0
TAKE-OUT					
lentil loaf	1 slice (1.6 oz)	83	4	tr	–
middle eastern lentil salad	1 serv (4.5 oz)	158	3	tr	–

FOOD	PORTION	CALS	FAT	SAT FAT	TRANS FAT
yemiser selatta ethiopian lentil salad	1 serv (3 oz)	115	7	1	–
LETTUCE (see also SALAD)					
arugula	6 leaves (0.4 oz)	3	tr	tr	0
arugula shredded	1 cup	5	tr	tr	0
boston	1 head (5.7 oz)	21	tr	tr	0
boston chopped	6 leaves	7	tr	tr	0
cornsalad field salad	1 cup (1.9 oz)	7	tr	–	–
iceberg	1 lg head (26.5 oz)	106	1	tr	0
iceberg	6 med leaves	7	tr	tr	0
iceberg shredded	1 cup	10	tr	tr	0
looseleaf outer leaves	6 (5 oz)	22	tr	tr	0
looseleaf shredded	1 cup	5	tr	tr	0
red leaf	6 leaves (3.6 oz)	16	tr	tr	0
red leaf shredded	1 cup	4	tr	tr	0
romaine	3 leaves (3 oz)	14	tr	tr	0
romaine heart	6 leaves (1.3 oz)	6	tr	tr	0
romaine shredded	1 cup	8	tr	tr	0
Andy Boy					
Romaine Hearts	6 leaves (3 oz)	20	1	0	0
Dole					
Classic Romaine	1½ cups (3 oz)	15	0	0	0
Shredded	1½ cups (3 oz)	15	0	0	0
Earthbound Farm					
Organic Baby Romaine Salad	2 cups	15	0	0	0
Frieda's					
Limestone	⅔ cup	10	0	0	0
Green Giant					
Hearts Of Romaine	6 leaves (3 oz)	14	0	0	0
Mann's					
Romaine Jumbo Hearts	3 oz	15	0	0	0
Ocean Mist					
Romaine Hearts	6 leaves	20	1	0	0
Ready Pac					
Baby Arugula	4 cups	20	1	0	–
Bella Romaine	1½ cups	15	0	0	0
River Ranch					
Romaine Chopped	1½ cups	10	0	0	0
Romaine Hearts	1½ cups	10	0	0	0

FOOD	PORTION	CALS	FAT	SAT FAT	TRANS FAT
LILY ROOT					
dried	1 oz	89	1	–	–
fresh	1 oz	32	tr	–	–
LIMA BEANS					
CANNED					
lima beans	½ cup	95	tr	tr	0
Allens					
Medium Green	½ cup	140	1	0	0
Del Monte					
Green	½ cup	80	0	0	0
Hanover					
Butter Beans In Sauce	½ cup	100	0	0	0
S&W					
Small Green	½ cup (4.4 oz)	80	0	0	0
DRIED					
cooked	½ cup	150	tr	tr	0
FROZEN					
C&W					
Baby	½ cup	110	0	0	0
Fresh Like					
Baby	3.5 oz	138	1	–	–
Green Giant					
Baby & Butter Sauce as prep	⅔ cup	100	2	1	0
LIME					
fresh	1 (2.4 oz)	20	tr	tr	0
wedge	1 (8 g)	2	tr	tr	0
Sunkist					
Fresh	1 (2 oz)	20	0	0	0
LIME JUICE					
bottled	1 oz	6	tr	tr	0
fresh	1 oz	8	tr	tr	0
from 1 lime	1.1 oz	11	tr	tr	0
Adina					
Lime Mint Mojita	8 oz	70	0	0	0
Honest Ade					
Limeade	8 oz	50	0	0	0
Minute Maid					
Light Limeade	8 oz	15	0	0	0

FOOD	PORTION	CALS	FAT	SAT FAT	TRANS FAT
Newman's Own					
Virgin Limeade	8 oz	140	0	0	0
Sabor Latino					
Limeade	8 oz	160	0	0	0
Simply					
Limeade	8 oz	120	0	0	0
LING					
blue raw	3.5 oz	83	1	–	–
fresh baked	3 oz	95	1	–	–
fresh fillet baked	5.3 oz	168	1	–	–
LINGCOD					
baked	3 oz	93	1	tr	–
fillet baked	5.3 oz	164	2	tr	–
LIQUOR/LIQUEUR (*see also* BEER AND ALE, CHAMPAGNE, MALT, WINE)					
7&7	1 serv	178	0	0	0
alabama slammer	1 serv	103	tr	0	–
amaretto sour	1 serv	295	tr	tr	–
angel's kiss	1 serv	85	1	1	–
anisette	1 oz	111	0	0	0
antifreeze	1 serv	177	tr	tr	–
apricot brandy	1 oz	96	0	0	0
apricot sour	1 serv	164	tr	0	–
aquavit	1 oz	65	0	0	0
b 52	1 serv	247	4	2	–
b&b	1 serv	75	0	0	0
bahama breeze	1 serv	70	tr	0	–
bahama mama	1 serv	153	tr	tr	–
bailey's & amaretto	1 serv	184	5	3	–
banana colada	1 serv	376	1	tr	–
bay breeze	1 serv	173	tr	tr	–
bend me over	1 serv	242	tr	tr	–
benedictine	1 oz	104	0	0	0
betsy ross	1 serv	206	0	0	0
black devil	1 serv	220	tr	tr	–
black russian	1 serv	184	tr	tr	–
bloody mary	1 serv	150	tr	tr	–
blue whale	1 serv	222	tr	0	–
bourbon & soda	1 serv (4 oz)	105	0	0	0

FOOD	PORTION	CALS	FAT	SAT FAT	TRANS FAT
bourbon sour	1 serv	166	tr	0	–
brandy alexander	1 serv	266	6	4	–
brandy sour	1 serv	164	tr	0	–
bushwacker	1 serv	286	5	2	–
coffee liqueur	1 serv (1.5 oz)	175	tr	tr	–
cognac	1 oz	67	0	0	0
cosmopolitan martini	1 serv	126	tr	0	–
creme de menthe	1 serv (1.5 oz)	186	tr	tr	–
curacao liqueur	1 oz	81	0	0	0
daiquiri	1 serv (2 oz)	112	tr	tr	–
daiquiri banana	1 serv	277	tr	tr	–
dark & stormy	1 serv	64	0	0	0
doctor pepper	1 serv	95	0	0	0
frozen daiquiri	1 serv	393	2	–	–
frozen daiquiri pineapple	1 serv	186	tr	tr	–
frozen tequila screwdriver	1 serv	159	tr	tr	–
fuzzy navel	1 serv	247	tr	tr	–
gin	1 serv (1.5 oz)	110	0	0	0
gin & tonic	1 serv (7.5 oz)	171	0	0	0
gin ricky	1 serv	114	tr	0	–
grasshopper	1 serv	275	5	3	–
happy hawaiian	1 serv	434	8	5	–
harvey wallbanger	1 serv	198	tr	tr	–
head banger	1 serv	165	0	0	0
hot buttered rum	1 serv	219	4	3	–
hot toddy	1 serv	188	1	tr	–
hurricane	1 serv	205	tr	0	–
kamikaze	1 serv	136	0	0	0
long island iced tea	1 serv	292	tr	0	–
lynchburg lemonade	1 serv	465	tr	tr	–
mai tai	1 serv	165	tr	tr	–
manhattan	1 serv	171	tr	0	–
margarita	1 serv	173	0	0	0
margarita strawberry	1 serv	106	tr	tr	–
martini	1 serv (3 oz)	206	0	0	0
martini apple	1 serv	147	tr	tr	–
martini rum	1 serv	131	0	0	0
mellow yellow	1 serv	95	0	0	0
mexican grasshopper	1 serv	638	19	12	–
mint julep	1 serv	136	tr	tr	–

FOOD	PORTION	CALS	FAT	SAT FAT	TRANS FAT
mississippi mud	1 serv	496	12	7	–
mudslide	1 serv	566	10	6	–
narragansett	1 serv	168	0	0	0
nutcracker	1 serv	730	10	6	–
old fashioned	1 serv	223	tr	0	–
orange crush	1 serv	461	tr	tr	–
pain killer	1 serv	277	tr	tr	–
peppermint pattie	1 serv	344	tr	tr	–
pina colada	1 serv (4.5 oz)	245	3	2	–
planter's cocktail	1 serv	105	0	0	0
planter's punch	1 serv	233	tr	tr	–
presbyterian	1 serv	170	0	0	0
purple passion	1 serv	215	tr	tr	–
rob roy	1 serv	171	0	0	0
rum	1 serv (1.5 oz)	97	0	0	0
rum boogie	1 serv	134	tr	0	–
rum cola	1 serv	209	tr	0	–
rum highball	1 serv	170	0	0	0
rum punch	1 serv	448	1	tr	–
rum sour	1 serv	156	tr	0	–
rum swizzle	1 serv	187	0	0	–
rusty nail	1 serv	159	0	0	0
sake	1 serv (1 oz)	39	0	0	0
salty dog	1 serv	210	tr	tr	–
scotch & soda	1 serv	104	0	0	0
screwdriver rum	1 serv	166	tr	tr	–
sea breeze	1 serv	207	tr	tr	–
sex on the beach	1 serv	190	tr	tr	–
slippery nipple	1 serv	142	2	2	–
sloe gin fizz	1 serv (2.5 oz)	132	0	0	0
snake bite	1 serv	362	0	0	0
tequila gimlet	1 serv	150	tr	0	–
tequila sour	1 serv	156	tr	0	–
tequila stinger	1 serv	221	tr	0	–
tequila sunrise	1 serv (6.8 oz)	232	tr	tr	–
tom collins	1 serv (7.5 oz)	121	0	0	0
vermouth cassis	1 serv	97	tr	0	–
vodka	1 serv (1.5 oz)	97	0	0	0
vodka gimlet	1 serv	150	tr	0	–
vodka sour	1 serv	138	tr	0	–

FOOD	PORTION	CALS	FAT	SAT FAT	TRANS FAT
vodka stinger	1 serv	378	tr	tr	–
whiskey	1 serv (1.5 oz)	105	0	0	0
whiskey sour	1 serv (3.5 oz)	162	tr	tr	–
white russian	1 serv	290	8	5	–
zombie	1 serv	235	tr	tr	–

LITCHI JUICE
Ceres
Litchi	8 oz	120	0	0	0

LIVER (see also PATÉ)
beef braised	1 slice (2.4 oz)	130	4	1	0
beef pan fried	1 slice (2.8 oz)	142	4	1	0
chicken fried	3 oz	146	5	2	0
chicken simmered	3 oz	142	6	2	0
lamb braised	3 oz	187	7	3	0
lamb fried	3 oz	202	11	4	–
moose braised	3 oz	132	4	–	0
pork braised	3 oz	140	4	1	0
turkey simmered	1 liver (2.9 oz)	227	17	6	0
veal braised	1 slice (2.8 oz)	154	5	2	0
veal pan fried	1 slice (2.4 oz)	129	4	1	0

Organic Prairie
Beef	2 oz	80	2	1	–

TAKE-OUT
calves liver w/ onions	1 serv (5 oz)	177	4	1	0

LLAMA
llama	3 oz	120	3	–	–

LOBSTER
northern cooked	1 cup	142	1	tr	–
northern cooked	3 oz	83	1	tr	–
northern raw	1 lobster (5.3 oz)	136	1	–	–
northern raw	3 oz	77	1	–	–
spiny steamed	1 (5.7 oz)	233	3	tr	–
spiny steamed	3 oz	122	2	tr	–

Phillips Seafood
Lobster Cake	1 (3 oz)	230	15	2	0

TAKE-OUT
newburg	1 cup	485	27	–	–

FOOD	PORTION	CALS	FAT	SAT FAT	TRANS FAT
LOGANBERRIES					
frzn	1 cup	80	tr	–	–
LONGANS					
fresh	1	2	0	0	0
LOQUATS					
fresh	1	5	tr	tr	–
LOTUS					
root raw sliced	10 slices	45	tr	tr	–
root sliced cooked	10 slices	59	tr	tr	–
seeds dried	1 oz	94	1	tr	–
Eden					
Dried Sliced	5 slices (0.3 oz)	35	0	0	0
Frieda's					
Lotus Root Fresh	1 cup	50	0	0	0
LOX (see SALMON)					
LUPINES					
dried cooked	1 cup	197	5	1	–
LYCHEES					
fresh	1	6	tr	–	–
Frieda's					
Fresh	6–8 (3.5 oz)	60	0	0	0
MACA ROOT					
Navitas Naturals					
Powder Geletanized	1 tsp (5 g)	20	0	0	0
Raw Powder	1 tsp (5 g)	20	0	0	0
MACADAMIA NUTS					
dry roasted w/ salt	11 nuts (1 oz)	200	22	4	–
oil roasted	1 oz	204	22	3	–
Hawaiian Host					
White Choco	3 pieces (1.4 oz)	230	15	9	0
Keto					
Chocolate Covered	1 oz	171	19	5	–
Maranatha					
Macadamia Butter	2 tbsp	230	24	–	–
Mauna Loa					
Chocolate Trio	9 pieces	200	15	7	–

FOOD	PORTION	CALS	FAT	SAT FAT	TRANS FAT
Dry Roasted Salted	¼ cup	200	21	4	–
Dry Roasted Unsalted	¼ cup	200	21	4	–
Honey Roasted	¼ cup	210	21	3	–
Kona Coffee Glazed	¼ cup	190	15	3	–
Maui Onion & Garlic	1 pkg (1.2 oz)	230	23	4	0
Milk Chocolate Coated	3 pieces	230	16	6	0
Milk Chocolate Toffee	7 pieces	210	13	5	–

MACE
ground	1 tsp	8	1	tr	0

MACKEREL
CANNED
jack	1 can (12.7 oz)	563	23	7	–
jack	1 cup	296	12	4	–

Brunswick
Jack In Water	2 oz	100	5	2	–

Chicken Of The Sea
Jack In Tomato Sauce	¼ cup	70	3	1	–
Jack In Water	⅓ cup	90	4	2	–

Orleans
Jack	¼ cup	90	4	2	–

DRIED
Eden
Bonito Flakes	2 tbsp	5	0	0	0

FRESH
atlantic cooked	3 oz	223	15	4	–
atlantic raw	3 oz	174	12	3	–
jack baked	3 oz	171	9	2	–
jack fillet baked	6.2 oz	354	18	5	–
king baked	3 oz	114	2	tr	–
king fillet baked	5.4 oz	207	4	1	–
pacific baked	3 oz	171	9	2	–
pacific fillet baked	6.2 oz	354	18	5	–
spanish cooked	1 fillet (5.1 oz)	230	9	3	–
spanish cooked	3 oz	134	5	2	–
spanish raw	3 oz	118	5	2	–

SMOKED
atlantic	3.5 oz	296	24	5	–

MAHI MAHI
fresh baked	4 oz	192	13	4	0

FOOD	PORTION	CALS	FAT	SAT FAT	TRANS FAT
Phillips Seafood					
Coconut Mahi Mahi w/ Sauce	3 pieces	290	13	4	0
MALANGA					
dasheen mashed	1 cup	226	tr	tr	–
dasheen pieces boiled	1 cup	212	tr	tr	–
pieces fried	1 cup	304	11	2	–
root raw	1 (10.7 oz)	299	1	tr	–
Frieda's					
Malanga	⅔ cup	90	0	0	0
MALT					
malt liquor	1 bottle (12 oz)	148	0	0	0
nonalcoholic	1 bottle (12 oz)	133	tr	tr	–
MALTED MILK					
chocolate as prep w/ milk	1 cup	179	5	3	–
chocolate flavor powder	3 heaping tsp (0.7 oz)	79	1	tr	–
natural flavor as prep w/ milk	1 cup	186	6	3	–
natural flavor powder	3 heaping tsp (0.7 oz)	87	2	1	–
MAMMY-APPLE					
fresh	1	431	4	–	–
MANGO					
fresh	1	135	1	tr	–
C&W					
Chunks	¾ cup	90	0	0	0
Peeled Snacks					
Fruit Picks Go-Mango-Man-Go	1 pkg (1.4 oz)	120	0	0	0
Sunsweet					
Philippine dried	6 pieces (1.5 oz)	130	0	0	0
Thailand dried	⅓ cup (1.4 oz)	140	0	0	0
Tomorrow's Tropicals					
Fresh	½ (3.6 oz)	70	1	0	–
MANGO JUICE					
Ceres					
Mango	8 oz	120	0	0	0
Naked Juice					
Mighty Mango	8 oz	120	0	0	0

FOOD	PORTION	CALS	FAT	SAT FAT	TRANS FAT
Old Orchard					
Nectar Cocktail	8 oz	120	0	0	0
MANGOSTEEN					
canned in syrup	1 cup	143	1	–	0
MARGARINE					
squeeze	1 tsp	34	4	1	–
stick corn	1 stick (4 oz)	815	91	15	–
stick corn	1 tsp	34	4	1	–
tub corn	1 tsp	34	4	1	–
tub diet	1 tsp	17	2	tr	–
Benecol					
Spread Light	1 tbsp	50	5	1	0
Spread Regular	1 tbsp	70	8	1	0
Blue Bonnet					
Light Stick	1 tbsp	50	5	1	–
Soft Spread	1 tbsp	60	7	1	0
Soft Spread Light	1 tbsp	40	5	1	0
Stick	1 tbsp	80	9	2	–
Brummel & Brown					
Creamy Fruit Spread Strawberry	1 tbsp	50	4	1	0
Spread w/ Yogurt	1 tbsp	45	5	1	0
Crystal Farms					
60/40 Margarine Butter	1 tbsp	100	11	5	1
Margarine	1 tbsp	100	11	2	3
Fleischmann's					
Soft Spread Light	1 tbsp	40	5	0	0
Soft Spread Original	1 tbsp	70	8	2	0
Soft Spread Unsalted	1 tbsp	70	8	2	0
Soft Spread w/ Olive Oil	1 tbsp	70	8	2	0
I Can't Believe Its Not Butter					
Regular Stick	1 tbsp	90	10	2	0
Soft Fat Free	1 tbsp	5	0	0	0
Soft Light	1 tbsp	50	5	1	0
Soft Regular	1 tbsp	80	9	2	0
Soft w/ Calcium	1 tbsp	50	5	1	0
Spray	5 sprays	0	0	0	0
Squeeze	1 tbsp	60	7	1	0
Stick Light	1 tbsp	50	6	1	0

FOOD	PORTION	CALS	FAT	SAT FAT	TRANS FAT
Parkay					
Light Spread	1 tbsp	50	5	1	0
Original Spread	1 tbsp	60	7	2	0
Original Stick	1 tbsp	90	10	2	–
Spray	5 sprays	0	0	0	0
Spread + Calcium	1 tbsp	45	5	1	0
Squeeze	1 tbsp	70	8	2	0
Stick Light	1 tbsp	50	5	1	–
Promise					
Buttery Spread	1 tbsp	80	8	2	0
Stick	1 tbsp	90	10	2	–
Smart Balance					
37% Light	1 tbsp	45	5	2	0
67% Light	1 tbsp	80	9	3	0
Omega Plus w/ Flax Oil	1 tbsp	80	9	3	0
Spectrum					
Essential Omega	1 tbsp	80	10	1	0
Spread	1 tbsp	88	10	1	0
Take Control					
Light	1 tbsp	45	5	1	–
Spread	1 tbsp (0.5 oz)	80	8	1	–

MARJORAM

dried	1 tsp	2	tr	tr	0

MARINADE (see SAUCE)

MARLIN

raw	3 oz	110	3	–	–

MARSHMALLOW

marshmallow	1 cup (1.6 oz)	146	tr	–	–
marshmallow	1 reg (0.3 oz)	23	0	0	0
Gol D Lite					
Sugar Free	⅓ pkg (0.9 oz)	51	0	0	0

MATZO

brie	1 piece (0.5 oz)	54	3	1	0
egg	1 (1 oz)	109	1	tr	0
matzo ball	1 med (1.2 oz)	48	2	tr	0
plain	1 (1 oz)	111	tr	tr	0
whole wheat	1 (1 oz)	98	tr	tr	0

FOOD	PORTION	CALS	FAT	SAT FAT	TRANS FAT
Eddyleon					
Dark Chocolate Coated Egg Matzo	1 oz	97	3	2	–
Milk Chocolate Coated Egg Matzo	1 oz	97	4	3	–
Horowitz Margareten					
Egg	1 (1.2 oz)	130	1	1	0
Manischewitz					
Dark Chocolate Coated Egg	½ (1.5 oz)	90	5	3	–
Egg	1 (1.2 oz)	120	1	0	–
Egg & Onion	1 (1 oz)	100	1	0	0
Matzo Ball Mix	2 tbsp	50	0	0	0
Thin Unsalted	1 (0.8 oz)	90	0	0	0
Streit's					
Egg	1 (1.1 oz)	120	1	1	–
Egg & Onion	1 (1 oz)	100	1	0	0
Passover	1 (1 oz)	110	1	0	–
MAYONNAISE					
diet	1 tbsp	36	3	1	0
imitation	1 tbsp	35	3	tr	0
mayonnaise	1 tbsp	99	11	2	0
Blue Plate					
Squeeze	1 tbsp	100	11	2	–
Cains					
All Natural	1 tbsp	100	11	2	0
Light	1 tbsp	50	5	0	0
Carb Options					
Whipped Dressing	1 tbsp	50	5	1	–
Hellman's					
Light	1 tbsp	45	5	1	0
Real	1 tbsp	90	10	2	0
Real Canola No Cholesterol	1 tbsp	90	10	1	0
Reduced Fat	1 tbsp	20	2	0	0
Hollywood					
Canola	1 tbsp	100	11	1	–
Safflower	1 tbsp	100	11	2	–
Kraft					
Mayo	1 tbsp	90	10	2	0

FOOD	PORTION	CALS	FAT	SAT FAT	TRANS FAT
Miracle Whip					
Free	1 tbsp	15	0	0	0
Light	1 tbsp	25	2	0	0
Original	1 tbsp	40	3	0	0
Nasoya					
Fat Free Nayonaise	1 tbsp	10	0	0	0
Nayonaise	1 tbsp	35	4	1	–
Smart Balance					
Omega	1 tbsp	120	14	1	0
Omega Plus	1 tbsp	50	5	0	0
Spectrum					
Canola Squeeze	1 tbsp	100	11	1	0
Canola Squeeze Light Eggless Vegan	1 tbsp	35	4	0	0
Organic Dijon	1 tbsp	90	10	2	0
Organic Olive Oil	1 tbsp	100	11	2	0
Organic Roasted Garlic	1 tbsp	100	11	2	0
Organic Squeeze	1 tbsp	100	11	2	0
Organic Wasabi	1 tbsp	100	11	2	0
MEAT STICKS					
jerky beef	1 piece (0.7 oz)	82	5	2	–
pork jerky	1 strip (0.5 oz)	62	4	2	0
venison jerky	1 strip (0.5 oz)	55	3	1	0
Jack Link's					
Beef Jerky Teriyaki	1 oz	80	1	0	0
Organic Prairie					
Beef Jerky	1 oz	75	2	1	0
Pemmican					
Homestyle Tender All Flavors	1 oz	80	2	1	–
Kippered Beef Original	1 pkg (1 oz)	60	1	0	–
Kippered Beef Peppered	1 pkg (1 oz)	60	1	0	–
Kippered Beef Sweet & Hot	1 pkg (1 oz)	70	1	0	–
Kippered Beef Teriyaki	1 pkg (1 oz)	60	1	0	–
Long Lasting Hot & Spicy	1 oz	60	1	0	–
Long Lasting Original	1 oz	60	1	0	–
Long Lasting Peppered	1 oz	60	1	0	–
Long Lasting Teriyaki	1 oz	70	1	0	–
Premium Cut Beef Jerky	1 oz	80	1	0	–
Premium Cut Turkey Peppered	1 oz	70	1	0	–

FOOD	PORTION	CALS	FAT	SAT FAT	TRANS FAT
Premium Cut Turkey Sweet Smoked	1 oz	70	1	0	–
Shredded Beef Jerky All Flavors	¼ cup	80	2	1	–
Steak Tips All Flavors	1 oz	70	2	1	–
Slim Jim					
Beef Jerky	7 pieces	130	8	4	1
Beef Jerky Hickory Smoked	1 oz	80	2	1	0
Classic Handipack	1 box	210	19	7	–
Giant Caddy Pepperoni	1 pkg	150	13	5	1
Twin Pack Cheese & Pepperoni	1 pkg	150	12	7	–
Tanka					
Natural Buffalo Cranberry Bar	1 (1 oz)	70	2	1	0
Natural Buffalo Cranberry Bite	1 (0.5 oz)	35	1	0	0
Tofurky					
Jurky Original	4 pieces (1 oz)	100	2	–	–
Wellshire					
Matt's Select Pepperoni	1 stick (0.9 oz)	90	7	3	–
Tom Tom Snack Hot n' Spicy Turkey	1 stick (0.8 oz)	50	3	1	–

MEAT SUBSTITUTES (*see also* BACON SUBSTITUTES, CANADIAN BACON SUBSTITUTES, CHICKEN SUBSTITUTES, HAMBURGER SUBSTITUTES, SAUSAGE SUBSTITUTES, TURKEY SUBSTITUTES)

FOOD	PORTION	CALS	FAT	SAT FAT	TRANS FAT
Fantastic					
Sloppy Joe Mix not prep	¼ cup	70	1	0	–
Taco Filling not prep	¼ cup	80	1	0	–
Gardenburger					
BBQ Riblets w/ Sauce	1 serv (5 oz)	240	5	0	0
Helen's Kitchen					
GardenSteak Tofu Steak	1 (3 oz)	150	2	0	0
Lightlife					
Balogna	4 slices (2 oz)	60	0	0	0
Gimme Lean Ground Beef	1 serv (2 oz)	50	0	0	0
Smart BBQ	¼ cup	70	0	0	0
Smart Cutlet Salisbury Steak	1 (4.5 oz)	130	1	0	–
Smart Deli Country Ham	4 slices (2 oz)	90	0	0	0
Smart Deli Pastrami Style	4 slices (2 oz)	60	0	0	0
Smart Deli Pepperoni Style	13 slices (1 oz)	45	0	0	0
Smart Ground Original	⅓ cup (1.9 oz)	80	1	0	–
Smart Ground Taco Burrito	⅓ cup (2 oz)	70	0	0	0

FOOD	PORTION	CALS	FAT	SAT FAT	TRANS FAT
Smart Menu Crumbles	⅓ cup	80	1	0	–
Smart Menu Meatless Meatballs	5	160	7	1	–
Smart Menu Steak Strips	1 serv (3 oz)	80	0	0	0
Smart Tex Mex	¼ cup	50	0	0	0
Loma Linda					
Dinner Cuts	2 slices (3.2 oz)	90	1	0	0
Swiss Steak	1 piece (3.2 oz)	130	6	1	0
Morningstar Farms					
Meal Starters Steak Strips	12 pieces (3 oz)	140	3	1	0
Quorn					
Grounds	⅔ cup (3 oz)	80	3	1	–
Soy7					
Burger Bits as prep	½ cup	60	1	0	–
Burger Mix as prep	1 serv (3.2 oz)	120	3	0	–
Recipe Strips as prep	¾ cup	70	1	1	–
Taco Mix as prep	¼ cup	70	1	0	–
VeggieLand					
Crumbles Beef	½ cup	70	0	0	0
Veg-T-Balls	3 (3 oz)	113	3	0	–
Viana					
Cowgirl Veggie Steaks	1 (3.7 oz)	260	14	3	1
Veggie Cevapcici	4 pieces (2.8 oz)	240	14	2	1
Veggie Gyros	24 strips (3 oz)	220	11	2	1
Veggie Kebab	½ cup	210	14	3	1
Worthington					
Bolono	3 slices (2 oz)	80	3	1	0
Choplets	2 slices (3.2 oz)	90	1	0	0
Corned Beef Vegetarian	3 slices (2 oz)	140	9	1	0
Dinner Roast	1 slice (3 oz)	180	11	2	0
Multigrain Cutlets	2 slices (3.2 oz)	100	1	1	0
Prime Steaks	1 piece (3.2 oz)	120	6	1	0
Vegetable Skallops	½ cup (3 oz)	90	1	0	0
Wham	2 slices (2 oz)	110	7	1	0
Yves					
Meatless Beef Skewers	1 (2.8 oz)	100	1	0	0
Meatless Bologna	4 slices	60	3	0	0
Meatless Pepperoni	6 slices	90	1	0	0
Meatless Ground Round Original	⅓ cup	60	1	0	0

FOOD	PORTION	CALS	FAT	SAT FAT	TRANS FAT
MEATBALL SUBSTITUTES					
meatless	2 (1.3 oz)	71	3	1	–
Gardenburger					
Mama Mia Meatballs	6 (3 oz)	110	5	1	0
Loma Linda					
Tender Rounds	6 (2.8 oz)	120	5	1	0
Quorn					
Meatballs	4 (2.4 oz)	110	3	1	–
MEATBALLS					
beef	1 lg (1.5 oz)	111	7	3	–
beef	1 med (1 oz)	74	5	2	–
beef cocktail	1 (0.2 oz)	18	1	tr	–
turkey	1 med (1 oz)	47	2	tr	–
Honeysuckle White					
Turkey Italian Style frzn	3 (3 oz)	190	10	3	–
Ian's					
Italian	3 (2.2 oz)	145	4	1	–
Mama Lucia					
Homestyle	4	207	20	8	1
Italian Style	4	280	23	10	1
Sausage Beef	8	220	17	7	1
Organic Classics					
Italian Beef	3 (3 oz)	180	11	5	–
Shady Brook					
Italian Beef	3 oz	260	20	8	–
Turkey Meatballs Appetizer Size + Sweet & Sour Sauce	6 + 2 tbsp sauce	235	10	3	0
Turkey Meatballs Italian Style	3 (3 oz)	190	10	3	0
Tyson					
Italian Style Chicken	6 (3 oz)	180	11	3	–
TAKE-OUT					
albondigas w/ sauce	3 + sauce (5.3 oz)	372	27	8	–
porcupine + tomato sauce	3 + sauce	160	7	3	–
swedish w/ cream sauce	3 + sauce (4.7 oz)	215	12	5	–
sweet & sour	3 + sauce (4.5 oz)	188	11	3	–
MELON					
sprite	1 (10.6 oz)	110	0	0	0
Frieda's					
Camouflage	1 cup (5 oz)	50	0	0	0

FOOD	PORTION	CALS	FAT	SAT FAT	TRANS FAT
SpriteMelon	1 (10.5 oz)	115	0	0	0
Temptation	¹⁄₁₀ melon (4.7 oz)	55	0	0	0

MEXICAN FOOD (see SALSA, SPANISH FOOD, TORTILLA)

MILK
CANNED

FOOD	PORTION	CALS	FAT	SAT FAT	TRANS FAT
condensed sweetened	1 cup	982	27	17	–
condensed sweetened	1 oz	123	3	2	–
evaporated	½ cup	169	10	6	–
evaporated skim	½ cup	99	tr	tr	–
Carnation					
Evaporated	2 tbsp	40	2	2	0
Evaporated Fat Free	2 tbsp	25	0	0	0
Evaporated Lowfat 2%	2 tbsp	25	1	0	0
Meyenberg					
Evaporated Goat Milk	8 oz	145	8	5	–
Pet					
Evaporated	2 tbsp	40	2	2	–
DRIED					
buttermilk	1 tbsp	25	tr	tr	–
nonfat instantized	1 pkg (3.2 oz)	244	tr	tr	–
Alba					
Instant Non-Fat as prep	1 cup	80	0	0	0
Bob's Red Mill					
Buttermilk Sweet Cream as prep	8 oz	60	1	1	0
Non Fat as prep	8 oz	80	0	0	0
Carnation					
Instant Nonfat as prep	1 cup	80	0	0	0
Meyenberg					
Instant Goat Milk as prep	1 cup	142	7	4	–
Organic Valley					
Buttermilk	3 tbsp	110	1	0	0
Nonfat	3 tbsp	90	0	0	0
REFRIGERATED					
1%	1 cup	102	3	2	–
1%	1 qt	409	10	6	–
1% protein fortified	1 cup	119	3	2	–
1% protein fortified	1 qt	477	12	7	–
2%	1 cup	121	5	3	–

FOOD	PORTION	CALS	FAT	SAT FAT	TRANS FAT
2%	1 qt	485	19	12	–
buffalo	7 oz	224	16	–	–
buttermilk	1 cup	99	2	1	–
buttermilk	1 qt	396	9	5	–
camel	7 oz	160	8	–	–
donkey	7 oz	86	2	–	–
goat	1 cup	168	10	7	–
goat	1 qt	672	40	26	–
human	1 cup	171	11	5	–
indian buffalo	1 cup	236	17	11	–
low sodium	1 cup	149	8	5	–
mare	7 oz	98	4	–	–
nonfat	1 cup	86	tr	tr	–
nonfat protein fortified	1 qt	400	2	2	–
sheep	1 cup	264	17	11	–
whole	1 cup	150	8	5	–
Active Lifestyle					
Fat Free w/ Plant Sterols	8 oz	90	0	0	0
Borden					
Fat Free Skim	1 cup	80	0	0	0
Farmland					
Buttermilk	8 oz	160	4	3	–
Fat Free	8 oz	80	0	0	0
Special Request 1% Plus Omega-3	8 oz	130	3	2	–
Special Request Skim Plus	8 oz	110	0	0	0
Special Request Skim Plus 100% Lactose Free	8 oz	110	0	0	0
Whole	8 oz	160	4	3	–
Hood					
1%	1 cup	110	3	2	0
2%	1 cup	130	5	3	0
Buttermilk Fat Free	1 cup	90	0	0	0
Calorie Countdown 2%	8 oz	90	5	3	0
Calorie Countdown Fat Free	8 oz	45	0	0	0
Fat Free	1 cup	80	0	0	0
Simply Smart 0% Fat	1 cup	90	0	0	0
Simply Smart 1% Fat	1 cup	120	3	2	0
Whole	1 cup	150	8	5	0

FOOD	PORTION	CALS	FAT	SAT FAT	TRANS FAT
Horizon Organic					
Fat Free	8 oz	90	0	0	0
Lactaid					
1% Lowfat	1 cup	110	3	2	–
2% Reduced Fat	1 cup	130	5	3	–
Calcium Fortified	1 cup	80	0	0	0
Fat Free	1 cup	90	0	0	0
Whole	1 cup	150	8	5	–
Meyenberg					
Goat Milk	8 oz	142	7	4	–
Goat Milk Low Fat	8 oz	89	2	2	–
Organic Valley					
Fat Free	1 cup	90	0	0	0
Lactose Free Fat Free	1 cup	90	0	0	0
Whole Nonhomogenized	1 cup	150	8	5	0
SunMilk					
Heart Healthy 1% Sunflower Oil	8 oz	120	2	0	0
Heart Healthy 2% Sunflower Oil	8 oz	120	3	0	0
Tuscan					
Whole	8 oz	150	8	5	0
Welsh Farms					
Fat Free	8 oz	80	0	0	0
SHELF-STABLE					
Parmalat					
2% Reduced Fat	8 oz	130	5	3	–
Fat Free	8 oz	80	0	0	0
Lactose Free 2% Reduced Fat	8 oz	130	5	3	–
MILK DRINKS					
chocolate milk	1 cup	208	8	5	–
chocolate milk	1 qt	833	34	21	–
chocolate milk 1%	1 cup	158	3	2	–
chocolate milk 2%	1 cup	179	5	3	–
Bravo!					
Blenders Creamy Double Chocolate	1 bottle (11 oz)	180	4	3	0
Blenders Creamy French Vanilla	1 bottle (11 oz)	160	4	3	0

FOOD	PORTION	CALS	FAT	SAT FAT	TRANS FAT
Cal-C					
Orange Tangerine	8 oz	70	0	0	0
Peach Mango	8 oz	70	0	0	0
Strawberry Citrus	8 oz	70	0	0	0
Cocio					
Chocolate Milk	1 bottle	225	7	–	–
CocoaVia					
Indulgence Rice Chocolate	1 bottle (5.65 oz)	150	3	1	0
Dove					
Bravo! Dark Chocolate	1 bottle	310	16	–	–
Bravo! Milk Chocolate	1 bottle	310	16	–	–
Farmland					
Really Really Good! Chocolate Milk	8 oz	160	3	2	–
Garelick					
Colossal Coffee	1 cup	145	3	2	–
Ultimate Chocolate	1 cup	150	3	2	–
Hershey's					
Chocolate Milk Fat Free	1 bottle	160	0	0	0
Chocolate Milk Reduced Fat	1 bottle	200	5	3	–
Hood					
Calorie Countdown Chocolate 2%	8 oz	90	5	3	0
Chocolate Lowfat	1 cup	170	3	2	0
Chocolate Milk	1 cup	230	9	5	0
Coffee Lowfat Milk	1 cup	170	3	2	0
Horizon Organic					
Lowfat Chocolate Milk	8 oz	170	3	2	0
Strawberry	8 oz	200	5	3	0
Keto					
Chocolate Milk Mix	1 scoop	36	1	–	–
Lifeway					
La Fruta All Flavors	8 oz	180	2	2	–
Nesquik					
Chocolate as prep w/ lowfat milk	1 cup	210	5	3	–
Chocolate No Sugar as prep w/ lowfat milk	1 cup	130	1	1	–
Double Chocolate as prep w/ lowfat milk	1 cup	210	5	3	–

FOOD	PORTION	CALS	FAT	SAT FAT	TRANS FAT
Ready-To-Drink Banana	1 cup	200	5	3	–
Ready-To-Drink Chocolate	1 cup	200	5	3	–
Ready-To-Drink Double Chocolate	1 cup	200	5	3	–
Ready-To-Drink Fat Free Chocolate	1 cup	160	0	0	0
Ready-To-Drink Strawberry	1 cup	200	5	3	–
Ready-To-Drink Very Vanilla	1 cup	200	5	3	–
Strawberry as prep w/ lowfat milk	1 cup	210	4	3	–
Vanilla as prep w/ lowfat milk	1 cup	210	4	3	–
Organic Valley					
Buttermilk Lowfat 1%	1 cup	100	3	2	0
Parmalat					
Chocolate Milk 2% Reduced Fat	1 cup	190	5	3	–
Quaker					
Chocolate	8 oz	140	5	–	–
Strawberry	8 oz	130	5	–	–
Vanilla	8 oz	130	5	–	–
Rosa's Original					
Horchata All Flavors	8 oz	160	2	–	–
Sipahh					
Straw Banana	1 straw	15	0	0	0
Straw Cookies and Cream	1 straw	15	0	0	0

MILK SUBSTITUTES

FOOD	PORTION	CALS	FAT	SAT FAT	TRANS FAT
imitation milk	1 cup	150	8	2	–
imitation milk	1 qt	600	33	7	–
soy milk	1 cup	79	5	1	–
8th Continent					
Soymilk Chocolate	8 oz	140	3	1	0
Soymilk Original	8 oz	80	3	1	0
Soymilk Vanilla	8 oz	100	3	1	0
Soymilk Fat Free Original	8 oz	60	0	0	0
Soymilk Fat Free Vanilla	8 oz	70	0	0	0
Soymilk Light Chocolate	8 oz	90	2	1	0
Soymilk Light Original	8 oz	50	2	0	0
Soymilk Light Vanilla	8 oz	60	1	0	0

FOOD	PORTION	CALS	FAT	SAT FAT	TRANS FAT
Almond Breeze					
Chocolate	8 oz	115	3	tr	0
Original	8 oz	57	3	tr	0
Original Unsweetened	8 oz	40	3	0	0
Vanilla	8 oz	91	3	tr	0
Brazsoy					
Condensed Soy Milk	1 serv (0.7 oz)	54	1	0	0
Soy Cream	1 tbsp (0.5 oz)	27	3	tr	0
DariFree					
Fat Free as prep	8 oz	70	0	0	0
Fat Free Chocolate as prep	8 oz	110	0	0	0
EdenBlend					
Organic	8 oz	120	3	1	0
Edensoy					
Organic Carob	8 oz	170	4	1	0
Organic Chocolate	8 oz	180	4	1	0
Organic Original	8 oz	140	5	1	0
Organic Original Unsweetened	8 oz	120	6	1	0
Organic Original Light	8 oz	100	2	0	0
Organic Vanilla	8 oz	150	3	1	0
Organic Light Vanilla	8 oz	110	1	0	0
Keto					
Low Carb Mix	1 scoop	54	2	–	–
Lifeway					
SoyTreat All Flavors	8 oz	160	4	0	–
Living Harvest					
Hempmilk Original	1 cup	130	3	1	0
Hempmilk Vanilla	1 cup	130	3	1	0
Lundberg					
Organic Drink Rice Original	8 oz	120	3	0	0
Manitoba Harvest					
Hemp Bliss Chocolate	8 oz	160	7	1	0
Hemp Bliss Original	1 cup	110	7	1	0
Hemp Bliss Vanilla	8 oz	150	7	1	0
Odwalla					
Soy Smart Chai	8 oz	150	4	1	–
Soy Smart Vanilla	8 oz	120	4	1	–
Soymilk Plain	8 oz	110	4	1	0
Soymilk Vanilla Being	8 oz	100	3	0	0

FOOD	PORTION	CALS	FAT	SAT FAT	TRANS FAT
Organic Valley					
Soy Original	1 cup	100	3	1	0
Soy Unsweetened	1 cup	80	4	1	0
Pacific Foods					
Almond Low Fat Original	1 cup	70	3	0	0
Almond Low Fat Vanilla	1 cup	100	3	0	0
Multi Grain Low Fat Original	1 cup	160	2	1	0
Oat Organic Low Fat Original	1 cup	130	3	0	0
Oat Organic Low Fat Vanilla	1 cup	130	3	0	0
Rice Low Fat Plain	1 cup	130	2	0	0
Rice Low Fat Vanilla	1 cup	130	2	0	0
Soy Organic Unsweetened Original	1 cup	90	5	1	0
Soy Select Low Fat Plain	1 cup	70	3	0	0
Soy Select Low Fat Vanilla	1 cup	80	3	0	0
Soy Ultra	1 cup	130	4	1	0
Soy Ultra Plain	1 cup	120	4	1	0
Rice Dream					
Carob	8 oz	150	3	0	0
Heartwise Vanilla	8 oz	140	2	0	0
Horchata	8 oz	130	4	1	0
Original	8 oz	120	3	0	0
Original Enriched	8 oz	120	3	0	0
Vanilla Enriched	8 oz	130	3	0	0
Silk					
Chocolate	1 cup	140	4	0	–
Vanilla	1 bottle (11 oz)	140	5	1	–
Sno*e					
Tofu as prep	8 oz	80	5	2	–
Tofu Low Fat as prep	8 oz	70	3	0	–
Soy Dream					
Classic Vanilla	8 oz	140	4	1	0
Original Enriched	8 oz	100	4	1	0
Vitamite					
Non-Dairy	1 cup (8 oz)	110	5	2	–
Vitasoy					
Classic Original	8 oz	120	5	1	–
Complete Original	8 oz	70	2	0	–
Complete Vanilla	8 oz	50	1	0	–
Creamy Original	8 oz	110	4	1	–

FOOD	PORTION	CALS	FAT	SAT FAT	TRANS FAT
Green Tea Soymilk	8 oz	120	4	1	–
Light Original	8 oz	60	2	1	–
Light Chocolate	8 oz	100	2	1	–
Lite Vanilla	8 oz	70	2	1	–
Original Unsweetened	8 oz	80	4	1	–
Rich Chocolate	8 oz	160	4	1	–
Smooth Vanilla	8 oz	120	4	1	–
Vanilla Delight	8 oz	120	4	1	–
White Wave					
Mocha	1 cup	140	4	0	–
WildWood					
Organic Soymilk Plain	8 oz	100	4	1	0
Organic Soymilk Unsweetened	8 oz	72	4	1	0
MILKFISH (AWA)					
baked	3 oz	162	7	–	–
MILKSHAKE					
chocolate	1 serv (10 oz)	393	14	8	–
malted milk shake	1 serv (10 oz)	402	14	8	–
vanilla	1 serv (10 oz)	379	13	8	–
Ben & Jerry's					
Cherry Garcia	1 bottle (8 oz)	320	12	–	–
Chocolate Fudge Brownie	1 bottle (8 oz)	340	12	–	–
Chunky Monkey	1 bottle (8 oz)	330	10	–	–
Breyers					
Quick Vanilla	1 serv (10 oz)	320	17	11	–
Carb Options					
Chocolate Delite	1 can (11 oz)	190	9	2	–
Creamy Vanilla	1 can (11 oz)	190	9	2	–
Hershey's					
Chocolate	1 bottle	270	8	5	–
Cookies 'N' Cream	1 bottle	280	7	5	–
Strawberry	1 bottle	280	7	5	–
Vanilla Cream	1 bottle	320	7	5	–
Nesquik					
Ready-To-Drink Chocolate	1 cup	170	5	3	–
MILLET					
cooked	1 cup (6.1 oz)	207	2	tr	–
Arrowhead Mills					
Organic Hulled not prep	¼ cup	150	2	0	0

FOOD	PORTION	CALS	FAT	SAT FAT	TRANS FAT
MINERAL WATER (see WATER)					
MISO					
dried	1 oz	86	3	–	–
miso	½ cup	284	8	1	–
Eden					
Hacho	1 tbsp	40	2	tr	0
Organic Genmai	1 tbsp	25	1	0	0
Organic Mugi	1 tbsp	25	1	0	0
Organic Shiro	1 tbsp	30	1	0	0
Tekka	1 tsp	5	0	0	0
MOLASSES					
blackstrap	1 cup (11.5 oz)	771	tr	–	–
blackstrap	1 tbsp (0.7 oz)	47	0	0	0
molasses	1 cup (11.5 oz)	873	1	–	–
molasses	1 tbsp (0.7 oz)	53	0	0	0
Brer Rabbit					
Dark	1 tbsp	60	0	0	0
Grandma's					
Robust	1 tbsp	60	0	0	0
MONKFISH					
baked	3 oz	82	2	–	–
MOOSE					
roasted	4 oz	142	1	tr	0
MOTH BEANS					
dried cooked	1 cup	207	1	tr	–
MOUSSE					
TAKE-OUT					
chocolate	½ cup (7.1 oz)	447	33	19	–
orange	½ cup	87	5	–	–
MUFFIN					
MIX					
blueberry	1 (1.75 oz)	149	4	1	–
corn	1 (1.75 oz)	160	5	1	–
wheat bran as prep	1 (1.75 oz)	138	5	1	–
Betty Crocker					
Apple Cinnamon as prep	1	170	7	2	–
Apple Streusel as prep	1	210	8	1	–

FOOD	PORTION	CALS	FAT	SAT FAT	TRANS FAT
Banana Nut as prep	1	170	6	1	–
Cranberry Orange as prep	1	150	5	1	–
Double Chocolate as prep	1	220	11	4	–
Golden Corn as prep	1	160	5	1	–
Lemon Poppyseed as prep	1	180	8	1	–
Sunkist Lemon Poppyseed as prep	1	190	7	1	–
Twice The Blueberries as prep	1	140	3	1	–
Wild Blueberry as prep	1	170	5	1	–
Carbsense					
Honey Bran not prep	1 serv (1.3 oz)	120	4	0	–
Glory					
Golden Sweet Corn as prep	1	170	5	1	–
Jiffy					
Apple Cinnamon as prep	1	190	7	3	–
Banana Nut as prep	1	180	7	4	–
Blueberry as prep	1	190	7	3	–
Bran w/ Dates as prep	1	170	6	3	–
Corn as prep	1	180	6	2	–
Raspberry as prep	1	180	7	3	–
Ketogenics					
Apple Cinnamon Bran as prep	1	190	10	0	–
Chocolate Chip as prep	1	215	14	0	–
Wild Blueberry as prep	1	190	14	0	–
King Arthur					
Cranberry Orange Whole Grain not prep	¼ cup	180	1	0	0
MiniCarb					
Apple Cinnamon as prep	1	225	16	2	–
Sweet Corn as prep	1	225	16	1	–
Miracle Maize					
Country Style as prep	1	155	6	1	–
Sweet as prep	1	180	6	1	–
Miracle Muffins					
Banana w/ Splenda as prep	1	86	3	0	–
Sweet Rewards					
Low Fat Apple Cinnamon as prep	1	140	2	0	–
READY-TO-EAT					
blueberry	1 (2 oz)	158	4	1	–

FOOD	PORTION	CALS	FAT	SAT FAT	TRANS FAT
oat bran wheat free	1 (2 oz)	154	4	1	–
toaster type blueberry	1	103	3	tr	–
toaster type corn	1	114	4	1	–
toaster type wheat bran w/ raisins	1 (1.3 oz)	106	3	1	–
Fred's Incredible Muffins					
All Flavors	1 (2.5 oz)	100	3	0	0
Natural Ovens					
Blueberry	1 (2.5 oz)	180	5	1	–
Carrot Nut	1 (2.5 oz)	170	6	1	–
Raisin Bran	1 (2.5 oz)	170	3	0	–
Otis Spunkmeyer					
Apple Cinnamon	1 (4 oz)	420	22	4	–
Cheese Streusel	½ muffin (2 oz)	220	10	3	–
Low Fat Wild Blueberry	1 (2.25 oz)	200	4	1	–
Uncle Wally's					
Chocolate Passion	1 (2 oz)	130	0	0	0
Cranberry Orange Supreme	1 (2 oz)	130	0	0	0
Fat Free Apple Cinnamon Delight	1 (2 oz)	110	0	0	0
Fat Free Wild Blueberry Bliss	1 (2 oz)	120	0	0	0
Golden Waves Of Corn	1 (2 oz)	120	0	0	0
Honey Raisin Bran	1 (2 oz)	130	0	0	0
No Nut Banana	1 (2 oz)	130	0	0	0
VitaMuffin					
AppleBerryBran	1 (2 oz)	100	0	0	0
BlueBran	1 (2 oz)	100	0	0	0
CranBran	1 (2 oz)	100	0	0	0
Sugar Free Low Carb Banana Nut	1 (2 oz)	90	2	1	0
VitaTops Dark Chocolate Pomegranate	1 (2 oz)	100	2	1	0
VitaTops Deep Chocolate	1 (2 oz)	100	2	1	–
VitaTops Golden Corn	1 (2 oz)	100	1	0	0
VitaTops MultiBran	1 (2 oz)	100	1	0	0
TAKE-OUT					
corn	1 lg (2.5 oz)	214	7	1	–
raisin bran lowfat	1 (4 oz)	270	1	0	–

MULBERRIES

FOOD	PORTION	CALS	FAT	SAT FAT	TRANS FAT
fresh	1 cup	61	1	–	–

FOOD	PORTION	CALS	FAT	SAT FAT	TRANS FAT
Navitas Naturals					
Dried	1 oz	91	0	0	0
MULLET					
striped cooked	3 oz	127	4	1	–
striped raw	3 oz	99	3	1	–
MUNG BEANS					
dried cooked	1 cup	213	1	tr	–
MUNGO BEANS					
dried cooked	1 cup	190	1	tr	–
MUSHROOMS					
CANNED					
caps	8 (1.6 oz)	12	tr	tr	0
caps pickled	6 (0.8 oz)	5	tr	tr	0
chanterelle	3.5 oz	12	1	–	–
pickled	1 cup	33	tr	tr	0
pieces	½ cup	20	tr	tr	0
straw	1 cup	58	1	tr	0
Green Giant					
Pieces & Stems	½ cup	25	0	0	0
Sunny Dell					
Portabella Sliced	½ cup	20	0	0	0
DRIED					
chanterelle	1 oz	25	tr	–	–
shiitake	1 (3.6 g)	11	tr	tr	0
tree ear	½ cup (0.4 oz)	36	tr	–	–
wood ear mok yee	½ cup (0.4 oz)	25	tr	–	–
Eden					
Maitake Sliced	10 pieces (0.3 oz)	35	0	0	0
Shitake	3 (0.4 oz)	35	0	0	0
Shitake Sliced	3 pieces (0.3 oz)	35	0	0	0
Frieda's					
Chanterelle	2 pieces (4 g)	15	0	0	0
Wood Ear	3 pieces (4 g)	15	0	0	0
FRESH					
brown italian or crimini sliced	1 cup	19	tr	tr	0
brown italian or crimini whole	1 (0.7 oz)	5	tr	tr	0
chanterelle	3.5 oz	11	tr	–	–
enoki raw	1 lg (5 g)	2	tr	tr	0

FOOD	PORTION	CALS	FAT	SAT FAT	TRANS FAT
enoki sliced	1 cup	29	tr	tr	0
enoki whole	1 cup	28	tr	tr	0
maitake diced	1 cup	26	tr	tr	0
maitake whole	1 (6.6 g)	2	tr	tr	0
morel	3.5 oz	9	tr	–	–
oyster	1 sm (0.5 oz)	5	tr	tr	0
oyster sliced	1 cup	30	tr	tr	0
portabella raw	1 cap (3 oz)	22	tr	tr	0
portabella sliced grilled	1 cup (4.2 oz)	42	1	tr	0
raw sliced	½ cup	8	tr	tr	0
shiitake cooked	4 (2.5 oz)	40	tr	tr	0
shiitake pieces cooked	1 cup	81	tr	tr	0
white	1 (0.6 oz)	4	tr	tr	0
white sliced cooked	1 cup	28	tr	tr	0
Frieda's					
Enoki	¼ pkg (1 oz)	10	0	0	0
Golden Gourmet					
Beech Brown	4 oz	20	1	–	0
Beech White	4 oz	13	1	–	0
King Trumpet	4 oz	20	0	0	0
Maitake	4 oz	20	1	–	0
FROZEN					
Alexia					
Mushroom Bites	1 serv (2 oz)	110	4	1	0
Farm Rich					
Breaded	5 (3 oz)	120	2	0	0
TAKE-OUT					
battered fried	1 lg (0.6 oz)	39	3	tr	–
creamed	1 cup	171	11	3	–
stuffed	1 (0.8 oz)	67	4	1	–
MUSKRAT					
roasted	3 oz	199	10	–	–
MUSSELS					
blue raw	1 cup	129	3	1	–
blue raw	3 oz	73	2	tr	–
fresh blue cooked	3 oz	147	4	1	–
MUSTARD					
dry mustard	1 tsp	15	1	tr	–

FOOD	PORTION	CALS	FAT	SAT FAT	TRANS FAT
hot chinese	1 tsp	3	tr	tr	0
organic yellow	1 tsp	5	0	0	0
seed	1 tsp	15	1	tr	0
yellow prepared	1 tbsp	3	tr	tr	0
Annie's Naturals					
Organic Horseradish Mustard	1 tsp	5	0	0	0
Boar's Head					
Delicatessen Style	1 tsp (5 g)	0	0	0	0
Honey	1 tsp (5 g)	10	0	0	0
Bone Suckin'					
Fat Free Gluten Free	1 tbsp	25	0	0	0
Country Cupboard					
Smokey Garlic or Horseradish	1 tsp	10	0	0	0
D'Oni					
Bold As Love Honey Habanero	1 tsp	5	0	0	0
Eden					
Organic Brown	1 tsp	0	0	0	0
Yellow	1 tsp	0	0	0	0
Emeril's					
Horseradish	1 tbsp	5	0	0	0
Smooth Honey	1 tbsp	10	0	0	0
French's					
Classic Yellow	1 tsp	0	0	0	0
Honey	1 tsp	10	0	0	0
Honey Dijon	1 tsp	10	0	0	0
Horseradish	1 tsp	5	0	0	0
Spicy Brown	1 tsp	5	0	0	0
Gulden's					
Spicy Brown	1 tsp	5	0	0	0
Hebrew National					
Deli	1 tsp	4	0	0	0
Hellman's					
Deli	1 tsp	5	0	0	0
Dijonnaise	1 tsp	5	0	0	0
Honey Mustard	1 tsp	10	0	0	0
Kosciusko					
Spicy Brown	1 tsp	0	0	0	0
Luzianne					
Creole Mustard	1 tbsp	10	0	0	0

FOOD	PORTION	CALS	FAT	SAT FAT	TRANS FAT
Robert Rothchild Farm					
Champagne Garlic	1 tsp	6	0	0	0
Sara Lee					
Country Honey	1 tbsp	10	0	0	0
Cranberry Honey	1 tbsp	10	0	0	0
School House Kitchen					
Sweet Smooth Hot	1 tsp	15	1	0	–
MUSTARD GREENS					
fresh chopped cooked	½ cup	11	tr	tr	–
fresh raw chopped	½ cup	7	tr	tr	–
frozen chopped cooked	½ cup	14	tr	tr	–
Allen's					
Seasoned Southern Style	½ cup	30	0	0	0
Glory					
Seasoned canned	½ cup	35	0	0	0
NATTO					
natto	½ cup	187	10	1	–
NAVY BEANS					
CANNED					
navy	1 cup	296	1	tr	–
Eden					
Organic	½ cup	110	0	0	0
DRIED					
cooked	1 cup	259	1	tr	–
NECTARINE					
fresh	1	67	1	–	–
Chiquita					
Fresh	1 med (4.9 oz)	70	1	0	–
Sunsweet					
Dried	3 pieces (1.4 oz)	100	0	0	0
NECTARINE JUICE					
Sun Shower					
100% Juice	8 oz	93	0	0	0
NEUFCHATEL					
neufchatel	1 oz	74	7	4	–
neufchatel	1 pkg (3 oz)	221	20	13	–

FOOD	PORTION	CALS	FAT	SAT FAT	TRANS FAT
Back To Nature					
Organic	⅛ pkg (1 oz)	70	6	4	–
Organic Valley					
Soft	2 tbsp	70	6	4	0

NONI JUICE
Lakewood
Noni Pure Juice	2 oz	8	0	0	0

NOODLES
FOOD	PORTION	CALS	FAT	SAT FAT	TRANS FAT
cellophane	1 cup	492	tr	tr	–
chow mein	1 cup (1.6 oz)	237	14	2	–
egg	1 cup (38 g)	145	2	tr	–
egg cooked	1 cup (5.6 oz)	213	2	tr	–
japanese soba cooked	1 cup (4 oz)	113	tr	tr	–
japanese somen cooked	1 cup (6.2 oz)	231	tr	tr	–
korean acorn noodles not prep	2 oz	195	tr	–	–
rice cooked	1 cup (6.2 oz)	192	tr	tr	–
spinach/egg cooked	1 cup (5.6 oz)	211	3	1	–
A Taste Of Thai					
Rice Wide	2 oz	200	0	0	0
Annie Chun's					
Chow Mein	2 oz	200	1	0	0
Noodle Bowl Teriyaki	1 pkg	310	3	0	–
Noodle Express Chinese Chow Mein	½ pkg	160	4	1	–
Noodle Express Singapore Curry	½ pkg	160	3	0	–
Noodle Express Spicy Szechuan	½ pkg	170	3	0	–
Noodle Express Teriyaki	½ pkg	160	2	0	–
Noodle Express Thai Peanut	½ pkg	200	7	1	–
Rice	2 oz	210	0	0	0
Rice Pad Thai	2 oz	210	0	0	0
Azumaya					
Asian Style Thin Cut	1 cup	210	1	0	–
Catelli					
Egg	3 oz	317	3	–	–
Hodgson Mill					
Egg Whole Wheat not prep	2 oz	190	2	1	–
Light 'N Fluffy					
Egg Extra Wide cooked	1½ cups	210	3	1	0

FOOD	PORTION	CALS	FAT	SAT FAT	TRANS FAT
Manischewitz					
Egg Medium	1¼ cups	220	3	1	–
Fine Yolk Free	1½ cups	210	1	0	–
Fine Egg	1½ cups	220	3	1	–
Wide Yolk Free	1¾ cups	210	1	0	–
Nasoya					
Chinese	1 cup	210	1	0	–
Japanese	1 cup	210	1	0	–
Spinach	1 cup	210	1	0	–
No Yolks					
Extra Broad	2 oz	210	1	0	0
Pennsylvania Dutch					
Yolk Free Ribbons as prep	1½ cups	210	1	0	–

NUTMEG

ground	1 tsp	12	1	1	0

NUTRITION SUPPLEMENTS (see also CEREAL BARS, ENERGY BARS, ENERGY DRINKS)

FOOD	PORTION	CALS	FAT	SAT FAT	TRANS FAT
Amino Vital					
Jel All Flavors	1 pkg (4.9 oz)	70	0	0	0
Boost					
Breeze	8 oz	160	0	0	0
Diabetic	8 oz	250	12	–	–
Clif					
Shot Energy Gel All Flavors	1 pkg (1.1 oz)	100	0	0	0
DiabetiTrim					
Shake French Vanilla	1 pkg	90	1	0	–
Ensure					
Shake Creamy Milk Chocolate	1 bottle (8 oz)	250	6	1	0
Shake Strawberries & Cream	1 bottle (8 oz)	250	6	1	0
GeniSoy					
Soy Natural Protein Powder	1 scoop (1 oz)	100	0	0	0
Glucerna					
Shake Creamy Chocolate Delight	1 bottle (8 oz)	200	7	1	0
Shake Homemade Vanilla	1 bottle (8 oz)	200	7	1	0
Jelly Belly					
Sport Beans Berry Blue	1 pkg (1 oz)	100	0	0	0
Joint Juice					
Tropical Fruit	1 can (8 oz)	30	0	0	0

FOOD	PORTION	CALS	FAT	SAT FAT	TRANS FAT
Kindercal					
Vanilla	1 can (8 oz)	250	11	3	–
Nutribar					
Shake Chocolate Supreme as prep w/ 2% milk	1 serv (10 oz)	262	8	4	–
Shake Vanilla as prep w/ 2% milk	1 (10 oz)	259	7	4	–
PermaLean					
Protein Powder Bodacious Berry	1 scoop (1 oz)	104	tr	0	–
Protein Powder Chocoholic Chocolate	1 scoop (1 oz)	104	tr	0	–
PowerBar					
Powergel All Flavors	1 pkg (1.4 oz)	120	2	–	0
Pria					
Complete Shake Creamy Milk Chocolate	1 pkg (11.6 oz)	170	5	1	0
Complete Shake French Vanilla	1 pkg (11.6 oz)	170	5	1	0
Resource					
Beneprotein Protein Powder	1 scoop	25	0	0	0
Optisource High Protein Drink	1 box (4 oz)	100	3	0	0
Slim-Fast					
Optima Ready-To-Drink Creamy Milk Chocolate	1 can (11 oz)	190	6	3	0
Optima Shake Mix Chocolate Royale as prep w/ fat free milk	1 serv	190	5	1	0
Optima Shake Mix French Vanilla as prep w/ fat free milk	1 serv	200	4	1	0
Vitasoy					
Weight Management Meal All Flavors	1 bottle (10 oz)	200	1	0	0
NUTS MIXED (see also individual names)					
dry roasted w/ peanuts salted	¼ cup	203	18	2	0
dry roasted w/ peanuts w/o salt	¼ cup	203	18	2	0
oil roasted w/o peanuts salted	¼ cup	221	20	3	0

FOOD	PORTION	CALS	FAT	SAT FAT	TRANS FAT
oil roasted w/o peanuts w/o salt	¼ cup	221	20	3	0
Estee					
Chocolate Covered Fruit & Nut Mix Fructose Sweetened	¼ cup	210	12	7	–
Good Sense					
Deluxe Mix	¼ cup	180	13	2	–
Here's Howe					
Royal Mixed Nuts	1 oz	180	17	3	–
Judy's					
Sugar Free Mixed Nut Brittle	¼ piece (1 oz)	120	7	2	–
Maranatha					
Tamari Organic	¼ cup	160	14	2	–
Tamari Roasted	¼ cup	160	14	2	–
Mauna Loa					
Macadamia Mixed	¼ cup	190	15	2	–
Macadamias & Cashews	¼ cup	180	15	3	–
Organic Trails					
Tamari Roasted Nuts & Seeds	¼ cup	190	15	2	0
Peanut Better					
Mixed Nut Butter Creamy & Crunchy	2 tbsp	190	17	2	0
Planters					
NUT-rition Energy Mix	¼ cup	180	14	2	0
NUT-rition Heart Healthy Mix	¼ cup	170	16	2	0

OCA
Frieda's

FOOD	PORTION	CALS	FAT	SAT FAT	TRANS FAT
Oca	½ cup	70	0	0	0

OCTOPUS

FOOD	PORTION	CALS	FAT	SAT FAT	TRANS FAT
dried boiled	3 oz	144	2	tr	–
fresh steamed	3 oz	139	2	tr	–
smoked	1 oz	40	1	tr	–
TAKE-OUT					
ensalada de pulpo	1 cup	299	21	3	–

OHELOBERRIES

FOOD	PORTION	CALS	FAT	SAT FAT	TRANS FAT
fresh	1 cup	39	tr	–	–

OIL

FOOD	PORTION	CALS	FAT	SAT FAT	TRANS FAT
almond	1 cup	1927	218	1	–

FOOD	PORTION	CALS	FAT	SAT FAT	TRANS FAT
almond	1 tbsp	120	14	1	–
apricot kernel	1 cup	1927	218	14	–
apricot kernel	1 tbsp	120	14	1	–
avocado	1 cup	1927	218	25	–
avocado	1 tbsp	124	14	2	–
babassu palm	1 tbsp	120	14	11	–
butter oil	1 cup	1795	204	127	–
butter oil	1 tbsp	112	13	8	–
canola	1 cup	1927	218	15	–
canola	1 tbsp	124	14	2	–
coconut	1 tbsp	117	14	12	0
corn	1 cup	1927	218	28	–
corn	1 tbsp	120	14	2	–
cottonseed	1 cup	1927	218	56	–
cottonseed	1 tbsp	120	14	4	–
cupu assu	1 tbsp	120	14	7	–
garlic oil	1 tbsp	150	17	1	1
grapeseed	1 tbsp	120	14	1	0
hazelnut	1 cup	1927	218	1	–
hazelnut	1 tbsp	120	14	1	–
mustard	1 cup	1927	218	25	–
mustard	1 tbsp	124	14	2	–
oat	1 tbsp	120	14	3	–
olive	1 cup	1909	216	26	–
olive	1 tbsp	119	14	2	–
palm	1 cup	1927	218	107	–
palm	1 tbsp	120	14	7	–
palm kernel	1 cup	1879	218	178	–
palm kernel	1 tbsp	117	14	11	–
peanut	1 cup	1909	216	36	–
peanut	1 tbsp	119	14	2	–
peppermint	1 tsp	42	4	–	–
poppyseed	1 tbsp	120	14	2	–
pumpkin seed	1 oz	217	29	–	–
rice bran	1 tbsp	120	14	3	–
safflower	1 cup	1927	218	20	–
safflower	1 tbsp	120	14	1	–
sesame	1 tbsp	120	14	2	–
sheanut	1 tbsp	120	14	6	–
soybean	1 cup	1927	218	31	–

FOOD	PORTION	CALS	FAT	SAT FAT	TRANS FAT
soybean	1 tbsp	120	14	2	–
soybean organic	1 tbsp	120	14	2	–
sunflower	1 cup	1927	218	23	–
sunflower	1 tbsp	120	14	1	–
teaseed	1 tbsp	120	14	3	–
tomatoseed	1 tbsp	120	14	3	–
vegetable	1 cup	1927	218	2	–
vegetable	1 tbsp	120	14	2	–
walnut	1 cup	1927	218	20	–
walnut	1 tbsp	120	14	1	–
wheat germ	1 tbsp	120	14	3	–
Alpha					
Hazelnut	1 oz	257	29	2	–
Asoyia					
Soybean Ultra Low Lin	1 tbsp	129	14	2	0
Botticelli					
Olive	1 tbsp	120	14	2	0
Carapelli					
Grapeseed	1 tbsp	120	14	1	–
Olive Extra Virgin	1 tbsp	120	14	2	–
Consorzio					
Dipping Oil	1 tbsp	120	14	2	0
Olive Basil	1 tbsp	120	14	2	–
Olive Roasted Pepper	1 tbsp	120	14	2	–
Organic Extra Virgin Olive Meyer Lemon	1 tbsp	120	14	2	–
Eden					
Olive Extra Virgin	1 tbsp	120	14	2	0
Organic Safflower	1 tbsp	120	14	1	0
Organic Soybean	1 tbsp	120	14	2	0
Toasted Sesame	1 tbsp	120	14	2	0
Enova					
Oil	1 tbsp	120	14	1	0
Hollywood					
Canola Enriched	1 tbsp	120	14	1	–
Peanut Enriched Gold	1 tbsp	120	14	2	–
Safflower Expeller Pressed	1 tbsp	120	14	1	0
House Of Tsang					
Mongolian Fire	1 tsp	45	5	1	–
Wok Oil	1 tbsp	130	14	3	0

FOOD	PORTION	CALS	FAT	SAT FAT	TRANS FAT
Iowa Natural					
Soybean 1% Linolenic	1 tbsp	129	14	2	0
Kinloch Plantation					
100% Virgin Pecan	1 tbsp	130	14	2	0
Living Harvest					
Organic Hemp Oil	2 tbsp	250	28	3	0
Loriva					
Avocado	1 tbsp	120	14	2	–
Basil Flavored	1 tbsp	120	14	1	–
Canola	1 tbsp	120	14	1	–
Canolive	1 tbsp	120	14	1	–
Garlic Flavored	1 tbsp	120	14	1	–
Grapeseed	1 tbsp	120	14	1	–
Olive	1 tbsp	120	14	2	–
Olive Organic Extra Virgin	1 tbsp	120	14	1	–
Peanut	1 tbsp	120	14	2	–
Rice Bran	1 tbsp	120	14	2	–
Safflower	1 tbsp	120	14	1	–
Sesame	1 tbsp	120	14	2	–
Sunflower	1 tbsp	120	14	2	–
Toasted Sesame	1 tbsp	120	14	2	–
Walnut	1 tbsp	120	14	2	–
Manitoba Harvest					
Hemp Seed Oil	1 tbsp	126	14	2	0
Mazola					
Corn	1 tbsp	120	14	2	0
No Stick Spray	⅓ sec spray	0	0	0	0
Pure Cooking Spray Canola All Flavors	¼ sec spray	0	0	0	0
Right Blend	1 tbsp	120	14	1	0
Vegetable	1 tbsp	120	14	2	0
Monini					
Olive Extra Virgin	1 tbsp	118	13	2	–
Nutiva					
Organic Coconut Extra Virgin	1 tbsp	120	14	13	–
Organic Hemp Cold Pressed	1 tbsp	120	14	1	–
Nutrium					
Soybean Low Linolenic	1 tbsp	129	14	2	0
Olivo					
Spray Olive Oil 100% Extra Virgin	⅓ sec spray	0	0	0	0

FOOD	PORTION	CALS	FAT	SAT FAT	TRANS FAT
Orville Redenbacher's					
Popping & Topping	1 tbsp	120	14	2	–
Pacifica Culinaria					
Avocado	1 tbsp	120	14	2	0
Avocado Blood Orange	1 tbsp	120	14	2	0
Pam					
Cooking Spray All Types	⅓ sec spray	0	0	0	0
Organic Canola	⅓ second spray	0	0	0	0
Pompeian					
Olive	1 tbsp	130	14	–	–
Robert Rothchild Farm					
Basil Infused	1 tbsp	120	14	2	0
Smart Balance					
Omega Oil	1 tbsp	120	14	1	0
Spectrum					
Almond	1 tbsp	120	14	1	0
Apricot Kernel	1 tbsp	120	14	1	0
Avocado	1 tbsp	120	14	2	0
Canola Organic	1 tbsp	120	14	1	0
Coconut Organic	1 tbsp	120	14	12	0
Corn	1 tbsp	120	14	0	0
Grapeseed	1 tbsp	120	14	0	0
Grapeseed Oil Spray	⅓ sec spray	0	0	0	0
Hazelnut Toasted Organic	1 tbsp	120	14	1	0
Mediterranean Olive Organic	1 tbsp	120	14	2	0
Organic Extra Virgin Oil Spray	⅓ sec spray	0	0	0	0
Peanut	1 tbsp	120	14	3	0
Pumpkin Seed Organic	1 tbsp	120	14	3	0
Sesame Organic	1 tbsp	120	14	2	0
Sesame Toasted Organic	1 tbsp	120	14	2	0
Soy Organic	1 tbsp	120	14	2	0
Sunflower Organic	1 tbsp	120	14	2	0
Walnut	1 tbsp	120	14	2	0
Walnut Organic	1 tbsp	120	14	1	0
Vistive					
Soybean Low Linolenic	1 tbsp	129	14	2	0
Wesson					
Canola	1 tbsp	120	14	4	–

OKRA
CANNED

FOOD	PORTION	CALS	FAT	SAT FAT	TRANS FAT
pickled	6 pods (2.3 oz)	18	tr	tr	0

FOOD	PORTION	CALS	FAT	SAT FAT	TRANS FAT
Glory					
Cut	½ cup	25	0	0	0
McIlhenny					
Spicy Pickled	1 oz	10	0	0	0
FRESH					
cooked w/ salt	8 pods	19	tr	tr	0
luffa chinese okra cooked	1 cup	39	tr	tr	0
sliced cooked w/ salt	½ cup	18	tr	tr	0
FROZEN					
McKenzie's					
Breaded Okra	1 serv (2.8 oz)	90	1	0	–
Cut	1 serv (3 oz)	25	0	0	0
TAKE-OUT					
batter dipped fried	10 pieces (2.6 oz)	142	10	1	–
OLIVES					
green	4 med	15	2	tr	–
green	3 extra lg	15	2	tr	–
green olive tapenade	1 tbsp	25	3	0	–
ripe	1 sm	4	tr	tr	–
ripe	1 lg	5	tr	tr	–
ripe	1 colossal	12	1	tr	–
ripe	1 jumbo	7	1	tr	–
spanish stuffed	5 (0.5 oz)	15	1	0	–
Peloponnese					
Amfissa	3	45	5	0	–
Ionian Green	3	25	3	0	–
Kalamata Pitted	5	45	5	0	–
Kalamata Spread	1 tsp	15	2	0	–
Stonewall Kitchen					
Mixed Olive Spread	1 tbsp	35	2	0	0
ONION					
CANNED					
cocktail	½ cup	41	tr	tr	–
Boar's Head					
Sweet Vidalia In Sauce	1 tbsp	10	0	0	0
French's					
Original French Fried	2 tbsp	45	4	2	0
DRIED					
flakes	1 tbsp	17	tr	tr	–

FOOD	PORTION	CALS	FAT	SAT FAT	TRANS FAT
powder	1 tsp	7	tr	tr	–
shallots	1 tbsp	3	0	0	0
Bob's Red Mill					
Minced	1 tbsp	40	1	0	0
FRESH					
cooked w/o salt	1 sm (2 oz)	26	tr	tr	–
cooked w/o salt	1 med (3.3 oz)	41	tr	tr	–
cooked w/o salt	1 lg (4.5 oz)	56	tr	tr	–
cooked w/o salt chopped	1 tbsp	7	tr	tr	–
raw chopped	1 tbsp	4	tr	tr	–
raw chopped	½ cup	32	tr	tr	–
raw sliced	1 (0.5 oz)	6	tr	tr	–
raw sliced	½ cup	23	tr	0	–
scallions raw	1 med (0.5 oz)	5	tr	tr	–
scallions raw chopped	¼ cup	8	tr	tr	–
shallots raw chopped	¼ cup	29	tr	tr	–
sweet whole raw	1 (11.6 oz)	106	tr	tr	–
whole raw	1 sm (2.5 oz)	28	tr	tr	–
whole raw	1 med (4 oz)	44	tr	tr	–
whole raw	1 lg (5.3 oz)	60	tr	tr	–
Antioch Farms					
Vidalia	1 med	60	0	–	0
Arrowfarms					
Cipoline	2 (1.1 oz)	20	0	0	0
Blue Ribbon					
Yellow	1 med (5.2 oz)	60	0	0	0
Christopher Ranch					
Shallots	1 (1 oz)	20	0	0	0
Earthbound Farm					
Organic Green Onions	¼ cup	10	0	0	0
Organic Red	1 med (5.2 oz)	60	0	0	0
Frieda's					
Cipolline	3 (3 oz)	30	0	0	0
Maui	⅓ cup (1.1 oz)	10	0	0	0
Pearl	⅔ cup (3 oz)	30	0	0	0
Shallots	1 tbsp (1 oz)	20	0	0	0
Nature's Harvest					
Onion	1 med (5.2 oz)	60	0	0	0
OsoSweet					
Onion	1 med (5 oz)	60	0	0	0

FOOD	PORTION	CALS	FAT	SAT FAT	TRANS FAT
FROZEN					
Alexia					
Onion Rings	6 (3 oz)	230	12	1	0
C&W					
Petite Whole	⅔ cup (3 oz)	30	0	0	0
Farm Rich					
Petals Breaded + Sauce	10 (3 oz)	200	12	2	0
Ian's					
Rings & Strings	5-9 pieces (2.5 oz)	152	7	1	–
TAKE-OUT					
creamed	1 cup	187	9	2	–
fried	½ cup	57	5	–	–
rings breaded & fried	8–9 (3 oz)	276	16	7	–
OPOSSUM					
roasted	3 oz	188	9	–	–
ORANGE					
CANNED					
Del Monte					
SunFresh Mandarin	½ cup	80	0	0	0
Dole					
Fruit Bowls Mandarin Oranges	1 pkg	70	0	0	0
FRESH					
california navel	1	65	tr	tr	–
california valencia	1	59	tr	tr	–
florida	1	69	tr	tr	–
peel	1 tbsp	6	tr	tr	–
sections	1 cup	85	tr	tr	–
Frieda's					
Cara Cara	1 med (5 oz)	70	0	0	0
Mandarin Delite	1 cup (5 oz)	60	0	0	0
Mandarin Page	1 cup (5 oz)	60	0	0	0
Mandarin Pixie	1 cup (5 oz)	60	0	0	0
Mandarin Satsuma	1 (5 oz)	60	0	0	0
Melogold	½ (6 oz)	50	0	0	0
Seville	1 (3 oz)	40	0	0	0
Sunkist					
Cara Cara Navel	1 med	80	0	0	0
Minneola Tangelo	1 (3.8 oz)	70	0	0	0
Moro	1 (5.4 oz)	70	0	0	0

FOOD	PORTION	CALS	FAT	SAT FAT	TRANS FAT
Orange	1 med	80	0	0	0
Satsuma Mandarin	1 (3.8 oz)	50	0	0	0
ORANGE JUICE					
canned	1 cup	104	tr	tr	–
chilled	1 cup	110	1	tr	–
fresh	1 cup	111	tr	tr	–
frzn as prep	1 cup	112	tr	tr	–
frzn not prep	6 oz	339	tr	tr	–
mandarin orange	7 oz	94	tr	–	–
orange drink	6 oz	94	0	0	0
After The Fall					
24 Karrot Orange	8 oz	120	0	0	0
Bright & Early					
Orange Drink	8 oz	110	0	0	0
Crystal Light					
Sunrise Sunrise Sugar Free Mix as prep	1 serv	5	0	0	0
Dole					
100% Juice	8 oz	110	0	0	0
Florida's Natural					
Calcium & Vitamin D	8 oz	110	0	0	0
Hood					
100% Juice	1 cup	120	0	0	0
Italian Volcano					
Blood Orange Organic	1 serv (6.75 oz)	84	0	0	0
Minute Maid					
Country Style	8 oz	110	0	0	0
Heart Wise	8 oz	110	0	0	0
Kids+	8 oz	110	0	0	0
Light	8 oz	50	0	0	0
Original	8 oz	110	0	0	0
Plus Calcium	8 oz	110	0	0	0
W/ Extra Vitamin C & E Plus Zinc	8 oz	110	0	0	0
Naked Juice					
Just OJ	8 oz	110	0	0	0
NutraBalance					
Fortified	1 pkg (4 oz)	60	0	0	0
Ocean Spray					
100% Juice	8 oz	120	0	0	0

FOOD	PORTION	CALS	FAT	SAT FAT	TRANS FAT
Odwalla					
100% Juice	8 oz	110	0	0	0
Organic Valley					
W/ Calcium	1 cup	110	0	0	0
Simply					
Orange Calcium Fortified	8 oz	110	0	0	0
Orange Original	8 oz	110	0	0	0
Snapple					
Orangeade	8 oz	120	0	0	0
SSips					
Orangeade	8 oz	120	0	0	0
Tang					
Orange Drink as prep	1 serv	90	0	0	0
Sugar Free Orange as prep	1 serv (8 oz)	5	0	0	0
Tree Ripe					
100% Juice + Calcium & Vitamins	8 oz	120	0	0	0
Organic 100% Juice	6 oz	90	0	0	0
Tropicana					
Antioxidant Advantage	8 oz	110	0	0	0
Calcium + Vitamin D	8 oz	110	0	0	0
Fiber	8 oz	120	0	0	0
Healthy Heart	8 oz	120	0	0	0
Healthy Kids	8 oz	110	0	0	0
Light 'n Healthy w/ Calcium	8 oz	50	0	0	0
Light 'n Healthy w/ Pulp	8 oz	50	0	0	0
No Pulp	8 oz	110	0	0	0
Orangeade	8 oz	111	0	0	0
Organic	8 oz	120	0	0	0
Uncle Matt's					
Organic 100% Juice Pulp Free	8 oz	110	0	0	0
Organic 100% Juice w/ Pulp	8 oz	110	0	0	0
Welsh Farms					
Juice	8 oz	110	0	0	0
TAKE-OUT					
orange julius	1 serv (24 oz)	443	tr	tr	–

ORGAN MEATS (*see* BRAINS, GIBLETS, GIZZARDS, HEART, KIDNEY, LIVER, SWEETBREADS)

FOOD	PORTION	CALS	FAT	SAT FAT	TRANS FAT
OREGANO					
crumbled	1 tsp	3	tr	tr	0
ground	1 tsp	6	tr	tr	0
OSTRICH					
cooked	3 oz	120	3	–	–
OYSTERS					
canned eastern	1 cup	112	4	1	0
eastern baked	6 med	47	1	tr	0
eastern raw	6 med	50	1	tr	0
eastern sauteed	6 med	76	5	1	0
smoked	6	33	1	tr	0
Brunswick					
Smoked	1 can (3 oz)	140	8	2	–
Bumble Bee					
Smoked	¼ cup	120	7	2	–
Whole	¼ cup	70	3	1	0
Chicken Of The Sea					
Smoked In Oil	1 can (3.75 oz)	140	8	2	–
Smoked In Water	1 can (3.75 oz)	120	3	1	–
Smoked Teriyaki	1 can (3.75 oz)	120	3	1	–
Whole	½ can (2 oz)	80	3	1	–
TAKE-OUT					
breaded & fried	6	368	18	5	0
fritter	1 (1.4 oz)	121	6	1	0
oysters rockefeller	1 cup	302	17	8	0
stew	1 cup	208	13	8	0
PANCAKE/WAFFLE SYRUP					
lite	¼ cup	98	0	0	0
pancake syrup	1 pkg (2 oz)	156	tr	tr	–
pancake syrup	¼ cup	209	tr	tr	–
Country Cupboard					
Boysenberry	¼ cup	0	0	0	0
Maple Butter	¼ cup	0	0	0	0
Strawberry	¼ cup	0	0	0	0
Eggo					
Lite	¼ cup	110	0	0	0
Original	¼ cup	240	0	0	0

FOOD	PORTION	CALS	FAT	SAT FAT	TRANS FAT
Estee					
Maple	¼ cup	30	0	0	0
Hungry Jack					
Lite	¼ cup	100	0	0	0
Original	¼ cup	210	0	0	0
Karo					
Pancake Syrup	¼ cup	240	0	0	0
Keto					
Maple Butter	¼ cup	0	0	0	0
Ketogenics					
Zero Carb	¼ cup	0	0	0	0
Log Cabin					
Lite	¼ cup	100	0	0	0
Original	¼ cup	210	0	0	0
Mrs. Butterworth's					
Lite	¼ cup	100	0	0	0
Original	¼ cup (2 oz)	230	0	0	0
Smucker's					
Breakfast Syrup Sugar Free	¼ cup	30	0	0	0
Stonewall Kitchen					
Maine Maple	¼ cup	210	0	0	0

PANCAKES
FROZEN

FOOD	PORTION	CALS	FAT	SAT FAT	TRANS FAT
Aunt Jemima					
Buttermilk	3 (3 oz)	210	4	1	0
Buttermilk Low Fat	3 (3 oz)	210	4	1	0
Whole Grain	3 (3 oz)	230	6	1	0
Eggo					
Buttermilk	3	280	9	2	0
Minis	11	260	8	1	0
Golden					
Potato Latkes	1 (1.3 oz)	70	3	0	0
Ian's					
Blueberry	1 (1.3 oz)	100	2	0	–
Pancake	1 (1.3 oz)	100	2	0	–
Inland Valley					
Potato	1 (2 oz)	120	8	4	–
McCain					
Homestyle BabyCakes	4 pieces (2.6 oz)	150	9	2	0

FOOD	PORTION	CALS	FAT	SAT FAT	TRANS FAT
Ratner's					
Potato Latkes	2 (3 oz)	160	7	0	0
MIX					
Arrowhead Mills					
Gluten Free Pancake & Waffle as prep	2 (5 in)	240	6	1	0
Aunt Paula's					
Pancake & Waffle Mix as prep	2	132	8	–	–
Betty Crocker					
Buttermilk as prep	3	200	3	1	–
Original as prep	3	200	3	1	–
Big Train					
Low Carb Pancake & Waffle Mix as prep	3	190	10	5	–
Bisquick					
Shake 'N Pour Blueberry as prep	3	210	4	1	–
Carbolite					
Low Carb Mix not prep	⅓ cup	100	tr	–	–
Carbsense					
Buckwheat not prep	½ cup	140	3	0	–
Buttermilk not prep	½ cup	140	3	0	–
Don's Chuck Wagon					
Buckwheat Mix	⅓ cup	160	1	0	–
Hodgson Mill					
Buckwheat not prep	⅓ cup	140	1	0	–
Whole Wheat Buttermilk not prep	⅓ cup	120	1	0	–
Hungry Jack					
Buttermilk Pancake & Waffle not prep	⅓ cup	150	2	–	–
Easy Pack Blueberry not prep	½ cup	200	3	–	–
Pancake & Waffle Extra Light & Fluffy not prep	⅓ cup	150	2	–	–
Potato not prep	2 tbsp	70	0	0	0
Keto					
Banana not prep	⅓ cup	114	2	–	–
Original not prep	⅓ cup	114	2	–	–
Ketogenics					
Low Carb not prep	⅔ cup	185	4	2	–

FOOD	PORTION	CALS	FAT	SAT FAT	TRANS FAT
King Arthur					
Multi-Grain Buttermilk not prep	6 tbsp	160	2	0	0
MiniCarb					
Apple Cinnamon as prep	2	150	6	1	–
TAKE-OUT					
buckwheat	1 (7 in)	142	5	1	0
plain	1 (7 in)	183	3	1	0
potato	1 (1.3 oz)	70	4	1	0
w/ butter & syrup	2 (8.1 oz)	520	14	6	–
whole wheat	1 (7 in)	183	8	2	0

PANCREAS (see SWEETBREAD)

PANINI (see SANDWICHES)

PAPAYA

FOOD	PORTION	CALS	FAT	SAT FAT	TRANS FAT
fresh	1	117	tr	tr	–
fresh cubed	1 cup	54	tr	tr	–
Del Monte					
In Extra Light Syrup w/ Passion Fruit Puree	½ cup	70	0	0	0
Frieda's					
Mexican	1 cup (5 oz)	50	0	0	0

PAPAYA JUICE

FOOD	PORTION	CALS	FAT	SAT FAT	TRANS FAT
nectar	1 cup	142	tr	tr	–
Ceres					
Papaya	8 oz	120	0	0	0
Lakewood					
Red	8 oz	80	0	0	0
Yellow	8 oz	105	0	0	0
Langers					
Papaya Delight 100% Juice	8 oz	130	0	0	0
Old Orchard					
Nectar Cocktail	8 oz	120	0	0	0

PAPRIKA

FOOD	PORTION	CALS	FAT	SAT FAT	TRANS FAT
dried	1 tsp	1	tr	tr	0
Bob's Red Mill					
Hungarian	½ tsp	11	0	0	0

FOOD	PORTION	CALS	FAT	SAT FAT	TRANS FAT
PARSLEY					
dried	1 tbsp	4	tr	tr	0
freeze dried	1 tbsp	1	tr	–	0
fresh chopped	1 tbsp	1	tr	tr	0
fresh chopped	½ cup	5	tr	tr	0
fresh sprigs	5 (1.8 oz)	18	tr	tr	0
Dorot					
Chopped Cubes frzn	1 cube (4 g)	5	tr	tr	0
Frieda's					
Parsley Root	⅔ cup	10	1	0	–
PARSNIPS					
fresh cooked	1 (5.6 oz)	130	tr	tr	–
fresh sliced cooked	½ cup	63	tr	tr	–
raw sliced	½ cup	50	tr	tr	–
Frieda's					
Sliced	1 cup	100	0	0	0
PASSION FRUIT					
purple fresh	1	18	tr	–	–
PASSION FRUIT JUICE					
purple	1 cup	126	tr	–	–
yellow	1 cup	149	tr	–	–
Ceres					
Passion Fruit	8 oz	120	0	0	0
PASTA (see also NOODLES, PASTA DINNERS, PASTA SALAD)					
DRY					
corn cooked	1 cup (4.9 oz)	176	1	tr	–
elbows	1 cup	389	2	tr	–
elbows cooked	1 cup (4.9 oz)	197	1	tr	–
shells small cooked	1 cup (4 oz)	162	1	tr	–
spaghetti cooked	1 cup (4.9 oz)	197	1	tr	–
spinach spaghetti cooked	1 cup (4.9 oz)	182	1	tr	–
spirals cooked	1 cup (4.7 oz)	189	tr	tr	–
vegetable cooked	1 cup (4.7 oz)	172	tr	tr	–
whole wheat all shapes cooked	1 cup	174	tr	tr	–
Annie Chun's					
Soba Noodles	2 oz	200	1	0	–
Barilla					
Pastina	2 oz	210	2	1	–

FOOD	PORTION	CALS	FAT	SAT FAT	TRANS FAT
Penne	1 cup (2 oz)	200	1	0	0
Plus Penne	2 oz	200	1	0	0
Plus Rotini not prep	2 oz	210	2	0	0
Tortelloni Porcini Mushroom	¾ cup	240	8	5	–
Tortelloni Ricotta & Asparagus	¾ cup	240	8	5	–
Tortelloni Ricotta & Spinach	¾ cup	240	8	7	–
Bella Vita					
Low Carb Penne Rigate	2 oz	190	1	0	–
Catelli					
All Shapes	3 oz	301	1	–	–
Bistro Cracked Black Pepper Fettuccine	¼ pkg	320	1	tr	0
Bistro Italian Herb Fettuccine	¼ pkg	310	2	tr	0
Bistro Lemon Pepper Linguine	¼ pkg	320	2	1	0
Bistro Rainbows	3 oz	320	1	tr	0
Bistro Spinach Lasagne	3 oz	320	2	1	0
Bistro Sun Dried Tomato & Basil Spaghettini	¼ pkg	320	2	tr	0
Bistro Vegetable Fusilli	3 oz	320	1	tr	0
Healthy Harvest Flax Omega-3	3 oz	290	3	1	0
Healthy Harvest Multigrain	3 oz	310	2	tr	0
Healthy Harvest Organic Whole Wheat	3 oz	320	2	0	0
Healthy Harvest Whole Wheat All Shapes	3 oz	310	2	tr	0
Darielle					
All Shapes not prep	2 oz	160	1	0	–
DaVinci					
Rotini	1 cup	210	1	0	–
Spaghetti	2 oz	210	1	0	–
DeBoles					
Angel Hair Rice Pasta	¼ pkg (2 oz)	210	1	0	–
Elbow Corn Pasta Wheat Free	⅙ pkg (2 oz)	200	2	0	–
Fettuccini	¼ pkg (2 oz)	210	1	0	–
Organic Angel Hair Whole Wheat	¼ pkg (2 oz)	210	2	0	0
Organic Eggless Ribbon	1 cup (2 oz)	210	1	0	–
Organic Fettucini Spinach	¼ pkg (2 oz)	210	1	0	–
Organic Lasagna	¼ pkg (2.5 oz)	260	1	0	–
Organic Rigatoni Whole Wheat	1 cup (2 oz)	210	2	0	–
Rigatoni	¼ pkg (2 oz)	210	1	0	–

FOOD	PORTION	CALS	FAT	SAT FAT	TRANS FAT
DeCecco					
Spaghetti w/ Spinach	⅛ pkg (2 oz)	200	1	0	–
Dreamfields					
Lasagna not prep	2 pieces (2 oz)	190	1	0	0
Rotini not prep	⅔ cup (2 oz)	190	1	0	0
Due Amici					
Pasta Lite Low Carb Fusilli	2 oz	160	1	0	–
Eden					
Bifun Pasta not prep	2 oz	200	1	0	0
Harusame Pasta not prep	2 oz	190	0	0	0
Kudzu	2 oz	200	0	0	0
Organic Gemelli Spelt & Buckwheat not prep	½ cup (2 oz)	210	2	tr	0
Organic Ribbons Artichoke not prep	½ cup (2 oz)	210	2	0	0
Organic Rigatoni Kamut & Buckwheat not prep	½ cup (2 oz)	200	2	tr	0
Organic Spaghetti 100% Whole Wheat not prep	2 oz	210	2	0	0
Organic Spirals Flax Rice not prep	½ cup (2 oz)	200	2	0	0
Organic Spirals Kamut Vegetable not prep	½ cup (2 oz)	210	2	0	0
Organic Spirals Rye not prep	½ cup (2 oz)	200	0	0	0
Organic Spirals Spinach not prep	½ cup (2 oz)	210	1	0	0
Organic Udon not prep	¼ pkg	200	2	0	0
Organic Udon Spelt not prep	¼ pkg	200	1	0	0
Organic Vegetable Alphabets not prep	½ cup (2 oz)	210	2	0	0
Organic Vegetable Shells not prep	½ cup (2 oz)	210	2	0	0
Organic Ziti Rigati Spelt not prep	½ cup (2 oz)	210	2	0	0
Soba Japanese 100% Buckwheat not prep	2 oz	200	1	0	0
Soba Japanese Lotus Root not prep	2 oz	190	1	0	0
Soba Japanese Mugwort not prep	2 oz	190	1	0	0

FOOD	PORTION	CALS	FAT	SAT FAT	TRANS FAT
Soba Japanese Wild Yam not prep	2 oz	190	1	0	0
Udon Japanese not prep	2 oz	190	2	0	0
Udon Japanese Brown Rice not prep	2 oz	190	1	0	0
Food For Life					
Ezekiel 4:9 Sprouted Grain	2 oz	210	2	1	0
Hodgson Mill					
Lasagna Whole Wheat not prep	2 oz	190	1	0	–
Organic Fettuccine Whole Wheat w/ Milled Flax Seed not prep	2 oz	200	2	0	–
Pasta Ribbons Whole Wheat not prep	2 oz	190	1	0	–
Spaghetti Whole Wheat not prep	2 oz	190	1	0	–
Veggie Bows not prep	2 oz	200	1	0	–
Wagon Wheels Veggie not prep	2 oz	200	1	0	–
Keto					
Elbows not prep	1.6 oz	108	0	0	0
Spaghetti not prep	1.3 oz	130	1	0	–
LifeStream					
Organic All Shapes	2 oz	208	4	1	0
Lundberg					
Organic Spaghetti Brown Rice	2 oz	210	2	1	0
Maddy's					
Gluten Free not prep	4 oz	310	2	2	0
Mueller's					
Elbow Macaroni not prep	½ cup	210	1	0	0
Multigrain Rotini not prep	1 cup (2 oz)	190	2	0	0
Notta Pasta					
Rice Pasta All Shapes	2 oz	200	0	0	0
Pastalia					
Heart Health Low Carb not prep	2 oz	176	2	–	–
Real Torino					
Tirali not prep	1 cup (2 oz)	210	1	0	–
Revival					
Soy Penne	⅙ box	200	2	0	–
Soy Thin Spaghetti	⅙ box	200	2	0	–

FOOD	PORTION	CALS	FAT	SAT FAT	TRANS FAT
Rice Select					
Orzo Original not prep	⅓ cup	210	1	–	–
Ronzoni					
Elbows not prep	½ cup (2 oz)	210	1	0	–
Healthy Harvest Multigrain Spaghetti	1/7 pkg (2 oz)	190	2	0	0
Healthy Harvest Whole Wheat Blend Spaghetti	1/7 pkg (2 oz)	180	1	0	0
Lasagne	2½ pieces (2 oz)	210	1	0	–
Smart Pasta not prep	2 oz	180	1	0	0
San Giorgio					
Elbows not prep	½ cup	210	1	0	–
Soy7					
Pasta All Shapes	2 oz	200	1	0	–
Whey Cool					
High Protein Xtreme Rotini	1 serv (2 oz)	210	2	0	–
FRESH					
cooked	2 oz	75	1	tr	–
spinach cooked	2 oz	74	1	tr	–
REFRIGERATED					
Buitoni					
Angel Hair	1¼ cups	230	3	1	–
Fettuccine	1¼ cups	240	3	1	–
Fettuccine Spinach	1¼ cups	260	3	1	–
Linguine	1¼ cups	240	3	1	–
Ravioletti Three Cheese	1 cup	270	6	3	–
Ravioli Doublestuffed Mozzarella & Herb	1½ cups	340	12	6	–
Ravioli Four Cheese 100% Whole Wheat	1¼ cups	320	10	6	0
Ravioli Chicken & Roasted Garlic	1¼ cups	340	11	3	–
Ravioli Chicken Parmesan	1¼ cups	310	8	2	–
Ravioli Classic Beef	1¼ cups	340	10	3	–
Ravioli Garden Vegetable	1 cup	250	5	2	–
Ravioli Light Four Cheese	1¼ cups	230	4	2	–
Tortellini Herb Chicken	1 cup	340	9	3	–
Tortellini Mixed Cheese	1 cup	320	7	4	–
Tortellini Spinach Cheese	1 cup	320	7	4	0
Tortellini Three Cheese	1 cup	320	7	4	–

FOOD	PORTION	CALS	FAT	SAT FAT	TRANS FAT
Tortelloni Cheese & Roasted Garlic	1 cup	270	8	4	–
Tortelloni Chicken & Prosciutto	1 cup	320	9	3	0
Tortelloni Mozzarella & Herb	1 cup	330	9	4	0
Tortelloni Mozzarella & Pepperoni	1 cup	330	10	5	–
Tortelloni Portabello Mushroom & Cheese	1 cup	290	6	2	0
Tortelloni Sun Dried Tomato	1 cup	310	9	2	–
Tortelloni Sweet Italian Sausage	1 cup	330	9	3	–
Pasta Prima					
Ravioli Spinach & Mozzarella	1 cup	200	5	2	–
Ravioli Sun Dried Tomato & Mozzarella	1 cup	200	5	2	–

PASTA DINNERS (see also PASTA SALAD)
CANNED
Annie's Homegrown

FOOD	PORTION	CALS	FAT	SAT FAT	TRANS FAT
Organic All Stars	1 cup	150	1	0	–
Organic BernieOs	1 cup	150	1	0	–
Organic Cheesy Ravioli	1 cup	180	4	2	–
Organic P'sghetti Loops	1 cup	190	4	1	–
Chef Boyardee					
99% Fat Free Beef Ravioli	1 cup	170	2	1	0
Beef Ravioli	1 cup	240	8	3	0
Beefaroni	1 cup	260	10	5	0
Mini Ravioli	1 cup	250	9	4	0
Spaghetti & Meat Balls	1 cup	270	10	5	0
SpaghettiOs					
A to Z's w/ Meatballs	1 cup	260	9	4	1
A to Z's w/ Sliced Franks	1 cup	230	6	3	0
Mini Beef Ravioli In Meat Sauce	1 cup	260	5	2	0
Pasta	1 cup	180	1	0	0
Plus Calcium	1 cup	170	1	1	0
FROZEN					
Amy's					
Cannelloni w/ Vegetables	1 pkg (9 oz)	330	12	8	–
Lasagna Cheese	1 pkg (10.25 oz)	330	12	7	–
Lasagna Garden Vegetable	1 pkg (10.25 oz)	290	9	4	–
Macaroni & Cheese	1 pkg (9 oz)	410	16	10	–
Macaroni & Soy Cheese	1 pkg (9 oz)	370	15	2	–

FOOD	PORTION	CALS	FAT	SAT FAT	TRANS FAT
Pasta & Vegetable Alfredo	1 cup	220	8	4	–
Pasta Primavera	1 pkg (9 oz)	300	11	6	–
Ravioli w/ Sauce	1 pkg (8 oz)	340	12	5	–
Rice Mac & Cheese	1 pkg (9 oz)	140	16	10	–
Skillet Meals	1 cup	250	11	3	–
Tofu Vegetable Lasagna	1 pkg (9.5 oz)	300	10	2	–
Vegetable Lasagna	1 pkg (9.5 oz)	280	12	5	–
Banquet					
Family Size Egg Noodles w/ Beef & Brown Gravy	1 serv	150	5	3	–
Family Size Macaroni & Cheese	1 cup	230	7	3	–
Lasagna w/ Meat Sauce	1 meal (9.5 oz)	260	8	3	–
Bertolli					
Meatballs Pomodoro & Penne	1 serv (12 oz)	600	31	8	0
Boca					
Lasagna Meatless	1 pkg (9.4 oz)	290	5	2	0
Cedarlane					
Zone Chicken & Vegetables Pasta & Ginger	1 pkg (10 oz)	340	12	5	0
Zone Lasagna Vegetable	1 pkg (10.9 oz)	310	12	5	0
Celentano					
Cheese Ravioli	4 (4.3 oz)	230	4	2	0
Contessa					
Ravioli Portobello	6 (6.7 oz)	360	17	8	0
Glory					
Macaroni & Cheese	1 pkg	480	23	6	2
Glutino					
Gluten Free Duo Mushroom Penne	1 pgk (10.5 oz)	380	6	2	0
Gluten Free Macaroni & Cheese	1 pkg (8.8 oz)	430	20	9	1
Gluten Free Penne Alfredo	1 pkg (9.1 oz)	340	8	4	0
Golden Cuisine					
Cheese Manicotti	1 pkg	360	12	6	tr
Spaghetti & Meatballs	1 pkg	490	22	9	1
Tuna Casserole	1 pkg	386	8	3	0
Green Giant					
Skillet Meal Chicken & Cheesy Pasta as prep	1¼ cups	270	6	3	0

FOOD	PORTION	CALS	FAT	SAT FAT	TRANS FAT
Healthy Choice					
Breaded Chicken Breast w/ Mac & Cheese	1 pkg	290	5	2	–
Creamy Garlic Shrimp w/ Bow Tie Pasta	1 pkg (11.5 oz)	280	5	2	0
Fettuccini Alfredo	1 pkg	280	7	3	–
Fettuccini Alfredo Chicken	1 pkg	290	7	3	–
Lasagna Bake	1 pkg	270	7	3	–
Macaroni & Cheese	1 meal (9 oz)	240	5	3	–
Macaroni & Cheese	1 pkg	290	7	3	–
Manicotti	1 pkg	280	5	3	–
Manicotti w/ Three Cheeses	1 meal (11 oz)	300	9	3	–
Rigatoni w/ Broccoli & Chicken	1 pkg	270	7	3	–
Spaghetti & Sauce w/ Seasoned Beef	1 meal (10 oz)	260	8	2	–
Spaghetti w/ Meat Sauce	1 pkg	310	6	3	–
Stuffed Pasta Shells	1 pkg	290	6	3	–
Helen's Kitchen					
Farfalle & Basil Pasta w/ Tofu Steaks	1 pkg (9 oz)	320	11	4	0
Joseph's Pasta					
Grilled Chicken Ravioli w/ Roasted Red Pepper Sauce	1 pkg (14 oz)	540	15	8	–
Kashi					
Chicken Pasta Promodoro	1 pkg (10 oz)	280	6	2	0
Kid Cuisine					
Cheese Blaster Mac & Cheese	1 meal	380	11	5	0
Twist & Twirl Spaghetti w/ Mini Meatballs	1 meal	460	14	4	0
Lean Cuisine					
Cafe Classics Bow Tie Pasta & Chicken	1 pkg (9.5 oz)	240	5	1	0
Cafe Classics Bowl Three Cheese Stuffed Rigatoni	1 pkg (10 oz)	260	7	4	0
Cafe Classics Cheese Lasagna w/ Chicken Breast Scallopini	1 pkg (10 oz)	290	8	2	0
Cafe Classics Four Cheese Cannelloni	1 pkg (9.1 oz)	260	7	4	0
Cafe Classics Grilled Chicken & Penne Pasta	1 pkg (12 oz)	320	5	2	0

FOOD	PORTION	CALS	FAT	SAT FAT	TRANS FAT
Cafe Classics Jumbo Rigatoni w/ Meatballs	1 pkg (15.4 oz)	400	8	3	0
Cafe Classics Lasagna w/ Meat Sauce	1 pkg (10.5 oz)	310	7	3	0
Cafe Classics Macaroni & Beef	1 pkg (9.5 oz)	270	5	2	0
Cafe Classics Macaroni & Cheese	1 pkg (10 oz)	300	7	4	0
Cafe Classics Penne Pasta w/ Tomato Basil Sauce	1 pkg (10 oz)	270	3	1	0
Cafe Classics Roasted Chicken w/ Lemon Pepper Fettuccini	1 pkg (8.1 oz)	250	6	2	0
Cafe Classics Shrimp & Angel Hair Pasta	1 pkg (10 oz)	240	5	1	0
Cafe Classics Spaghetti w/ Meat Sauce	1 pkg (11.5 oz)	280	4	1	0
Cafe Classics Spaghetti w/ Meatballs	1 pkg (9.5 oz)	270	5	2	0
Dinnertime Selects Chicken Fettuccini	1 pkg (12 oz)	360	7	3	0
One Dish Favorites Alfredo Pasta w/ Chicken & Broccoli	1 pkg (10 oz)	270	6	3	0
One Dish Favorites Angel Hair Pasta Marinara	1 pkg (10 oz)	260	4	2	0
One Dish Favorites Cheese Ravioli	1 pkg (8.5 oz)	250	6	4	0
One Dish Favorites Chicken Fettuccini	1 pkg (9.25 oz)	280	7	3	0
One Dish Favorites Lasagna Cheese Florentine Bake	1 pkg (10 oz)	270	6	2	0
One Dish Favorites Lasagna Chicken Florentine	1 pkg (10 oz)	270	6	2	0
One Dish Favorites Lasagna Classic Five Cheese	1 pkg (11.5 oz)	330	7	3	0
Skillet Chicken Alfredo	1 serv	180	4	2	0
Marie Callender's					
Cheese Ravioli In Marinara Sauce w/ Spirals & Garlic Bread	1 meal (16 oz)	750	29	9	–
Macaroni & Cheese	1 meal (12 oz)	540	24	15	–
Meat Lasagna	1 cup	240	9	5	0

FOOD	PORTION	CALS	FAT	SAT FAT	TRANS FAT
Skillet Meal Chicken Alfredo	½ pkg	490	29	14	–
Skillet Meal Penne Pasta & Meatballs	½ pkg	600	31	11	–
Skillet Meal Rigatoni Vegetables In Cheese Sauce	1 cup	290	12	7	–
Spaghetti w/ Meat Sauce & Garlic Bread	1 meal (17 oz)	670	25	11	–
Stuffed Pasta Trio	1 meal (10.5 oz)	380	16	9	–
Michelina's					
Lasagna w/ Meat Sauce	1 pkg (9 oz)	340	12	5	0
Milton's					
Lasagna Vegetable w/ Multigrain Pasta	1 cup (8 oz)	340	16	9	0
Mon Cuisine					
Vegetarian Spaghetti & Meatballs	1 pkg (10 oz)	360	4	0	–
Morton					
Macaroni & Cheese	1 serv (8 oz)	240	8	4	–
Spaghetti w/ Meat Sauce	1 meal (8.5 oz)	200	6	3	–
Organic Classics					
Cajun Chicken Tetrazzini w/ Penne Pasta	1 pkg (10 oz)	370	10	5	0
Chicken Cacciatore w/ Penne Pasta	1 pkg (10 oz)	270	4	1	0
Macaroni & Meat Sauce	1 pkg (10 oz)	340	9	3	–
Savvy Faire					
Lasagna Florentine	1 pkg (9.2 oz)	300	19	4	–
Seeds Of Change					
Chicken Fettuccine Alfredo	1 pkg (10 oz)	340	10	5	0
Lasagna Creamy Spinach	1 pkg (11 oz)	370	16	11	1
Lasagna Vegetable	1 pkg (11 oz)	310	9	4	0
Penne Marinara	1 pkg (11 oz)	290	7	3	0
Slim-Fast					
Fettuccine Alfredo	1 pkg	240	6	3	–
Rotini w/ Tomato & Italian Herb	1 pkg	240	2	1	–
Shells & Creamy Cheese Sauce	1 pkg	240	6	3	–
South Beach					
Penne & Chicken In Roasted Red Pepper Sauce w/ Broccoli	1 pkg	290	13	4	0

FOOD	PORTION	CALS	FAT	SAT FAT	TRANS FAT
Stouffer's					
Cheesy Spaghetti Bake	1 pkg (12 oz)	460	24	9	1
Chicken Parmigiana	1 pkg (13.13 oz)	460	18	4	0
Escalloped Chicken & Noodles	1 pkg (8 oz)	330	18	4	0
Homestyle Chicken & Noodles	1 pkg (12 oz)	340	12	3	0
Italian Sausage Stuffed Rigatoni	1 pkg (9.13 oz)	380	14	8	0
Lasagna Vegetable	1 pkg (10.5 oz)	390	18	7	0
Lasagna Bake w/ Meat Sauce	1 pkg (11.5 oz)	380	13	6	1
Macaroni & Cheese	1 cup (6 oz)	350	17	7	0
Macaroni & Beef	1 pkg (11.5 oz)	330	11	5	1
Manicotti Cheese	1 pkg (9 oz)	360	14	6	0
Shrimp Scampi	1 pkg (14 oz)	410	11	5	0
Tuna Noodle Casserole	1 pkg (10 oz)	350	15	5	0
Turkey Tetrazzini	1 pkg (10 oz)	380	20	8	0
Taste Above					
Meatless Thai Peanut Coconut Sauce w/ Veggie Chicken & Vermicelli	1 pkg (10 oz)	320	19	2	0
Meatless Tuscan Marinara Sauce w/ Veggie Chicken & Penne Pasta	1 pkg (10 oz)	320	19	2	0
Weight Watchers					
Smart Ones Lasagna w/ Meat Sauce	1 pkg (10.5 oz)	300	6	3	0
Yves					
Meatless Lasagna	1 pkg (10.5 oz)	300	3	1	0
MIX					
A Taste Of Thai					
Coconut Ginger	1 cup	280	7	7	–
Pad Thai For Two	½ pkg	345	1	tr	–
Peanut Noodles as prep	1 cup	330	10	5	–
Red Curry Noodles as prep	1 cup	280	8	4	–
Annie's Homegrown					
Gluten Free Rice Pasta & Cheddar as prep	1 cup	330	5	2	0
Organic Shells & Real Aged Wisconsin Cheddar as prep	1 cup	370	15	9	–
Organic Whole Wheat Shells & Cheddar as prep	1 cup	360	15	9	–

FOOD	PORTION	CALS	FAT	SAT FAT	TRANS FAT
Organic Skillet Meals Beef Stroganoff as prep	1 cup	320	13	6	0
Organic Skillet Meals Cheddar & Herb Chicken as prep	1 cup	310	7	4	0
Organic Skillet Meals Cheese Lasagna as prep	1 cup	280	9	4	0
Organic Skillet Meals Cheeseburger Macaroni as prep	1 cup	350	13	6	0
Organic Skillet Meals Chicken Fettucine as prep	1 cup	330	8	4	0
Organic Skillet Meals Creamy Tuna Spirals as prep	1 cup	260	7	4	0
Shells & Real Aged Wisconsin Cheddar as prep	1 cup	290	5	3	0
Shells & White Cheddar as prep	1 cup	290	5	3	0
Aramana					
Cheddar Cheeseburger as prep	1 cup	260	17	10	–
Creamy Chicken Alfredo as prep	1 cup	260	16	10	–
Mild Mexican as prep	1 cup	260	16	10	–
Back To Nature					
Alfredo & Gemelli as prep	1 cup	340	11	6	–
Macaroni & Cheese as prep	1 cup	320	10	6	–
White Cheddar & Spirals as prep	1 cup	330	12	7	–
Carapelli					
Penne Alfredo as prep	1 cup	240	1	1	–
Spirals Creamy Tomato as prep	1 cup	240	1	0	–
DeBoles					
Organic Macaroni & Cheese Whole Wheat as prep	1 cup	410	14	8	–
Pasta & Cheese as prep	1 cup	420	15	9	–
Rice Shells & Cheddar as prep	½ cup	260	8	5	–
Keto					
Macaroni & Cheese not prep	1 serv	112	10	–	–
Knorr					
Pasta & Sauce Jalapeno Jack as prep	1 cup	230	3	1	–

FOOD	PORTION	CALS	FAT	SAT FAT	TRANS FAT
Pasta Sides w/ Whole Grains Alfredo as prep	⅔ cup	300	11	5	–
Kraft					
Bistro Deluxe Sundried Tomato Parmesan as prep	1 cup	300	10	6	0
Near East					
Angel Hair w/ Spicy Tomato as prep	1 cup	240	6	1	–
Radiatore Basil & Herb as prep	1 cup	240	6	1	–
Vermicelli Garlic & Oil as prep	1 cup	310	9	2	–
Pasta Roni					
Angel Hair w/ Herbs as prep	1 cup	310	13	4	2
Chicken as prep	1 cup	300	12	4	2
Chicken Quesadilla as prep	1 cup	310	13	3	2
Fettuccine Alfredo as prep	1 cup	450	25	7	4
Nature's Way Mushrooms In Cream Sauce as prep	1 cup	280	10	3	0
Sour Cream & Chives as prep	1 cup	310	15	5	2
Stroganoff as prep	1 cup	350	14	5	2
Road's End Organics					
Mac & Cheese Dairy Free Gluten Free as prep	1 cup	310	1	0	0
Shells & Cheese as prep	1 cup	330	1	0	0
Whey Cool					
High Protein Macaroni & Cheese as prep	1 serv	260	5	2	–
REFRIGERATED					
Country Crock					
Elbow Macaroni & Cheese	1 cup	380	17	8	0
SHELF-STABLE					
It's Pasta Anytime					
Penne With Tomato Italian Sausage Sauce	1 pkg (15.25 oz)	540	8	1	–
TastyBite					
Peanut Sauce w/ Noodles	1 pkg (10 oz)	530	19	6	0
TAKE-OUT					
bami goreng indonesian noodle dish	1 cup	170	3	1	–
lasagna meatless	1 piece (9 oz)	356	11	7	0
lasagna w/ meat	1 piece (8 oz)	362	14	7	0

FOOD	PORTION	CALS	FAT	SAT FAT	TRANS FAT
lasagna w/ vegetables	1 serv (9 oz)	315	10	6	–
macaroni & cheese w/ ham	1 cup	542	33	13	0
manicotti cheese filled marinara sauce	1 (5 oz)	229	10	6	0
manicotti cheese filled w/ meat sauce	1 (5 oz)	239	11	6	0
pasta w/ pesto sauce	1 cup	370	25	4	0
ravioli cheese & spinach filled w/ cream sauce	1 cup	362	17	6	0
ravioli meat filled w/ marinara sauce	1 cup	372	16	5	0
ravioli cheese w/ tomato sauce	1 cup	335	14	6	–
rigatoni w/ sausage sauce	¾ cup	260	12	4	–
spaghetti w/ red clam sauce	1 cup	285	8	1	0
spaghetti w/ sauce & meatballs	2 cups	670	26	8	0
spaghetti w/ white clam sauce	1 cup	456	20	3	–
tortellini cheese w/ tomato sauce	1 cup	332	14	6	–
tortellini meat filled w/ marinara sauce	1 cup	281	10	3	0
tortellini spinach filled w/ marinara sauce	1 cup	238	8	2	0

PASTA SALAD
MIX
Dole

FOOD	PORTION	CALS	FAT	SAT FAT	TRANS FAT
Veggie Pasta Salads Broccoli Ranch	1½ cups	230	13	2	0
Veggie Pasta Salads Cheddar Bacon Ranch	1½ cups	370	22	5	0
Veggie Pasta Salads Garden Vegetable	1½ cups	240	14	2	0
Veggie Pasta Salads Italian Herb	1½ cups	270	12	3	0

TAKE-OUT

FOOD	PORTION	CALS	FAT	SAT FAT	TRANS FAT
pasta salad w/ crab vegetables mayonnaise	1 cup	317	16	2	–
tortellini salad cheese filled w/ vinaigrette dressing	1 cup	333	18	7	0

FOOD	PORTION	CALS	FAT	SAT FAT	TRANS FAT
PATÉ					
chicken liver canned	1 tbsp	26	2	1	0
duck paté	1 oz	96	8	–	–
fish paté	1 oz	76	7	–	–
liver w/ truffle	1 serv (2 oz)	183	16	6	0
mushroom anchovy paté	1 can (2.25 oz)	130	11	2	–
paté de foie gras smoked canned	1 tbsp	60	6	2	0
pork paté	1 oz	107	10	4	–
pork paté en croute	1 oz	91	7	3	–
rabbit paté	1 oz	66	5	3	–
shrimp	1 can (2.25 oz)	140	10	2	–
PEACH					
CANNED					
halves in heavy syrup	1 half	60	tr	tr	–
halves in light syrup	1 half	44	tr	tr	–
halves juice pack	1 half	34	tr	tr	–
halves water pack	1 half	18	tr	tr	–
peach sauce	½ cup	120	0	0	0
spiced in heavy syrup	1 cup	180	tr	tr	–
spiced in heavy syrup	1 fruit	66	tr	tr	–
Del Monte					
Carb Clever Sliced	½ cup	30	0	0	0
Freestone Lite Slices	½ cup	60	0	0	0
Freestone Sliced	½ cup	100	0	0	0
Fruit Cup Diced Extra Light Syrup	1 pkg (4 oz)	50	0	0	0
Fruit Cup Diced In Heavy Syrup	1 serv (4 oz)	80	0	0	0
Fruit Naturals Chunks	½ cup	70	0	0	0
Fruit To Go Banana Berry Peaches	1 pkg (4 oz)	70	0	0	0
Fruit To Go Peachy Peaches	1 pkg (4 oz)	70	0	0	0
Halves In Heavy Syrup	½ cup	100	0	0	0
Orchard Select Sliced Cling	½ cup	80	0	0	0
Sliced In 100% Juice	½ cup	60	0	0	0
Sliced Light Syrup Raspberry Flavor	½ cup	80	0	0	0
Dole					
All Natural Yellow Cling Sliced	½ cup	80	0	0	0

FOOD	PORTION	CALS	FAT	SAT FAT	TRANS FAT
Liberty Gold					
Sliced Cling In Heavy Syrup	½ cup	100	0	0	0
S&W					
Slices Lightly Sweetened Juice	½ cup	80	0	0	0
Yellow Cling In Heavy Syrup	½ cup	100	0	0	0
DRIED					
halves	1 cup	383	1	tr	–
halves	10	311	1	tr	–
halves cooked w/ sugar	½ cup	139	tr	tr	–
halves cooked w/o sugar	½ cup	99	tr	tr	–
Crispy Green					
Crispy Peaches	1 pkg (0.36 oz)	38	0	0	0
Mrs. May's					
Fruit Chips	1 pkg	35	0	0	0
FRESH					
peach	1	37	tr	tr	–
sliced	1 cup	73	tr	tr	–
Chiquita					
Peach	1 med (3.4 oz)	40	0	0	0
FROZEN					
slices sweetened	1 cup	235	tr	tr	–
C&W					
Ultimate Sliced	¾ cup	50	0	0	0
PEACH JUICE					
nectar	1 cup	134	tr	tr	–
After The Fall					
Georgia Peach	8 oz	130	0	0	0
Ceres					
Peach	8 oz	120	0	0	0
Froose					
Playful Peach	1 box (4.2 oz)	80	0	0	0
PEANUT BUTTER					
chunky	2 tbsp	188	16	3	–
chunky	1 cup	1520	129	25	–
chunky w/o salt	2 tbsp	188	16	3	–
chunky w/o salt	1 cup	1520	129	25	–
smooth	2 tbsp	188	16	3	–
smooth	1 cup	1517	128	25	–
smooth w/o salt	2 tbsp	188	16	3	–
smooth w/o salt	1 cup	1517	129	25	–

FOOD	PORTION	CALS	FAT	SAT FAT	TRANS FAT
Arrowhead Mills					
Organic Creamy	2 tbsp	190	17	3	0
Organic Honey Sweetened Creamy	2 tbsp	190	16	3	0
Organic Natural Crunchy	2 tbsp	190	17	3	0
Carb Options					
Creamy	2 tbsp	190	17	4	–
Cream-Nut					
Natural	2 tbsp	190	16	3	0
Estee					
Creamy Low Sodium	2 tbsp	180	16	3	–
Jif					
Creamy	2 tbsp	190	16	3	0
Creamy To Go	1 pkg (2.25 oz)	270	32	6	0
Extra Crunchy	2 tbsp	190	16	3	–
Peanut Butter & Honey	2 tbsp	190	15	3	0
Reduced Fat Creamy	2 tbsp	190	12	3	–
Reduced Fat Crunchy	2 tbsp	190	12	3	–
Simply	2 tbsp	190	16	3	–
Kettle					
Organic Unsalted	2 tbsp	170	14	3	0
Maranatha					
Crunchy	2 tbsp	190	16	–	–
Salted	2 tbsp	190	16	3	–
Peanut Better					
Cinnamon Currant	2 tbsp	180	14	2	–
Deep Chocolate	2 tbsp	170	13	3	–
Hickory Smoked	2 tbsp	190	16	3	–
Onion Parsley	2 tbsp	180	15	3	–
Peanut Praline	2 tbsp	180	15	3	–
Rosemary Garlic	2 tbsp	180	15	3	–
Spicy Southwestern	2 tbsp	190	17	3	–
Sweet Molasses	2 tbsp	180	14	2	–
Thai Ginger & Red Pepper	2 tbsp	180	15	3	–
Vanilla Cranberry	2 tbsp	170	13	2	–
Peanut Butter & Co.					
Cinnamon Raisin Swirl	2 tbsp	143	7	1	–
Crunch Time	2 tbsp	200	16	2	–
Dark Chocolate Dreams	2 tbsp	175	12	3	–
Smooth Operator	2 tbsp	200	16	2	–

FOOD	PORTION	CALS	FAT	SAT FAT	TRANS FAT
The Heat Is On	2 tbsp	164	10	2	–
White Chocolate Wonderful	1 tbsp	165	12	3	–
Reese's					
Creamy	2 tbsp	200	15	2	0
Peanut Butter Chips	1 tbsp	80	4	4	–
Skippy					
Creamy	2 tbsp	190	17	4	–
Creamy w/ 2 slices white bread	1 sandwich	340	19	3	–
Reduced Fat Creamy	2 tbsp	190	12	3	–
Roasted Honey Nut	2 tbsp	190	17	4	–
Roasted Honey Nut Super Chunk	2 tbsp	190	17	4	–
Squeeze Stix	1 pkg	140	12	3	–
Squeeze Stix Chocolate	1 pkg	140	10	3	–
Squeez'It	2 tbsp	190	17	4	–
Super Chunk	2 tbsp	190	17	4	–
Super Chunk Reduced Fat	2 tbsp	190	12	3	–
Smart Balance					
Chunky Omega	2 tbsp	200	17	3	0
Smucker's					
Goober All Flavors	3 tbsp	240	13	3	–
Natural Chunky	2 tbsp	210	16	3	–
Natural Creamy	2 tbsp	210	16	3	–
Natural Honey	2 tbsp	200	16	3	–
Natural No Salt Added Creamy	2 tbsp	210	16	3	–
Natural Reduced Fat Creamy	2 tbsp	200	12	2	–
Teddies					
Old Fashioned	2 tbsp	190	16	2	0

PEANUTS

FOOD	PORTION	CALS	FAT	SAT FAT	TRANS FAT
chocolate coated	¼ cup	193	12	5	0
cooked w/ salt	½ cup	286	20	3	0
dry roasted w/ salt	28 nuts (1 oz)	164	14	2	0
dry roasted w/o salt	¼ cup	214	18	3	0
dry roasted w/o salt	28 (1 oz)	164	14	2	0
honey roasted	¼ cup	191	16	3	0
milk chocolate coated	1	21	1	1	0
sugar coated	¼ cup	203	13	2	0
yogurt coated	¼ cup	230	16	7	0

FOOD	PORTION	CALS	FAT	SAT FAT	TRANS FAT
A Taste Of Thai					
Spicy Peanut Bake	¼ pkg	45	2	1	–
At Last!					
Chocolate Covered	1 pkg (0.9 oz)	150	11	5	–
Brach's					
Double Dippers	15 pieces	210	12	6	–
Chocolate Covered					
Estee					
Chocolate Coated	¼ cup	170	9	4	–
Fructose Sweetened					
Frito Lay					
Salted	1 oz	160	14	2	0
Salted w/ Shells	½ cup	160	14	2	0
Judy's					
Sugar Free	¼ piece (1 oz)	90	5	2	–
Coconut Peanut Brittle					
Low Carb Creations					
Soft Peanut Brittle	2 pieces (1 oz)	140	10	2	–
Nuts Are Good					
Buffalo	1 oz	120	6	1	0
Pina Colada	1 oz	130	7	1	0
Raspberry	1 oz	130	7	1	0
Vanilla Rum	1 oz	130	7	1	0
Planters					
Cocktail	1 oz	170	14	2	–
Dry Roasted	1 oz	170	14	2	0
Sunfood					
Organic Wild Jungle	1 oz	174	14	2	0
Sweet Delight					
Peanut Roasters	⅓ pkg (1 oz)	160	12	–	–
PEAR					
CANNED					
halves in heavy syrup	1 cup	188	tr	tr	–
halves in heavy syrup	1 half	68	tr	tr	–
halves in light syrup	1 half	45	tr	tr	–
halves juice pack	1 cup	123	tr	tr	–
halves water pack	1 half	22	tr	tr	–
Del Monte					
Carb Clever Sliced	½ cup	40	0	0	0

FOOD	PORTION	CALS	FAT	SAT FAT	TRANS FAT
Fruit Cup Diced In Heavy Syrup	1 pkg (4 oz)	80	0	0	0
Fruit Cup Diced Extra Light Syrup	1 pkg (4 oz)	50	0	0	0
Halves In 100% Juice	½ cup	60	0	0	0
Halves In Light Syrup	½ cup	60	0	0	0
Orchard Select Sliced Bartlett	½ cup	80	0	0	0
S&W					
Halves In Lightly Sweetened Juice	½ cup	80	0	0	0
DRIED					
halves	10	459	1	tr	–
halves	1 cup	472	1	tr	–
halves cooked w/ sugar	½ cup	196	tr	tr	–
halves cooked w/o sugar	½ cup	163	tr	tr	–
Bare Fruit					
Organic	1 pkg (0.6 oz)	46	0	0	0
FRESH					
asian	1 (4.3 oz)	51	tr	tr	–
pear	1	98	1	tr	–
sliced w/ skin	1 cup	97	1	tr	–
Chiquita					
Pear	1 med (5.8 oz)	100	1	0	–

PEAR JUICE

FOOD	PORTION	CALS	FAT	SAT FAT	TRANS FAT
nectar	1 cup	149	tr	tr	–
Ceres					
Pear	8 oz	120	0	0	0
Froose					
Perfect Pear	1 box (4.2 oz)	80	0	0	0
Izze					
Sparkling Pear	8 oz	130	0	0	0
Langers					
Kid's 100% Juice	4 oz	60	0	0	0

PEAS

FOOD	PORTION	CALS	FAT	SAT FAT	TRANS FAT
CANNED					
green	½ cup	59	tr	tr	–
green low sodium	½ cup	59	tr	tr	–
Del Monte					
Sweet	½ cup	60	0	0	0

FOOD	PORTION	CALS	FAT	SAT FAT	TRANS FAT
Sweet No Salt Added	½ cup	60	0	0	0
Sweet Very Young Small	½ cup	60	0	0	0
Green Giant					
50% Less Sodium Young Tender Sweet	½ cup	60	0	0	0
Young Tender Sweet	½ cup	60	0	0	0
Le Sueur					
50% Less Sodium Young Tender	½ cup	60	0	0	0
Libby's					
No Salt No Sugar Added	½ cup	70	1	0	0
S&W					
Petite	½ cup (4.4 oz)	70	0	0	0
Small	½ cup (4.4 oz)	70	0	0	0
Tillen Farms					
Crispy Snapper Pickled	¼ cup	15	0	0	0
DRIED					
split cooked	1 cup	231	1	tr	–
Arrowhead Mills					
Organic Green Split not prep	¼ cup	160	1	0	0
Snapea Crisps					
Baked Original	22 (1 oz)	70	8	1	0
FRESH					
green cooked	½ cup	67	tr	tr	–
green raw	½ cup	58	tr	tr	–
snap peas cooked	½ cup	34	tr	tr	–
snap peas raw	½ cup	30	tr	tr	–
Frieda's					
Snow Peas	1 cup	35	0	0	0
Sugar Snap	⅔ cup (3 oz)	35	0	0	0
River Ranch					
Sugar Snap	1½ cups	35	0	0	0
FROZEN					
green cooked	½ cup	63	tr	tr	–
snap peas cooked	½ cup	42	tr	tr	–
Birds Eye					
Steamfresh Garlic Baby Peas & Mushrooms	¾ cup	80	2	0	0
Steamfresh Sweet Peas	⅓ cup	70	0	0	0

FOOD	PORTION	CALS	FAT	SAT FAT	TRANS FAT
C&W					
Alfredo	½ cup	110	5	3	0
Early Harvest Petite No Salt Added	⅔ cup	70	0	0	0
Sugar Snap	⅔ cup	40	0	0	0
Fresh Like					
Garden	3.5 oz	85	1	–	–
Green Giant					
Early June No Sauce	⅔ cup	50	1	0	0
La Choy					
Snow Pea Pods	½ pkg (3 oz)	35	2	0	–
Pictsweet					
Green Peas	⅔ cup	70	0	0	0
SHELF-STABLE					
TastyBite					
Agra Peas & Greens	½ pkg (5 oz)	138	10	2	0
PECANS					
candied	1 oz	190	17	3	–
dry roasted	1 oz	187	18	1	–
dry roasted salted	1 oz	187	18	1	–
halves dry roasted w/ salt	20 (1 oz)	200	21	2	–
halves dried	1 cup	721	73	6	–
oil roasted	1 oz	195	20	2	–
oil roasted salted	1 oz	195	20	2	–
Emerald					
Glazed Pecan Pie	¼ cup	150	11	1	0
Keto					
Chocolately Covered	1 oz	207	19	4	–
Sweet Delights					
Pecan Roasters	⅓ pkg (1 oz)	210	21	2	–
PECTIN					
liquid	1 oz	3	0	0	0
powder	1 pkg (1.75 oz)	162	tr	tr	0
PEPEAO					
dried	¼ cup	18	tr	–	0
raw sliced	1 cup	25	tr	–	0
PEPPER					
black	1 tsp	5	tr	tr	0

FOOD	PORTION	CALS	FAT	SAT FAT	TRANS FAT
cayenne	1 tsp	6	tr	tr	0
white	1 tsp	7	tr	tr	0
Emeril's					
Kicked Up Red Sauce	1 tsp	0	0	0	0
McCormick					
Lemon & Pepper Seasoning Salt	¼ tsp	0	0	0	0

PEPPERMINT

fresh chopped	2 tbsp	2	tr	tr	0

PEPPERS
CANNED

FOOD	PORTION	CALS	FAT	SAT FAT	TRANS FAT
chili green	1 cup (5.5 oz)	29	tr	tr	–
chili green hot chopped	½ cup	17	tr	tr	–
chili pepper paste	1 tbsp	6	1	–	–
chili red hot	1 (2.6 oz)	18	tr	tr	–
chili red hot chopped	½ cup	17	tr	tr	–
green halves	½ cup	13	tr	tr	–
jalapeno chopped	½ cup	17	tr	tr	–
red halves	½ cup	13	tr	tr	–
B&G					
Cherry Hot	1 (1 oz)	10	0	0	0
Cherry Sweet	1 (1 oz)	10	0	0	0
Hot Pepper Rings	7 pieces (1 oz)	0	0	0	0
Pepperoncini	3 pieces (1 oz)	10	0	0	0
Roasted w/ Balsamic Vinegar	½ piece (1 oz)	10	0	0	0
Sweet Fried	1 oz	25	2	–	–
Gertie's Finest					
Piquillo	1 oz	10	0	0	0
Las Palmas					
Diced Green Chiles	2 tbsp	5	0	0	0
Jalapenos Sliced	3 tbsp	10	0	0	0
Old El Paso					
Green Chiles Chopped	2 tbsp (1 oz)	5	0	0	0
Pace					
Green Chiles Diced	2 tbsp	10	0	0	0
Tillen Farms					
Bell Peppers Pickled Sweet	¼ cup	25	0	0	0
DRIED					
ancho	1 (0.6 oz)	48	1	tr	–
ancho	1 tsp	3	tr	–	0

FOOD	PORTION	CALS	FAT	SAT FAT	TRANS FAT
casabel	1 tsp	3	tr	–	0
chipotle smoked	1 tsp	3	tr	–	0
green	1 tbsp	1	tr	tr	–
guajillo	1 tsp	3	tr	–	0
mulato	1 tsp	3	tr	–	0
pasilla	1 (7 g)	24	1	–	–
pasilla	1 tsp	3	tr	–	0
red	1 tbsp	1	tr	tr	–
Frieda's					
California Chili	2 tbsp	15	0	0	0
FRESH					
banana	1 (4 in) (1.2 oz)	9	tr	tr	–
banana	1 cup (4.4 oz)	33	1	tr	–
chili green hot	1	18	tr	tr	–
chili green hot chopped	½ cup	30	tr	tr	–
chili red chopped	½ cup	30	tr	tr	–
chili red hot	1 (1.6 oz)	18	tr	tr	–
green	1 (2.6 oz)	20	tr	tr	–
green chopped	½ cup	13	tr	tr	–
green chopped cooked	½ cup	19	tr	tr	–
green cooked	1 (2.6 oz)	20	tr	tr	–
habanero	1 tsp	9	tr	–	–
hungarian	1 (0.9 oz)	8	tr	tr	–
jalapeno	1 (0.5 oz)	4	tr	tr	–
jalapeno sliced	1 cup (3.2 oz)	27	1	tr	–
red	1 (2.6 oz)	20	tr	tr	–
red chopped	½ cup	13	tr	tr	–
red chopped cooked	½ cup	19	tr	tr	–
red cooked	1 (2.6 oz)	20	tr	tr	–
serrano	1 (6 g)	2	tr	0	–
serrano chopped	1 cup (3.7 oz)	34	tr	tr	–
yellow	1 (6.5 oz)	50	tr	–	–
yellow	10 strips	14	tr	–	–
Chiquita					
Pepper	1 med (5.2 oz)	30	0	0	0
Frieda's					
Peppadew	⅓ cup	40	0	0	0
FROZEN					
green chopped	1 oz	6	tr	tr	–
red chopped	1 oz	6	tr	tr	–

FOOD	PORTION	CALS	FAT	SAT FAT	TRANS FAT
C&W					
Strips	¾ cup	25	0	0	0
Roast Works					
Flame Roasted Red	1 serv (3 oz)	45	1	0	0
PERCH					
FRESH					
cooked	1 fillet (1.6 oz)	54	1	tr	–
cooked	3 oz	99	1	tr	–
ocean perch atlantic cooked	1 fillet (1.8 oz)	60	1	tr	–
ocean perch atlantic cooked	3 oz	103	2	tr	–
ocean perch atlantic raw	3 oz	80	1	tr	–
raw	3 oz	77	1	tr	–
red raw	3.5 oz	114	4	–	–
PERSIMMONS					
dried japanese	1 (1.2 oz)	93	tr	–	0
fresh	1 (6 oz)	118	tr	tr	0
Frieda's					
Dried Fuyu	⅓ cup (1.4 oz)	140	0	0	0
PHEASANT					
breast cooked	½ breast (4.5 oz)	312	15	4	0
leg cooked	1 (2.6 oz)	184	9	3	0
PHYLLO					
sheet	1 (0.7 oz)	57	1	tr	–
Ekizian					
Sheets	¼ lb	433	9	4	0
Fillo Factory					
Kataifi Shredded Fillo	1 (2 oz)	180	2	0	0
Organic	2 sheets (1.5 oz)	130	1	0	0
Organic Whole Wheat	2 sheets (1.8 oz)	140	1	0	0
Shells Large	1 (0.7 oz)	80	2	0	–
PICANTE (see SALSA)					
PICKLES					
bread & butter	6 slices	39	tr	tr	0
dill	1 lg (4.7 oz)	24	tr	tr	0
dill low sodium	1 med (2.3 oz)	12	tr	tr	0
dill sliced	6 slices	7	tr	tr	0
sweet gherkin	1 (1.2 oz)	41	tr	tr	0

FOOD	PORTION	CALS	FAT	SAT FAT	TRANS FAT
tsukemono japanese pickles sliced	¼ cup	10	tr	tr	0
B&G					
Bread & Butter	3 slices (1 oz)	25	0	0	0
Kosher Dill	⅓ (1 oz)	0	0	0	0
Kosher Dill No Salt	½ (1 oz)	10	0	0	0
Sour	½ (1 oz)	0	0	0	0
Sweet Gerkins	1 (1 oz)	35	0	0	0
Claussen					
Kosher Dills Whole	½ (1 oz)	5	0	0	0
Del Monte					
Dill Halves	1 piece (1 oz)	5	0	0	0
Hamburger Dill Chips	1 serv (1 oz)	0	0	0	0
Sweet	1 serv (1 oz)	40	0	0	0
Sweet Gerkins	1 serv (1 oz)	40	0	0	0
Tiny Kosher Dill	1 serv (1 oz)	5	0	0	0
Hebrew National					
Dill	1	23	0	0	0
Mt Olive					
Bread & Butter No Sugar Added	1 oz	0	0	0	0

PIE (see also PIE CRUST, PIE FILLING)
FROZEN

FOOD	PORTION	CALS	FAT	SAT FAT	TRANS FAT
Amy's					
Apple	1 serv (4 oz)	240	8	5	–
Edwards					
Pie Slices Chocolate Creme	1 slice (2.7 oz)	290	17	9	2
Pie Slices Key Lime	1 slice (3.2 oz)	330	16	10	2
Pie Slices Oreo Cream	1 slice (2.6 oz)	290	17	9	3
Mrs. Smith's					
Bake & Serve No Sugar Added Apple	1 slice (4.6 oz)	310	16	7	0
Blueberry Crumb	1 slice (4.2 oz)	320	14	6	0
Cherry	1 slice (4.6 oz)	330	16	7	0
Cinnabon Apple Crumb	1 slice (4.6 oz)	350	16	7	0
Classic Cream Key Lime	1 slice (4.2 oz)	410	19	13	0
Coconut Custard	1 slice (4.4 oz)	300	17	9	0
Deep Dish Berry Burst	1 slice (4.2 oz)	340	15	7	0
Dutch Apple Crumb	1 slice (4.6 oz)	370	17	7	0

FOOD	PORTION	CALS	FAT	SAT FAT	TRANS FAT
Pumpkin Custard	1 slice (4.6 oz)	300	15	7	0
Soda Shoppe Boston Cream	1 slice (2.7 oz)	220	9	3	0
Soda Shoppe Chocolate Cream	1 slice (4.6 oz)	350	17	8	3
Soda Shoppe Lemon Meringue	1 slice (4.2 oz)	300	10	2	3
Sara Lee					
Apple	1 slice (4.6 oz)	340	16	4	–
Cherry	1 slice (4.6 oz)	320	14	3	–
Coconut Cream	1 slice (4.8 oz)	330	19	11	–
French Silk	1 slice (4.8 oz)	340	21	12	–
Key West Lime	1 slice (4.2 oz)	400	25	12	–
Lemon Meringue	1 slice (5 oz)	220	5	3	–
Mince	1 slice (4.6 oz)	370	15	3	–
Pumpkin	1 slice (4.6 oz)	260	11	3	–
Southern Pecan	1 slice (4.2 oz)	520	24	5	–
Southern Sweet Potato	1 slice (4.6 oz)	280	10	3	–
Sulce de Leche Caramel Swirl	1 slice (4.4 oz)	400	26	15	–
READY-TO-EAT					
Entenmann's					
Peach Raspberry Melba	⅛ pie (2.6 oz)	250	9	4	0
SNACK					
Lifestream					
Pie Oh-My Apple	1 (3.5 oz)	280	11	5	0
Pie Oh-My Pineapple	1 (3.5 oz)	280	11	5	0
TAKE-OUT					
apple	⅛ of 9 in pie (5.4 oz)	411	19	5	–
banana cream	⅛ of 9 in pie (5.2 oz)	398	20	6	–
blueberry	⅛ of 9 in pie (5.2 oz)	360	18	4	–
butterscotch	⅛ of 9 in pie (4.5 oz)	355	18	5	–
cherry	⅛ of 9 in pie (6.3 oz)	486	22	5	–
chocolate creme	1 slice (4 oz)	344	22	6	–
coconut creme	⅛ of 9 in pie (4.7 oz)	396	21	8	–
coconut custard	⅙ of 8 in pie (3.6 oz)	271	14	6	–

FOOD	PORTION	CALS	FAT	SAT FAT	TRANS FAT
custard	⅛ of 9 in pie (4.5 oz)	262	11	4	–
key lime	1 slice (5 oz)	420	14	6	0
lemon meringue	1 slice (4.5 oz)	303	10	2	–
mince	⅛ of 9 in pie (5.8 oz)	477	18	4	–
pecan	1 slice (4 oz)	452	21	4	–
pumpkin	1 slice (3.8 oz)	229	10	2	–
vanilla cream	⅛ of 9 in pie (4.4 oz)	350	18	5	–
PIE CRUST					
FROZEN					
baked	⅛ of 9 in pie	113	7	2	–
baked	9 in crust	884	56	18	–
puff pastry shell	1 (1.4 oz)	223	15	2	0
tart shell	1 (1 oz)	149	10	3	–
Mrs. Smith's					
Deep Dish Shell	1 slice (1 oz)	130	7	4	0
Pepperidge Farm					
Puff Pastry Sheets	⅙ sheet	170	11	3	5
Puff Pastry Shell	1	190	13	4	5
Pet-Ritz					
Deep Dish	⅛ pie (0.7 oz)	90	5	2	–
MIX					
Betty Crocker					
Pie Crust as prep	⅛ crust	110	8	2	–
Jiffy					
Pie Crust Mix	1/7 crust	180	10	4	–
MiniCarb					
Pie Crust Mix	1 slice	105	7	4	–
READY-TO-EAT					
chocolate crumb	9 in crust	1063	65	14	0
chocolate crumb	⅛ of 9 in pie	132	8	2	0
graham cracker	9 in crust	1037	52	11	0
graham cracker	⅛ of 9 in pie	109	5	1	0
graham cracker dessert shell	1 (1.1 oz)	148	7	2	0
Keebler					
Reduced Fat Graham	⅛ pie (0.7 oz)	90	4	0	–

FOOD	PORTION	CALS	FAT	SAT FAT	TRANS FAT
Nilla Wafers					
Pie Crust	1/6 (1 oz)	140	8	2	–
PIE FILLING					
apple	1/8 can (2.6 oz)	74	tr	tr	–
apple	1 can (21 oz)	599	1	tr	–
cherry	1/8 can (2.6 oz)	85	tr	tr	–
cherry	1 can (21 oz)	683	1	tr	–
pumpkin pie mix	1 cup	282	tr	tr	–
Colac					
All Flavors	1 tbsp	19	0	0	0
Comstock					
Blueberry	1/3 cup	100	0	0	0
Country Cherry	1/3 cup	90	0	0	0
Light Cherry	1/3 cup	60	0	0	0
Farmer's Market					
Organic Pumpkin Pie Mix	1/2 cup	100	0	0	0
PIEROGI					
pierogi	3/4 cup (4.4 oz)	307	19	7	–
Mrs. T's					
Broccoli & Cheddar	3 (4.2 oz)	200	5	1	–
Potato & American Cheese	3 (4.2 oz)	220	4	2	–
Potato & 4 Cheese Blend	3 (4.2 oz)	230	7	2	0
Potato & Cheddar	3 (4.2 oz)	180	3	1	0
Rogies Jalapeno & Cheddar	7 (3 oz)	120	2	1	–
PIGEON PEAS					
dried cooked	1 cup	204	1	tr	–
dried cooked	1/2 cup	102	tr	tr	–
PIGNOLIA (*see* PINE NUTS)					
PIG'S FEET					
cooked	1	201	14	4	0
pickled	1	177	14	5	0
PIKE					
northern cooked	1/2 fillet (5.4 oz)	176	1	tr	–
northern cooked	3 oz	96	1	tr	–
northern raw	3 oz	75	1	tr	–
roe raw	1 oz	37	tr	–	–

FOOD	PORTION	CALS	FAT	SAT FAT	TRANS FAT
walleye baked	3 oz	101	1	tr	–
walleye fillet baked	4.4 oz	147	2	tr	–

PILLNUTS
canarytree dried	1 oz	204	23	9	–

PIMIENTOS
canned	1 slice	0	0	0	0
canned	1 tbsp	3	tr	tr	–

PINE NUTS
pignolia dried	1 oz	146	14	2	–
pignolia dried	1 tbsp	51	5	1	–
pinyon dried	1 oz	161	17	3	–
Frieda's					
Pine Nuts	¼ cup	150	15	2	–
Good Sense					
Pignolias	¼ cup	190	15	4	–

PINEAPPLE
CANNED
chunks in heavy syrup	1 cup	199	tr	tr	–
chunks juice pack	1 cup	150	tr	tr	–
crushed in heavy syrup	1 cup	199	tr	tr	–
slices in heavy syrup	1 slice	45	tr	tr	–
slices in light syrup	1 slice	30	tr	tr	–
slices juice pack	1 slice	35	tr	tr	–
slices water pack	1 slice	19	tr	tr	–
tidbits in heavy syrup	1 cup	199	tr	tr	–
tidbits in juice	1 cup	150	tr	tr	–
tidbits in water	1 cup	79	tr	tr	–
Del Monte					
Chunks In Heavy Syrup	½ cup	90	0	0	0
Chunks In Its Own Juice	½ cup	70	0	0	0
Crushed In Heavy Syrup	½ cup	90	0	0	0
Crushed In Its Own Juice	½ cup	70	0	0	0
Fruit Cup Tidbits	1 pkg (4 oz)	50	0	0	0
Fruit Naturals Chunks	½ cup	70	0	0	0
Dole					
All Natural Chunks	½ cup	60	0	0	0
Chunks Juice Pack	½ cup	60	0	0	0

FOOD	PORTION	CALS	FAT	SAT FAT	TRANS FAT
Liberty Gold					
Crushed No Sugar Added	½ cup	80	0	0	0
Slices Natural Juice	½ cup	80	0	0	0
DRIED					
Mrs. May's					
Fruit Chips	1 pkg	35	0	0	0
Sunsweet					
Pineapples	⅓ cup (1.4 oz)	130	0	0	0
FRESH					
diced	1 cup	77	tr	tr	–
slice	1 slice	42	tr	tr	–
Cala Fruit					
Golden Sliced	1 serv (3.5 oz)	50	0	0	0
Frieda's					
Zululand Queen	1 cup (5 oz)	70	1	0	–
Frosty Fresh					
Peeled & Cored	½ cup	60	0	0	0
FROZEN					
chunks sweetened	½ cup	104	tr	tr	–
Europe's Best					
Aloha Gold	1 cup	70	0	0	0
Roast Works					
Flame Roasted	1 serv (3 oz)	80	0	0	0
PINEAPPLE JUICE					
canned	1 cup	139	tr	tr	–
frzn as prep	1 cup	129	tr	tr	–
frzn not prep	6 oz	387	tr	tr	–
Adina					
Pineapple Ginger Gin-Jah	8 oz	80	0	0	0
Ceres					
Pineapple	8 oz	120	0	0	0
Langers					
100% Juice	8 oz	130	0	0	0
Sundia					
Purely	½ cup	60	0	0	0
Walnut Acres					
Organic	8 oz	130	0	0	0
PINK BEANS					
dried cooked	1 cup	252	1	tr	–

FOOD	PORTION	CALS	FAT	SAT FAT	TRANS FAT
PINTO BEANS					
dried cooked	1 cup	245	1	tr	0
Arrowhead Mills					
Organic Dried not prep	¼ cup	150	0	0	0
Eden					
Organic Spicy	½ cup	120	1	0	0
Organic Spicy Refried	½ cup	90	1	0	0
TAKE-OUT					
stewed w/ viandas	1 cup	222	8	2	–
PISTACHIOS					
dry roasted w/ salt	49 nuts (1 oz)	161	13	2	0
dry roasted w/o salt	49 nuts (1 oz)	162	13	2	0
in shells	½ cup	165	13	2	0
Love'n Bake					
Pistachio Paste	2 tbsp	160	11	1	–
Sweet Delights					
Pistachio Roasters	⅓ pkg (1 oz)	190	14	–	–
PITANGA					
fresh	1	2	tr	–	–
fresh	1 cup	57	1	–	–
PIZZA (see also PIZZA CRUST)					
Alexia					
Pizza Snack Sweet Italian Sausage Roasted Peppers & Parmesan	6 pieces (3 oz)	210	10	3	0
Pizza Snacks Pesto Chicken w/ Fresh Mozzarella	6 pieces (3 oz)	220	11	3	0
Amy's					
Cheese	⅓ pie	300	13	4	–
Pocket Sandwich Cheese Pizza	1 (4.5 oz)	300	9	4	–
Pocket Sandwich Vegetarian Pizza	1 (4.5 oz)	250	6	3	–
Roasted Vegetable	⅓ pie	260	8	2	–
Soy Cheese	⅓ pie	290	11	1	–
Spinach	⅓ pie	300	12	4	–
Banquet					
Pepperoni	1 pie (6.75 oz)	490	23	7	–

FOOD	PORTION	CALS	FAT	SAT FAT	TRANS FAT
Boca					
Supreme w/ Rising Crust Sausage & Pepperoni	⅓ pkg (4.3 oz)	280	8	3	0
Cedarlane					
Zone Cheese	1 (6.5 oz)	380	14	5	0
Celeste					
4 Cheese	1 (5.7 oz)	360	16	8	2
Ellio's					
All Cheesy	1 slice	160	5	2	0
Cheese	1 slice	150	4	2	0
Microwave Single Slice	1 slice	360	8	4	0
Pepperoni	1 slice	160	5	3	0
Farm Rich					
Slices Pepperoni	2 (3.5 oz)	280	14	7	0
Freschetta					
Pepperoni	½ pie (5.8 oz)	470	21	9	–
Glutino					
Gluten Free Duo Cheese	1 (6.1 oz)	420	12	5	0
Gluten Free Spinach & Feta	1 (6.1 oz)	430	16	5	0
Healthy Choice					
French Bread Cheese	1 pie	340	5	2	–
French Bread Pepperoni	1 pie	340	5	2	–
French Bread Supreme	1 pie	340	5	2	–
French Bread Vegetable	1 pie	320	5	2	–
Ian's					
Cheese	1 slice (1.5 oz)	100	3	2	–
Jeno's					
Crisp 'N Tasty Cheese	1 pie (6.8 oz)	460	19	6	–
Kid Cuisine					
Cheese Pizza Painter	1 meal	320	6	3	0
Dip & Dunk Cheese Pizza Strips	1 meal	510	14	6	0
Primo Pepperoni Pizza	1 meal	400	7	3	0
Lean Cuisine					
Casual Eating Deluxe	1 pkg (6 oz)	370	9	4	0
Casual Eating Four Cheese	1 pkg (6 oz)	400	9	4	0
Casual Eating French Bread Cheese	1 serv (6 oz)	320	7	4	0

FOOD	PORTION	CALS	FAT	SAT FAT	TRANS FAT
Casual Eating French Bread Deluxe	1 pkg (6.1 oz)	310	9	4	0
Casual Eating French Bread Pepperoni	1 pkg (5.25 oz)	300	7	3	0
Casual Eating Margherita	1 pkg (6 oz)	320	9	3	0
Casual Eating Pepperoni	1 pkg (6 oz)	380	9	4	0
Casual Eating Roasted Vegetable	1 pkg (6 oz)	330	5	2	0
Casual Eating Spinach & Mushroom	1 pkg (6.1 oz)	310	7	4	0
Casual Eating Three Meat	1 pkg (6.4 oz)	350	9	4	0
Lean Pockets					
Pepperoni	1 (4.5 oz)	280	7	4	–
Sausage & Pepperoni	1 (4.5 oz)	280	7	3	–
Lunchables					
Maxed Deep Dish	1 pkg	510	13	5	0
Mini Pizza	1 pkg	480	14	5	0
Pepperoni Sausage	1 pkg	440	12	5	0
Marie Callender's					
French Bread Cheese	1 (7.2 oz)	530	24	14	–
French Bread Pepperoni	1 (7.5 oz)	570	28	14	–
French Bread Supreme	1 (7.5 oz)	510	23	11	–
Mr. P's					
Cheese	1 pie (6.5 oz)	410	11	5	0
Red Baron					
Classic Crust 4 Cheese	1 pie (8.6 oz)	740	39	19	1
Deep Dish Single Pepperoni	1 pizza	460	22	9	–
French Bread Supreme	1 pie (5.8 oz)	370	15	6	–
South Beach					
Deluxe w/ Wheat Crust	1 pie	340	11	4	0
Four Cheese w/ Wheat Crust	1 pie	340	11	4	0
Grilled Chicken & Vegetable w/ Wheat Crust	1 pie	330	10	4	0
Pepperoni w/ Wheat Crust	1 pie	350	12	4	0
Stouffer's					
Corner Bistro Flatbread Chicken Bacon & Spinach	1 pkg (9.13 oz)	640	29	14	0
Corner Bistro Flatbread Margherita	1 pkg (9.13 oz)	540	22	9	0

FOOD	PORTION	CALS	FAT	SAT FAT	TRANS FAT
Corner Bistro Flatbread Shrimp & Roasted Garlic	1 pkg (9.33 oz)	600	19	10	0
French Bread Grilled Vegetable	1 pkg (11.63 oz)	340	12	5	0
French Bread Sausage	1 pkg (4.2 oz)	420	21	7	0
French Bread Sausage & Pepperoni	1 pkg (4.2 oz)	460	24	8	0
French Bread White Pizza	1 pkg (10.13 oz)	470	23	7	0
Tony's					
Pizza For One Cheese	1 (6.5 oz)	500	22	12	0
Totino's					
Crisp Crust Cheese	½ pie	320	14	5	–
TAKE-OUT					
cheese	⅛ of 16 in pie	423	18	8	–
cheese	16 in pie	3384	144	61	–
cheese deep dish individual	1 (5.5 oz)	460	24	9	–
cheese & vegetables	⅛ of 16 in pie	428	16	6	–
ground beef	16 in pie	3753	172	68	–
ham & pineapple	⅛ of 16 in pie	439	16	6	–
no cheese	⅛ of 16 in pie	262	7	2	–
pepperoni	⅛ of 16 in pie	469	22	9	–
white pizza	⅛ of 16 in pie	484	17	9	–

PIZZA CRUST

FOOD	PORTION	CALS	FAT	SAT FAT	TRANS FAT
crust	1 slice (1.7 oz)	130	2	0	–
whole wheat	⅛ crust	140	1	0	0
Alvarado Street Bakery					
Sprouted Wheat California Style	⅛ pie	190	3	1	0
Betty Crocker					
Italian Herb Crust Mix	¼ crust (1.6 oz)	180	2	1	–
Boboli					
Thin Crust	⅕ crust (2 oz)	160	4	1	–
Carbsense					
Garlic & Herb as prep	1 slice	100	1	1	–
Jiffy					
Crust Mix as prep	⅕ crust	180	4	3	–
Keto					
Dough Mix as prep	1 slice	79	1	–	–
MiniCarb					
Parmesan Herb Mix as prep	1 slice	130	5	1	–

FOOD	PORTION	CALS	FAT	SAT FAT	TRANS FAT
PLANTAINS					
cooked mashed	1 cup	232	tr	tr	–
sliced cooked	1 cup	179	tr	tr	–
Chester's					
Chips	1 oz	150	9	1	0
Grab Em Snacks					
Chips Black Pepper	1 oz	150	8	1	0
TAKE-OUT					
mofongo	1 serv	320	3	1	–
ripe fried	2.8 oz	214	7	–	–
sweet baked w/ ice cream	1 serv	285	8	5	–
PLUM JUICE					
Sunsweet					
PlumSmart Light	8 oz	60	0	0	0
PLUMS					
canned in heavy syrup	1 cup	163	tr	tr	0
canned purple juice pack	1 cup	146	tr	tr	0
canned purple water pack	1 cup	102	tr	tr	0
dried japanese	1	9	tr	tr	0
fresh	1	30	tr	tr	0
pickled	1	34	tr	tr	0
Chiquita					
Fresh	2 med (4.6 oz)	80	1	0	–
Eden					
Umeboshi Plum Paste	1 tsp	5	0	0	0
Umeboshi Plums	1 (8 g)	5	0	0	0
POI					
poi	1 cup	240	0	0	0
POKEBERRY SHOOTS					
cooked	½ cup	16	tr	–	–
fresh	½ cup	18	tr	–	–
POLENTA					
Bob's Red Mill					
Corn Grits Polenta not prep	¼ cup	130	1	0	0
Frieda's					
Organic	2 slices (3.5 oz)	70	0	0	0

FOOD	PORTION	CALS	FAT	SAT FAT	TRANS FAT
POLLACK					
altantic fillet baked	5.3 oz	178	2	tr	–
atlantic baked	3 oz	100	1	tr	–
POMEGRANATE					
fresh	1 (5.4 oz)	105	tr	tr	0
POMEGRANATE JUICE					
Apple & Eve					
Organic	8 oz	130	0	0	0
Frutzzo					
Organic 100% Juice	1 bottle (12 oz)	130	0	0	0
Izze					
Sparkling Pomegranate	8 oz	80	0	0	0
Langers					
100% Juice	8 oz	150	0	0	0
Naked Juice					
Pomegranate Passion	8 oz	150	0	0	0
Odwalla					
PomaGrand 100% Juice	8 oz	160	0	0	0
Old Orchard					
100% Pure	8 oz	140	0	0	0
POM					
100% Juice	8 oz	140	0	0	0
Pomegranate Blueberry	8 oz	140	0	0	0
Pomegranate Cherry	8 oz	140	0	0	0
Pomegranate Mango	8 oz	140	0	0	0
Pomegranate Tangerine	8 oz	150	0	0	0
POMPANO					
broiled	4 oz	192	13	4	0
smoked	2 oz	109	6	2	0
steamed	4 oz	232	13	5	0
TAKE-OUT					
battered & fried	4 oz	304	21	6	0
breaded & fried	4 oz	361	22	6	0
POPCORN (see also POPCORN CAKES)					
air popped	1 cup (0.3 oz)	31	tr	tr	–
caramel coated	1 cup (1.2 oz)	152	5	1	–
caramel coated w/ peanuts	⅔ cup (1 oz)	114	2	tr	–

FOOD	PORTION	CALS	FAT	SAT FAT	TRANS FAT
cheese	1 cup (0.4 oz)	58	4	1	–
oil popped	1 cup (0.4 oz)	55	3	1	–
Cape Cod					
White Cheddar	2⅓ cups	170	12	3	0
Chester's					
Microwave Butter	3 cups	170	12	2	–
Microwave Cheddar Cheese	3 cups	200	13	3	–
Cracker Jack					
Butter Toffee	¾ cup	140	4	2	–
Original	½ cup	120	2	0	0
Dale & Thomas					
Caramel	½ cup	75	4	1	0
Hall Of Fame Kettlecorn	½ cup	34	1	0	0
North Country Cheddar	½ cup	73	5	1	0
Peanut Butter & White Chocolate Drizzlecorn	½ cup	115	6	3	1
Purepopped Natural	½ cup	26	2	0	0
Sweet Georgia Pecan	½ cup	96	3	1	0
Toffee Crunch Drizzlecorn	½ cup	107	5	2	1
Jay's					
Caramel	¾ cup	110	0	0	0
Ok-Ke-Doke Cheese	1 oz	160	11	3	–
Jolly Time					
American's Best 94% Fat Free	5 cups	100	2	0	–
American's Best White	5 cups	100	1	0	–
American's Best Yellow	5 cups	90	2	0	0
Blast O Butter Light	4 cups	120	6	1	–
Butter Licious Light	5 cups	130	5	1	–
Crispy'n White Light	5 cups	125	5	1	–
Healthy Pop 94% Fat Free	5 cups	100	2	0	–
Healthy Pop Caramel Apple	5 cups	110	2	0	–
Healthy Pop Kettle	4 cups	100	2	0	–
Healthy Pop Minis	4 cups	90	2	0	0
Mallow Magic	2.5 cups	180	13	3	–
The Big Cheez	3.5 cups	140	9	2	–
White	5 cups	100	1	0	–
Yellow	5 cups	100	1	0	–
Judy's					
Sugar Free Popcorn Nut Brittle	¼ piece (1 oz)	100	5	1	–

FOOD	PORTION	CALS	FAT	SAT FAT	TRANS FAT
LesserEvil					
Black&White	1 cup	120	2	1	0
KettleCorn	1 cup	120	2	1	0
MaplePecan	1 cup	120	2	0	0
PeanutButter & Choco	1 cup	120	2	1	0
SinNamon	1 cup	120	2	1	0
Mauna Loa					
Macadamia Nut Butter Corn Crunch	1 oz	150	8	4	–
Newman's Own					
Microwave 94% Fat Free	3½ cups	110	2	0	0
Microwave Butter	3½ cups	130	5	2	0
Microwave Butter Boom	3½ cups	130	5	2	0
Microwave Light Butter	3½ cups	120	4	2	0
Microwave Low Sodium Butter	3½ cups	130	5	2	0
Microwave Natural	3½ cups	130	5	2	0
Organic Pop's Corn Butter	3½ cups	160	9	5	–
Organic Pop's Corn No Butter No Salt 94% Fat Free	3½ cups	120	2	1	–
Oogie's					
Romano & Pesto	1 oz	138	6	1	0
Smoked Gouda	1 oz	132	7	1	0
Spicy Chipotle & Lime	1 oz	143	7	1	0
White Cheddar	1 oz	142	7	1	0
Orville Redenbacher's					
Hot Air	1 cup	15	0	0	0
Kernel Original	1 cup	15	0	0	0
Microwave Butter Light	1 cup	20	1	0	–
Microwave Kettle Korn Sweet	1 cup	35	3	1	–
Microwave Movie Theater Butter Light	1 cup	20	1	tr	–
Microwave Movie Theater Extra Butter	1 cup	35	3	1	–
Microwave Natural Light	1 cup	20	1	0	–
Microwave Pour Over Butter	1 cup	40	3	1	–
Microwave Pour Over Cheddar	1 cup	50	3	1	–
Microwave Regular Butter	1 cup	35	2	1	–
Microwave Regular Corn On The Cob	1 cup	35	3	1	–
Microwave Regular Natural	1 cup	15	2	0	–

FOOD	PORTION	CALS	FAT	SAT FAT	TRANS FAT
Microwave Regular Old Fashioned Butter	1 cup	35	2	1	–
Microwave Regular Tender White	1 cup	40	3	1	–
Microwave Smart Pop Butter	1 cup	15	0	0	0
Microwave Smart Pop Kettle Korn	1 cup	20	0	0	0
Microwave Smart Pop Movie Theater Butter	1 cup	20	0	0	0
Microwave Sweet Caramel	1 cup	90	5	1	–
Microwave Sweet Cinnabon	1 cup	50	3	1	–
Microwave Sweet Honey Butter	1 cup	35	3	1	–
Microwave Sweet 'N Buttery	1 cup	40	3	1	–
Microwave Ultimate Butter	1 cup	30	3	1	–
White	1 cup	15	0	0	0
Poppycock					
The Original	½ cup	160	8	2	–
Smart Balance					
Light as prep	4 cups	120	5	2	0
Low Fat as prep	5 cups	120	2	0	0
Movie Style as prep	3.5 cups	170	9	4	0
Smartfood					
Reduced Fat White Cheddar	3 cups	140	6	2	0
White Cheddar	1 pkg	160	10	2	–
Snyder's Of Hanover					
Butter	⅝ oz	100	8	1	0
Utz					
Butter	2 cups	170	12	3	0
Cheese	2 cups	160	11	2	0
Puff'n Corn Original Hulless	2 cups	150	17	3	4
Wise					
Butter	1 pkg (0.5 oz)	80	5	1	0
Hot Cheese	1 oz	150	10	2	0

POPCORN CAKES
Orville Redenbacher's

FOOD	PORTION	CALS	FAT	SAT FAT	TRANS FAT
Butter	2	60	1	0	–
Caramel	1	40	0	0	0
Chocolate	1	45	0	0	0
Mini Butter	8	60	1	0	–
Mini Caramel	7	50	0	0	0

FOOD	PORTION	CALS	FAT	SAT FAT	TRANS FAT
Mini Peanut Caramel Crunch	6	60	1	0	–
Mini Peanut Crunch	6	60	1	0	–
Mini Sour Cream & Onion	8	60	1	0	–
White Cheddar	2	60	1	0	–

POPOVER

home recipe as prep w/ 2% milk	1 (1.4 oz)	87	3	1	–
home recipe as prep w/ whole milk	1 (1.4 oz)	90	3	1	–
mix as prep	1 (1.2 oz)	67	2	tr	–

POPPY SEEDS

poppy seeds	1 tbsp	47	4	tr	0
Bob's Red Mill					
Poppy Seeds	3 tbsp	170	14	2	0
Love'n Bake					
Poppy Seed Filling	2 tbsp	120	5	0	–

PORGY

fresh	3 oz	77	tr	–	–

PORK (see also HAM, MEAT STICKS, PORK DISHES)
FRESH

boneless loin lean & fat roasted	3.5 oz	195	9	3	tr
center loin chop bone in broiled	1 (3 oz)	178	9	3	tr
center rib chop lean & fat bone in broiled	1 (3 oz)	189	11	4	tr
country style ribs bone in lean & fat braised	3.5 oz	288	19	7	tr
dehydrated oriental style	1 cup (0.8 oz)	135	14	5	0
fresh ham rump half lean & fat roasted	4 oz	278	16	6	0
fresh ham shank half lean & fat roasted	4 oz	319	22	8	0
fresh ham whole lean & fat roasted	4 oz	302	19	7	0
ground cooked	4 oz	328	23	9	0
ham hock cooked	1	167	12	4	0
shoulder chop bone in braised	1 (3 oz)	229	15	6	tr

FOOD	PORTION	CALS	FAT	SAT FAT	TRANS FAT
sirloin roast lean & fat bone in roasted	4 oz	231	13	4	tr
spareribs bone in roasted	3 oz	304	26	8	tr
tail simmered	3 oz	336	30	11	–
tenderloin roast boneless lean & fat roasted	4 oz	145	4	1	tr
top loin chop boneless lean & fat broiled	1 (3.5 oz)	195	9	3	tr
Boar's Head					
Smoked Shoulder Butt Roast	3 oz	170	13	5	–
Freirich					
Porkette	4 oz	220	18	7	–
Organic Prairie					
Ground	4 oz	300	24	9	–
Smithfield					
Smoked Pork Chop	3 oz	100	3	1	0
Tyson					
Baby Back Ribs Buffalo	4 oz	300	24	9	0
Ground Reduced Fat	4 oz	260	20	7	–
Half Loin Boneless	4 oz	190	12	5	–
Loin Chops Bone-In Center Cut	4 oz	190	13	5	–
Spareribs	4 oz	290	24	9	–
Stew Meat	4 oz	130	5	2	–
FROZEN					
Organic Prairie					
Chop	1 (3.3 oz)	220	13	5	–
READY-TO-EAT					
Sara Lee					
Oven Roasted	2 oz	70	3	1	–
TAKE-OUT					
chicharrones pork cracklings fried	1 cup	492	38	13	–
chop breaded & fried	1 lg (5 oz)	441	26	8	–
chop breaded & fried	1 med (3.4 oz)	304	18	5	–
chop stewed	1 lg (4.6 oz)	315	18	7	0

PORK DISHES

A La Carte Gourmet

Pork Loin w/ Cream Spinach Feta Stuffing	1 serv (5 oz)	200	9	5	–

FOOD	PORTION	CALS	FAT	SAT FAT	TRANS FAT
Hormel					
Center Cut Loin Lemon Garlic	1 serv (4 oz)	130	5	2	–
Extra Lean Apple Bourbon	1 serv (4 oz)	140	5	2	0
Extra Lean Teriyaki	4 oz	140	4	2	–
Pork Roast Au Jus	1 serv (5 oz)	180	7	3	–
Morton's Of Omaha					
Tender Pork Roast w/ Gravy & Vegetables	1 serv (5 oz)	210	10	3	0
Smithfield					
Tenderloin Garlic & Herb	3 oz	100	3	1	–
Tenderloin Hickory Sweet	4 oz	110	3	1	–
Tyson					
Roast Pork w/ Vegetables	1 serv (4 oz)	190	4	2	0
Wellshire					
Baby Back Ribs w/ Sauce	2 ribs (5 oz)	260	18	7	–
Shredded Pork In BBQ Sauce	¼ cup	90	2	1	–
TAKE-OUT					
kalua pork	1 cup (7 oz)	497	34	13	–
spareribs barbecued w/ sauce	2 med (2.8 oz)	248	18	6	–
tourtiere	1 piece (4.9 oz)	451	34	10	–

PORK RINDS (see SNACKS)

POT PIE
Amy's

FOOD	PORTION	CALS	FAT	SAT FAT	TRANS FAT
Broccoli	1 (7.5 oz)	430	22	10	–
Country Vegetable	1 (7.5 oz)	370	16	9	–
Shepherd's	1 (8 oz)	160	4	0	–
Vegetable	1 (7.5 oz)	420	19	12	–
Vegetable Non-Dairy	1 (7.5 oz)	320	9	1	–
Banquet					
Beef	1 (7 oz)	400	23	11	–
Cheesy Potato & Broccoli w/ Ham	1 (7 oz)	410	23	10	–
Family Size Hearty Chicken	1 cup	460	29	11	–
Macaroni & Cheese	1 pkg (6.5 oz)	210	5	3	–
Turkey	1 (7 oz)	370	20	8	–
Vegetable Cheese	1 (7 oz)	340	17	7	–
Hot Pockets					
Pot Pie Express Chicken	1 piece (4.5 oz)	350	17	4	–

FOOD	PORTION	CALS	FAT	SAT FAT	TRANS FAT
Ian's					
Chicken	1 pkg (9.4 oz)	510	23	10	0
Marie Callender's					
Chicken	1 (9.5 oz)	680	48	21	–
Chicken & Broccoli	1 (9.5 oz)	670	43	12	–
Chicken Au Gratin	1 (9.5 oz)	690	46	21	–
Turkey	1 (9.5 oz)	680	46	19	–
Mon Cuisine					
Vegan	1 pkg (9 oz)	650	39	6	–
Morton					
Macaroni & Cheese	1 (6.5 oz)	210	5	3	–
Vegetable w/ Beef	1 (7 oz)	340	21	9	–
Vegetable w/ Chicken	1 (7 oz)	320	18	7	–
Vegetable w/ Turkey	1 (7 oz)	310	18	9	–
Pepperidge Farm					
Chili Beans & Cornbread	1 cup	360	17	5	–
Reduced Fat Roasted White Meat Chicken	1 cup	470	21	7	–
Roasted White Meat Chicken	1 cup	510	32	9	–
Stouffer's					
Chicken White Meat	1 pkg (10 oz)	660	37	14	1
TAKE-OUT					
beef	8 in pie (14.6 oz)	938	57	13	–
chicken	8 in pie (14.6 oz)	897	52	16	–
ham	1 serv (11 oz)	752	45	10	–
oyster	1 serv (11.5 oz)	817	53	15	0
st. stephen's day pie	1 serv (16.7 oz)	549	29	16	–

POTATO (see also CHIPS, KNISH, PANCAKES)

FOOD	PORTION	CALS	FAT	SAT FAT	TRANS FAT
CANNED					
potatoes	½ cup	54	tr	tr	–
Del Monte					
New Whole	2 med (5.5 oz)	60	0	0	0
Savory Sides Au Gratin	½ cup	80	3	1	0
S&W					
Whole Small	2 (5.5 oz)	60	0	0	0
FRESH					
baked skin only	1 skin (2 oz)	115	tr	tr	–
baked w/ skin	1 (6.5 oz)	220	tr	tr	–
baked w/o skin	1 (5 oz)	145	tr	tr	–

FOOD	PORTION	CALS	FAT	SAT FAT	TRANS FAT
baked w/o skin	½ cup	57	tr	tr	–
boiled	½ cup	68	tr	tr	–
microwaved	1 (7 oz)	212	tr	tr	–
microwaved w/o skin	½ cup	78	tr	tr	–
raw w/o skin	1 (3.9 oz)	88	tr	tr	–
Arrowfarms					
Yukon Gold	1 med (5 oz)	100	0	0	0
Dole					
Idaho	1 (5.3 oz)	100	0	0	0
Frieda's					
Fingerling	4 (5 oz)	100	0	0	0
Green Giant					
Red Potatoes	1 med (5 oz)	100	0	0	0
Lucinda's					
Red "C"	1 med (5.2 oz)	100	0	0	0
SunLite					
SunLite	1 (5 oz)	87	0	0	0
FROZEN					
french fries	10 strips	111	4	2	–
french fries thick cut	10 strips	109	4	2	–
hash browns	½ cup	170	9	4	–
potato puffs	½ cup	138	7	3	–
potato puffs as prep	1	16	1	tr	–
Alexia					
Hashed Browns	1 serv (3 oz)	80	0	0	0
Mashed Red w/ Garlic & Parmesan	½ cup	150	6	4	0
Mashed Yukon Gold & Sea Salt	½ cup	150	6	4	0
Oven Crinkles Classic	1 serv (3 oz)	120	4	1	0
Oven Crinkles Salt & Pepper	1 serv (3 oz)	120	4	1	0
Oven Fries Garlic	12 pieces	140	6	1	0
Oven Reds	1 serv (3 oz)	120	4	1	0
Waffle Fries	8 pieces	150	5	1	0
Yukon Gold Fries w/ Sea Salt	1 serv (3 oz)	130	4	0	0
Cascadian Farm					
Organic Country Style	¾ cup	50	0	0	0
Organic Hash Browns	1 cup	60	0	0	0
Funster					
BBQ Lite	14 pieces (3 oz)	140	3	0	0

FOOD	PORTION	CALS	FAT	SAT FAT	TRANS FAT
Cheddar	14 pieces (3 oz)	135	3	0	0
Original	14 pieces (3 oz)	135	3	0	0
Green Giant					
Roasted Potatoes w/ Garlic & Herb Sauce as prep	½ cup	90	2	1	0
Healthy Choice					
Cheddar Broccoli Potatoes	1 pkg	270	7	3	–
Ian's					
Alphatots	1 serv (3.5 oz)	156	7	5	0
Fries Sweet Potato	7 (2.5 oz)	70	3	1	0
Inland Valley					
Crinkle Cuts	15 (3 oz)	150	5	1	–
Crisscut Fries	13 (3 oz)	160	7	2	–
Curly QQQ's	1⅓ cups (3 oz)	180	8	2	–
Fajita Fries	17 (3 oz)	170	8	2	–
French Fries	15 (3 oz)	130	4	1	–
Hash Browns	⅔ cup	70	0	0	0
Home Browns	1 patty (2.2 oz)	130	7	2	–
Mashed Homestyle	⅔ cup	160	6	3	–
Simply Shreds	1 cup	70	0	0	0
Stix	5 (3 oz)	170	10	3	–
Stuffed Spudz w/ Cheese	5 pieces	210	11	5	–
Tater Babies	8 (3 oz)	130	5	1	–
Tater Puffs	10	160	7	2	–
Twice Baked	1 (5.2 oz)	230	12	7	–
Twice Baked Sour Cream Bacon & Chives	1 (5.2 oz)	240	8	3	–
Twice Baked Triple Cheese	1 (5.2 oz)	250	10	5	–
Larry's					
Mashed Broccoli & Cheddar Cheese	1 serv (5 oz)	180	8	2	0
Mashed Cheddar Cheese	1 serv (5 oz)	190	8	2	0
Mashed Old Fashioned Butter	1 serv (5 oz)	190	9	3	0
Mashed Sour Cream & Chives	1 serv (5 oz)	180	8	2	0
Mashed Sweet Potatoes	1 serv (4 oz)	140	4	2	0
Lean Cuisine					
One Dish Favorites Deluxe Cheddar	1 pkg (10.4 oz)	260	7	4	0
McCain					
French Fries Crinkle Cut	18 (3 oz)	130	4	0	0

FOOD	PORTION	CALS	FAT	SAT FAT	TRANS FAT
Mash-Bites	1 serv (3 oz)	50	7	1	0
Roasters All American	1 serv (3 oz)	120	3	0	0
Roasters Grilled Garlic & Onion	1 serv (3 oz)	120	3	0	0
Seasoned Wedges Skin On	1 serv (3 oz)	120	5	0	0
Shoestring French Fries	45 (3 oz)	140	5	1	0
Smiles	6 (3 oz)	160	6	1	0
Steak Fries	8 (3 oz)	120	3	0	0
Tasti Tater	1 serv (3 oz)	160	7	1	0
Oh Boy!					
Stuffed w/ Onion Sour Cream & Chives	1 (5 oz)	110	2	0	–
Roast Works					
Roasted Seasoned Wedge	1 serv (3 oz)	100	2	0	0
Roasted Wedges Rosemary Redskin	1 serv (3 oz)	110	3	0	0
Roasted Wedges Yukon Gold	1 serv (3 oz)	110	3	0	0
MIX					
au gratin as prep	½ cup	160	9	6	–
instant mashed flakes as prep w/ whole milk & butter	½ cup	118	6	4	–
instant mashed flakes not prep	½ cup	78	tr	tr	–
instant mashed granules as prep w/ whole milk & butter	½ cup	114	5	3	–
instant mashed granules not prep	½ cup	372	1	tr	–
scalloped	½ cup	105	5	3	–
Betty Crocker					
Mashed Butter & Herb	½ cup	160	7	2	–
Hungry Jack					
Casserole Potatoes Au Gratin as prep	½ cup	100	1	–	–
Casserole Potatoes Creamy Scalloped as prep	½ cup	150	1	–	–
Casserole Potatoes Four Cheese as prep	½ cup	150	1	–	–
Easy Mash'd Cheesy Homestyle not prep	¼ cup	150	2	–	–
Easy Mash'd Creamy Butter not prep	¼ cup	150	2	–	–

FOOD	PORTION	CALS	FAT	SAT FAT	TRANS FAT
Easy Mash'd Premium Homestyle not prep	¼ cup	150	2	–	–
Original Mashed not prep	⅓ cup	80	0	0	0
Idahoan					
AuGratin as prep	½ cup	150	6	1	–
Hash Browns as prep	½ cup	160	8	1	–
Hash Browns Cheesy not prep	½ cup	120	2	1	–
Mashed Baked as prep	½ cup	110	3	1	–
Mashed Butter & Herb as prep	½ cup	110	3	1	–
Mashed Buttery Homestyle as prep	½ cup	110	3	1	–
Mashed Four Cheese as prep	½ cup	100	3	1	–
Mashed Southwest as prep	½ cup	110	3	1	–
Roasted Garlic as prep	½ cup	600	3	1	–
Scalloped as prep	½ cup	150	7	1	–
REFRIGERATED					
Country Crock					
Garlic Mashed	⅔ cup	160	7	3	0
Homestyle Mashed	⅔ cup	190	10	5	0
Diner's Choice					
Mashed	⅔ cup	110	5	3	0
PurelyIdaho					
Cheddar Crusted	¾ cup	120	1	0	–
Simply Potatoes					
Diced w/ Onion	⅔ cup	60	0	0	0
Homestyle Slices	⅔ cup	70	0	0	0
Mashed	⅔ cup	170	10	5	1
Mashed Sweet Potatoes	⅔ cup	160	3	1	1
Red Potato Wedges	½ cup	50	0	0	0
Shredded Hash Browns	½ cup	50	0	0	0
SHELF-STABLE					
TastyBite					
Bombay Potatoes	½ pkg (5 oz)	105	4	tr	0
TAKE-OUT					
au gratin w/ cheese	½ cup	178	10	4	–
baked topped w/ cheese sauce	1	475	29	11	–
baked topped w/ cheese sauce & bacon	1	451	26	10	–
baked topped w/ cheese sauce & broccoli	1	402	14	9	–

FOOD	PORTION	CALS	FAT	SAT FAT	TRANS FAT
baked topped w/ cheese sauce & chili	1	481	22	13	–
baked topped w/ sour cream & chives	1	394	22	10	–
french fries	1 reg	235	12	4	–
hash browns	½ cup (2.5 oz)	151	9	4	–
indian yogurt potatoes	1 serv	315	9	4	–
mashed	½ cup	111	4	1	–
o'brien	1 cup	157	3	2	–
potato dumpling	3.5 oz	334	1	–	–
potato pancake	1 (1.3 oz)	101	7	1	–
potato salad	½ cup	179	10	2	–
red new boiled	5 sm (5 oz)	120	0	0	0
scalloped	½ cup	127	5	–	–
twice baked w/ cheese	1 half (10 oz)	392	18	10	–

POTATO STARCH

potato starch	1 oz	96	tr	–	–

Bob's Red Mill

Potato Starch	1 tbsp	40	0	0	0

POUT

ocean baked	3 oz	86	1	tr	–
ocean fillet baked	4.8 oz	139	2	1	–

PRETZELS

chocolate covered	1 (0.4 oz)	47	1	tr	0
soft	1 lg (5 oz)	483	4	1	0
twists salted	10 (2.1 oz)	229	2	tr	–
twists w/o salt	10 (2.1 oz)	229	2	tr	–
whole wheat	2 sm (1 oz)	103	1	tr	–
yogurt covered	1 (4 g)	19	1	1	0
yogurt covered	1 cup (3 oz)	391	13	11	0

Aramana

Soy Pretzels	15 (1 oz)	100	3	2	–

Cape Cod

Pretzels	25	130	1	0	0

Combos

Cheddar Cheese Cracker	1 pkg (1.7 oz)	240	11	5	0
Nacho Cheese	1 pkg (1.7 oz)	230	8	5	0
Pizzeria Pretzel	1 pkg (1.7 oz)	230	8	5	0

FOOD	PORTION	CALS	FAT	SAT FAT	TRANS FAT
Glenny's					
Organic Original Salted	8 (1 oz)	110	0	0	0
Organic Sourdough	6 (1 oz)	110	0	0	0
Glutino					
Gluten Free All Shapes	44 (1.4 oz)	190	8	4	0
Goodniks					
Yogurt Pretzels	15	180	7	6	0
Handi-Snack					
Mister Salty Pretzels 'N Cheese	1 pkg	90	4	1	0
Healthy Handfuls					
Python Pretzels	1 box (1.5 oz)	170	1	0	0
Landies Candies					
Sugar Free Chocolate	4 (1.5 oz)	220	12	7	–
New York Style					
Pretzel Flatz Original Salt	12	110	1	0	0
Newman's Own					
Organic Bavarian Sour Dough	1	90	0	0	0
Organic Hi Protein	22	120	1	0	–
Organic Salt & Pepper Rounds	8	100	1	0	–
Organic Salt & Pepper Thins	10	120	1	0	–
Organic Salted Nuggets	20	120	2	0	–
Organic Salted Rods	4	120	2	0	–
Organic Salted Rounds	8	110	1	0	–
Organic Salted Sticks	13	110	1	0	–
Organic Salted Thins	10	110	1	0	–
Organic Spelt	20	120	1	0	–
Organic Unsalted Rounds	8	110	1	0	–
Quinlan					
Low Fat Mini	1 oz	110	1	0	0
Rold Gold					
Braided Twists	8	110	1	0	0
Braided Twists Honey Wheat	8	110	1	0	0
Checkers	20	110	2	0	0
Rods	3	110	1	0	0
Sourdough Hard	1	100	1	0	0
Sourdough Specials	5	110	1	0	0
Sticks	48	100	0	0	0
Thins	9	110	1	0	0
Tiny Twists	18	110	0	0	0
Tiny Twists Cheddar	20	110	1	0	0

FOOD	PORTION	CALS	FAT	SAT FAT	TRANS FAT
Tiny Twists Honey Mustard	13	110	1	0	0
Snyder's Of Hanover					
100 Calorie Pack Snaps	1 pkg (0.9 oz)	100	1	0	0
100 Calorie Pack Stick	1 pkg (0.9 oz)	100	1	0	0
Dips Milk Chocolate	1 oz	140	6	4	0
Dips Special Dark Chocolate	1 oz	140	5	3	0
Mini Unsalted	1 oz	110	0	0	0
MultiGrain Sticks Lightly Salted	1 oz	120	2	0	0
MultiGrain Twists	1 oz	120	2	0	0
Nibblers Sourdough	1 oz	120	0	0	0
Old Tyme	1 oz	120	1	0	0
Organic Honey Wheat	1 oz	130	2	0	0
Organic Oat Bran	1 oz	120	0	0	0
Pieces Garlic Bread	1 oz	140	7	3	0
Pieces Honey Mustard & Onions	1 oz	140	7	3	0
Pieces Hot Buffalo Wing	1 oz	140	7	3	0
Pretzel Sandwich Peanut Butter	1 oz	140	7	2	0
Rods	1 oz	120	1	0	0
Snaps	1 oz	120	1	0	0
Sourdough Unsalted	1 oz	100	0	0	0
Sticks 12 Multi Grain	1 oz	130	2	0	0
Spinzels					
Braided	1 pkg (0.5 oz)	55	1	0	–
Superpretzel					
Mozzarella	2 (1.8 oz)	130	4	2	0
Pretzelfils Pizza	2 (1.8 oz)	130	2	1	0
Soft	1 (2.25 oz)	160	1	0	0
Soft Bites	5 (1.9 oz)	150	1	0	0
Softstix	2 (1.8 oz)	130	3	2	0
Utz					
Braided Twists Baked Honey Wheat	1 oz	110	2	0	0
Chocolate Covered	6 (1.1 oz)	140	5	5	0
Hard	1	90	0	0	0
Special	1 oz	110	1	0	0
Special Multigrain	1 oz	110	1	0	0
Sticks Organic Whole Grain	1 oz	120	2	0	0
Wege					
Honey Wheat	1 (0.8 oz)	120	2	0	–

FOOD	PORTION	CALS	FAT	SAT FAT	TRANS FAT
Wise					
Fat Free Sticks	1 oz	100	0	0	0
Low Fat Honey Wheat Braided Twists	1 oz	110	1	0	0

PRUNE JUICE

jarred	1 cup	182	tr	tr	–
L&A					
100% Juice	8 oz	180	0	0	0
Lakewood					
Organic	8 oz	165	0	0	0
Langers					
Plus 100% Juice	8 oz	180	0	0	0
Ocean Spray					
100% Juice	8 oz	180	0	0	0
Old Orchard					
Healthy Balance	8 oz	70	0	0	0
Sunsweet					
100% Juice	8 oz	180	0	0	0
PlumSmart	8 oz	160	0	0	0

PRUNES

cooked w/o sugar	½ cup	133	tr	tr	0
dried	1	20	tr	tr	0
Earthbound Farm					
Organic Dried Plums	5	110	0	0	0
Love'n Bake					
Prune Lekvar	2 tbsp	90	0	0	0
Newman's Own					
Organic	½ cup	110	0	0	0
St Dalfour					
French Prunes	3	100	0	0	0
Sunsweet					
Pitted Dried	5	100	0	0	0

PUDDING

MIX
Keto

Banana not prep	½ scoop	62	3	–	–
Chocolate not prep	½ scoop	66	3	–	–
French Vanilla not prep	½ scoop	62	3	–	–

FOOD	PORTION	CALS	FAT	SAT FAT	TRANS FAT
Uncle Ben's					
Rice Pudding Cinnamon & Raisins as prep	½ cup	160	1	0	–
Rice Pudding French Vanilla as prep	½ cup	120	0	0	0
READY-TO-EAT					
Boost					
Vanilla	1 pkg (5 oz)	240	9	1	–
Hunt's					
Dessert Favorites Banana Cream Pie	1 serv (3.5 oz)	140	6	2	–
Dessert Favorites Chocolate Brownie	1 serv (3.5 oz)	190	7	2	–
Dessert Favorites Chocolate Mud Pie	1 serv (3.5 oz)	170	7	2	–
Dessert Favorites Chocolate Peanut Butter Pie	1 serv (3.5 oz)	190	8	2	–
Dessert Favorites Dulce De Leche Caramel Cream	1 serv (3.5 oz)	140	5	2	–
Dessert Favorites Lemon Meringue Pie	1 serv (3.5 oz)	130	3	1	–
Snack Pack Butterscotch	1 serv (3.5 oz)	130	5	2	–
Snack Pack Chocolate	1 serv (3.5 oz)	104	5	2	–
Snack Pack Chocolate Fudge	1 serv (3.5 oz)	150	5	2	–
Snack Pack Chocolate Marshmallow	1 serv (3.5 oz)	130	5	2	–
Snack Pack Fat Free Chocolate	1 serv (3.5 oz)	90	0	0	0
Snack Pack Fat Free Tapioca	1 serv (3.5 oz)	80	0	0	0
Snack Pack Fat Free Vanilla	1 serv (3.5 oz)	80	0	0	0
Snack Pack Lemon	1 serv (3.5 oz)	120	3	1	–
Snack Pack Swirl Chocolate Caramel	1 serv (3.5 oz)	140	5	2	–
Snack Pack Swirl S'mores	1 serv (3.5 oz)	140	5	2	–
Snack Pack Tapioca	1 serv (3.5 oz)	130	5	2	–
Snack Pack Vanilla	1 serv (3.5 oz)	130	5	2	–
Jell-O					
100 Calorie Pack Fat Free Chocolate Vanilla Swirl	1 pkg (4 oz)	100	0	0	0
100 Calorie Pack Fat Free Tapioca	1 pkg (4 oz)	100	0	0	0

FOOD	PORTION	CALS	FAT	SAT FAT	TRANS FAT
Fat Free Chocolate Fudge & Caramel	1 serv (4 oz)	100	0	0	0
Fat Free Vanilla Caramel	1 serv (4 oz)	100	0	0	0
Sugar Free Dulce De Leche	1 pkg (3.7 oz)	60	1	1	0
Tapioca	1 serv (4 oz)	110	2	2	0
Kozy Shack					
Black Forest	1 pkg (4 oz)	120	3	2	0
Chocolate	1 pkg (4 oz)	139	4	2	–
Chocolate No Sugar Added	1 pkg (4 oz)	93	3	2	–
Rice	1 pkg (4 oz)	135	3	2	–
Tapioca	1 pkg (4 oz)	130	3	2	0
Tapioca No Sugar Added	1 pkg	90	3	2	0
Vanilla	1 pkg (4 oz)	130	3	2	–
Vanilla No Sugar Added	1 pkg (4 oz)	90	2	2	–
Lifeway					
Organic Chocolate	½ cup	170	4	–	–
Organic Rice	½ cup	140	4	–	–
Organic Vanilla	½ cup	150	4	–	–
Swiss Miss					
Lemon Meringue Pie	1 pkg (4 oz)	150	3	1	–
Low Fat Tapioca	1 pkg (4 oz)	130	3	1	1
Low Fat Vanilla	1 serv (4 oz)	120	2	1	–
TAKE-OUT					
blancmange	1 serv (4.7 oz)	154	5	–	–
bread w/ raisins	1 cup	306	9	3	0
coconut	1 cup	291	9	7	0
corn	1 cup	328	13	6	–
indian pudding	½ cup	156	4	2	0
noodle pudding kugel	1 cup	297	10	2	0
plum pudding	1 slice (1.5 oz)	125	5	3	0
queen of puddings	1 serv (4.4 oz)	266	10	–	–
rice pudding	1 cup	302	4	2	0
sweet potato	1 cup	215	6	1	0
tapioca	1 cup	236	7	3	0
yorkshire	1 serv (3 oz)	177	8	–	–

PUFFERFISH

FOOD	PORTION	CALS	FAT	SAT FAT	TRANS FAT
raw	3 oz	72	0	0	0

FOOD	PORTION	CALS	FAT	SAT FAT	TRANS FAT
PUMMELO					
fresh	1	228	tr	–	–
sections	1 cup	71	tr	–	–
Sunkist					
Fresh	¼	90	1	0	0
PUMPKIN					
butter	1 tbsp	32	0	0	0
canned	½ cup	41	tr	tr	–
cooked mashed	½ cup	24	tr	tr	–
flowers cooked	½ cup	10	tr	tr	–
flowers raw	1	0	0	0	0
leaves cooked	½ cup	7	tr	tr	–
leaves raw	½ cup	4	tr	tr	–
raw cubed	½ cup	15	tr	tr	–
Farmer's Market					
Organic Puree	½ cup	50	0	0	0
Libby's					
Puree	½ cup	40	1	0	–
PUMPKIN SEEDS					
dried	1 oz	154	13	2	–
roasted	¼ cup	296	24	5	–
salted & roasted	¼ cup	296	24	5	–
whole roasted	1 oz	127	6	1	–
whole roasted	¼ cup	71	3	1	–
whole salted roasted	¼ cup	71	3	1	–
David					
All Natural	¼ cup	160	13	3	–
Eden					
Dry Roasted & Salted	¼ cup	200	16	3	0
Good Sense					
Roasted & Salted	½ cup	160	13	3	0
Mrs. May's					
Pumpkin Crunch	1 oz	164	11	2	0
PURSLANE					
cooked	1 cup	21	tr	–	–
fresh	1 cup	7	tr	–	–
QUAIL					
cooked bone removed	1 (2.7 oz)	177	11	3	0

FOOD	PORTION	CALS	FAT	SAT FAT	TRANS FAT
QUICHE					
Mrs. Smith's					
Pour-A-Quiche Bacon & Onion	1 serv (4.3 oz)	230	16	8	0
TAKE-OUT					
cheese	⅛ of 9 in pie	566	44	21	–
lorraine	⅛ of 9 in pie	568	44	20	–
mushroom	1 slice (3 oz)	256	18	–	–
spinach	⅛ of 9 in pie	342	26	12	–
QUINCE					
fresh	1	53	tr	tr	–
QUINOA					
quinoa not prep	1 cup (6 oz)	636	10	1	–
Alti Plano Gold					
Natural	1 pkg	170	3	0	–
Eden					
Quinoa not prep	¼ cup	180	4	0	0
Seeds Of Change					
French Herb Quinoa Blend as prep	1 cup	290	4	1	0
RABBIT					
domestic w/o bone roasted	3 oz	167	7	2	–
wild w/o bone stewed	3 oz	147	3	1	–
RACCOON					
roasted	3 oz	217	12	–	–
RADICCHIO					
raw shredded	½ cup	5	tr	–	–
RADISHES					
chinese dried	½ cup	157	tr	tr	–
chinese raw	1 (12 oz)	62	tr	tr	–
chinese raw sliced	½ cup	8	tr	tr	–
chinese sliced cooked	½ cup	13	tr	tr	–
daikon dried	½ cup	157	tr	tr	–
daikon raw	1 (12 oz)	62	tr	tr	–
daikon raw sliced	½ cup	8	tr	tr	–
daikon sliced cooked	½ cup	13	tr	tr	–
red raw	10	7	tr	tr	–
red sliced	½ cup	10	tr	tr	–

FOOD	PORTION	CALS	FAT	SAT FAT	TRANS FAT
white icicle raw	1 (0.5 oz)	2	tr	tr	–
white icicle raw sliced	½ cup	7	tr	tr	–
Eden					
Daikon Dried Shredded	2 tbsp	45	0	0	0
Daikon Pickled	2 slices (0.5 oz)	5	0	0	0
Frieda's					
Black	¾ cup	15	0	0	0
Chinese Lo Bok	⅔ cup	25	0	0	0
Daikon	½ cup	15	1	0	–
Korean Moo	⅔ cup	15	0	0	0
TAKE-OUT					
korean kimchee	½ cup	31	1	–	–
moo namul saengche korean salad	1 serv (3.7 oz)	34	tr	tr	–

RAISINS

FOOD	PORTION	CALS	FAT	SAT FAT	TRANS FAT
cinnamon coated	¼ cup	108	tr	tr	0
cooked	¼ cup	162	tr	tr	0
golden seedless	¼ cup	109	tr	tr	0
jumbo golden	¼ cup	130	0	0	0
milk chocolate coated	¼ cup	176	7	4	0
milk chocolate coated	28 (1 oz)	109	4	2	0
seedless	55 (1 oz)	86	tr	tr	0
sultanas	1 oz	88	0	–	0
Amazin'					
Raisin All Flavors	1 oz	84	0	0	0
Bob's Red Mill					
Unsulfured	⅓ cup	130	0	0	0
Brach's					
California Chocolate Covered	35	170	6	5	–
Earthbound Farm					
Organic Jumbo Flame Seedless	¼ cup	120	0	0	0
Estee					
Chocolate Covered Fructose Sweetened	¼ cup	180	6	5	–
Fool					
Cinnamon Raisin Spread	1 tbsp	20	0	0	0
Godiva					
Milk Chocolate Covered	1 pkg (1.2 oz)	150	7	4	0

FOOD	PORTION	CALS	FAT	SAT FAT	TRANS FAT
Goodniks					
Yogurt Raisins	3 tbsp	145	5	5	0
Newman's Own					
Organic	¼ cup	130	0	0	0
Sun-Maid					
California Golden	¼ cup	130	0	0	0
California Seedless	¼ cup	130	0	0	0
Sunsweet					
Red Flame	¼ cup	130	0	0	0
Tree Of Life					
Organic	¼ cup (1.4 oz)	130	0	0	–
RASPBERRIES					
canned in heavy syrup	½ cup	117	tr	tr	–
fresh	1 cup	61	1	tr	–
fresh	1 pint	154	2	tr	–
frzn sweetened	1 cup	256	tr	tr	–
frzn sweetened	1 pkg (10 oz)	291	tr	tr	–
frzn unsweetened	¾ cup	130	0	0	0
C&W					
Ultimate Red	¾ cup	70	0	0	0
Cascadian Farm					
Organic frzn	1¼ cup	60	0	0	0
Europe's Best					
Raspberries frzn	¾ cup	60	0	0	0
Frieda's					
Dried	⅓ cup (1.4 oz)	145	1	0	0
Oregon					
In Heavy Syrup	½ cup	120	0	0	0
RASPBERRY JUICE					
Crystal Light					
Raspberry Ice Sugar Free	8 oz	5	0	0	0
Naked Juice					
Raspberry Ade	8 oz	90	0	0	0
Nantucket Nectars					
Organic Very Raspberry	8 oz	120	0	0	0
Newman's Own					
Razz-Ma-Tazz Raspberry	8 oz	120	0	0	0
Old Orchard					
Organic 100% Juice	8 oz	120	0	0	0

FOOD	PORTION	CALS	FAT	SAT FAT	TRANS FAT
RELISH					
hamburger	1 tbsp	19	tr	tr	–
hamburger	½ cup	158	1	tr	–
hot dog	1 tbsp	14	tr	tr	–
hot dog	½ cup	111	1	tr	–
piccalilli	1.4 oz	13	tr	–	–
sweet	1 tbsp	19	tr	tr	–
sweet	½ cup	159	1	tr	–
B&G					
India	1 tbsp	15	0	0	0
Piccalilli	1 tbsp	20	0	0	0
Sweet	1 tbsp	15	0	0	0
Del Monte					
Hamburger	1 tbsp	20	0	0	0
Hot Dog	1 tbsp	15	0	0	0
Sweet Pickle	1 tbsp	20	0	0	0
Frieda's					
Kim Chee	¼ cup	15	0	0	0
Matouk's					
Hot Chow	2 tbsp	20	0	0	0
Kuchela	1 tsp	9	1	0	–
Patak's					
Brinjal Eggplant Sweet Spicy	1 tbsp	70	4	1	–
Garlic	1 tbsp	45	3	0	–
Lime Mild	1 tbsp	30	3	0	–
Mango Mild	1 tbsp	40	4	0	–
Peloponnese					
Sun Dried Tomato	1 tbsp	25	2	0	–
RENNIN					
tablet	1 (0.9 g)	1	0	–	0
RHUBARB					
fresh	½ cup	13	tr	–	–
frzn	½ cup	60	tr	–	–
frzn as prep w/ sugar	½ cup	139	tr	–	–
RICE (see also RICE CAKES, WILD RICE)					
arborio	½ cup	100	0	–	0
brown long grain cooked	1 cup (6.8 oz)	216	2	tr	–
brown medium grain cooked	1 cup (6.8 oz)	218	2	tr	–

FOOD	PORTION	CALS	FAT	SAT FAT	TRANS FAT
glutinous cooked	1 cup (6.1 oz)	169	tr	tr	–
starch	1 oz	98	0	0	0
white long grain cooked	1 cup (5.5 oz)	205	tr	tr	–
white long grain instant cooked	1 cup (5.8 oz)	162	tr	tr	–
white medium grain cooked	1 cup (6.5 oz)	242	tr	tr	–
white short grain cooked	1 cup (6.5 oz)	242	tr	tr	–
A Taste Of Thai					
Coconut Garlic Basil as prep	¾ cup	160	0	0	0
Coconut Ginger as prep	¾ cup	190	0	0	0
Jasmine not prep	¼ cup	160	0	0	0
Yellow Curry as prep	¾ cup	180	2	1	–
Arrowhead Mills					
Organic Brown Basmati not prep	¼ cup	140	2	0	0
Organic Long Grain Brown not prep	¼ cup	160	1	0	0
Buitoni					
Risotto Garden Vegetable	1 serv	210	1	0	–
Risotto Portobello Mushrooms	1 serv	210	0	0	0
Risotto Rosemary & Potatoes	1 serv	210	1	0	–
Risotto Tomato Basil	1 serv	210	1	0	–
Carolina					
Black Beans & Rice Mix as prep	1 serv	200	2	0	–
Gold as prep	1 cup	160	0	0	0
Spanish Rice Mix as prep	1 serv	180	1	0	–
Country Crock					
Chicken Rice w/ Herbs	1 cup	210	4	1	0
Fantastic					
Arborio not prep	¼ cup	160	4	0	0
Basmati not prep	¼ cup	160	0	0	0
Jasmine not prep	¼ cup	160	0	0	0
Gourmet House					
Brown & White not prep	¼ cup	160	10	0	0
Green Giant					
Rice Pilaf	1 pkg (9.9 oz)	200	3	2	0
White & Wild & Green Beans	1 pkg (9.9 oz)	260	5	1	1
Knorr					
Asian Side Dish Chicken Fried Rice as prep	1 cup	240	1	0	–
Rice Sides Rice Medley as prep	1 cup	250	5	1	0

FOOD	PORTION	CALS	FAT	SAT FAT	TRANS FAT
Rice Sides Sesame Chicken w/ Whole Grains as prep	⅔ cup	300	9	2	–
Lundberg					
Eco-Farmed Black Japonica not prep	¼ cup	170	2	0	0
Eco-Farmed California Brown Basmati not prep	¼ cup	160	2	0	0
Eco-Farmed White California Arborio not prep	¼ cup	10	0	0	0
Organic Brown Golden Rose not prep	¼ cup	160	1	0	0
Organic Rice Sensations Ginger Miso not prep	½ cup	116	1	0	0
Organic Risotto Porcini Mushroom not prep	½ cup	143	1	1	0
Organic White Sushi Rice no prep	¼ cup	150	0	0	0
Organic Wild Blend not prep	¼ cup	150	2	0	0
RiceXpress Chicken Herb	½ pkg (4.4 oz)	250	5	1	0
RiceXpress Santa Fe Grill	½ pkg (4.4 oz)	260	5	1	0
Risotto Butternut Squash not prep	½ cup	143	1	1	0
Mahatma					
Jambalaya as prep	1 cup	190	1	0	–
Nacho Cheese Mix as prep	1 serv	250	3	2	–
Thai Jasmine as prep	¾ cup	160	0	0	0
Marrakesh Express					
Pilaf Tomato & Basil as prep	1 cup	190	0	0	0
Risotto Parmesan as prep	1 cup	200	1	0	–
Near East					
Creative Grains Chicken & Herb as prep	1 cup	270	6	1	–
Creative Grains Creamy Parmesan as prep	1 cup	280	8	4	–
Creative Grains Roasted Garlic as prep	1 cup	220	5	1	–
Creative Grains Roasted Pecan as prep	1 cup	240	8	1	–

FOOD	PORTION	CALS	FAT	SAT FAT	TRANS FAT
Long Grain & Wild Rice Roasted Vegetable & Chicken as prep	1 cup	220	5	2	–
Long Grain & Wild Rice Garlic & Herb as prep	1 cup	220	5	2	–
Pilaf Brown Rice as prep	1 cup	210	5	2	–
Pilaf Chicken as prep	1 cup	220	5	2	–
Pilaf Mix Curry as prep	1 cup	220	5	2	–
Pilaf Mix Garlic & Herb as prep	1 cup	220	3	tr	–
Pilaf Mix Long Grain & Wild as prep	1 cup	220	5	2	–
Pilaf Mix Rice as prep	1 cup	220	5	2	–
Pilaf Mix Roasted Chicken & Garlic as prep	1 cup	220	4	1	–
Pilaf Mix Spanish Rice as prep	1 cup	310	8	5	–
Pilaf Mix Toasted Almond as prep	1 cup	230	6	2	–
Pilaf Mix Wild Mushroom & Herb as prep	1 cup	220	5	2	–
Nueva Cocina					
Arroz A La Mexicana	1 cup	190	1	–	–
Arroz Con Pollo	1 cup	150	0	0	0
Gallo Pinto	1/3 pkg	220	0	0	0
Moros Y Cristianos	1/3 pkg	220	0	0	0
Paella	1/5 pkg	160	0	0	0
Pacific Foods					
Ready-To-Serve Lemon & Herb	1/2 pkg	240	3	0	0
Ready-To-Serve Roasted Chicken	1/2 pkg	240	6	1	0
Ready-To-Serve Spanish Style	1/2 pkg	230	3	0	–
Ready-To-Serve Wild Rice & Mushroom	1/2 pkg	230	3	0	0
Patak's					
Basmati	1 pkg	430	5	2	–
Coconut	1 pkg	500	12	9	–
Yellow	1 pkg	440	5	2	–
Rice A Roni					
Beef as prep	1 cup	310	9	2	2
Chicken as prep	1 cup	310	9	2	2
Express Asian Fried	1 cup	280	6	1	0

FOOD	PORTION	CALS	FAT	SAT FAT	TRANS FAT
Fried Rice as prep	1 cup	320	11	2	2
Garden Vegetable as prep	1 cup	270	10	3	2
Long Grain & Wild as prep	1 cup	250	7	1	0
Lower Sodium Chicken as prep	1 cup	270	5	1	1
Parmesan Chicken as prep	1 cup	370	15	5	2
Red Beans & Rice as prep	1 cup	290	7	2	1
Savory Whole Grain Blends Spanish as prep	1 cup	250	8	1	0
Spanish as prep	1 cup	260	7	2	1
Rice Expressions					
Indian Basmati	1 cup	180	tr	0	–
Organic Brown	1 cup	160	1	0	–
Organic Long Grain	1 cup	180	tr	0	–
Organic Rice Pilaf	1 cup	170	3	0	–
Organic Tex Mex	1 cup	190	2	0	–
Rice Select					
Jasmati	1 serv	150	0	0	0
Kasmati	1 serv	150	1	–	–
Risotto	1 serv	150	0	0	0
Royal Blend	1 serv	160	1	–	0
Royal Blend w/ Lentils	1 serv	130	1	0	0
Royal Blend w/ Red Beans	1 serv	130	1	0	0
Sushi Rice not prep	¼ cup	190	0	0	0
Teriyaki Fried Rice not prep	¼ cup	160	1	0	–
Texmati Brown	1 serv	170	1	–	–
Texmati Light Brown	1 serv	170	1	–	–
Texmati White	1 serv	150	1	–	–
Texmati Royal Blend Brown & Wild	1 serv	160	2	0	0
River Rice					
Brown Long Grain not prep	¼ cup	150	1	0	–
S&W					
Arborio as prep	¾ cup	150	0	0	0
Basmati Mix as prep	¾ cup	160	0	0	0
Brown Long Grain not prep	¼ cup	150	1	0	–
Long Grain Organic not prep	¼ cup	150	0	0	0
Seeds Of Change					
Moroccan Lentil Rice Pilaf as prep	1 cup	180	1	0	0
Tuscan Rice & Beans as prep	1 cup	180	1	0	0

FOOD	PORTION	CALS	FAT	SAT FAT	TRANS FAT
Success					
Boil-In-Bag Brown as prep	1 cup	150	1	0	0
Boil-In-Bag Jasmine as prep	¾ cup	150	0	0	0
Boil-In-Bag White as prep	1 cup	190	0	0	0
Ready To Serve Brown	1 cup	170	5	1	0
Ready To Serve White	1 pkg	190	4	0	0
Ready To Serve Yellow Rice Mix	1 pkg	190	4	0	0
Whole Grain Herb Roasted Chicken as prep	1 cup	290	10	2	0
Whole Grain Multigrain Pilaf as prep	1 cup	230	3	1	0
Whole Grain Portobello Mushroom as prep	1 cup	220	2	0	0
TastyBite					
Pilaf Multigrain	½ pkg (5 oz)	200	5	1	0
Pilaf Tandoori	½ pkg (5 oz)	183	3	0	0
Uncle Ben's					
Boil-In-Bag	1 cup	190	1	0	–
Brown Natural as prep	1 cup	170	1	–	–
Country Inn Chicken & Broccoli as prep	1 cup	190	1	0	–
Country Inn Chicken & Vegetables as prep	1 cup	200	2	1	–
Country Inn Mexican Fiesta as prep	1 cup	200	1	0	–
Country Inn Oriental Fried as prep	1 cup	200	1	0	–
Country Inn Three Cheese as prep	1 cup	200	2	1	–
Country Inn Wheat	1 cup	200	1	0	–
Fast & Natural	1 cup	190	2	0	–
Flavorful Four Cheese as prep	1 cup	190	1	0	–
Flavorful Garlic & Butter as prep	1 cup	200	1	0	–
Flavorful Lemon & Herb as prep	1 cup	200	1	0	–
Flavorful Spanish as prep	1 cup	200	1	0	–
Instant	1 cup	190	1	0	–
Long Grain & Wild Butter Herb as prep	1 cup	190	1	0	–

FOOD	PORTION	CALS	FAT	SAT FAT	TRANS FAT
Long Grain & Wild Fast Cook as prep	1 cup	200	1	0	–
Long Grain & Wild Original as prep	1 cup	200	0	0	0
Long Grain & Wild Roasted Garlic as prep	1 cup	200	1	0	–
Ready Rice Long Grain & Wild as prep	1 cup	240	4	0	–
Ready Rice Original as prep	1 cup	230	4	0	–
Ready Rice Roasted Chicken as prep	1 cup	230	4	0	–
Ready Rice Teriyaki as prep	1 cup	190	4	0	–
Ready Rice Whole Grain Brown	1 cup	220	4	1	–
White Original as prep	1 cup	170	0	0	0
Water Maid					
White Medium Grain not prep	¼ cup	160	0	0	0
TAKE-OUT					
coconut rice	1 serv	500	42	–	–
nasi goreng (fried rice)	1 serv	206	4	–	–
nasi goreng indonesian rice & vegetables	1 cup (4.9 oz)	130	0	0	–
pea palau rice & peas fried in ghee	1 serv	144	5	3	–
pilaf	½ cup	84	3	1	–
risotto	1 serv (6.6 oz)	426	18	–	–
spanish	¾ cup	363	27	10	–

RICE CAKES (see also POPCORN CAKES)
Lundberg

FOOD	PORTION	CALS	FAT	SAT FAT	TRANS FAT
Eco-Farmed Apple Cinnamon	1 (0.7 oz)	80	1	0	0
Eco-Farmed Brown Rice Salt Free	1 (0.7 oz)	70	0	0	0
Eco-Farmed Toasted Sesame	1 (0.7 oz)	70	0	0	0
Organic Caramel Corn	1 (0.7 oz)	80	1	0	0
Organic Green Tea w/ Lemon	1 (0.7 oz)	80	0	0	0
Organic Mochi Sweet	1 (0.7 oz)	70	0	0	0
Mr. Krispers					
Baked Rice Krisps Barbecue	37	110	3	0	0
Baked Rice Krisps Nacho	37	120	3	0	0

FOOD	PORTION	CALS	FAT	SAT FAT	TRANS FAT
Baked Rice Krisps Sea Salt & Pepper	37	110	4	0	0
Baked Rice Krisps Sour Cream & Onion	37	110	4	0	0
Quaker					
Mini Delights Chocolatey Drizzle	1 pkg (0.7 oz)	90	4	4	0
Riceworks					
Sweet Chili	10 (1 oz)	140	6	1	0
Wasabi	10 (1 oz)	140	6	1	0
Tastemorr					
Rice Crisps Caramel	7	55	0	0	0

ROCKFISH

FOOD	PORTION	CALS	FAT	SAT FAT	TRANS FAT
pacific cooked	3 oz	103	2	tr	–
pacific cooked	1 fillet (5.2 oz)	180	3	1	–
pacific raw	3 oz	80	1	tr	–

ROE (see also individual fish names)

FOOD	PORTION	CALS	FAT	SAT FAT	TRANS FAT
fresh baked	1 oz	58	2	1	0

ROLL
FROZEN
Alexia

FOOD	PORTION	CALS	FAT	SAT FAT	TRANS FAT
Ciabatta	1 (1.5 oz)	100	2	0	0
French	1 (1.5 oz)	100	0	0	0
Three Cheese Focaccia	1 (1.5 oz)	110	2	1	0
Whole Grain	1 (1.5 oz)	90	1	0	0
Eggo					
Toaster Swirlz Cinnamon Roll Minis	4 (1.6 oz)	120	3	1	0
Pillsbury					
Dinner Rolls Crusty French	1	110	2	0	–
Sara Lee					
Deluxe Cinnamon Rolls w/ Icing	1 (2.7 oz)	320	15	9	–
READY-TO-EAT					
bialy	1 (2.2 oz)	138	0	0	0
brioche sweet roll	1 (3.5 oz)	410	23	14	–
brown & serve	1 (1 oz)	85	2	tr	–
cheese	1 (2.3 oz)	238	12	4	–

FOOD	PORTION	CALS	FAT	SAT FAT	TRANS FAT
cinnamon raisin	1 (2¾ in)	223	10	3	–
dinner	1 (1 oz)	85	2	tr	–
egg	1 (2½ in)	107	2	1	–
french	1 (1.3 oz)	105	2	tr	–
hamburger	1 (1½ oz)	123	2	1	–
hamburger multigrain	1 (1½ oz)	113	2	1	–
hamburger reduced calorie	1 (1½ oz)	84	1	tr	–
hard	1 (3½ in)	167	2	tr	–
hot cross bun	1	202	4	–	–
hot dog	1 (1½ oz)	123	2	1	–
hot dog reduced calorie	1 (1½ oz)	84	1	tr	–
hot dog whole wheat	1 (1.5 oz)	110	2	0	–
kaiser	1 (3½ in)	167	2	tr	–
oat bran	1 (1.2 oz)	78	2	tr	–
rye	1 (1 oz)	81	1	tr	–
submarine	1 (4.7 oz)	155	2	tr	–
wheat	1 (1 oz)	77	2	tr	–
whole wheat	1 (1 oz)	75	1	tr	–
Alvarado Street Bakery					
Sprouted Wheat Burger Bun	1 (2.2 oz)	140	2	0	0
Country Kitchen					
Wheat Light	1	80	2	0	–
Natural Ovens					
Best Burger Bun	1	178	4	0	–
Better Wheat Buns	1	140	2	0	–
Gourmet Dinner	1	70	1	0	–
Nature's Own					
100% Whole Grain Sugar Free	1 (1.9 oz)	110	2	1	0
Butter Buns	1 (1.7 oz)	120	2	2	0
Pepperidge Farm					
Hamburger 100% Whole Wheat	1	120	2	0	0
Hoagie Soft w/ Sesame Seeds	1	210	6	2	0
Hot & Crusty Sourdough	1	100	1	0	0
Hot Dog	1	140	3	1	0
Hot Dog Whole Grain White	1	110	1	0	0
Parker House Dinner	1	80	2	1	0
Premium Wheat	1	220	5	1	0
Rudi's Organic Bakery					
100% Whole Wheat	1 (2.3 oz)	160	2	0	0

FOOD	PORTION	CALS	FAT	SAT FAT	TRANS FAT
Hot Dog Spelt	1 (2 oz)	140	2	0	0
Hot Dog Wheat	1 (2 oz)	150	2	0	0
Hot Dog White	1 (2 oz)	150	2	0	0
Sara Lee					
Hamburger Bun Classic	1 (2.6 oz)	200	3	1	–
Hamburger Bun Classic Wheat	1 (2.6 oz)	200	4	1	–
Heart Healthy Hamburger Bun Wheat	1 (2.6 oz)	190	3	1	0
Hot Dog Gourmet	1 (1.5 oz)	120	2	0	–
Stroehmann					
Hot Dog Wheat	1 (1.8 oz)	140	3	1	0
Super Bakery					
Daily Donut Reduced Fat	1 (2.2 oz)	200	6	2	0
Organic Sandwich Bun	1 (3.6 oz)	250	3	0	0
Sub Roll	1 (3.6 oz)	250	3	0	0
REFRIGERATED					
cinnamon w/ frosting	1	109	4	1	–
crescent	1 (1 oz)	98	4	1	–
Pillsbury					
Crescent	1 (1.7 oz)	170	10	3	3
Crescent Reduced Fat	1 (1 oz)	100	5	1	–

ROSE APPLE

FOOD	PORTION	CALS	FAT	SAT FAT	TRANS FAT
fresh	3.5 oz	32	tr	–	–

ROSE HIP

fresh	1 oz	26	0	0	0

ROSELLE

fresh	1 cup	28	tr	–	–

ROSEMARY

dried	1 tsp	4	tr	tr	0
fresh	1 tbsp	1	tr	tr	0

ROUGHY

orange baked	3 oz	75	1	tr	–

RUBS (see HERBS/SPICES)

RUTABAGA

cooked mashed	½ cup	41	tr	tr	–
raw cubed	½ cup	25	tr	tr	–

FOOD	PORTION	CALS	FAT	SAT FAT	TRANS FAT
Glory					
Cut Fresh	1 cup	50	0	0	0
SABLEFISH					
baked	3 oz	213	17	3	–
fillet baked	5.3 oz	378	30	6	–
smoked	1 oz	72	6	1	–
smoked	3 oz	218	17	4	–
SAFFLOWER					
seeds dried	1 oz	147	11	1	–
SAFFRON					
dried	1 tsp	2	tr	tr	0
SAGE					
ground	1 tsp	2	tr	tr	0
SALAD (see also SALAD TOPPINGS)					
Dole					
American Blend	1½ cups	15	0	0	0
Baby Spinach Salad	1½ cups (3 oz)	20	0	0	0
Butter & Red Leaf	1½ cups (3 oz)	10	0	0	0
Classic Iceberg	1½ cups (3 oz)	15	0	0	0
Classic Romaine	1½ cups (3 oz)	15	0	0	0
European Blend	1½ cups (3 oz)	15	0	0	0
Field Greens	1½ cups (3 oz)	15	0	0	0
French Blend	1½ cups (3 oz)	15	0	0	0
Greener Selection	1½ cups (3 oz)	15	0	0	0
Hearts Delight	1½ cups (3 oz)	15	0	0	0
Italian Blend	1½ cups (3 oz)	15	0	0	0
Kits Asian Crunch	1½ cups (3.5 oz)	120	6	1	0
Kits Bacon Lettuce Toss	1½ cups (3.5 oz)	130	9	2	0
Kits Caesar	1½ cups (3 oz)	170	15	2	–
Kits Caesar Light	1½ cups (3 oz)	100	7	2	–
Kits Fall Harvest	1½ cups (3.5 oz)	150	11	2	0
Kits Romano	1½ cups (3 oz)	150	12	2	–
Kits Spring Garden	1½ cups (3.5 oz)	140	11	2	0
Kits Sunflower Ranch	1½ cups (3 oz)	160	16	2	–
Mediterranean Blend	1½ cups	15	0	0	0
Very Veggie Blend	1½ cups (3 oz)	20	0	0	0

FOOD	PORTION	CALS	FAT	SAT FAT	TRANS FAT
Earthbound Farm					
Organic Baby Arugula	2 cups	20	0	0	0
Organic Baby Lettuce	2 cups	15	0	0	0
Organic Baby Spinach	2 cups	10	0	0	0
Organic Fresh Herb	2 cups	15	0	0	0
Organic Mixed Baby Greens	2 cups	15	0	0	0
Fresh Express					
Baby Spinach Trio	4 cups (3 oz)	20	0	0	0
Mann's					
Rainbow	3 oz	25	0	0	0
Ready Pac					
All American	2.5 cups	15	0	0	0
Bordeaux	1 pkg (5 oz)	35	0	0	0
Bowl Salad Chef	1 pkg	350	25	8	–
Bowl Salad Chicken Caesar	1 pkg	380	27	7	–
Bowl Salad Greek	1 pkg	400	35	8	–
Bowl Salad Spinach Bacon	1 pkg	300	17	6	–
Bowl Salad Spring Mix Veggie	1 pkg	330	23	5	–
Caesar Romaine	1½ cups	15	0	0	0
Classic Crisp Salad	2¼ cups	10	0	0	0
Continental	3 cups	20	0	0	0
Costa Brava	3 cups	15	0	0	0
Hearty Green Salad	2½ cups	10	0	0	0
Lafayette	3 cups	10	0	0	0
Milano	3 cups	15	0	0	0
Organic Caesar Romaine	2¼ cups	15	0	0	0
Organic Mesclun Blend	1 pkg (4.5 oz)	35	0	0	0
Organic Monterey	3 cups	15	0	0	0
Parisian	2 cups	20	0	0	0
Portofino	1 pkg (5 oz)	25	0	0	0
Santa Barbara	3½ cups	15	0	0	0
Spring Mix	1 pkg (5 oz)	35	0	0	0
River Ranch					
American Blend	1½ cups	15	0	0	0
Caesar Kit	1½ cups	110	12	2	–
European Blend	1¾ cups	10	0	0	0
Garden	1½ cups	15	0	0	0
Garden Supreme	1½ cups	15	0	0	0
Italian Blend	1¾ cups	15	0	0	0
Raspberry Vinaigrette Kit	1¾ cups	130	8	0	–

FOOD	PORTION	CALS	FAT	SAT FAT	TRANS FAT
Riviera Blend	1½ cups	10	0	0	0
TAKE-OUT					
7-layer salad	2 cups	557	51	11	–
caesar	4 cups	734	61	11	–
chef salad w/o dressing	3 cups	535	32	16	–
cobb w/ dressing	4 cups	645	49	13	0
greek w/ dressing	4 cups	424	29	14	0
mixed salad greens shredded	1 cup	9	tr	tr	0
somen w/ lettuce egg fish pork	2 cups	550	17	5	–
spinach no dressing	4 cups	429	19	6	–
tossed w/o dressing	2 cups	22	tr	tr	0
tossed w/ avocado w/o dressing	2 cups	90	6	1	0
tossed w/ chicken w/o dressing	3 cups	194	4	1	0
tossed w/ egg w/o dressing	2 cups	93	5	1	0
tossed w/ seafood w/o dressing	3 cups	120	1	tr	0
tossed w/ shrimp & egg w/o dressing	3 cups	185	5	1	0
waldorf	1 cup	242	21	3	–
wilted lettuce w/ bacon dressing	1 cup	99	8	3	–

SALAD DRESSING (see also SALAD TOPPINGS)
MIX
A Taste Of Thai

FOOD	PORTION	CALS	FAT	SAT FAT	TRANS FAT
Peanut Dressing as prep	2 tbsp	40	2	1	–
Good Seasons					
Italian as prep	2 tbsp	130	14	2	–
Italian not prep	⅛ pkg (3 g)	5	0	0	0
READY-TO-EAT					
blue cheese	1 tbsp	77	8	2	–
french	1 tbsp	67	6	2	–
french reduced calorie	1 tbsp	22	1	tr	–
italian	1 tbsp	69	7	1	–
italian reduced calorie	1 tbsp	16	2	tr	–
russian	1 tbsp	76	8	1	–
russian reduced calorie	1 tbsp	23	1	tr	–
sesame seed	1 tbsp	68	7	1	–

FOOD	PORTION	CALS	FAT	SAT FAT	TRANS FAT
thousand island	1 tbsp	59	6	1	–
thousand island reduced calorie	1 tbsp	24	2	tr	–
Annie's Naturals					
Cilantro & Lime	2 tbsp	100	10	1	–
French	2 tbsp	90	9	1	–
Goddess Dressing	2 tbsp	130	13	1	–
Low Fat Mustard Vinaigrette	2 tbsp	45	2	0	–
Organic Buttermilk	2 tbsp	70	7	1	–
Organic Papaya Poppy Seed	2 tbsp	120	11	2	–
Organic Red Wine	2 tbsp	160	17	3	–
Organic No Fat Yogurt w/ Dill	2 tbsp	20	0	0	0
Sea Veggie & Sesame	2 tbsp	110	11	1	–
Tuscany Italian	2 tbsp	80	7	1	–
Bernstein's					
Chunky Blue Cheese	2 tbsp	120	13	2	0
Creamy Caesar	2 tbsp	120	13	1	0
Italian Restaurant Recipe	2 tbsp	120	12	1	0
Light Fantastic Roasted Garlic Balsamic	2 tbsp	45	4	0	0
Red Wine & Garlic Italian	2 tbsp	110	1	0	0
Cains					
Caesar Creamy	2 tbsp	170	19	3	0
Caesar Fat Free	2 tbsp	30	0	0	0
Caesar Light	2 tbsp	70	6	1	0
Chianti Vinaigrette	2 tbsp	130	12	2	0
Creamy Dill Cucumber Fat Free	2 tbsp	35	0	0	0
French	2 tbsp	120	11	2	0
French Light	2 tbsp	80	5	1	0
Greek	2 tbsp	160	17	3	0
Italian Fat Free	2 tbsp	15	0	0	0
Ranch	2 tbsp	180	19	3	0
Ranch Light	2 tbsp	80	6	1	0
Carb Options					
Italian	2 tbsp	70	8	1	–
Ranch	2 tbsp	150	17	3	–
Consorzio					
Balsamic Vinaigrette	2 tbsp	60	1	1	–
Caesar Parmesan & Romano	2 tbsp	120	7	1	–
Honey Mustard	2 tbsp	100	8	0	–

FOOD	PORTION	CALS	FAT	SAT FAT	TRANS FAT
Italian	2 tbsp	60	7	1	–
Mango	1 tbsp	15	0	0	0
Raspberry & Balsamic	1 tbsp	15	0	0	0
Strawberry Balsamic	1 tbsp	10	0	0	0
David Burke					
Flavor Spray Ranch	2 sprays	0	0	0	0
Drew's					
Low Carb Garlic Italian	1 tbsp	80	9	1	–
Low Carb Lemon Tahini Goddess	1 tbsp	80	9	1	–
Low Carb Sesame Orange	1 tbsp	80	9	1	–
Emeril's					
Bleu Cheese	2 tbsp	110	12	2	–
Honey Mustard	2 tbsp	100	9	1	–
House Herb Vinaigrette	2 tbsp	100	10	1	–
Kicked Up French	2 tbsp	80	5	1	–
Girard's					
White Balsamic Vinaigrette	2 tbsp	140	13	2	0
Ken's					
Bacon Ranch	2 tbsp	140	15	2	0
Caesar	2 tbsp	170	18	3	0
Country French w/ Vermont Honey	2 tbsp	150	12	2	0
Fat Free Italian	2 tbsp	25	0	0	0
Fat Free Raspberry Pecan	2 tbsp	50	0	0	0
Honey Mustard	2 tbsp	130	11	2	0
Italian w/ Aged Romano	2 tbsp	110	12	2	0
Lite Italian	2 tbsp	50	5	1	0
Lite Ranch	2 tbsp	80	6	1	0
Lite Red Wine Vinegar & Olive Oil	2 tbsp	50	5	1	0
Lite Vinaigrette Balsamic & Basil	2 tbsp	50	5	1	0
Lite Chunky Blue Cheese	2 tbsp	80	7	2	0
Red Wine Vinegar & Olive Oil	2 tbsp	120	12	2	0
Russian	2 tbsp	140	14	2	0
Thousand Island	2 tbsp	140	13	2	0
Kraft					
Free French	2 tbsp	50	0	0	0

FOOD	PORTION	CALS	FAT	SAT FAT	TRANS FAT
Free Ranch	2 tbsp	50	0	0	0
Free Thousand Island	2 tbsp	45	0	0	0
LaMartinique					
Blue Cheese Vinaigrette	2 tbsp	160	17	6	–
Poppy Seed	2 tbsp	170	15	4	–
Marie's					
Blue Cheese Lite Chunky	2 tbsp	80	6	2	0
Blue Cheese Vinaigrette	2 tbsp	120	11	3	0
Caesar	2 tbsp	170	19	4	0
Coleslaw	2 tbsp	120	13	2	0
Creamy Ranch	2 tbsp	170	19	3	0
Red Wine Vinaigrette	2 tbsp	60	5	1	0
Sesame Ginger	2 tbsp	70	8	2	0
Nasoya					
Creamy Dill	1 tbsp	30	3	0	–
Creamy Italian	2 tbsp	70	7	1	–
Garden Herb	2 tbsp	60	7	1	–
Sesame Garlic	2 tbsp	60	7	1	–
Newman's Own					
Balsamic Vinaigrette	2 tbsp	90	9	1	0
Caesar	2 tbsp	150	16	2	0
Creamy Caesar	2 tbsp	150	16	15	–
Family Recipe Italian	2 tbsp	120	13	1	–
Lighten Up Balsamic Vinaigrette	2 tbsp	45	4	1	–
Lighten Up Caesar	2 tbsp	70	6	1	0
Lighten Up Honey Mustard	2 tbsp	70	4	1	0
Lighten Up Italian	2 tbsp	60	6	1	–
Lighten Up Low Fat Sesame Ginger	2 tbsp	35	2	0	0
Lighten Up Raspberry & Walnut	2 tbsp	70	5	1	0
Lighten Up Red Wine Vinegar & Olive Oil	2 tbsp	110	10	2	–
Olive Oil & Vinegar	2 tbsp	150	16	3	–
Parmesan & Roasted Garlic	2 tbsp	110	11	2	–
Ranch	2 tbsp	140	15	–	–
Two Thousand Island	2 tbsp	140	14	2	–
Old Dutch					
Sweet & Sour	2 tbsp	50	0	0	0

FOOD	PORTION	CALS	FAT	SAT FAT	TRANS FAT
San-J					
Tamari Mustard	2 tbsp	25	0	0	0
Tamari Peanut	2 tbsp	60	2	–	–
Tamari Sesame	2 tbsp	45	2	–	–
School House Kitchen					
Balsamic Vinaigrette Basico	2 tbsp	160	17	1	0
Seeds Of Change					
Vinaigrette Balsamic	2 tbsp	60	4	0	0
Vinaigrette Greek Feta	2 tbsp	60	5	1	0
Vinaigrette Roasted Garlic	2 tbsp	60	4	0	0
Vinaigrette Sweet Basil	2 tbsp	60	5	0	0
Sonoma					
Creamy Tomato Bacon	2 tbsp	150	15	3	0
South Beach					
Balsamic Vinaigrette	2 tbsp	50	4	0	0
Italian	2 tbsp	60	4	0	–
Ranch	2 tbsp	70	7	1	–
Spectrum					
Honey Dijon	2 tbsp	35	2	0	0
Organic Creamy Dill	2 tbsp	25	0	0	0
Organic Creamy Garlic	2 tbsp	20	0	0	0
Organic Greek Goddess	2 tbsp	110	11	2	0
Organic Omega 3 Balsamic Vinaigrette	2 tbsp	80	8	1	0
Organic Omega 3 Ginger Garlic Vinaigrette	2 tbsp	80	8	1	0
Organic Omega 3 Raspberry Vinaigrette	2 tbsp	80	8	1	0
Organic Porcini Mushroom Vinaigrette	2 tbsp	70	6	1	0
Organic Rocky Mountain Ranch	2 tbsp	130	14	2	0
Organic Sweet Onion & Garlic	2 tbsp	15	0	0	0
Organic Toasted Sesame	2 tbsp	15	0	0	0
Provencal Garlic Lover's	2 tbsp	50	5	0	0
Zesty Italian	2 tbsp	30	2	0	0
Steel's					
Honey Mustard	1 tbsp	90	7	1	–
Sweet Ginger Lime	1 tbsp	68	7	0	–

FOOD	PORTION	CALS	FAT	SAT FAT	TRANS FAT
Vino De Milo					
Gorgonzola Pear Riesling	2 tbsp	80	7	1	0
Pomegranate Port	2 tbsp	90	7	1	0
Wishbone					
Blue Cheese w/ Gorgonzola	2 tbsp	140	15	3	0
Caesar w/ Aged Romano	2 tbsp	80	8	1	–
Classic Ranch Extra Thick	2 tbsp	140	15	3	–
Creamy Caesar	2 tbsp	170	18	3	–
Creamy Italian	2 tbsp	110	10	2	0
Deluxe French	2 tbsp	50	2	0	–
Fat Free Chunky Blue Cheese	2 tbsp	35	0	0	0
Fat Free Italian	2 tbsp	20	0	0	0
Fat Free Ranch	2 tbsp	30	0	0	0
Fat Free Western	2 tbsp	45	0	0	0
Five Cheese Italian	2 tbsp	120	10	2	–
Italian	2 tbsp	90	8	1	0
Just 2 Good Blue Cheese	2 tbsp	45	2	1	–
Just 2 Good Creamy Caesar	2 tbsp	50	2	1	–
Just 2 Good Deluxe French	2 tbsp	50	2	0	–
Just 2 Good Italian	2 tbsp	35	2	0	–
Just 2 Good Ranch	2 tbsp	40	2	0	–
Just 2 Good Thousand Island	2 tbsp	50	2	0	–
Just 2 Good Western	2 tbsp	70	2	0	–
Light Vinaigrette Asian Sesame	2 tbsp	70	5	1	–
Light Vinaigrette Raspberry Walnut	2 tbsp	80	5	1	0
Light Ranch Extra Thick	2 tbsp	70	6	1	0
Ranch	2 tbsp	160	17	3	–
Russian	2 tbsp	110	6	1	–
Salad Spritzers Balsamic Breeze	10 sprays	10	1	0	0
Salad Spritzers Italian	10 sprays	10	1	0	0
Salad Spritzers Red Wine Mist	10 sprays	10	1	0	0
Thousand Island	2 tbsp	130	12	2	–
Vinaigrette Berry	2 tbsp	50	5	1	–
Vinaigrette Lemon Garlic & Herb	2 tbsp	70	5	1	–
Vinaigrette Olive Oil	2 tbsp	60	5	1	–
Western	2 tbsp	160	12	2	–

FOOD	PORTION	CALS	FAT	SAT FAT	TRANS FAT
TAKE-OUT					
vinegar & oil	1 tbsp	72	8	2	–
SALAD TOPPINGS					
Fresh Gourmet					
Crispy Onions Garlic Pepper	1½ tbsp	35	2	0	0
Tortilla Strips Lightly Salted	2 tbsp	35	2	0	0
Wonton Strips Wasabi Ranch	2 tbsp	35	2	0	0
Salad Pizazz!					
Asian Medley	1 tbsp	40	3	0	–
Cherry Cranberry Pecano	1 tbsp	35	2	0	–
Honey Toasted Delites	1 tbsp	40	3	0	–
Orange Cranberry Almondine	1 tbsp	35	2	0	–
Raspberry Cranberry Walnut Frisco	1 tbsp	30	2	0	–
Tomato 'N Bacon Parmesano	1 tbsp	30	1	0	–
Tomato Pinenut Tuscano	1 tbsp	130	2	0	–
SALMON					
CANNED					
w/ bone	½ cup	106	5	1	0
Bumble Bee					
Blueback	¼ cup	110	7	2	–
Keta	¼ cup	90	4	1	–
Pink	¼ cup	90	5	1	0
Red	¼ cup	110	7	2	0
Skinless & Boneless	¼ cup	50	1	0	0
Smoked Fillets In Oil	⅓ cup	150	9	2	–
Chicken Of The Sea					
Pink	1 pkg (3 oz)	90	3	1	–
Pink Skinless Boneless	¼ cup	60	2	1	–
Red	¼ cup	110	7	2	–
Smoked Pacific	1 pkg (3 oz)	120	4	1	–
Libby's					
Alaskan Sockeye Red	¼ cup	110	7	2	–
Pink Skinless Boneless	¼ cup	50	1	0	–
Red	¼ cup	110	7	2	–
FRESH					
atlantic farmed baked	4 oz	233	14	3	0
cloudberry native alaska	3.5 oz	51	1	–	0
coho wild poached	4 oz	209	9	2	0

FOOD	PORTION	CALS	FAT	SAT FAT	TRANS FAT
pink baked	4 oz	169	5	1	0
roe raw	1 oz	59	3	–	–
sockeye baked	4 oz	245	12	2	0
FROZEN					
Phillips Seafood					
Salmon Cakes	1 (3 oz)	180	13	3	0
SMOKED					
lox	1 oz	33	1	tr	0
TAKE-OUT					
guisado salmon stew	1 serv (7.4 oz)	320	16	3	0
roulette w/ spinach stuffing	1 serv (4 oz)	160	6	2	–
salmon cake	1 (4.2 oz)	264	16	4	0
salmon loaf	1 slice (3.7 oz)	206	11	3	0
SALSA					
black bean & corn	2 tbsp	15	0	0	0
citrus	2 tbsp (1 oz)	10	0	0	0
peach	2 tbsp	15	0	0	0
tomato-less corn & chile	2 tbsp	45	0	0	0
Bone Suckin'					
Fat Free Gluten Free	2 tbsp	40	0	0	0
Cape Cod					
Medium & Mild	2 tbsp	15	0	0	0
Chi-Chi's					
Fiesta Mild	2 tbsp	10	0	0	0
Del Salsa					
Fire Roasted All Flavors	2 tbsp	8	0	0	0
Emeril's					
Original Recipe	2 tbsp	10	0	0	0
Gringo Billy's					
Salsa Mix	1 tsp	5	1	0	–
Muir Glen					
Organic Medium	2 tbsp	10	0	0	0
Newman's Own					
Bandito Pineapple	2 tbsp	15	0	0	0
Bandito Mild	2 tbsp	10	0	0	0
Bandito Peach	2 tbsp	25	0	0	0
Bandito Roasted Garlic	2 tbsp	10	0	0	0
Bandito Tequila Lime	2 tbsp	15	0	0	0

FOOD	PORTION	CALS	FAT	SAT FAT	TRANS FAT
Ortega					
Garden Style Mild	2 tbsp	10	0	0	0
Picante Mild	2 tbsp	10	0	0	0
Pace					
Black Bean & Corn	2 tbsp	25	0	0	0
Organic Picante	2 tbsp	10	0	0	0
Thick & Chunky	2 tbsp	10	0	0	0
Robert Rothchild Farm					
Tomatillo & Pepper	2 tbsp	20	0	0	0
Seeds Of Change					
Black Bean & Tomato Mild	2 tbsp	15	0	0	0
Garlic & Cilantro Mild	2 tbsp	15	0	0	0
Snyder's Of Hanover					
Sweet	2 tbsp	20	0	0	0
Tostitos					
All Natural	2 tbsp	15	0	0	0
Con Queso	2 tbsp	40	3	1	–
Monterey Jack Queso	2 tbsp	40	3	1	0
Restaurant Style	2 tbsp	15	0	0	0
Tree Of Life					
Medium	2 tbsp (1 oz)	10	0	0	–
Mild	2 tbsp (1 oz)	10	0	0	–
Utz					
Sweet	2 tbsp	10	0	0	0
Walnut Acres					
Organic Fiesta Cilantro	2 tbsp	10	0	0	0
Organic Sweet Southwestren Peach	2 tbsp	20	0	0	0
SALSIFY					
fresh sliced cooked	½ cup	46	tr	–	–
Frieda's					
Salsify	¾ cup	70	0	0	0
SALT/SEASONED SALT					
salt	1 tbsp	0	0	0	0
salt	1 tsp	0	0	0	0
sea salt coarse	¼ tsp	0	0	0	0
sea salt fine	¼ tsp	0	0	0	0

FOOD	PORTION	CALS	FAT	SAT FAT	TRANS FAT
BaconSalt					
Original	¼ tsp	0	0	0	0
Peppered	¼ tsp	0	0	0	0
Bob's Red Mill					
Garlic Salt Blend	¼ tsp	0	0	0	0
Sea Salt	¼ tsp	0	0	0	0
Eden					
French Celtic Salt	¼ tsp	0	0	0	0
Portuguese Coast Salt	¼ tsp	0	0	0	0
Maine Coast					
Sea Salt w/ Sea Veg	¼ tsp	0	0	0	0
McCormick					
Celery Salt	¼ tsp	0	0	0	0
Morton					
Iodized	¼ tsp	0	0	0	0
Kosher	1 tsp	0	0	0	0
Spice Hunter					
Celery Salt	¼ tsp	0	0	0	0
Garlic Salt	¼ tsp	0	0	0	0

SALT SUBSTITUTES

FOOD	PORTION	CALS	FAT	SAT FAT	TRANS FAT
gomasio sesame salt	2 tsp	34	3	–	0
AlsoSalt					
Butter Flavored	¼ tsp	1	0	0	0
Garlic Flavored	¼ tsp	1	0	0	0
Salt Substitute	¼ tsp	tr	0	0	0
Chef Paul Prudhomme's					
Magic Salt Free Seasoning	¼ tsp	0	0	0	0
Eden					
Organic Seaweed Gomasio Sesame Salt	1 tsp	15	2	0	0
Organic Gomasio Sesame Salt	1 tsp	15	2	0	0
French's					
No Salt	¼ cup	0	0	0	0
Molly McButter					
Lite Sodium	1 tsp	5	0	0	0

SANDWICHES

FOOD	PORTION	CALS	FAT	SAT FAT	TRANS FAT
Amy's					
Pocket Sandwich Broccoli & Cheese	1 (4.5 oz)	270	10	4	–

FOOD	PORTION	CALS	FAT	SAT FAT	TRANS FAT
Pocket Sandwich Roasted Vegetables	1 (4.5 oz)	220	8	2	–
Pocket Sandwich Spinach Feta	1 (4.5 oz)	250	9	5	–
Pocket Sandwich Tofu Scramble	1 (4 oz)	160	6	0	–
Pocket Sandwich Vegetable Pie	1 (5 oz)	300	9	2	–
Toaster Pops Grilled Cheese	1	180	8	4	–
Aunt Jemima					
Biscuit Sausage Egg & Cheese	1 (4 oz)	340	21	7	3
Croissant Sausage Egg & Cheese	1 (4 oz)	350	23	7	2
Griddlecake Sausage Egg & Cheese	1 (4.4 oz)	350	20	7	–
Aunt Trudy's					
Classic Samosa Fillo Pocket	1 (5 oz)	280	10	1	0
Fillo Pocket Cheese & Tomato	1 (5 oz)	320	15	5	0
Fillo Pocket Mediterranean Olive & Veggies	1 (5 oz)	270	10	1	0
Organic Fillo Pocket Roasted Sweet Potato	1 (5 oz)	310	12	2	0
Cedarlane					
Wrap Low Fat Couscous & Vegetable Veggie	1 (6 oz)	220	3	0	0
Fillo Factory					
Organic Fillo Pocket Asian Vegetable	1 (5 oz)	240	10	2	0
Gardenburger					
100% Meatless Maraherita Pizza Wrap	1 (4.7 oz)	240	8	3	0
Wrap Black Bean Chipotle	1 (4.7 oz)	240	8	2	0
Guiltless Gourmet					
Wrap California Veggie	1 (5.7 oz)	270	5	0	0
Wrap Mediterranean Spinach	1 (5.7 oz)	270	5	1	0
Ian's					
Mini Chicken Patty	2 (5.3 oz)	368	10	2	0
Lean Pockets					
Bacon Egg & Cheese	1 (4.5 oz)	150	5	1	–
Barbecue Sauce w/ Beef	1 (4.5 oz)	290	7	2	–
Chicken Cheddar & Broccoli	1 (4.5 oz)	260	7	2	–
Chicken Fajita	1 (4.5 oz)	260	7	3	–
Chicken Parmesan	1 (4.5 oz)	280	7	2	–

FOOD	PORTION	CALS	FAT	SAT FAT	TRANS FAT
Ham & Cheese	1 (4.5 oz)	280	7	4	–
Meatballs & Mozzarella	1 (4.5 oz)	290	7	3	–
Philly Steak & Cheese	1 (4.5 oz)	280	7	3	–
Sausage Egg & Cheese	1 (4.5 oz)	140	5	2	–
Steak Fajita	1 (4.5 oz)	260	7	2	–
Three Cheese & Chicken Quesadilla	1 (4.5 oz)	280	7	2	–
Turkey & Ham w/ Cheddar	1 (4.5 oz)	280	7	2	–
Turkey Broccoli & Cheese	1 (4.5 oz)	270	7	3	–
Lunchables					
Chicken Dunks	1 pkg	310	6	2	0
Stackers Ham & American	1 pkg	430	17	8	1
Stackers Turkey & American	1 pkg	420	17	8	1
Madalena's Masterpiece					
Calzone Artichoke Parmesan	1 (10 oz)	570	29	11	–
Calzone Grilled Chicken	1 (10 oz)	520	22	10	–
Calzone Sausage Pepperoni	1 (10 oz)	640	36	15	–
Panini Garlic Chicken	1 (8 oz)	450	25	11	–
Panini Honey Ham	1 (8 oz)	520	25	9	–
Panini Turkey Pesto	1 (8 oz)	500	26	10	–
Panini Veggie	1 (8 oz)	480	26	9	–
Quesabake Mexican Sausage	1 (7 oz)	510	26	12	–
Quesabake Roasted Veggie	1 (7 oz)	460	24	13	–
Oscar Mayer					
Deli Creations Honey Ham & Swiss	1 pkg (6.8 oz)	440	14	5	0
Deli Creations Steakhouse Cheddar	1 pkg (7.1 oz)	450	15	6	1
Deli Creations Turkey & Cheddar Dijon	1 pkg (6.7 oz)	430	15	5	1
PBJammerz					
Peanut Butter & Jelly All Flavors	1 (2 oz)	220	13	3	0
Smucker's					
Uncrustables Grilled Cheese	1 (1.8 oz)	150	6	3	–
Uncrustables Peanut Butter & Grape Jelly	1 (2 oz)	210	9	2	–
Uncrustables Peanut Butter & Strawberry Jam	1 (2 oz)	210	9	2	–
South Beach					
Breakfast Wraps All American	1 serv (4.6 oz)	200	9	4	0

FOOD	PORTION	CALS	FAT	SAT FAT	TRANS FAT
Breakfast Wraps Denver	1 serv (4.6 oz)	180	7	3	–
Wrap Kit Deli Ham & Turkey	1 pkg	220	10	5	0
Wrap Kit Grilled Chicken Caesar	1 pkg	230	10	4	0
Wrap Kit Southwestern Style Chicken	1 pkg	250	10	5	0
Wrap Kit Turkey & Bacon Club	1 pkg	250	13	4	0
Stouffer's					
Corner Bistro Panini Southwestern Chicken	1 pkg (6 oz)	360	16	7	0
Corner Bistrol Panini Philly Style Steak & Cheese	1 pkg (6 oz)	340	16	6	0
TAKE-OUT					
bacon & egg	1 (6.2 oz)	388	21	6	–
bacon lettuce & tomato w/ mayo	1 (5.8 oz)	344	17	4	–
beef barbecue w/ bun	1 (6.7 oz)	417	12	4	–
calzone beef & cheese	1 (14 oz)	1476	76	27	–
calzone cheese	1 (15 oz)	1632	93	44	–
chicken salad	1 (5 oz)	333	16	3	–
crab cake w/ bun	1	308	8	2	–
croque monsieur	1 (12.4 oz)	765	46	26	–
egg salad	1 (5.6 oz)	485	35	7	–
french dip w/ roll	1 (6.8 oz)	357	13	5	–
fried egg	1 (3.4 oz)	226	9	2	–
grilled cheese	1 (2.9 oz)	290	16	6	–
gyro	1 (13.7 oz)	593	12	4	–
ham & egg	1 (4.4 oz)	272	11	3	0
ham w/ cheese w/ lettuce & mayo	1 (5.4 oz)	369	18	7	–
hot turkey w/ gravy	1	389	10	3	–
peanut butter & jelly	1 (3.3 oz)	327	14	3	–
reuben w/ sauerkraut & cheese	1 (6.4 oz)	463	29	10	–
roast beef w/ gravy	1 (7.8 oz)	386	16	6	–
sloppy joe pork on bun	1 (6.5 oz)	318	9	3	–
tuna melt	1 (5.3 oz)	350	16	5	–
tuna salad w/ lettuce	1 (5.9 oz)	289	7	1	–
turkey w/ mayo	1 (5 oz)	329	11	3	–

FOOD	PORTION	CALS	FAT	SAT FAT	TRANS FAT
SAPODILLA					
fresh	1	140	2	–	–
fresh cut up	1 cup	199	3	–	–
SAPOTES					
fresh	1	301	1	–	–
SARDINES					
CANNED					
atlantic in oil w/ bone	1 can (3.2 oz)	192	11	1	–
atlantic in oil w/ bone	2	50	3	tr	–
pacific in tomato sauce w/ bone	1	68	5	1	–
pacific in tomato sauce w/ bone	1 can (13 oz)	658	44	11	–
Beach Cliff					
In Louisiana Hot Sauce	1 can (3.7 oz)	150	8	2	0
In Mustard Sauce	1 can (3.7 oz)	150	8	2	0
In Olive Oil	1 can (3.7 oz)	200	14	2	0
In Tomato Sauce	1 can (3.7 oz)	140	6	2	0
In Water	1 can (3.7 oz)	150	8	2	0
Small In Soybean Oil	1 can (3.7 oz)	200	12	3	0
w/ Hot Green Chilies	1 can (3.7 oz)	180	12	3	0
Brunswick					
In Louisiana Hot Sauce	1 can (3.7 oz)	150	8	2	0
In Mustard Sauce	1 can (3.7 oz)	150	8	2	0
In Soybean Oil	1 can (3.7 oz)	110	12	3	0
In Spring Water	1 can (3.7 oz)	150	8	2	0
In Tomato Sauce	1 can (3.7 oz)	150	8	2	0
W/ Hot Tabasco Peppers	1 can (3.7 oz)	110	12	3	0
Bumble Bee					
In Hot Sauce	¼ cup	90	6	1	–
In Mustard	¼ cup	70	4	1	–
In Oil	1 can (3.7 oz)	130	9	2	0
In Water	1 can (3.7 oz)	120	7	2	0
Chicken Of The Sea					
In Hot Sauce	1 can (3.75 oz)	130	6	2	–
In Mustard Sauce	1 can (3.75 oz)	150	8	4	–
In Oil	1 can (3.75 oz)	190	14	6	–
In Tomato Sauce	1 can (3.75 oz)	130	6	2	–
In Water	1 can (3.75 oz)	100	4	2	–

FOOD	PORTION	CALS	FAT	SAT FAT	TRANS FAT
Goya					
In Tomato Sauce	2 pieces (2.2 oz)	50	1	0	–
King Oscar					
In Olive Oil	1 can (3.75 oz)	150	11	3	0
Skinless Boneless In Soya Oil	3 pieces (1.9 oz)	120	7	2	–
Season					
Brisling In Water	1 can (3.75 oz)	145	10	4	–
FRESH					
raw	3.5 oz	135	5	–	–
SAUCE (see also BARBECUE SAUCE, GRAVY, SPAGHETTI SAUCE)					
adobo fresco	2 tbsp	81	8	1	–
bearnaise	1 oz	177	19	12	–
cheese mix as prep w/ milk	1 cup	307	17	9	–
curry mix as prep	1 cup	120	6	1	–
curry mix as prep w/ milk	1 cup	270	15	6	–
enchilada sauce green	¼ cup	46	4	2	–
enchilada sauce red	¼ cup	79	8	4	–
fish sauce chinese	1 tbsp	9	0	0	0
fish sauce vietnamese nuoc mam	1 tbsp	6	0	0	0
hoisin	1 tbsp	35	1	–	–
morroccan tagine	½ cup (4 oz)	70	3	0	–
mushroom mix as prep w/ milk	1 cup	228	10	5	–
oyster	1 tbsp	8	0	0	0
plum sauce	0.5 oz	42	0	0	–
satay peanut sauce	1 oz	77	6	2	–
sour cream mix as prep w/ milk	1 cup	509	30	16	–
stroganoff mix as prep	1 cup	271	11	7	–
sweet & sour mix as prep	1 cup	294	tr	tr	–
teriyaki	1 tbsp	15	0	0	0
teriyaki mix as prep	1 cup	131	1	tr	–
white sauce mix as prep w/ milk	1 cup	241	13	6	–
A Taste Of Thai					
Chili Sauce Garlic Pepper	1 tsp	10	0	0	0
Chili Sauce Sweet Red	1 tsp	10	0	0	0
Fish Sauce	1 tbsp	15	0	0	0

FOOD	PORTION	CALS	FAT	SAT FAT	TRANS FAT
Pad Thai Sauce Mix	2 tbsp	90	1	1	–
Peanut Satay	2 tbsp	80	5	4	–
Peanut Sauce Mix	¼ pkg	45	2	1	–
A1					
Bold Steak Sauce	1 tbsp	20	0	0	0
Annie Chun's					
Marinade & Dressing Lemongrass Herb	1 tbsp	25	2	0	–
Noodle Sauce & Dressing Sesame Cilantro	1 tbsp	60	4	0	–
Shiitake Mushroom	1 tbsp	15	0	0	0
Annie's Naturals					
Marinade Organic Spicy Ginger	2 tbsp	35	2	–	–
Marinade Organic Teriyaki	1 tbsp	30	1	–	0
Organic Worcestershire	1 tbsp	20	0	0	0
Asian Creations					
Marvelous Mango	¼ cup	20	0	0	0
Pad Thai Pizzazz	2 oz	110	6	1	–
Peanut Passion	¼ cup	130	9	4	–
Asian Gourmet					
Duck Sauce Peking Style	2 tbsp	40	0	0	0
Boar's Head					
Ham Glaze Sugar & Spice	2 tbsp	120	0	0	0
Bone Suckin'					
Hiccuppin' Hot	1 tsp	10	0	0	0
Yaki Stir Fry	1 tbsp	30	0	0	0
Cains					
Tartar	2 tbsp	160	16	3	0
Carb Options					
Alfredo	¼ cup	110	10	4	–
Asian Teriyaki Marinade	1 tbsp	5	1	–	–
Cheese	¼ cup	90	8	3	–
Garden Style	½ cup	80	5	1	–
Steak Sauce	1 tbsp	5	0	0	0
Consorzio					
Marinade Baja Lime	1 tbsp	60	6	0	–
Marinade California Teriyaki	1 tbsp	40	2	0	–
Marinade Dijon Peppercorn	1 tbsp	15	0	0	0
Marinade Jamaican Jerk	1 tbsp	10	0	0	0

FOOD	PORTION	CALS	FAT	SAT FAT	TRANS FAT
Marinade Lemon Pepper	1 tbsp	60	6	0	–
Marinade Roasted Garlic	1 tbsp	35	2	0	–
Marinade Sesame Ginger	1 tbsp	25	1	0	–
Marinade Southwestern Chipotle	1 tbsp	30	2	0	–
Marinade Tropical Grill	1 tbsp	40	3	0	–
Del Monte					
Seafood Cocktail	¼ cup	100	0	0	0
Sloppy Joe Hickory Flavor	¼ cup	60	0	0	0
Sloppy Joe Original	¼ cup	50	0	0	0
D'Oni					
Happy Together Orange Chili Garlic	2 tbsp	50	0	0	0
Moondance Marinade	1 tbsp	10	0	0	0
Eden					
Ponzu Sauce	1 tbsp	5	0	0	0
Emeril's					
Marinade Hickory Maple Chipotle	1 tbsp	35	3	–	–
Marinade Lemon Rosemary Gaaahlic	1 tbsp	70	8	1	–
Marinade Orange Herb Poppyseed	1 tbsp	150	15	2	–
Steak Sauce	1 tbsp	20	0	0	0
Fage					
Tzatziki	2 tbsp	30	2	1	0
Frank's					
Buffalo Wing	1 tbsp	5	0	0	0
RedHot Chile & Lime	1 tsp	0	0	0	0
RedHot Original Cayenne Pepper	1 tsp	0	0	0	0
RedHot X-tra Hot	1 tsp	0	0	0	0
French's					
Worchestershire	1 tsp	0	0	0	0
Good Clean Food					
Simmer Sauce Balsamic Mushroom	⅜ cup (3 oz)	100	6	1	–
Simmer Sauce Cacciatore	⅜ cup (3 oz)	70	4	1	–
Simmer Sauce Creole	⅜ cup (3 oz)	45	2	1	–
Simmer Sauce Dill	⅜ cup (3 oz)	60	4	1	–

FOOD	PORTION	CALS	FAT	SAT FAT	TRANS FAT
Simmer Sauce French Tarragon	⅜ cup (3 oz)	90	6	1	–
Simmer Sauce Mediterranean	⅜ cup (3 oz)	50	3	–	–
Gringo Billy's					
Chipotle Dipping & Grilling Sauce	1 tsp	5	0	0	0
House Of Tsang					
General Tsao	1 tsp	45	1	0	–
Hoisin	1 tsp	15	0	0	0
Kobe Steak Grill	1 tbsp	50	4	1	–
Korean Teriyaki Stir Fry	1 tbsp	35	2	0	–
Peanut Sauce Bangkok Padang	1 tbsp	45	3	1	–
Spicy Brown Bean	1 tbsp	15	0	0	0
Sweet & Sour	1 tbsp	35	0	0	0
Sweet Ginger Sesame	1 tbsp	40	1	0	–
Thai Peanut	1 tbsp	50	3	1	–
Jok'n'Al					
Cocktail	¼ cup	29	0	0	0
Plum	1 tbsp	10	0	0	0
Ken's					
Marinade Herb & Garlic	1 tbsp	20	1	0	0
Marinade Lemon & Pepper	1 tbsp	10	0	0	0
Marinade Teriyaki	1 tbsp	20	0	0	0
Kikkoman					
Teriyaki	1 tbsp	15	0	0	0
Knorr					
Alfredo Mix as prep	2 oz	60	3	2	1
Bearnaise Mix as prep	2 oz	35	1	tr	tr
Curry Indian Madras	1 oz	30	2	2	tr
Curry Thai	1 oz	35	3	2	0
Demi-Glace Mix as prep	2 oz	30	1	tr	tr
Green Peppercorn Mix as prep	2 oz	35	1	tr	tr
Hollandaise Mix as prep	2 oz	35	1	tr	tr
Mango Habanero	1 oz	20	0	0	0
Sweet Red Chili	1 oz	80	0	0	0
White Mix as prep	2 oz	20	1	tr	tr
Las Palmas					
Enchilada Green	¼ cup	25	2	0	0
Enchilada Mild	¼ cup	20	1	0	0
Red Chili	¼ cup	20	1	0	0

FOOD	PORTION	CALS	FAT	SAT FAT	TRANS FAT
Latino Chef					
Chimichurri Sun Dried Tomato	2 tbsp	120	10	1	0
Sofrito	2 tbsp	20	1	–	–
Lea & Perrins					
Worcestershire	1 tsp	5	0	0	0
Lee Kum Kee					
Plum Sauce	2 tbsp	100	0	0	0
Lollipop Tree					
Grilling & Glazing Chipotle	1 tbsp	50	0	0	0
Grilling & Glazing Mango Garlic	2 tbsp	60	0	0	0
Matouk's					
Calypso	1 tsp	0	0	0	0
Flambeau Sauce	1 tsp	0	0	0	0
Milo's					
Simmer Sauce Bombay Cabernet	3 oz	35	0	0	0
Mrs. Dash					
10 Minute Marinade Lemon Herb Peppercorn	1 tbsp	25	2	–	–
10 Minute Marinade Mesquite Grille	1 tbsp	25	2	–	–
10 Minute Marinade Southwestern Chipotle	1 tbsp	20	2	–	–
10 Minute Marinade Zesty Garlic Herb	1 tbsp	25	2	–	–
Nando's					
Curry Coconut	¼ cup	71	5	1	–
Fresh Lemon	¼ cup	61	5	1	–
Marinade Lime & Cilantro	1 tbsp	27	2	0	–
Marinade Sundried Tomato	1 tbsp	15	1	0	–
Peri-Peri Pepper Extra Hot	1 oz	17	1	tr	–
Peri-Peri Pepper Garlic	1 oz	12	1	tr	–
Peri-Peri Pepper Hot	1 oz	16	1	tr	–
Peri-Peri Pepper Wild Herb	1 oz	14	1	tr	–
Roasted Red	¼ cup	70	5	0	–
Sweet Apricot	¼ cup	51	0	0	0
Newman's Own					
Fra Diavolo	½ cup	70	3	0	–
Steak Sauce	1 tbsp	20	1	0	–

FOOD	PORTION	CALS	FAT	SAT FAT	TRANS FAT
Old El Paso					
Enchilada Mild	¼ cup	25	1	0	0
Ortega					
Enchilada	¼ cup	15	1	0	0
Taco	1 tbsp	10	0	0	0
Pace					
Taco Sauce Green	1 tbsp	5	0	0	0
Taco Sauce Red	2 tbsp	10	0	0	0
Patak's					
Dopiaza	½ cup	90	5	0	–
Jalfrezi Sweet Peppers & Coconut	½ cup	140	8	3	–
Korma Rich Creamy Coconut	½ cup	240	20	12	–
Rogan Josh Spicy Tomato & Cardamom	½ cup	90	4	0	–
Tikka Masala Tangy Lemon & Cilantro	½ cup	120	8	1	–
Road's End Organics					
Alfredo Style Dairy Free Gluten Free	⅓ pkg	35	0	0	0
Cheddar Style Dairy Free	⅓ pkg	35	0	0	0
Robert Rothchild Farm					
Anne Mae's Smoky Sweet Chipotle	2 tbsp	35	0	0	0
San-J					
Japanese Steak	1 tbsp	13	0	0	0
Sweet & Tangy	1 tbsp	50	0	0	0
Szechuan	1 tsp	5	0	0	0
Teriyaki	1 tbsp	10	0	0	0
Thai Peanut	2 tbsp	70	3	–	–
South Beach					
Steak Sauce	1 tbsp	5	0	0	0
Steel's					
Sugar Free Cocktail w/ Dill & Lemon	¼ cup	36	0	0	0
Sugar Free Hoisin	2 tbsp	15	0	0	0
Sugar Free Mango Curry	1 tbsp	13	0	0	0
Sugar Free Peanut Sauce	1 tbsp	34	2	–	–
Sugar Free Sweet & Sour	2 tbsp	10	0	0	0

FOOD	PORTION	CALS	FAT	SAT FAT	TRANS FAT
Tabasco					
Pepper Sauce	1 tsp	0	0	0	0
The Wizard's					
Organic Worcestershire Vegetarian Wheat Free	1 tsp	0	0	0	0
Ty Ling					
Duck	2 tbsp	70	0	0	0
Walden Farms					
Calorie Free Scampi Sauce	2 tbsp	0	0	0	0
Calorie Free Seafood Sauce	1 tbsp	0	0	0	0
WildWood					
Aioli	1 tbsp	80	9	1	0
Pesto Basil & Pine Nuts	¼ cup	230	23	4	0
Wingers					
Hotter Than Hot	1 tsp	0	0	0	0
TAKE-OUT					
cucumber yogurt sauce	1½ tbsp	20	0	0	0
SAUERKRAUT					
canned	½ cup	22	tr	tr	–
B&G					
Sauerkraut	2 tbsp (1 oz)	6	0	0	0
Boar's Head					
Sauerkraut	2 tbsp (1 oz)	5	0	0	0
Del Monte					
Bavarian Style	2 tbsp	15	0	0	0
Sauerkraut	2 tbsp	0	0	0	0
Eden					
Organic	½ cup	25	0	0	0
Hebrew National					
Sauerkraut	2 tbsp	5	0	0	0
S&W					
Canned	2 tbsp (1 oz)	5	0	0	0
Red Cabbage	2 tbsp (1 oz)	15	0	0	0
Silver Floss					
Sauerkraut	½ cup	20	0	0	0
SAUSAGE					
beef & pork	1 link (2.3 oz)	196	17	4	–
beef & pork w/ cheddar cheese	1 link (2.7 oz)	228	20	7	–
bierschinken	3.5 oz	174	11	–	–

FOOD	PORTION	CALS	FAT	SAT FAT	TRANS FAT
bierwurst	3.5 oz	258	21	–	–
blutwurst uncooked	3.5 oz	424	39	–	–
bockwurst	3.5 oz	276	25	–	–
bratwurst pork cooked	1 link (2.5 oz)	226	19	7	–
brotwurst pork & beef	1 link (2.5 oz)	226	19	7	–
chipolata	3.5 oz	342	32	12	–
chorizo	1 link (2.1 oz)	273	23	8	–
fleischwurst	3.5 oz	305	29	–	–
free range chicken breakfast	2 links (2.7 oz)	110	6	1	–
gelbwurst uncooked	3.5 oz	363	33	–	–
italian pork cooked	1 (2.4 oz)	230	18	6	–
jagdwurst	3.5 oz	211	16	–	–
knockwurst pork & beef	1 (2.5 oz)	221	20	7	–
mettwurst uncooked	3.5 oz	483	45	–	–
plockwurst uncooked	3.5 oz	312	45	–	–
polish kielbasa	2 oz	127	10	3	–
pork cooked	2 links (1.7 oz)	163	14	4	–
regensburger uncooked	3.5 oz	354	31	–	–
turkey italian smoked	1 (2 oz)	88	5	–	–
vienna canned	1 can (4 oz)	260	22	8	–
vienna canned	1 link (0.5 oz)	37	3	1	–
weisswurst uncooked	3.5 oz	305	27	–	–
zungenwurst (tongue)	3.5 oz	285	24	–	–
Al Fresco					
Apple Maple	1 (1.2 oz)	70	4	1	0
Buffalo Style	1 (3 oz)	160	8	3	0
Country Style	1 (1.2 oz)	60	4	1	0
Italian Sweet	1 (3 oz)	170	8	2	0
Roasted Garlic	1 (3 oz)	170	8	2	0
Spicy Jalapeno	1 (3 oz)	120	7	2	0
Sundried Tomato & Basil	1 (3 oz)	180	8	2	0
Sweet Apple	1 (3 oz)	160	8	3	0
Teriyaki Ginger	1 (3 oz)	180	8	2	0
Wild Blueberry	1 (1.2 oz)	90	4	1	0
Armour					
Brown'N Serve Lite Original	3	120	8	3	–
Brown'N Serve Turkey	3 links	120	8	3	–
Banquet					
Brown 'N Serve Lite Original	3 (2.1 oz)	120	9	3	0
Brown'N Serve Lite Maple	3 (2 oz)	130	9	3	0

FOOD	PORTION	CALS	FAT	SAT FAT	TRANS FAT
Bilinski's					
Chicken Bratwurst w/ Wild Rice	1 (2 oz)	70	2	1	–
Chicken Cajun-Style Andouille	2 oz	80	4	2	–
Chicken Italian w/ Peppers	1 (2 oz)	70	4	1	–
Chicken w/ Apples & Chardonnay	2 oz	70	6	2	–
Chicken w/ Cilantro	2 oz	70	4	1	–
Chicken w/ Jalapenos	2 oz	70	4	2	–
Chicken w/ Pesto	2 oz	90	5	2	–
Chicken w/ Spinach	2 oz	70	4	1	–
Chicken w/ Sun-Dried Tomato	2 oz	70	4	2	–
Boar's Head					
Bratwurst	1 (4 oz)	300	25	11	–
Hot Smoked	1 (3.2 oz)	250	22	9	–
Kielbasa	2 oz	120	10	4	–
Knockwurst Beef	1 (4 oz)	310	27	11	–
Healthy Ones					
Smoked	2 oz	80	3	1	0
Hebrew National					
Knockwurst Beef	1 (3 oz)	260	24	11	–
Honeysuckle White					
Turkey Roll Mild Italian	2.5 oz	100	5	2	–
Jennie-O					
Italian Hot	1 (3.9 oz)	160	10	3	–
Turkey Italian Sweet	1 link (3.9 oz)	160	10	3	–
Johnsonville					
Bratwurst Original	1 (3 oz)	270	22	8	0
Breakfast Patty Original	2 (2 oz)	180	15	5	0
Grilling Chorizo	1 (3 oz)	280	22	8	0
Italian Mild	1 (3 oz)	270	22	9	0
Original Summer	2 (2 oz)	170	15	6	0
Polish	1 (2.7 oz)	240	21	9	0
Pork	2 oz	180	15	5	0
Smoked Turkey	1 (3 oz)	110	6	2	0
Jones					
Light 50% Less Fat	2 (1.6 oz)	110	8	3	0
Little Pork	3	190	17	7	–
Murray's					
Chicken Hot Italian	3 oz	130	7	2	–
Chicken Spinach & Garlic	3 oz	100	5	2	–

FOOD	PORTION	CALS	FAT	SAT FAT	TRANS FAT
Chicken Sun Dried Tomato	3 oz	110	5	2	–
Chicken Sweet Italian	3 oz	130	7	2	–
Organic Prairie					
Bratwurst Pork	1 (3 oz)	210	19	6	–
Perdue					
Hot Italian Turkey Cooked	1 link (2.4 oz)	150	9	3	–
Sweet Italian Turkey Cooked	1 link (2.4 oz)	150	9	3	–
Shady Brook					
Turkey Breakfast	1 (2.3 oz)	80	4	2	–
Turkey Sweet Italian	1 (2.5 oz)	110	7	2	–
Turkey Bratwurt	3 oz	160	9	3	–
Soy Lean					
Pork Breakfast Patty	1 (2 oz)	75	3	1	–
Wellshire					
Andouille	1 link (3 oz)	197	9	4	–
Andouille Turkey	2 oz	59	3	2	–
Chorizo	1 piece (2 oz)	130	6	2	–
Chorizo Dried	1 oz	100	8	2	–
Italian Turkey Mild	1 link (2 oz)	70	4	0	–
Kielbasa Polska	1 piece (2 oz)	130	6	2	–
Kielbasa Turkey	1 piece (2 oz)	59	3	2	0
Turkey Maple Breakfast	1 link (2 oz)	70	4	0	–

SAUSAGE DISHES
TAKE-OUT

italian sausage w/ peppers & onions	1 cup	210	11	–	–
sausage roll	1 (2.3 oz)	311	24	–	–

SAUSAGE SUBSTITUTES

meatless	1 link (0.9 oz)	64	5	1	–
meatless	1 patty (1.3 oz)	98	7	1	–
Boca					
Bratwurst	1 (2.5 oz)	140	7	1	–
Breakfast Patties	1 (1.3 oz)	60	3	0	0
Breakfast Links	2 (1.6 oz)	70	3	1	0
Italian	1 (2.5 oz)	130	6	1	0
Gardenburger					
Veggie Breakfast	1 patty (1.5 oz)	45	3	0	0
Lightlife					
Gimme Lean	2 oz	50	0	0	0

FOOD	PORTION	CALS	FAT	SAT FAT	TRANS FAT
Smart Brats	1 (2 oz)	120	5	0	–
Smart Links Breakfast	2 (2 oz)	100	4	1	–
Smart Links Italian	1 (2 oz)	120	5	1	–
Smart Menu Breakfast Patty	1	45	2	0	–
Morningstar Farms					
Breakfast Links	2	60	2	1	–
Breakfast Patties	1 (1.3 oz)	80	3	1	0
Quorn					
Links	2 (1.6 oz)	70	3	0	–
Tofurky					
Turkey Beerbrats	1 (3.5 oz)	280	16	1	0
Turkey Breakfast Links	1 (1.6 oz)	130	6	0	0
Turkey Italian Sweet	1 (3.5 oz)	280	13	2	0
Turkey Kielbasa	1 (3.5 oz)	240	12	1	0
Worthington					
Saucettes Breakfast Links	1 (1.3 oz)	90	6	1	0
Yves					
Veggie Brats Classic	1 (3.3 oz)	160	5	0	0
SAVORY					
ground	1 tsp	4	tr	tr	0
SCALLOP					
raw	3 oz	75	1	tr	–
Mrs. Paul's					
Fried	13 (3.7 oz)	260	11	4	0
TAKE-OUT					
breaded & fried	2 lg	67	3	1	–
SCONE					
Finnegan's					
Irish Raisin	1 (2 oz)	170	4	1	–
King Arthur					
Cranberry Orange as prep	1	248	8	5	–
English Cream Tea Scone not prep	⅓ cup	180	1	0	–
TAKE-OUT					
apricot	1	232	7	–	–
blueberry	1 (3 oz)	270	9	4	–
cheese	1 (3.5 oz)	364	18	–	–
orange poppy	1 (3 oz)	260	6	4	–

FOOD	PORTION	CALS	FAT	SAT FAT	TRANS FAT
plain	1 (3.5 oz)	362	14	–	–
raisin	1 (3 oz)	270	8	3	–

SCUP
fresh baked	3 oz	115	3	–	–

SEA BASS (see BASS)

SEA CUCUMBER
dried	1 oz	74	1	–	–
fresh	1 oz	20	tr	–	–

SEA URCHIN
canned	1 oz	39	1	–	–
fresh	1 oz	36	1	–	–
roe paste	1 tbsp	19	tr	–	–

SEATROUT (see TROUT)

SEAWEED
agar dried	1 oz	87	tr	tr	–
agar fresh	1 oz	tr	tr	tr	–
hijiki dried	1 tbsp	9	0	0	0
irishmoss fresh	1 oz	14	tr	tr	–
kelp fresh	1 oz	12	tr	tr	–
kombu fresh	1 oz	12	tr	tr	–
laver fresh	1 oz	10	tr	tr	–
nori fresh	1 oz	10	tr	tr	–
nori sheet dried	1 (8 x 8 in)	5	0	0	0
seahair dried	1 tbsp	13	0	0	0
spirulina dried	1 oz	83	2	1	–
spirulina fresh	1 oz	7	tr	tr	–
tangle fresh	1 oz	12	tr	tr	–
wakame fresh	1 oz	13	tr	tr	–
Eden					
Agar Agar Bars	1 bar (7 g)	25	0	0	0
Agar Agar Flakes	1 tbsp	0	0	0	0
Arame Wild	½ cup	30	0	0	0
Hiziki Wild	½ cup	30	0	0	0
Kombu Wild	½ piece (3.3 g)	5	0	0	0
Nori Sheets	1 (2.5 g)	10	0	0	0
Organic Dulse Flakes	1 tsp	3	0	0	0

FOOD	PORTION	CALS	FAT	SAT FAT	TRANS FAT
Maine Coast					
Organic Alaria Whole Leaf	⅓ cup	18	tr	–	0
Organic Dulse Whole Leaf	½ cup	19	tr	–	0
Organic Kelp Whole Leaf	⅓ cup	17	tr	–	0
Organic Laver Whole Leaf	⅓ cup	22	tr	–	0
Organic Dulse Granules	1 tsp	6	0	0	0
Organic Kelp Granules	½ tsp	5	0	0	0
SEITAN (see WHEAT)					
SEMOLINA					
dry	1 cup (5.9 oz)	601	2	tr	–
SESAME					
seeds	1 tsp	16	2	–	–
sesame butter	1 tbsp	95	8	1	–
sesame crunch candy	1 oz	146	9	1	–
sesame crunch candy	20 pieces (1.2 oz)	181	12	2	–
tahini from roasted & toasted kernels	1 tbsp	89	8	1	–
tahini from stone ground kernels	1 tbsp	86	7	1	–
tahini from unroasted kernels	1 tbsp	85	8	1	–
Arrowhead Mills					
Organic Tahini	2 tbsp	190	18	3	0
Organic Seeds	¼ cup	210	19	3	0
Mrs. May's					
Black Sesame Crunch	1 oz	165	11	2	0
Peloponnese					
Tahini	1 tbsp	100	9	1	–
Sabra					
Tahini Sauce Taratore	1 oz	80	7	0	–
SESBANIA					
flower	1	1	0	0	0
flowers	1 cup	5	tr	–	0
flowers cooked	1 cup	23	tr	–	0
SHAD					
american baked	3 oz	214	15	–	–
cooked	1 oz	55	3	1	0
roe baked w/ butter & lemon	1 oz	36	1	–	–

FOOD	PORTION	CALS	FAT	SAT FAT	TRANS FAT
SHALLOTS (see ONION)					
SHARK					
fin dried	1 oz	32	tr	–	–
raw	3 oz	111	4	1	–
TAKE-OUT					
batter-dipped & fried	3 oz	194	12	3	–
SHEEPSHEAD FISH					
cooked	1 fillet (6.5 oz)	234	3	1	–
cooked	3 oz	107	1	tr	–
raw	3 oz	92	2	1	–
SHELLFISH (see individual names, SHELLFISH SUBSTITUTES)					
SHELLFISH SUBSTITUTES					
crab imitation	1 cup (4.4 oz)	144	1	tr	–
scallop imitation	3 oz	84	tr	–	–
shrimp imitation	3 oz	86	1	–	–
surimi	1 oz	28	tr	–	–
surimi	3 oz	84	1	–	–
Chicken Of The Sea					
Imitation Crab	1 pkg (2.5 oz)	40	0	0	0
Louis Kemp					
Crab Delights	½ cup (3 oz)	80	0	0	0
Crab Delights Chunk Style	½ cup (3 oz)	80	0	0	0
Crab Delights Easy Shred	½ cup (3 oz)	80	0	0	0
Crab Delights Leg Style	½ cup (3 oz)	80	0	0	0
Lobster Delights Chunk or Salad Style	½ cup (3 oz)	80	0	0	0
Scallop Delights Bay Style	½ cup (3 oz)	80	0	0	0
TAKE-OUT					
crab salad	1 cup	395	26	4	–
SHELLIE BEANS					
canned	½ cup	37	tr	tr	–
SHERBET					
orange	1 bar (2.75 oz)	91	1	1	–
orange	½ cup (4 oz)	132	2	1	–
orange	½ gal	2158	31	19	–

FOOD	PORTION	CALS	FAT	SAT FAT	TRANS FAT
Blue Bunny					
Cool Tubes Orange Sherbet	1 (3 oz)	110	1	1	0
Lime	½ cup	110	0	0	0
Rainbow	½ cup	110	0	0	0
Raspberry	½ cup	110	0	0	0
Breyers					
Orange	½ cup	120	2	1	–
Rainbow	½ cup	120	2	1	–
Hola Fruta					
Margarita	½ cup	140	1	1	0
Peach	½ cup	130	1	1	0
Pomegranate	½ cup	140	1	1	0
Hood					
Orange Burst	½ cup	120	1	1	0
Turkey Hill					
Fruit Rainbow	½ cup	120	1	–	–
Orange Grove	½ cup	120	1	–	–
SHRIMP					
CANNED					
canned	1 can (6 oz)	136	2	tr	0
chinese shrimp paste	1 tbsp	46	0	0	0
Bumble Bee					
Broken Shrimp	¼ cup	40	0	0	0
Medium or Large or Jumbo	¼ cup	40	0	0	0
Small	¼ cup	40	0	0	0
Tiny	¼ cup	40	0	0	0
Chicken Of The Sea					
Tiny Small or Medium	½ can (2 oz)	45	1	0	–
DRIED					
dried	10	15	tr	tr	0
FRESH					
broiled	6 med	46	2	tr	0
steamed	6 med	41	1	tr	0
FROZEN					
Chicken Of The Sea					
Cooked Large Peeled Deveined Tail On	3 oz	80	1	0	–
Large Raw Cleaned Tail Off	4 oz	120	2	0	–

FOOD	PORTION	CALS	FAT	SAT FAT	TRANS FAT
Contessa					
Orange Shrimp	11–13 (6 oz)	250	8	2	0
Ragin' Cajun	8–10 (4 oz)	170	10	3	3
Shrimp Scampi	8–10 (4 oz)	290	27	7	4
Margaritaville					
Calypso Coconut + Sauce	5 pieces	350	17	7	–
Island Lime	6 pieces	130	7	3	–
Jammin' Jerk	7 pieces	140	7	4	–
Paradise Cocktail + Sauce	5 pieces	85	0	0	0
Sunset Scampi	1 serv (½ pkg)	270	20	6	–
Surfside Skewers + Sauce	2 skewers	105	1	0	–
Mrs. Paul's					
Butterfly	7 (4 oz)	250	11	4	0
Phillips Seafood					
Breaded Shrimp	5 pieces	230	13	3	0
Buffalo Shrimp	5 pieces	260	13	3	0
Coconut Shrimp	5 pieces	330	20	7	0
Crab Stuffed Shrimp	3 pieces	160	10	2	0
Van de Kamp's					
Battered	6 (4 oz)	200	6	2	0
Breaded Popcorn	20 (4 oz)	260	11	5	0
TAKE-OUT					
breaded & fried	6 med (2.3 oz)	162	8	2	–
cocktail w/ sauce	4 shrimp	87	1	tr	0
curried	1 cup	295	14	4	–
gingered	4	80	tr	tr	–
jambalaya	1 cup	309	9	2	–
scampi	1 cup	310	22	13	–
shrimp newburg	1 serv (6.4 oz)	456	37	22	–
shrimp salad	¾ cup	212	12	2	–
shrimp w/ crab stuffing	5	158	8	2	–
SMELT					
rainbow cooked	3 oz	106	3	tr	–
rainbow raw	3 oz	83	2	tr	–

SMOOTHIES (*see also* FRUIT DRINKS, YOGURT DRINKS)

FOOD	PORTION	CALS	FAT	SAT FAT	TRANS FAT
8th Continent					
Refresher Orange Pineapple Banana	8 oz	150	0	0	0
Refresher Strawberry Banana	8 oz	150	0	0	0

FOOD	PORTION	CALS	FAT	SAT FAT	TRANS FAT
Bolthouse Farms					
Green Goodness	8 oz	140	0	0	0
Mango Lemonade	8 oz	120	0	0	0
Passion Fruit Apple Carrot Juice	8 oz	120	0	0	0
Strawberry Banana Fruit	8 oz	124	0	0	0
C&W					
Berry Blend	½ cup	90	2	1	0
Peach	½ cup	80	2	1	0
E4B					
100% Fruit Puree Blueberry Raspberry	4 oz	70	0	0	0
100% Fruit Puree Kiwi	4 oz	70	0	0	0
100% Fruit Puree Mango	4 oz	70	0	0	0
100% Fruit Puree Pear Caramel	4 oz	70	0	0	0
100% Fruit Puree Strawberry Banana	4 oz	70	0	0	0
Horizon Organic					
Tropical Punch	1 bottle (6.2 oz)	120	0	0	0
Jammin' Juice					
Mambo Mango	6 oz	92	0	0	0
C-Beta Carrot	6 oz	96	0	0	0
Ginger Party	6 oz	6	0	0	0
Guanabana Limbo	6 oz	78	0	0	0
Pure Passion	6 oz	78	0	0	0
Razz-Ade	6 oz	89	0	0	0
Kidz Dream					
Orange Cream	1 box	120	2	0	0
LightFull					
Satiety Smoothie Cafe Latte	1 (11 oz)	90	1	0	0
Satiety Smoothie Chocolate Fudge	1 (11 oz)	90	1	0	0
Satiety Smoothie Peaches & Cream	1 (11 oz)	100	0	0	0
Satiety Smoothie Strawberries & Cream	1 (11 oz)	90	0	0	0
Luna					
Berry Pomegranate	1 pkg	140	2	1	0
Orange Blossom	1 pkg	130	2	1	0
Vanilla Macadamia	1 pkg	150	4	1	0

FOOD	PORTION	CALS	FAT	SAT FAT	TRANS FAT
Naked Juice					
Chocolate Karma	8 oz	190	3	1	0
Vanilla Chai	8 oz	170	3	1	0
Nutiva					
Organic HempShake Amazon Acai not prep	4 tbsp	100	3	0	0
Organic HempShake Chocolate not prep	4 tbsp	80	2	tr	0
Odwalla					
Bluberry B Monster	8 oz	140	0	0	0
Citrus C Monster	8 oz	150	0	0	0
Mango Tango	8 oz	150	1	1	0
Sambazon					
Acai Amazon Cherry	8 oz	156	0	0	0
Acai Mango Banana	8 oz	190	5	1	0
Acai Mango Uprising	8 oz	190	5	1	0
Acai Protein Warrior Chocolate	8 oz	215	6	1	–
Acai Protein Warrior Vanilla	8 oz	215	6	1	0
Acai Shaman's Immunity	8 oz	90	0	0	0
Acai Soy Energy	8 oz	210	6	1	0
Acai Strawberry Sensation	8 oz	210	4	1	0
Acai Supergreens Revolution	8 oz	200	4	1	0
Organic Acai	1 bottle	155	3	1	0
Smooze					
Mango + Coconut	1 box (8.5 oz)	250	10	10	0
Passion Fruit + Coconut	1 box (8.5 oz)	225	8	8	0
Pineapple + Coconut	1 box (8.5 oz)	200	8	8	0
Soy Blendz					
Mango Orange Dream	1 bottle (10 oz)	220	3	1	–
Mixed Berry Medley	1 bottle (10 oz)	210	3	1	–
Orange Citrus Splash	1 bottle (10 oz)	220	4	1	–
Strawberry Banana Blast	1 bottle (10 oz)	230	3	0	–
Soy Fusion					
Berry	1 box (8.45 oz)	120	1	–	–
Matcha Green Tea	1 box (8.45 oz)	110	2	–	–
Tropicana					
Fruit Smoothie Mixed Berry	1 bottle (11 oz)	220	0	0	0
Fruit Smoothie Tropical Fruit	1 bottle (11 oz)	220	0	0	0
V8					
Splash Tropical Colada	8 oz	100	0	0	0

FOOD	PORTION	CALS	FAT	SAT FAT	TRANS FAT
WholeSoy & Co.					
Organic Soy Peach	8 oz	210	3	0	–
Organic Soy Raspberry	8 oz	210	3	0	–
Organic Soy Strawberry	8 oz	210	3	0	–
Yo On The Go					
All Flavors	1 box (8 oz)	180	3	2	0
Yoplait					
Go-Gurt All Fruit Flavors	1 bottle (5 oz)	120	1	0	0
Light All Flavors	1 bottle (8.3 oz)	90	0	0	0
Smoothie All Flavors	1 bottle (8.3 oz)	220	3	2	0
SNACKS					
cheese puffs	1 oz	157	10	2	–
corn puffs cheese	1 bag (8 oz)	1256	78	15	–
corn twists cheese	1 bag (8 oz)	1256	78	15	–
corn twists cheese	1 oz	157	10	2	–
oriental mix	1 oz	155	12	–	–
pork skins	1 oz	154	9	3	–
pork skins barbecue	1 oz	152	9	3	–
Baken-ets					
Fried Pork Skins	9 pieces	80	5	3	0
Fried Pork Skins Hot'n Spicy	9 pieces	80	5	2	0
Fried Pork Skins Sweet & Tangy BBQ	9 pieces	80	5	3	0
Pork Cracklins	8 pieces	90	6	2	–
Pork Cracklins Hot'n Spicy	8 pieces	80	5	2	–
Bowlby's					
Bits Almond	½ cup	100	19	3	–
Bits Pecan	½ cup	200	19	3	–
Bits Ranch	½ cup	170	16	2	–
Bits Salsa	½ cup	170	16	2	–
Bits Sour Cream Onion & Dill	½ cup	170	16	2	–
Bits'N'Pops	¾ cup	130	7	3	–
Bugles					
Baked Original	1⅓ cup	130	4	1	–
Chile Con Queso	1⅓ cups	160	9	7	–
Nacho	1½ cups	160	9	7	–
Original	1½ cups	160	9	8	–
Smokin'BBQ	1⅓ cups	150	8	7	–

FOOD	PORTION	CALS	FAT	SAT FAT	TRANS FAT
Carole's					
Soycrunch Cinnamon & Raisins	½ cup	110	1	0	–
Soycrunch Original	½ cup	120	2	0	–
Soycrunch Toffee	½ cup	110	2	0	–
Cheetos					
Asteriods Go Snack	¾ cup (1 oz)	160	10	2	0
Baked Crunchy	34 pieces (1 oz)	130	5	1	0
Crunchy	1 pkg (1.25 oz)	200	13	3	0
Natural White Cheddar	32 pieces (1 oz)	150	8	1	0
Puffs	13 pieces (1 oz)	160	10	2	0
Twisted	7 pieces (1 oz)	160	10	2	0
Chester's					
Puffcorn Butter	3 cups	160	11	2	0
Puffcorn Cheese	3 cups	160	11	2	0
Chex Mix					
Cheddar	⅔ cup	140	5	1	–
Hot 'N Spicy	⅔ cup	130	5	1	–
Nacho Fiesta	⅔ cup	120	4	1	–
Party Blend Bold	⅔ cup	140	6	1	–
Peanut Lovers	⅔ cup	140	6	1	–
Traditional	⅔ cup	130	4	1	–
Funyuns					
Mini Onion Rings Go Snacks	1 pkg	260	14	2	0
Onion Rings	13 pieces	140	7	1	0
Garden Of Eatin'					
Organic Baked Cheese Puffs	32 pieces	150	10	1	0
Organic Baked Chunchitos	35 pieces	140	7	1	0
Good Sense					
Snack Mix Cajun Corn 'N Sesame	¼ cup	150	8	1	–
Gram's Gourmet					
Crunchies Pork Rinds	⅛ pkg (0.5 oz)	70	5	2	–
Kangaroo					
Pita Snackers Crispy Cinnamon	10 pieces (1 oz)	90	2	0	–
Pita Snackers Sea Salt	10 pieces (1 oz)	90	2	0	–
Maranatha					
Organic Delight	¼ cup	150	10	2	–
Munchies					
Snack Mix Flamin' Hot	1 oz	140	6	1	–
Snack Mix Kids	1 oz	130	4	1	0

FOOD	PORTION	CALS	FAT	SAT FAT	TRANS FAT
Pumpkorn					
Caramel	⅓ cup	150	11	2	–
Chili	⅓ cup	150	11	2	–
Curry	⅓ cup	150	11	2	–
Maple Vanilla	⅓ cup	150	11	2	–
Mesquite	⅓ cup	150	11	2	–
Original	⅓ cup	150	11	2	–
Sabritones					
Chile & Lime	23 pieces	150	10	3	–
Snyder's Of Hanover					
CheddAirs	1 oz	130	5	1	0
MultiGrain Cheese Puffs	1 oz	130	6	1	0
Tumaro's					
Organic Krispy Crunchy Puffs Cheddar	22	120	3	0	–
Organic Krispy Crunchy Puffs Natural Corn	22	120	2	0	–
Organic Krispy Crunchy Puffs Ranch & Herb	22	130	4	0	–
Organic Krispy Crunchy Puffs Tangy BBQ	22	120	4	0	–
Utz					
Cheese Balls	50 (1 oz)	150	9	3	0
Cheese Curls	18 (1 oz)	150	9	3	0
Onion Rings	41 (1 oz)	130	5	1	0
Party Mix	1 oz	150	7	1	0
Pork Cracklins	0.5 oz	90	7	3	0
Pork Rinds Original	0.5 oz	80	5	2	0
Wise					
Cheez Doodles Crunchy	1 pkg (1 oz)	150	9	3	0
Cheese Doodles Crunchy Reduced Fat	1 oz	130	5	2	0
Cheez Doodles Puffed	1 pkg (0.7 oz)	110	6	2	0
Doodle O's	1 oz	160	11	3	0
Onion Rings	1 oz	140	6	2	0
Pork Rinds Original	1 oz	90	6	2	–
SNAIL					
cooked	3 oz	233	1	tr	–
raw	3 oz	117	tr	tr	–

FOOD	PORTION	CALS	FAT	SAT FAT	TRANS FAT
TAKE-OUT					
escargot cooked	5	25	0	0	0
SNAKE					
fresh	3 oz	78	tr	–	–
SNAPPER					
cooked	1 fillet (6 oz)	217	3	1	–
cooked	3 oz	109	1	tr	–
raw	3 oz	85	1	tr	–
SODA					
club	12 oz	0	0	0	0
cola	12 oz	151	tr	–	–
cream	12 oz	191	0	0	0
diet cola	12 oz	2	0	0	0
ginger ale	12 oz	124	0	–	0
grape	12 oz	161	0	0	0
lemon lime	12 oz	149	0	0	0
orange	12 oz	177	0	0	0
pepper type	12 oz	151	tr	–	–
quinine	12 oz	125	0	0	0
root beer	12 oz	152	0	0	0
shirley temple	1 serv	159	0	0	0
tonic water	12 oz	125	0	0	0
7 Up					
Diet	8 oz	0	0	0	0
Original	8 oz	100	0	0	0
Plus	12 oz	10	0	0	0
A&W					
Root Beer	12 oz	170	0	0	0
AJ Stephans					
Birch Beer	1 bottle	170	0	0	0
Black Cherry	1 bottle	180	0	0	0
Cream	1 bottle	170	0	0	0
Jamaican Style Ginger Beer	1 bottle	170	0	0	0
Lemon & Lime	1 bottle	190	0	0	0
Olde Style Root Beer	1 bottle	170	0	0	0
Barq's					
Diet French Vanilla Creme	8 oz	1	0	0	0
Diet Red Creme	8 oz	4	0	0	0

FOOD	PORTION	CALS	FAT	SAT FAT	TRANS FAT
Diet Root Beer	8 oz	1	0	0	0
Floatz	8 oz	127	0	0	0
French Vanilla Creme	8 oz	112	0	0	0
Red Creme	8 oz	115	0	0	0
Root Beer	8 oz	111	0	0	0
Big Red					
Vanilla Float	1 can	180	0	0	0
Blumers					
Black Cherry	12 oz	138	0	0	0
Blueberry Cream	12 oz	190	0	0	0
Cream	12 oz	181	0	0	0
Orange Cream	12 oz	187	0	0	0
Root Beer	12 oz	190	0	0	0
Bong Water					
Chronic Tonic	12 oz	144	0	0	0
Cottonmouth Quencher	12 oz	165	0	0	0
Green Dreams	12 oz	165	0	0	0
Purple Haze	12 oz	165	0	0	0
Briar's					
Black Cherry	12 oz	180	0	0	0
Cream	12 oz	180	0	0	0
Diet Root Beer	8 oz	4	0	0	0
Orange Cream	8 oz	120	0	0	0
Red Birch	8 oz	104	0	0	0
Root Beer	12 oz	168	0	0	0
Bubble Yum					
All Flavors	8 oz	110	0	0	0
Canada Dry					
Ginger Ale	12 oz	140	0	0	0
Cape Cod Dry					
Cranberry	8 oz	120	0	0	0
Diet Cranberry	8 oz	10	0	0	0
Capt'n Eli's					
Root Beer	8 oz	165	0	0	0
Carver's					
Ginger Ale	8 oz	94	0	0	0
Chronic 187					
Orange	12 oz	300	0	0	0
Coca-Cola					
Blak	8 oz	46	0	0	0

FOOD	PORTION	CALS	FAT	SAT FAT	TRANS FAT
C2	8 oz	45	0	0	0
Classic	8 oz	97	0	0	0
w/ Lime	8 oz	98	0	0	0
Coke					
Cherry	8 oz	104	0	0	0
Diet	8 oz	1	0	0	0
Diet Cherry	8 oz	1	0	0	0
Diet Plus	8 oz	0	0	0	0
Diet Vanilla	8 oz	1	0	0	0
Diet w/ Lime	8 oz	2	0	0	0
Vanilla	8 oz	100	0	0	0
Dr Pepper					
Original	12 oz	150	0	0	0
DRY					
Kumquat	12 oz	50	0	0	0
Lavender	12 oz	70	0	0	0
Lemongrass	12 oz	50	0	0	0
Rhubarb	12 oz	60	0	0	0
Fanta					
Apple	8 oz	121	0	0	0
Citrus	8 oz	91	0	0	0
Orange	8 oz	111	0	0	0
Firefighter					
Backdraft Root Beer	8 oz	90	0	0	0
Courageous Cola	8 oz	90	0	0	0
Flashover Orange	8 oz	20	0	0	0
Incendiary Citrus	8 oz	90	0	0	0
Rolling Code Black Cherry	8 oz	90	0	0	0
Fresca					
Soda	8 oz	2	0	0	0
Frostie					
Diet Cherry Limeade	12 oz	0	0	0	0
Diet Root Beer	12 oz	0	0	0	0
Vanilla Root Beer	12 oz	180	0	0	0
Hansen's					
Black Cherry	8 oz	110	0	0	0
Diet All Flavors	1 can	0	0	0	0
Ginger Beer	8 oz	100	0	0	0
Natural Black Cherry	1 can	160	0	0	0
Natural Cherry Vanilla	1 can	140	0	0	0

FOOD	PORTION	CALS	FAT	SAT FAT	TRANS FAT
Natural Creamy Root Beer	12 oz	160	0	0	0
Natural Ginger Ale	1 can	140	0	0	0
Natural Grapefruit	1 can	130	0	0	0
Natural Key Lime	1 can	130	0	0	0
Natural Kiwi Strawberry	1 can	130	0	0	0
Natural Mandarin Lime	1 can	130	0	0	0
Natural Orange Mango	1 can	170	0	0	0
Natural Raspberry	1 can	130	0	0	0
Natural Tangerine	1 can	160	0	0	0
Natural Tropical Passion	1 can	160	0	0	0
Natural Vanilla Cola	1 can	140	0	0	0
Hiball					
Club	10 oz	5	0	0	0
Tonic Water	10 oz	120	0	0	0
IBC					
Cream	12 oz	180	0	0	0
Inca Kola					
Diet	8 oz	1	0	0	0
Soda	8 oz	96	0	0	0
Jolt					
Blue	8 oz	120	0	0	0
Cherry Bomb	8 oz	90	0	0	0
Cola	8 oz	100	0	0	0
Red	8 oz	120	0	0	0
Ultra	8 oz	0	0	0	0
Jones Soda					
Blue Bubble Gum	12 oz	190	0	0	0
Cream	12 oz	190	0	0	0
Crushed Melon	12 oz	190	0	0	0
FuFu Berry	12 oz	190	0	0	0
Green Apple	12 oz	180	0	0	0
Orange Cream	12 oz	180	0	0	0
Kutztown					
Birch Beer	12 oz	160	0	0	0
Red Cream	12 oz	150	0	0	0
Sarsaparilla	12 oz	150	0	0	0
Lucozade					
Soda	7 oz	136	0	0	0
Maine Root					
All Flavors	12 oz	165	0	0	0

FOOD	PORTION	CALS	FAT	SAT FAT	TRANS FAT
Manzana Mia					
Soda	8 oz	99	0	0	0
Mello Yellow					
Diet	8 oz	3	0	0	0
Soda	8 oz	118	0	0	0
Mountain Dew					
Pitch Black	8 oz	110	0	0	0
Mr. Pibb					
Diet	8 oz	1	0	0	0
Nesbitt's					
Orange	12 oz	190	0	0	0
Northern Neck					
Diet Ginger Ale	8 oz	4	0	0	0
Ginger Ale	8 oz	94	0	0	0
Nuky					
Rose Soda	8 oz	120	0	0	0
Olde Brooklyn					
Coney Island Cream	8 oz	130	0	0	0
Flatbush Orange	8 oz	130	0	0	0
Williamsburg Root Beer	8 oz	120	0	0	0
Olde Philadelphia					
Black Cherry	12 oz	180	0	0	0
Cream	12 oz	190	0	0	0
Cream Diet	12 oz	0	0	0	0
Grape	12 oz	180	0	0	0
Orange Cream	12 oz	190	0	0	0
Pineapple	1 bottle	190	0	0	0
Root Beer	12 oz	180	0	0	0
Orangina					
Sparkling Citrus	8 oz	90	0	0	0
Pennsylvania Dutch					
Birch Beer	8 oz	110	0	0	0
Pepsi					
Blue Berry Cola Fusion	8 oz	100	0	0	0
Diet	12 oz	0	0	0	0
Edge	12 oz	70	0	0	0
Regular	12 oz	150	0	0	0
Vanilla	1 can	160	0	0	0
Vanilla Diet	1 can	0	0	0	0

FOOD	PORTION	CALS	FAT	SAT FAT	TRANS FAT
Polar					
Birch Beer	8 oz	110	0	0	0
Bitter Lemon Mixer	8 oz	120	0	0	0
Collins Mixer	8 oz	90	0	0	0
Cream	8 oz	120	0	0	0
Diet Pomegranate Dry	8 oz	10	0	0	0
Orange	8 oz	130	0	0	0
Pomegranate Dry	8 oz	120	0	0	0
Seltzer All Flavors	8 oz	0	0	0	0
Strawberry	8 oz	120	0	0	0
Tonic Water	8 oz	90	0	0	0
Vichy Water	8 oz	0	0	0	0
Prism					
Green Tea Soda Cola	8 oz	105	0	0	0
Lemon Lime	8 oz	117	0	0	0
Qibla					
Cola	18 oz	185	tr	–	–
Diet Cola	18 oz	1	0	0	0
Red Flash					
Soda	8 oz	105	0	0	0
Santa Cruz					
Organic Cherry	1 can	140	0	0	0
Organic Concord Grape	1 can	150	0	0	0
Organic Ginger Ale	1 can	150	0	0	0
Organic Lemon Lime	1 can	130	0	0	0
Organic Orange Mango	1 can	130	0	0	0
Organic Root Beer	1 can	150	0	0	0
Organic Vanilla Creme	1 can	160	0	0	0
Schweppes					
Ginger Ale	8 oz	120	0	0	0
Seagram's					
Ginger Ale	12 oz	130	0	0	0
Sex Kola					
All Flavors	12 oz	0	0	0	0
Diet All Flavors	12 oz	0	0	0	0
Sierra Mist					
Lemon Lime	12 oz	140	0	0	0
Ski					
Citrus	1 bottle (10 oz)	150	0	0	0

FOOD	PORTION	CALS	FAT	SAT FAT	TRANS FAT
Snow					
Sparkling Mint	8 oz	75	0	0	0
Souix City					
Cream	12 oz	180	0	0	0
Orange Cream	12 oz	200	0	0	0
Root Beer	12 oz	170	0	0	0
Sarsaparilla	12 oz	170	0	0	0
Sprite					
Diet Zero	8 oz	2	0	0	0
ReMix Aruba Jam	8 oz	97	0	0	0
Soda	8 oz	96	0	0	0
Steaz					
Organic Green Tea Soda Cola	8 oz	90	0	0	0
Organic Green Tea Soda Diet Black Cherry	8 oz	20	0	0	0
Organic Green Tea Soda Ginger Ale	8 oz	90	0	0	0
Organic Green Tea Soda Lemon	8 oz	90	0	0	0
Stewart's					
Cream	12 oz	180	0	0	0
Diet Cream	12 oz	0	0	0	0
Stirrings					
Club	6.3 oz	0	0	0	0
Ginger Ale	6.3 oz	100	0	0	0
Tonic Water	6.3 oz	85	0	0	0
Sunkist					
Diet Orange	8 oz	0	0	0	0
Orange	8 oz	130	0	0	0
Tab					
Soda	8 oz	1	0	0	0
Thomas Kemper					
Black Cherry	1 bottle	177	0	0	0
Old Fashioned Birch	1 bottle	170	0	0	0
Orange Cream	1 bottle	180	0	0	0
Pure Draft Honey Cola	1 bottle	140	0	0	0
Pure Draft Root Beer	1 bottle	160	0	0	0
Vanilla Cream	1 bottle	170	0	0	0
Three Drinks					
Citrus	12 oz	12	0	0	0

FOOD	PORTION	CALS	FAT	SAT FAT	TRANS FAT
Tommyknocker					
Almond Creme	12 oz	150	0	0	0
Key Lime Creme	12 oz	180	0	0	0
Orange Creme	12 oz	180	0	0	0
Root Beer	12 oz	150	0	0	0
Root Beer Float	12 oz	110	0	0	0
Strawberry Creme	12 oz	150	0	0	0
Uno Mas					
All Flavors	12 oz	130	0	0	0
Vermont Sweetwater					
Country Apple Jack	1 bottle	180	0	0	0
Kickin'Cow Cola	1 bottle	129	0	0	0
Mango Moonshine	1 bottle	180	0	0	0
Maple	1 bottle	101	0	0	0
Raspberry Rhubarb Ramble	1 bottle	180	0	0	0
Tangerine Cream Twister	1 bottle	180	0	0	0
Vermont Maple Seltzer	1 bottle	53	0	0	0
Vignette					
Wine Country Soda Chardonnay	12 oz	130	0	0	0
Wine Country Soda Pinot Noir	12 oz	130	0	0	0
Virgil's					
Micro Brewed Root Beer	12 oz	160	0	0	0
White Rock					
Organics Raspberry Creme	1 can (12.4 oz)	120	0	0	0
Organics Red Peach	1 can (12.4 oz)	120	0	0	0
White T					
All Flavors	12 oz	128	0	0	0
Diet All Flavors	12 oz	0	0	0	0
Windy City					
Root Beer	12 oz	170	0	0	0
Yoo-Hoo					
Original	9 fl oz	150	tr	tr	–
Z Cola					
No Artificial Sweeteners	8 oz	0	0	0	0
SOLE					
cooked	1 fillet (4.5 oz)	148	2	tr	–
cooked	3 oz	99	1	tr	–
lemon raw	3.5 oz	85	1	–	–

FOOD	PORTION	CALS	FAT	SAT FAT	TRANS FAT
TAKE-OUT					
breaded & fried	3.2 oz	211	11	3	–
SORGHUM					
sorghum	1 cup (6.7 oz)	651	6	1	–
SOUFFLE					
lemon chilled	1 cup	176	tr	–	–
raspberry chilled	1 cup	173	tr	–	–
spinach	1 cup	233	18	8	tr
SOUP					
CANNED					
Amy's					
Organic Barley	1 cup	50	1	0	–
Organic Black Bean Vegetable	1 cup	110	1	0	–
Organic Cream Of Mushroom	1 cup	120	9	2	–
Organic Cream Of Tomato	1 cup	100	2	2	–
Organic Lentil	1 cup	130	4	1	–
Organic Minestrone	1 cup	90	2	0	–
Organic No Chicken Noodle Soup	1 cup	90	3	0	–
Boston Market					
Chicken Broth Reduced Sodium	1 cup	15	1	0	–
Butterball					
Chicken Broth 99% Fat Free	1 cup	10	0	0	0
Campbell's					
25% Less Sodium Chicken Noodle as prep	1 cup	60	2	1	0
25% Less Sodium Cream Of Mushroom as prep	1 cup	110	8	1	0
98% Fat Free Cream Of Broccoli as prep	1 cup	70	2	1	0
98% Fat Free Cream Of Celery as prep	1 cup	60	3	1	0
98% Fat Free Cream Of Chicken as prep	1 cup	70	3	1	0
Cheddar Cheese as prep	1 cup	110	5	2	0
Chunky Beef and Country Vegetables	1 cup	150	3	1	0

FOOD	PORTION	CALS	FAT	SAT FAT	TRANS FAT
Chunky Chicken Mushroom Chowder	1 cup	210	12	3	0
Chunky Classic Chicken Noodle	1 cup	120	3	1	0
Chunky Grilled Chicken w/ Vegetables & Pasta	1 cup	100	2	1	0
Chunky Hearty Vegetable w/ Pasta	1 cup	120	2	1	0
Chunky New England Clam Chowder	1 cup	210	9	1	0
Chunky Old Fashioned Vegetable Beef	1 cup	130	3	1	0
Chunky Roadhouse Beef & Bean Chili	1 cup	230	8	4	1
Chunky Sirloin Burger w/ Country Vegetables	1 cup	180	7	3	0
Healthy Request Chicken Noodle as prep	1 cup	60	2	1	0
Healthy Request Chicken Rice as prep	1 cup	70	2	1	0
Healthy Request Cream Of Chicken as prep	1 cup	80	3	1	0
Healthy Request Italian Style Wedding	1 cup	120	3	1	0
Healthy Request Minestrone as prep	1 cup	80	1	1	0
Healthy Request Tomato as prep	1 cup	90	2	1	0
Low Sodium Chicken Broth	1 can	25	1	1	0
Microwavable Bowl Chicken Noodle	1 cup	70	2	1	0
Microwavable Bowl Vegetable	1 cup	110	1	0	0
Select Beef w/ Roasted Barley	1 cup	130	1	1	0
Select Blended Red Pepper Black Bean	1 cup	110	2	1	0
Select Chicken w/ Egg Noodles	1 cup	90	2	1	0
Select Harvest Tomato w/ Basil	1 cup	80	0	0	0
Select Honey Roasted Chicken w/ Golden Potatoes	1 cup	110	1	1	0
Select Italian Sausage w/ Pasta & Pepperoni	1 cup	150	6	3	0

FOOD	PORTION	CALS	FAT	SAT FAT	TRANS FAT
Select Italian Style Wedding	1 cup	110	3	1	0
Select Mexican Chicken Tortilla	1 cup	130	3	1	0
Select Potato Broccoli Cheese	1 cup	120	4	1	0
Select Savory Chicken & Long Grain Rice	1 cup	90	1	0	0
Select Split Pea w/ Roasted Ham	1 cup	160	1	0	0
Soup At Hand 25% Less Sodium Chicken w/ Mini Noodles	1 pkg (10.75 oz)	80	2	1	0
Soup At Hand Chicken & Stars	1 pkg	70	2	1	0
Soup At Hand Creamy Chicken	1 pkg (10.75 oz)	130	8	2	0
Soup At Hand Italian Style Wedding	1 pkg	90	5	1	0
Soup At Hand Vegetable Medley	1 pkg (10.75 oz)	100	2	1	0
Soup At Hand Velvety Potato	1 pkg (10.75 oz)	160	7	1	0
College Inn					
Beef Broth 99% Fat Free	1 cup	20	1	0	–
Beef Broth Fat Free Lower Sodium	1 cup	15	0	0	0
Chicken Broth Light & Fat Free	1 cup	5	0	0	0
Gold's					
Borscht Low Calorie	1 cup	20	0	0	0
Borscht Unsalted	1 cup	70	0	0	0
Hungarian Cabbage	6 oz	70	0	0	0
Schav	1 cup	15	1	–	–
Health Valley					
Organic Split Pea No Salt Added	1 cup	110	0	0	0
Healthy Choice					
Bean & Ham	1 cup	180	2	1	0
Beef & Potato	1 cup	110	1	0	–
Chicken & Dumplings	1 cup	140	3	1	0
Chicken & Pasta	1 cup	110	2	1	–
Chicken Corn Chowder	1 cup	140	2	1	–
Chicken Fiesta	1 cup	100	2	1	–
Chicken w/ Rice	1 cup	90	2	0	0
Chicken w/ Roasted Garlic	1 cup	120	2	1	–
Chili Beef	1 cup	170	2	1	–

FOOD	PORTION	CALS	FAT	SAT FAT	TRANS FAT
Clam Chowder	1 cup	110	2	1	–
Country Vegetable	1 cup	110	1	0	0
Creamy Tomato	1 cup	100	2	1	–
Garden Vegetable	1 cup	120	1	0	–
Hearty Chicken	1 cup	120	2	1	–
Italian Bean & Pasta	1 cup	100	2	1	–
Old Fashioned Chicken Noodle	1 cup	100	2	0	0
Roasted Italian Style Chicken	1 cup	120	2	1	–
Split Pea w/ Ham	1 cup	170	3	1	–
Turkey w/ Rice	1 cup	90	2	0	–
Vegetable Beef	1 cup	130	1	0	0
Vegetable Clam Chowder	1 cup	230	1	0	–
Zesty Gumbo	1 cup	100	2	1	0
Imagine					
Lobster Bisque	1 cup	130	5	3	0
Organic Creamy Butternut Squash	1 cup	90	2	0	0
Organic Creamy Chicken	1 cup	70	2	0	0
Organic Creamy Sweet Corn	1 cup	120	3	1	0
Organic Sweet Potato	1 cup	110	2	0	0
Organic Bistro Cuban Black Bean Bisque	1 cup	170	4	0	0
Organic Broth Beef	1 cup	20	1	0	0
Organic Broth Free Range Chicken	1 cup	10	0	0	0
Organic Broth Vegetable	8 oz	20	0	0	0
Manischewitz					
Clear Chicken Condensed	½ cup	15	1	0	–
Muir Glen					
Organic Garden Vegetable	1 cup	80	1	0	0
Organic Southwest Black Bean	1 cup	140	1	0	0
Pacific Foods					
Beef Broth	1 cup	20	0	0	0
Creamy Butternut Squash	1 cup	90	2	0	–
Creamy Roasted Carrot	1 cup	100	1	0	0
Creamy Roasted Red Pepper & Tomato	1 cup	100	2	2	0
Hearty Beef Barley	1 cup	110	2	2	0
Hearty Chicken Noodle	1 cup	80	1	0	0
Hearty Chicken Tortilla	1 cup	130	2	0	0

FOOD	PORTION	CALS	FAT	SAT FAT	TRANS FAT
Hearty Roasted Red Pepper & Corn Chowder	1 cup	210	12	7	0
Organic Creamy Tomato	1 cup	100	2	2	0
Organic Free Range Chicken Broth	1 cup	10	0	0	0
Organic French Onion	1 cup	35	0	0	0
Organic Low Sodium Chicken Broth	1 cup	10	0	0	0
Organic Mushroom Broth	1 cup	5	0	0	0
Organic Vegetarian Broth	1 cup	15	0	0	0
Progresso					
50% Less Sodium Chicken Gumbo	1 cup	110	2	1	0
50% Less Sodium Chicken Noodle	1 cup	90	2	0	0
50% Less Sodium Garden Vegetable	1 cup	100	0	0	0
50% Less Sodium Minestrone	1 cup	120	2	1	0
99% Fat Free Beef Barley	1 cup	120	2	1	0
Carb Monitor Chicken Vegetable	1 cup	70	2	0	–
Chicken Rice w/ Vegetable	1 cup	100	2	0	–
Rich & Hearty Beef Pot Roast	1 cup	130	2	1	–
Rich & Hearty Chicken & Homestyle Noodles	1 cup	110	2	1	0
Rich & Hearty Chicken Pot Pie	1 cup	170	6	2	0
Rich & Hearty Sirloin Steak & Vegetables	1 cup	130	2	1	0
Traditional Beef & Vegetable	1 cup	100	1	0	0
Traditional Beef Barley	1 cup	140	4	2	0
Traditional Chickarina	1 cup	120	5	2	0
Traditional Chicken & Herb Dumplings	1 cup	100	3	1	0
Traditional Chicken & Wild Rice	1 cup	100	2	1	0
Traditional Chicken Noodle	1 cup	100	2	1	0
Traditional Hearty Chicken & Rotini	1 cup	100	2	1	–
Traditional Homestyle Chicken	1 cup	100	2	0	0
Traditional Italian Style Wedding	1 cup	100	4	2	0

FOOD	PORTION	CALS	FAT	SAT FAT	TRANS FAT
Traditional New England Clam Chowder	1 cup	190	10	3	0
Traditional Split Pea w/ Ham	1 cup	140	1	0	0
Turkey Noodle	1 cup	90	2	0	–
Vegetable Classics 99% Fat Free Minestrone	1 cup	100	1	0	0
Vegetable Classics Creamy Mushroom	1 cup	130	3	0	0
Vegetable Classics French Onion	1 cup	50	2	1	0
Vegetable Classics Green Split Pea w/ Bacon	1 cup	170	1	1	0
Vegetable Classics Hearty Tomato	1 cup	110	1	0	0
Vegetable Classics Lentil	1 cup	150	2	1	0
Vegetable Classics Macaroni & Bean	1 cup	160	4	1	0
Vegetable Classics Tomato Rotini	1 cup	140	1	0	–
Vegetable Classics Vegetable	1 cup	80	1	0	0
Rienzi					
Chicken & Rice	1 cup	110	3	1	–
Italian Wedding Bell	1 cup	130	7	1	–
Snow's					
Clam Chowder	1 cup	200	15	4	–
Streit's					
Hearty Vegetarian Vegetable	1 cup	90	0	0	0
Mushroom Barley	1 cup	100	2	0	–
Swanson					
100% Fat Free Lower Sodium Beef Broth	1 cup	15	0	0	0
99% Fat Free Chicken Broth	1 cup	10	1	0	0
Organic Beef Broth	1 cup	15	1	1	0
Organic Chicken Broth	1 cup	15	1	0	0
Organic Vegetable Broth	1 cup	15	0	0	0
Valley Fresh					
Chicken Broth	1 cup	30	2	1	–
Chicken Broth 40% Less Sodium	1 cup	15	0	0	0

FOOD	PORTION	CALS	FAT	SAT FAT	TRANS FAT
Wolfgang Puck					
Chicken Parmesan w/ Pasta	1 cup	300	12	5	–
Hearty Lentil & Vegetable	1 cup	170	3	1	–
FROZEN					
Kettle Cuisine					
Gluten Free Angus Beef Steak Chili w/ Beans	1 pkg (10 oz)	250	12	5	0
Gluten Free Chicken w/ Rice Noodles	1 pkg (10 oz)	140	3	1	0
Gluten Free New England Clam Chowder	1 pkg (10 oz)	330	18	10	1
Nature's Entree					
Chowder	1 pkg (12 oz)	230	6	3	–
Tortellini Minestone	1 pkg (12 oz)	360	9	1	–
Phillips Seafood					
Cream Of Crab	1 cup	310	25	17	1
Shrimp Bisque	1 cup	280	18	12	0
Tabatchnick					
Barley Mushroom	1 serv (7.5 oz)	80	1	0	0
Chicken w/ Dumplings	1 serv (7.5 oz)	150	6	1	0
Cream Of Broccoli	1 serv (7.5 oz)	130	5	3	0
Macaroni & Cheese	1 serv (7.5 oz)	250	8	4	0
No Salt Pea	1 serv (7.5 oz)	140	0	0	0
Old Fashioned Potato	1 serv (7.5 oz)	100	2	0	0
Southwest Bean	1 serv (7.5 oz)	220	5	0	0
Vegetable	1 serv (7.5 oz)	90	2	0	0
Vegetarian Chili	1 serv (7.5 oz)	180	4	0	0
Wild Rice	1 serv (7.5 oz)	80	1	0	0
MIX					
beef broth cube	1 cube	6	tr	tr	–
chicken broth cube	1 cube (4.8 g)	9	tr	tr	–
A Taste Of Thai					
Coconut Ginger	2 tsp	15	1	0	–
Alpine Aire					
Low Carb Bay Shrimp Bisque	1 pkg	150	11	6	–
Low Carb Beefy Vegetable	1 pkg	100	4	2	–
Low Carb Broccoli Cheddar	1 pkg	140	10	6	–
Low Carb Mushroom & Chicken w/ Roasted Garlic	1 pkg	130	8	5	–

FOOD	PORTION	CALS	FAT	SAT FAT	TRANS FAT
Annie Chun's					
Noodle Bowl Chicken Noodle	1 pkg	260	2	0	–
Noodle Bowl Hot & Sour	1 pkg	280	3	0	–
Noodle Bowl Korean Kimchi	½ pkg	140	2	0	–
Noodle Bowl Miso	1 pkg	230	3	0	–
Noodle Bowl Thai Tom Yum	½ pkg	150	2	0	–
Noodle Bowl Udon	1 pkg	220	2	0	–
Azumaya					
Asian Style Thin Noodle	1 cup	120	0	0	0
Asian Style Wide Noodle	1 cup	120	0	0	0
Edward & Sons					
Bouillon Cubes Not-Beef	½ cube	20	2	1	0
Bouillon Cubes Not-Chicken	½ cube	15	2	1	0
Veggie Low Sodium	½ cup	20	2	1	0
Fantastic					
Noodle Bowl Hot & Sour as prep	2 cups	138	2	0	–
Noodle Bowl Miso w/ Tofu as prep	1 cup	100	1	0	–
Noodle Bowl Sesame Miso as prep	2 cups	90	1	0	0
Noodle Bowls Spring Vegetable as prep	2 cups	90	0	0	0
Noodle Soup Spicy Thai as prep	2 cups	110	1	0	–
Noodle Soup Cup Vegetarian Chicken as prep	1 cup	90	1	0	–
Soup Cup Italian Tomato as prep	2 cups	130	1	0	–
Soup Cup Mandarin Broccoli as prep	2 cups	110	0	0	0
Leahey Gardens					
No Beef Noodle	1½ cups	89	1	0	0
No Chicken Noodle	1½ cups	94	1	0	0
MiniCarb					
Miso w/ Tofu & Shiitake	1 pkg	33	1	0	–
Szechuan Beef	1 pkg	24	1	0	–
Thai Coconut Cream	1 pkg	100	6	4	–
Miso-Cup					
Golden Vegetable as prep	1 cup	30	1	0	0

FOOD	PORTION	CALS	FAT	SAT FAT	TRANS FAT
Japanese Restaurant Style as prep	1 cup	60	2	0	0
Organic Traditional w/ Tofu as prep	1 cup	35	1	0	0
Reduced Sodium as prep	1 cup	25	1	0	0
Savory Seaweed as prep	1 cup	30	1	0	0
Nissin					
Chicken Vegetable as prep	1 pkg	290	13	7	0
White Cheddar as prep	1 pkg	290	13	6	0
Nueva Cocina					
Frijoles Negros Con Chipotle Chile	1 cup	140	1	0	0
Sopa De Calabaza	1 cup	180	8	5	1
Sopa De Frijoles Colorados	1 cup	140	1	0	0
Sopa De Frijoles Negros	1 cup	140	0	0	0
Sopa De Maiz	1 cup	150	7	3	1
Sopa De Tortilla	1 cup	140	4	1	2
Ramen Noodle					
Beef as prep	1 pkg (2.2 oz)	280	11	6	–
Beef Low Fat as prep	1 pkg (2.2 oz)	216	1	tr	–
Chicken as prep	1 pkg (2.2 oz)	279	11	5	–
Chicken Low Fat as prep	1 pkg (2.2 oz)	216	1	tr	–
Oriental Low Fat as prep	1 pkg (2.2 oz)	217	1	tr	–
Shrimp as prep	1 pkg (2.2 oz)	294	13	4	–
Shrimp Low Fat as prep	1 pkg (2.2 oz)	218	1	tr	–
Tomato as prep	1 pkg (2.2 oz)	295	13	5	–
Rapunzel					
Cubes Vegetable Bouillon No Salt Added	½ cube	25	2	–	–
Cubes Vegetable Bouillon w/ Sea Salt	½ cube	15	1	–	–
Cubes Vegetable Bouillon w/ Sea Salt & Herbs	½ cube	15	2	–	–
San-J					
Miso Dark	1 pkg	40	2	–	–
Miso Mild	1 pkg	45	2	–	–
Simply Asia					
Soy Noodle Bowl	1 pkg	70	0	0	0
Slim-Fast					
Creamy Broccoli	1 pkg	210	5	2	–

FOOD	PORTION	CALS	FAT	SAT FAT	TRANS FAT
Creamy Chicken	1 pkg	220	5	2	–
Creamy Potato Cheddar & Chive	1 pkg	220	5	2	–
Thai Kitchen					
Instant Rice Noodle Bangkok Curry	1 pkg	192	5	0	–
Rice Noodle Bowl Spring Onion	1 bowl	170	2	0	–
Uncle Ben's					
Black Bean & Rice as prep	1 cup	150	2	0	–
Broccoli Cheese & Rice as prep	1 cup	110	2	0	–
REFRIGERATED					
Organic Classics					
French Onion w/ Croutons	1 cup	140	6	1	0
Seafood Chowder	1 cup	160	6	3	–
TAKE-OUT					
ban mein fish head	1 serv (10 oz)	277	10	4	–
beef stew soup	1 cup (8.8 oz)	221	5	2	–
black bean turtle soup	1 cup	241	1	tr	–
broccoli cheese	1 cup	165	9	3	–
brunswick stew soup	1 cup (8.5 oz)	232	6	2	–
caldo de res beef soup	1 cup	143	5	2	–
chinese velvet corn	1¼ cups	135	0	0	–
corn & cheese chowder	¾ cup	215	12	7	–
egg drop	1 cup	73	4	1	–
gazpacho	1 cup	46	tr	–	–
greek lemon	¾ cup	63	2	1	–
hot & sour	1 serv (14 oz)	173	8	2	–
matzo ball soup	1 cup	118	5	1	–
minestrone	1 cup	233	13	4	–
miso w/ tofu	1 cup	84	3	1	–
onion soup gratinee	1 serv	492	27	16	–
oxtail	1 cup	68	2	1	–
pasta e fagioll	1 cup (8.8 oz)	194	5	1	–
ratatouille	1 cup (7.5 oz)	266	25	3	–
shark fin	1 bowl (10 oz)	164	9	2	–
shrimp bisque	1 cup	263	14	4	–
sopa de albondigas	1 cup	171	11	4	–
thai lemon grass	1 bowl	100	4	–	–
vietnamese pho beef noodle	1 serv (7.8 oz)	480	12	5	–
wonton soup	1 cup	183	7	2	0
zupa koprowa polish dill soup	1 bowl	54	2	–	–

FOOD	PORTION	CALS	FAT	SAT FAT	TRANS FAT
SOUR CREAM					
sour cream	1 cup (8 oz)	493	48	30	–
sour cream	1 tbsp (0.4 oz)	26	3	2	–
Breakstone's					
Sour Cream	2 tbsp (1 oz)	60	5	4	–
Cabot					
Light	2 tbsp	35	3	2	
No Fat	2 tbsp	20	0	0	0
Sour Cream	2 tbsp	50	5	3	
Crowley					
Sour Cream	2 tbsp	60	5	4	–
Daisy					
No Fat	2 tbsp	20	0	0	0
Sour Cream	2 tbsp	60	5	4	0
Hood					
Fat Free	2 tbsp	20	0	0	0
Low Fat	2 tbsp	35	2	1	0
Sour Cream	2 tbsp	60	5	4	0
Horizon Organic					
Lowfat	2 tbsp	35	2	1	0
Sour Cream	2 tbsp	60	5	4	0
Organic Valley					
Lowfat	2 tbsp	40	2	2	0
SOUR CREAM SUBSTITUTES					
nondairy	1 cup	479	45	41	–
nondairy	1 oz	59	6	5	–
SOURSOP					
fresh	1	416	2	–	–
fresh cut up	1 cup	150	1	–	–

SOY (*see also* CHEESE SUBSTITUTES, ICE CREAM AND FROZEN DESSERTS, MILK SUBSTITUTES, MISO, SMOOTHIES, SOY SAUCE, SOYBEANS, TEMPEH, TOFU, YOGURT FROZEN)

FOOD	PORTION	CALS	FAT	SAT FAT	TRANS FAT
lecithin	1 tbsp	104	14	2	–
soya cheese	1.4 oz	128	11	–	–
Bob's Red Mill					
Lecithin Granules	1 tbsp	60	4	1	0
Protein Powder	1 tbsp	20	0	0	0
Fearn					
Granules	¼ cup	110	1	–	–

FOOD	PORTION	CALS	FAT	SAT FAT	TRANS FAT
Powder	¼ cup	100	5	–	–
Good Sense					
Soynuts Honey Roasted	⅓ cup	140	6	1	–
Soynuts Roasted & Salted	⅓ cup	140	7	1	–
Soynuts Roasted w/o Salt	⅓ cup	140	7	1	–
Health Trip					
Soynut Butter Honey Sweet	2 tbsp	170	13	2	–
Soynut Butter Original	2 tbsp	180	13	2	–
Soynut Butter Unsalted	2 tbsp	180	13	2	–
I.M. Healthy					
SoyNut Butter Original Creamy	2 tbsp (1.1 oz)	170	11	2	–
SoyNut Butter Unsweetened Chunky	2 tbsp (1.1 oz)	160	13	2	–
SoyNut Butter Unsweetened Creamy	2 tbsp (1.1 oz)	160	13	2	–
Revival					
Shake Chocolate Daydream Fructose	1 pkg	240	3	1	–
Shake Strawberry Smile Fructose	1 pkg	225	2	1	–
Shake Strawberry Smile Splenda	1 pkg	130	2	1	–
Shake Strawberry Smile Unsweetened	1 pkg	130	2	1	–
Soy Shake Plain	1 pkg	110	2	1	–
Soy Shake Vanilla Pleasure	1 pkg	220	2	1	–
Soy Shake Vanilla Pleasure Splenda	1 pkg	120	2	1	–
Soy Shake Vanilla Pleasure Unsweetened	1 pkg	120	2	1	–
Soynuts Chocolate Covered	⅙ cup	70	4	2	–
Soynuts Hot Jalapeno & Cheddar	⅙ cup	78	4	1	–
Soynuts Unsalted	⅙ cup	78	4	1	–
Soynuts Yogurt Covered	⅙ cup	720	4	3	–
Soy Juicy					
All Flavors	8 oz	160	3	1	–

FOOD	PORTION	CALS	FAT	SAT FAT	TRANS FAT

SOY DRINKS (see MILK SUBSTITUTES, SMOOTHIES)

SOY SAUCE

FOOD	PORTION	CALS	FAT	SAT FAT	TRANS FAT
shoyu	1 tbsp	9	tr	tr	–
soy sauce	1 tbsp	7	tr	tr	–
tamari	1 tbsp	11	tr	tr	–
Eden					
Organic Shoyu	1 tbsp	15	0	0	0
Organic Shoyu Reduced Sodium	1 tbsp	10	0	0	0
Organic Tamari	1 tbsp	15	0	0	0
House Of Tsang					
Ginger Soy Sauce	1 tbsp	20	0	0	0
Less Sodium	1 tbsp	5	0	0	0
Kikkoman					
Lite	1 tbsp (0.5 oz)	10	0	0	0
San-J					
Shoyu Organic	1 tbsp	15	0	0	0
Tamari	1 tbsp	15	0	0	0
Tamari Organic Wheat Free	1 tbsp	15	0	0	0
Tamari Organic Wheat Free Reduced Sodium	1 tbsp	20	0	0	0
Tamari Reduced Sodium	1 tbsp	20	0	0	0
Tree Of Life					
Shoyu	1 tbsp (0.5 oz)	15	0	0	–
Tamari Wheat Free	1 tbsp (0.5 oz)	15	0	0	–

SOYBEANS

FOOD	PORTION	CALS	FAT	SAT FAT	TRANS FAT
dried cooked	1 cup	298	15	2	–
dry roasted	½ cup	387	19	3	–
green cooked	½ cup	127	6	1	–
roasted	½ cup	405	22	3	–
roasted & toasted	1 cup	490	26	3	–
roasted & toasted salted	1 cup	490	26	3	–
sprouts raw	½ cup	43	2	tr	–
sprouts steamed	½ cup	38	2	tr	–
sprouts stir fried	1 cup	125	7	1	–
Arrowhead Mills					
Organic Dried not prep	¼ cup	160	8	1	0

FOOD	PORTION	CALS	FAT	SAT FAT	TRANS FAT
C&W					
In the Pod	½ cup	110	4	0	0
Eden					
Organic Blacksoy	½ cup	120	6	1	0
Frieda's					
Edamame	½ cup (2.6 oz)	100	3	0	–
South Beach					
Soy Nuts Dark Chocolate	1 pkg (0.7 oz)	100	6	3	0
Soyafarm					
Edamame Yuba Sticks	7 (2.5 oz)	123	6	–	–

SPAGHETTI (see PASTA, PASTA DINNERS, PASTA SALAD, SPAGHETTI SAUCE)

SPAGHETTI SAUCE
JARRED

FOOD	PORTION	CALS	FAT	SAT FAT	TRANS FAT
marinara sauce	1 cup	171	8	tr	–
spaghetti sauce	1 cup	272	12	2	–
Amy's					
Family Marinara	½ cup	50	1	0	–
Tomato Basil	½ cup	80	3	0	–
Barilla					
Arrabbiata Tomato & Spicy Pepper	½ cup	90	3	1	0
Basilico Tomato & Basil	½ cup	70	2	0	0
Boscaiola Mushrooms & Garlic	½ cup	90	3	1	0
Campagnola Roasted Garlic & Onion	½ cup	60	2	0	0
Garden Vegetable	½ cup	70	2	0	0
Restaurant Creations Cheese & Tomatoes	¼ cup	110	8	1	–
Restaurant Creations Pesto & Tomatoes	¼ cup	150	12	2	–
Rustica Sweet Peppers & Garlic	½ cup	70	3	0	0
Catelli					
Garden Select Country Mushroom	½ cup	80	2	tr	0
Garden Select Diced Tomatoes & Basil	½ cup	80	2	tr	0
Garden Select Fine Herbs	½ cup	80	2	tr	0
Garden Select Garlic & Onion	½ cup	80	2	tr	0

FOOD	PORTION	CALS	FAT	SAT FAT	TRANS FAT
Garden Select Parmesan & Romano	½ cup	80	3	1	tr
Garden Select Zucchini Primavera	½ cup	80	2	tr	0
Classico					
Italian Sausage	½ cup	90	2	1	–
Tomato & Basil	½ cup	60	1	0	0
Del Monte					
Chunky Garlic & Herb	½ cup	60	2	0	–
Chunky Italian Herb	½ cup	60	1	0	–
Garlic & Onion	½ cup	80	1	0	–
Tomato & Basil	½ cup	70	1	0	–
w/ Four Cheese	½ cup	70	2	0	–
w/ Green Peppers & Mushrooms	½ cup	80	1	0	–
w/ Meat	½ cup	60	1	0	–
w/ Mushrooms	½ cup	60	1	0	–
Eden					
Organic	½ cup	80	3	0	0
Organic No Salt	½ cup	80	3	0	0
Organic Pizza Pasta Sauce	½ cup	65	3	0	0
Emeril's					
Homestyle Marinara	½ cup	90	4	1	–
Roasted Gaaahlic	½ cup	70	3	0	–
Sicilian Gravy	½ cup	90	5	0	–
Vodka	½ cup	130	8	3	–
Francesco Rinaldi					
Alfredo	¼ cup (2.1 oz)	70	5	3	–
Chunky Garden Mushroom & Onion	½ cup (4.4 oz)	80	2	0	–
Chunky Garden Mushroom & Peppers	½ cup (4.4 oz)	80	2	0	–
Chunky Garden Tomato Garlic & Onion	½ cup	70	3	0	0
Dulce Super Mushroom	½ cup (4.4 oz)	110	5	1	–
Dulce Sweet & Tasty Tomato	½ cup (4.4 oz)	110	5	1	–
Hearty Diavolo	½ cup (4.4 oz)	70	4	1	–
Hearty Mushroom Pepper & Onion	½ cup	70	3	0	0
Hearty Tomato & Basil	½ cup (4.4 oz)	80	3	0	–

FOOD	PORTION	CALS	FAT	SAT FAT	TRANS FAT
Puttanesca	½ cup (4.3 oz)	70	4	1	–
Three Cheese	½ cup	80	2	1	0
Tomato Alfredo	¼ cup (2.1 oz)	60	4	2	–
Traditional Meat Flavored	½ cup (4.4 oz)	90	4	1	–
Traditional Mushroom	½ cup (4.4 oz)	90	4	1	–
Traditional No Salt Added	½ cup	70	3	0	0
Traditional Original	½ cup (4.4 oz)	90	4	1	–
Vodka Sauce	¼ cup (2.1 oz)	60	4	2	–
Hunt's					
Basil Garlic & Oregano	¼ cup	15	0	0	0
Cheese & Garlic	½ cup	50	1	0	0
Chunky Vegetable	½ cup	50	1	0	0
Family Favorites Lasagna	¼ cup	30	0	0	0
Family Favorites Pizza Sauce	¼ cup	25	0	0	0
Four Cheese	½ cup	50	1	0	0
Italian Sausage	½ cup	60	2	0	0
Light	½ cup	45	0	0	0
Meat	½ cup	60	1	0	0
No Added Sugar	½ cup	45	1	0	0
Roasted Garlic & Onion	½ cup	50	1	0	0
Traditional	½ cup	50	1	0	0
w/ Mushrooms	½ cup	45	1	0	0
Joey Pots & Pans					
Arrabbiata	½ cup	100	9	1	–
Marinara	½ cup	50	4	0	–
Vodka Sauce	½ cup	110	9	6	–
Knorr					
w/ Meat	4 oz	110	5	2	tr
Muir Glen					
Organic Chunky Tomato	¼ cup	15	0	0	0
Organic Garlic Roasted Garlic	½ cup	60	1	0	0
Organic Pizza Sauce	¼ cup	40	2	0	0
Organic Tomato Sauce No Salt Added	¼ cup	25	0	0	0
Newman's Own					
Bambolina	½ cup	90	5	1	0
Cabernet Marinara	½ cup	70	3	0	0
Five Cheese	½ cup	80	3	2	0
Italian Sausage & Peppers	½ cup	90	4	1	0
Marinara	½ cup	70	2	0	0

FOOD	PORTION	CALS	FAT	SAT FAT	TRANS FAT
Marinara w/ Mushrooms	½ cup	70	2	0	0
Pesto & Tomato Sauce	½ cup	80	4	1	0
Roasted Garlic & Green Peppers	½ cup	70	3	0	–
Sockarooni	½ cup	70	2	0	0
Tomato & Roasted Garlic	½ cup	70	3	0	0
Vodka Sauce	½ cup	110	5	2	–
Pomi					
Marinara	½ cup	80	4	0	–
Prego					
100% Natural Roasted Garlic Parmesan	½ cup	100	1	1	0
Heart Smart Traditional Italian	½ cup	100	3	1	0
Italian	½ cup	70	2	1	0
Italian Roasted Red Pepper & Garlic	½ cup	90	4	1	0
Italian Three Cheese	½ cup	80	2	1	0
Italian Tomato Basil & Garlic	½ cup	80	3	1	0
Italian Marinara	½ cup	100	5	1	0
Italian Meat	½ cup	130	4	1	0
Organic Mushroom	½ cup	90	3	0	0
Ragu					
Chunky Garden Style Tomato Garlic & Onion	½ cup (4.5 oz)	110	3	0	–
Fresh Italian	4 oz	110	3	1	0
Marinara	4 oz	100	3	tr	0
Pizza Quick Fresh Italian	2 oz	35	1	0	0
Robert Rothchild Farm					
Artichoke	½ cup	80	5	0	0
Seeds Of Change					
Balsamic Olive & Onion	½ cup	80	2	1	0
Garden Vegetable	½ cup	70	1	0	0
Mushroom & Onion	½ cup	70	2	0	0
Three Cheese Marinara	½ cup	70	2	1	0
Traditional Herb	½ cup	70	0	0	0
Tuttorosso					
Pasta Sauce Meat	½ cup	90	3	1	0
Vino De Milo					
Mediterranean Pinot Grigio	½ cup	90	4	1	0

FOOD	PORTION	CALS	FAT	SAT FAT	TRANS FAT
Portobella Shiraz	½ cup	40	1	0	0
Tuscan Merlot	½ cup	80	3	0	0
Walden Farms					
Alfredo Sauce Calorie Free	¼ cup	0	0	0	0
Marinara Calorie Free	⅓ cup	0	0	0	0
Walnut Acres					
Organic Garlic Garlic	½ cup	125	1	0	–
Organic Marinara & Zinfandel	½ cup	125	1	0	–
Organic Roasted Garlic	½ cup	125	1	0	–
Organic Tomato & Basil	½ cup	125	1	0	–
REFRIGERATED					
Buitoni					
Alfredo	¼ cup	140	12	7	–
Alfredo Portabello Mushroom	¼ cup	100	8	5	–
Alfredo Light	¼ cup	80	5	4	–
Marinara	½ cup	80	3	1	–
Marinara Roasted Garlic	½ cup	60	2	1	–
Pesto	¼ cup	330	27	5	–
Pesto w/ Basil	¼ cup	300	26	6	–
Pesto w/ Basil Reduced Fat	¼ cup	230	18	4	–
Pesto w/ Sun Dried Tomatoes	¼ cup	210	18	3	–
Tomato Herb Parmesan	½ cup	120	8	3	–
TAKE-OUT					
bolognese	5 oz	195	15	–	–

SPANISH FOOD
FROZEN

FOOD	PORTION	CALS	FAT	SAT FAT	TRANS FAT
Amy's					
Black Bean Vegetable Enchilada	1 (4.75 oz)	130	4	0	–
Burrito Bean & Cheese	1 (6 oz)	280	8	3	–
Burrito Bean & Rice Non-Dairy	1 (6 oz)	270	6	1	–
Burrito Black Bean Vegetable	1 (6 oz)	320	8	1	–
Burrito Breakfast	1 (6 oz)	210	6	tr	–
Cheese Enchilada	1 (4.75 oz)	210	12	6	–
Mexican Tamale Pie	1 (8 oz)	150	3	0	–
Banquet					
Enchilada Beef	1 pkg (11 oz)	370	12	5	–
Enchilada Cheese	1 pkg (11 oz)	360	10	4	–
Enchilada Chicken	1 pkg (11 oz)	350	10	3	–

FOOD	PORTION	CALS	FAT	SAT FAT	TRANS FAT
Cedarlane					
Organic Burrito Low Fat Rice & Cheese	1 (6 oz)	260	1	0	0
Organic Enchilada Low Fat Black Bean & Tofu	1 (9 oz)	220	3	0	0
Roasted Chile Relleno	1 pkg (10 oz)	400	20	12	0
Zone Burrito Beans & Cheese	1 (6 oz)	350	13	5	0
Contessa					
Fajitas Shrimp	2 (8 oz)	230	4	1	0
Paella w/ Chicken & Seafood	1½ cups	200	3	0	0
Seafood Veracruz not prep	1¾ cups	180	2	1	0
El Monterey					
Quesadillas Chicken Breast & Cheese	1 (5 oz)	280	13	6	0
Healthy Choice					
Chicken Enchiladas	1 pkg	360	7	3	–
Helen's Kitchen					
Cheese Enchiladas w/ Tofu Steaks In Spicy Red Sauce	½ pkg (5 oz)	150	9	1	0
Jose Ole					
Burrito Beef & Cheese	1 (5 oz)	300	10	4	0
Burrito Chicken	1 (5 oz)	270	7	2	0
Chimichanga Chicken & Cheese	1 (5 oz)	330	12	3	0
Chimichanga Shredded Beef	1 (5 oz)	350	15	5	1
Mini Burrito Chicken & Cheese	3	200	8	2	0
Mini Chimichanga Beef & Cheddar	3	240	12	3	0
Mini Quesadilla Grilled Chicken	3	220	8	3	0
Mini Tacos Beef & Cheese	4	200	11	4	0
Mini Taquitos Beef & Cheese	4	180	8	2	0
Soft Taco Beef & Cheese	1 (5 oz)	280	11	4	0
Taquitos Beef & Cheese Flour Tortilla	2	220	10	3	0
Taquitos Buffalo Chicken Flour Tortilla	2	200	10	2	0
Taquitos Chicken Flour Tortilla	3	180	8	1	0
Taquitos Chicken & Cheese Flour Tortilla	2	220	10	3	0

FOOD	PORTION	CALS	FAT	SAT FAT	TRANS FAT
Taquitos Pepperoni Pizza Flour Tortilla	2	240	14	4	0
Taquitos Shredded Beef Corn Tortilla	3	180	7	2	0
Lean Cuisine					
One Dish Favorites Chicken Enchilada	1 pkg (9 oz)	280	5	2	0
Patio					
Beef & Cheese Enchiladas Chili 'N Beans	1 meal (15.5 oz)	670	30	14	–
Burrito Bean & Cheese	1 (5 oz)	280	8	3	0
Burrito Beef & Bean Hot	1 (5 oz)	320	12	5	–
Burrito Beef & Bean Medium	1 (5 oz)	310	10	5	–
Burrito Beef & Bean Red Chili Pepper Red Hot	1 (5 oz)	320	12	5	–
Burrito Chicken	1 (5 oz)	280	8	2	0
Enchilada Beef	1 meal (12 oz)	320	12	5	–
Enchilada Cheese	1 meal (12 oz)	370	12	5	–
Enchilada Chicken	1 meal (12 oz)	400	12	4	–
Fiesta	1 meal (12 oz)	350	11	5	–
Mexican Style	1 meal (13.25 oz)	470	19	6	–
Stouffer's					
Chicken Enchilada w/ Cheese Sauce & Rice	1 pkg (7.13 oz)	280	12	7	1
Tyson					
Meal Kit Chicken Fajita	1 (3.8 oz)	130	4	1	–
Meal Kit Quesadilla Chicken	1 (4 oz)	250	10	5	–
READY-TO-EAT					
taco shell corn	1 (6.5 inch)	98	5	1	–
taco shell flour	1 (7 inch)	173	9	2	–
Ortega					
Tostada Shells	2 (1 oz)	140	6	1	2
SHELF-STABLE					
Fantastic					
Spanish Paella	1 pkg (8 oz)	280	5	1	–
TAKE-OUT					
arroz con coco	1 cup	532	38	33	–
burrito w/ beans	1 med (5 oz)	295	8	2	–
burrito w/ beans & rice	1 (3.5 oz)	221	5	1	–
burrito w/ beef	1 sm (3.4 oz)	297	13	5	–

FOOD	PORTION	CALS	FAT	SAT FAT	TRANS FAT
burrito w/ beef & beans	1 med (5 oz)	331	13	4	–
burrito w/ beef beans & cheese	1 med (5 oz)	379	19	9	–
burrito w/ chicken & beans	1 med (5 oz)	295	9	2	–
burrito w/ pork & beans	1 med (5 oz)	320	12	4	–
chiles rellenos meat & cheese filled	1 (5 oz)	213	16	5	0
chimichanga w/ bean cheese lettuce & tomato	1 (4.1 oz)	271	18	5	–
chimichanga w/ beef & rice	1 (10 oz)	634	36	8	–
chimichanga w/ beef beans lettuce & tomato	1 (4.1 oz)	254	15	3	–
chimichanga w/ beef cheese lettuce & tomato	1 (4.1 oz)	337	24	8	–
chimichanga w/ chicken sour cream lettuce & tomato	1 (4 oz)	277	20	6	–
enchilada w/ beans	1 (4.1 oz)	179	6	1	–
enchilada w/ beans & cheese	1 (4.6 oz)	233	11	5	–
enchilada w/ beef	1 (4 oz)	214	10	3	–
enchilada w/ beef & beans	1 (4 oz)	195	8	2	–
frijoles	1 cup	278	2	tr	–
frijoles w/ cheese	1 cup	225	8	4	–
nachos w/ beans & cheese	1 serv (9.4 oz)	616	33	13	–
nachos w/ beef beans cheese & sour cream	1 serv (19 oz)	1620	97	37	–
paella	1 serv (7 oz)	308	16	3	–
pupusa meat filled	1 (3.6 oz)	187	6	2	–
quesadilla w/ cheese	1 (5 oz)	498	28	14	–
quesadilla w/ meat & cheese	1 (6.5 oz)	605	35	16	–
taco de jueye w/ crab meat	1 (4.2 oz)	266	14	5	–
taco w/ beans lettuce tomato & salsa	1 (2.8 oz)	117	5	1	–
taco w/ chicken lettuce tomato & salsa	1 (2.5 oz)	114	5	1	–
taco w/ fish lettuce tomato & salsa	1 (2.7 oz)	101	4	1	–
tostada w/ beef lettuce tomato & salsa	1 (2.7 oz)	143	8	2	–

SPICES (*see individual names,* HERBS/SPICES)

FOOD	PORTION	CALS	FAT	SAT FAT	TRANS FAT
SPINACH					
CANNED					
drained	1 cup	49	1	tr	0
Del Monte					
Whole Leaf	½ cup	30	0	0	0
Popeye					
Spinach	½ cup	45	1	0	0
S&W					
Spinach	½ cup (4.5 oz)	30	0	0	0
FRESH					
baby raw	2 cups	20	0	0	0
cooked	1 cup	41	tr	tr	0
malabar cooked	1 cup	10	tr	–	–
mustard cooked	1 cup	29	tr	–	0
new zealand cooked	1 cup	22	tr	tr	–
raw	1 cup	7	tr	tr	–
Fresh Express					
Baby Spinach	3 cups	20	0	0	0
Spicy Spinach	3 cups (3 oz)	10	0	0	0
Ready Pac					
Baby	2 cups	20	0	0	0
Microwave Spinach as prep	½ cup	20	0	0	0
FROZEN					
chopped cooked	1 cup	30	tr	tr	0
Birds Eye					
Chopped	⅓ cup	20	0	0	0
C&W					
Baby Chopped	1 cup	30	0	0	0
Creamed	½ cup	100	7	2	0
Cascadian Farm					
Organic Cut	⅓ cup	25	0	0	0
Cedarlane					
Organic Spanakopita Spinach & Feta Pie	½ pkg (5 oz)	260	8	4	0
Fillo Factory					
Spanakopita Spinach & Cheese Fillo Appetizers	3 (3 oz)	190	9	5	0
Fresh Like					
Cut Leaf	3.5 oz	21	tr	–	–

FOOD	PORTION	CALS	FAT	SAT FAT	TRANS FAT
Green Giant					
No Sauce	½ cup	25	0	0	0
Stouffer's					
Creamed	½ pkg (4.5 oz)	200	16	4	0
Taverna					
Spinach Pie	1 piece (4.8 oz)	190	6	4	0
TAKE-OUT					
indian saag	1 serv	28	2	tr	–
spanakopita spinach pie	1 serv (3 oz)	148	11	5	–
SPINACH JUICE					
juice	7 oz	14	0	0	0
SPORTS DRINKS (see ENERGY DRINKS)					
SPOT					
baked	3 oz	134	5	2	–
SPROUTS					
kidney bean	½ cup	27	tr	tr	–
lentil sprouts	½ cup	40	tr	tr	–
mung bean	½ cup	16	tr	tr	–
mung bean canned	½ cup	8	tr	tr	–
mung bean cooked	½ cup	13	tr	tr	–
pea	½ cup	77	tr	tr	–
radish	½ cup	8	tr	tr	–
Brassica					
Broccoli Sprouts	½ cup (1 oz)	16	0	0	0
TAKE-OUT					
mung bean stir fried	½ cup	31	tr	tr	–
SQUAB					
boneless baked	1 (4 oz)	242	14	4	0
SQUASH (see also SQUASH SEEDS, ZUCCHINI)					
CANNED					
crookneck sliced	½ cup	14	tr	tr	–
Farmer's Market					
Organic Butternut	½ cup	50	tr	0	0
FRESH					
acorn cooked mashed	½ cup	41	tr	tr	–
acorn cubed baked	½ cup	57	tr	tr	–
butternut baked	½ cup	41	tr	tr	–

FOOD	PORTION	CALS	FAT	SAT FAT	TRANS FAT
crookneck sliced cooked	½ cup	18	tr	tr	–
hubbard baked	½ cup	51	tr	tr	–
hubbard cooked mashed	½ cup	35	tr	tr	–
scallop sliced cooked	½ cup	14	tr	tr	–
spaghetti cooked	½ cup	23	tr	tr	–
Frieda's					
Acorn	¾ cup (3 oz)	35	0	0	0
Baby Crookneck	⅔ cup (3 oz)	15	0	0	0
Baby Scallop	⅔ cup (3 oz)	15	0	0	0
Eight Ball	2 (4.4 oz)	18	0	0	0
Hubbard	¾ cup (3 oz)	35	0	0	0
Mini Pumpkin	¾ cup (3 oz)	20	0	0	0
Spaghetti	¾ cup (3 oz)	30	0	0	0
Star Spangled	⅔ cup (3 oz)	20	0	0	0
Turban	¾ cup (3 oz)	30	0	0	0
Glory					
Yellow Sliced	¾ cup	20	0	0	0
Martin Farms					
Butternut Fresh Cut	½ cup	40	0	0	0
FROZEN					
butternut cooked mashed	½ cup	47	tr	tr	–
crookneck sliced cooked	½ cup	24	tr	tr	–
C&W					
Butternut	½ cup	45	0	0	0
McKenzie's					
Southland Butternut	½ cup	70	3	1	0
TAKE-OUT					
fritter	1 (0.8 oz)	81	5	1	0

SQUASH SEEDS

roasted	1 oz	148	12	2	–
salted & roasted	1 oz	148	12	2	–
seeds dried	1 oz	154	13	2	–
seeds whole roasted	1 oz	127	6	1	–

SQUID

baked	1 cup	192	6	1	0
canned in its own ink	1 can (4 oz)	122	2	tr	0
dried	1 sm (1.5 oz)	147	2	1	0
pickled	1 oz	26	tr	tr	0
steamed	1 cup	147	2	1	0

FOOD	PORTION	CALS	FAT	SAT FAT	TRANS FAT
Contessa					
Calamari + Sauce	13 pieces + 2 tbsp sauce	160	6	2	0
Margaritaville					
Captain's Calamari Strips + Sauce	⅓ pkg	330	20	4	–
Van de Kamp's					
Fried Calamari	15 pieces (4 oz)	270	13	4	0
TAKE-OUT					
arroz con calamares	1 cup	400	17	2	–
calamari breaded & fried	1 cup	296	12	3	–

SQUIRREL

FOOD	PORTION	CALS	FAT	SAT FAT	TRANS FAT
roasted	3 oz	147	4	tr	–

STARFRUIT

FOOD	PORTION	CALS	FAT	SAT FAT	TRANS FAT
fresh	1	42	tr	–	–
Frieda's					
Dried	⅓ cup (1.4 oz)	120	0	0	0

STRAWBERRIES

FOOD	PORTION	CALS	FAT	SAT FAT	TRANS FAT
canned in heavy syrup	½ cup	117	tr	tr	0
fresh halves	1 cup	49	tr	tr	0
fresh whole	1 cup	46	tr	tr	0
fresh whole	1 pint	114	1	tr	0
frzn sweetened sliced	½ cup	122	tr	tr	0
frzn whole unsweetened	1 cup	77	tr	tr	0
organic fresh whole	8 med	45	0	0	0
whole sweetened frzn	1 cup	199	tr	tr	0
C&W					
Ultimate Sliced frzn	⅔ cup	50	0	0	0
Europe's Best					
Sliced frzn	¾ cup	40	1	0	0
Frieda's					
Dried	½ cup (1.4 oz)	150	0	0	0
Marie's					
Glaze	2 tbsp	40	0	0	0

STRAWBERRY JUICE

FOOD	PORTION	CALS	FAT	SAT FAT	TRANS FAT
Adina					
California Kiss Hibiscus Strawberry	8 oz	80	0	0	0

FOOD	PORTION	CALS	FAT	SAT FAT	TRANS FAT
Ceres					
Strawberry	8 oz	115	0	0	0
Giant Berry Farms					
Just Strawberries	1 bottle (12 oz)	140	0	0	0

STUFFING/DRESSING
FOOD	PORTION	CALS	FAT	SAT FAT	TRANS FAT
Fresh Gourmet					
All Natural Multi-Grain w/ Cranberries not prep	⅓ cup (1 oz)	110	3	0	0
Organic Seasoned not prep	⅓ cup (1 oz)	110	3	0	0
Kellogg's					
Stuffing Mix as prep	1 cup	240	13	3	4
Pepperidge Farm					
Corn Bread	¾ cup	170	2	0	0
Cube	¾ cup	140	1	0	0
Herb Seasoned	¾ cup	170	2	1	0
One Step Turkey	½ cup	170	7	1	0
Tofurky					
Wild Rice & Mushroom	½ cup	110	2	0	0
TAKE-OUT					
bread	1 cup	352	17	3	–
cornbread	½ cup	179	9	2	–
oyster	1 cup	304	18	4	0
sausage	½ cup	292	11	2	–

STURGEON
FOOD	PORTION	CALS	FAT	SAT FAT	TRANS FAT
broiled	3 oz	115	4	1	0
roe raw	1 oz	59	3	–	–
smoked	1 oz	49	1	tr	0
TAKE-OUT					
breaded & fried	4 oz	252	15	3	0

SUCKER
FOOD	PORTION	CALS	FAT	SAT FAT	TRANS FAT
white baked	3 oz	101	3	tr	–

SUGAR
FOOD	PORTION	CALS	FAT	SAT FAT	TRANS FAT
brown organic	1 tsp	17	0	0	0
brown packed	1 cup (7.7 oz)	828	0	0	0
brown unpacked	1 cup (5.1 oz)	547	0	0	0
cinnamon sugar	1 tsp	16	tr	tr	–
maple	1 piece (1 oz)	99	tr	tr	–
powdered	1 tbsp (0.3 oz)	31	0	0	0

FOOD	PORTION	CALS	FAT	SAT FAT	TRANS FAT
powdered unsifted	1 cup (4.2 oz)	467	tr	–	–
raw	1 pkg (5 g)	19	0	0	0
sugarcane stem	3 oz	54	0	0	0
white	1 cup (7 oz)	773	0	0	0
white	1 packet (3 g)	12	0	0	0
white	1 tsp (4 g)	15	0	0	0
Billington's					
Muscovado Light Brown	1 tsp	15	0	0	0
Bob's Red Mill					
Date Sugar	1 tsp	11	0	0	0
Turbinado	1 tsp	10	0	0	0
Domino					
Dark Brown	1 tsp	15	0	0	0
Organic Cane Sugar	1 tsp	15	0	0	0
White	1 tsp	15	0	0	0
Equinox					
Organic Maple Flakes	2 tsp	15	0	0	0
Gluco Burst					
Arctic Cherry	1 pkg (1.3 oz)	70	0	0	0
Princess Of Yum					
Citrus Lemon	2.5 tsp	40	0	0	0
French Vanilla	2.5 tsp	40	0	0	0

SUGAR SUBSTITUTES
Equal

FOOD	PORTION	CALS	FAT	SAT FAT	TRANS FAT
Flavor Sticks	1 pkg	0	0	0	0
Packet	1 pkg	0	0	0	0
Spoonful	1 tsp	0	0	0	0
Sugar Lite	1 tsp	8	0	0	0
Fran Gare's					
Miracle Sweet	1 tsp	10	0	0	0
Keto					
Sweet	½ tsp	0	0	0	0
Lo Han					
Sweet	2 scoops	2	0	0	0
Nature's Family					
Sun Crystals	1 pkg (4.5 g)	4	0	0	0
SomerSweet					
Sweetener	¼ tsp	0	0	0	0

FOOD	PORTION	CALS	FAT	SAT FAT	TRANS FAT
Splenda					
Flavor Blends All Flavors	1 pkg	0	0	0	0
No Calorie Granules	1 tsp	0	0	0	0
Sugar Blend For Baking	½ tsp	10	0	0	0
Sweetener	1 pkg	0	0	0	0
Steel's					
Brown	1 tsp	10	0	0	0
Sugar Substitute	1 tsp	10	0	0	0
Stevita					
Spoonable	⅓ tsp	0	0	0	0
Sugar Twin					
Packets	1	0	0	0	0
Spoonable Brown	1 tsp	0	0	0	0
Spoonable White	1 tsp	0	0	0	0
Sun Crystals					
Natural Sweetener	1 pkg (5 g)	4	0	0	0
Sweet Fiber					
All Natural	1 pkg	0	0	0	0
Sweet Simplicity					
Sweetener	1 pkg	0	0	0	0
Sweete					
Sugar Free	1 pkg	0	0	0	0
SweetLeaf					
SteviaPlus	1 pkg	0	0	0	0
Whey Low					
Gold	1 tsp	4	0	0	0
Granular	1 tsp	4	0	0	0
Maple Buzz	¼ cup	57	0	0	0
Powder	1 tsp	4	0	0	0
Zsweet					
All Natural	1 pkg (1 g)	0	0	0	0
SUGAR-APPLE					
fresh	1	146	tr	–	–
fresh cut up	1 cup	236	1	–	–
SUNCHOKE					
fresh raw sliced	½ cup	57	tr	0	–
Frieda's					
Sunchoke	½ cup (3 oz)	70	0	0	0

FOOD	PORTION	CALS	FAT	SAT FAT	TRANS FAT
SUNFISH					
pumpkinseed baked	3 oz	97	1	tr	–
SUNFLOWER					
seeds dry roasted w/ salt	¼ cup	186	16	2	0
seeds dry roasted w/o salt	¼ cup	186	16	2	0
seeds w/ hulls dried	¼ cup	66	6	1	0
Arrowhead Mills					
Organic Seeds	¼ cup	170	15	2	0
Bob's Red Mill					
Seeds Roasted & Salted	3 tbsp	186	15	2	0
David					
Kernels Original	¼ cup	200	17	2	–
Seeds BBQ	¼ cup	190	15	2	–
Seeds BBQ Sizzlin	¼ cup	190	16	2	–
Seeds Jalapeno	¼ cup	190	15	2	–
Seeds Nacho Cheese	¼ cup	180	15	2	–
Seeds Original	¼ cup	190	15	2	–
Seeds Ranch	¼ cup	190	15	2	–
Seeds Reduced Sodium	¼ cup	190	15	2	0
Frito Lay					
Seeds	3 tbsp	180	15	2	0
Good Sense					
Nuts Honey Roasted	¼ cup	190	15	2	–
Nuts Raw	¼ cup	170	15	2	–
Nuts Roasted & Salted	¼ cup	190	15	2	–
Seeds In Shell Roasted & Salted	½ cup	150	9	1	–
Sunflower Nuts Roasted w/o Salt	¼ cup	190	16	2	0
Maranatha					
Tamari Seeds	¼ cup	160	14	2	–
SunButter					
Creamy	2 tbsp	200	16	2	0
Organic	2 tbsp	203	16	1	0
SunGold					
Seeds Roasted Salted	1 oz	172	15	2	0
SUSHI					
TAKE-OUT					
california roll	1 piece (0.8 oz)	28	1	tr	–
fresh salmon rolls	4 pieces	250	7	1	–

FOOD	PORTION	CALS	FAT	SAT FAT	TRANS FAT
inari	1 sm	46	1	0	–
sashimi	1 serv (6 oz)	198	7	1	–
tuna roll	1 piece (0.7 oz)	23	tr	tr	–
vegetable roll	1 piece (1.2 oz)	27	1	tr	–
vinegared ginger	⅓ cup (1.6 oz)	48	tr	tr	–
wasabi	2 tsp (0.3 oz)	5	tr	0	–
yellowtail roll	1 piece (0.6 oz)	25	1	tr	–

SWAMP CABBAGE

FOOD	PORTION	CALS	FAT	SAT FAT	TRANS FAT
chopped cooked w/o salt	1 cup	20	tr	tr	0

SWEET POTATO (see also YAM)

FOOD	PORTION	CALS	FAT	SAT FAT	TRANS FAT
baked w/ skin	1 (3.5 oz)	118	tr	tr	–
canned in syrup	½ cup	106	tr	tr	–
canned pieces	1 cup	183	tr	tr	–
frzn cooked	½ cup	88	tr	tr	–
leaves cooked	½ cup	11	tr	tr	–
mashed	½ cup	172	tr	tr	–
Diner's Choice					
Mashed	⅔ cup	160	3	1	0
Farmer's Market					
Organic Puree	½ cup	96	0	0	0
Glory					
Casserole	½ cup	180	0	0	0
Cut Fresh	1 serv (5 oz)	140	0	0	0
Sweet Potatoes	⅔ cup	160	0	0	0
Green Giant					
Candied	¾ cup	240	7	1	2
Mrs. Paul's					
Candied	1 serv (5 oz)	300	1	1	0
Princella					
In Light Syrup	⅔ cup	160	0	0	0
Royal Prince					
Orange Pineapple	½ cup	160	0	0	0
Sugary Sam					
In Syrup	⅔ cup	160	0	0	0
TAKE-OUT					
candied	3.5 oz	144	3	1	–

SWEETBREAD (PANCREAS)

FOOD	PORTION	CALS	FAT	SAT FAT	TRANS FAT
beef braised	3 oz	230	15	5	0

FOOD	PORTION	CALS	FAT	SAT FAT	TRANS FAT
lamb braised	3 oz	199	13	6	0
pork braised	3 oz	186	9	3	0
testicles cooked	1 pair (6.8 oz)	241	6	2	0
veal braised	3 oz	218	12	4	0
SWISS CHARD					
cooked	½ cup	18	tr	–	–
raw chopped	½ cup	3	tr	–	–
Frieda's					
Bright Lights	1 cup (3 oz)	15	0	0	0
SWORDFISH					
cooked	3 oz	132	4	1	–
raw	3 oz	103	3	1	–
SYRUP					
corn dark & light	¼ cup	240	tr	0	–
date syrup	1 tbsp	63	tr	–	–
maple	1 cup (11.1 oz)	824	1	–	–
maple	1 tbsp	52	0	–	0
raspberry	1 oz	76	0	0	0
rose hip	1 oz	9	0	0	0
sorghum	1 cup (11.6 oz)	957	0	0	0
sorghum	1 tbsp (0.7 oz)	61	0	0	0
sugar syrup	¼ cup	76	0	0	0
Cary's					
Maple	¼ cup	210	0	0	0
DaVinci Gourmet					
Sugar Free All Flavors	1 tbsp	0	0	0	0
Eden					
Organic Barley Malt	1 tbsp	60	0	0	0
Estee					
Blueberry	¼ cup	30	0	0	0
Hershey's					
Strawberry	2 tbsp	100	0	0	0
Karo					
Corn Syrup Dark	2 tbsp	120	0	0	0
Corn Syrup Light	2 tbsp	120	0	0	0
Lundberg					
Organic Sweet Dreams Brown Rice	2 tbsp	110	0	0	0

FOOD	PORTION	CALS	FAT	SAT FAT	TRANS FAT
Navitas Naturals					
Yacon	2 tbsp	90	0	0	0
Nesquik					
Strawberry Calcium Fortified	2 tbsp	100	0	0	0
Pacifica Culinaria					
Pomegranate	1 tbsp	60	0	0	0
Watermelon	1 tbsp	60	0	0	0
Smucker's					
Blackberry	¼ cup	210	0	0	0
Blueberry	¼ cup	210	0	0	0
Boysenberry	¼ cup	210	0	0	0
Red Raspberry	¼ cup	210	0	0	0
Strawberry	¼ cup	210	0	0	0
Sundae Syrup 3 Musketeers	2 tbsp	110	2	1	–
Sundae Syrup Butterscotch	2 tbsp	100	0	0	0
Sundae Syrup Caramel	2 tbsp	100	0	0	0
Sundae Syrup Strawberry	2 tbsp	110	0	0	0
Spectrum					
Balsamic Organic	1 tbsp	35	0	0	0

TAHINI (see SESAME)

TAMARILLOS
Frieda's

FOOD	PORTION	CALS	FAT	SAT FAT	TRANS FAT
Gold or Red	2 (4.2 oz)	40	0	0	0

TAMARIND

FOOD	PORTION	CALS	FAT	SAT FAT	TRANS FAT
dried sweetened pulpitas	1 piece (0.8 oz)	56	tr	tr	0
dried sweetened pulpitas	½ cup	279	1	tr	0
fresh	1 (2 g)	5	tr	tr	0
fresh cut up	1 cup	143	tr	tr	0

TAMARIND JUICE

FOOD	PORTION	CALS	FAT	SAT FAT	TRANS FAT
nectar	1 cup	143	tr	–	0
Teptip					
Drink	1 can (11.2 oz)	210	3	0	–

TANGERINE
CANNED

FOOD	PORTION	CALS	FAT	SAT FAT	TRANS FAT
in light syrup	1 cup	154	tr	tr	0
juice pack	1 cup	92	tr	tr	0

FOOD	PORTION	CALS	FAT	SAT FAT	TRANS FAT
FRESH					
fresh	1 lg (4.2 oz)	64	tr	tr	0
fresh	1 med (3.1 oz)	47	tr	tr	0
fresh	1 sm (2.7 oz)	40	tr	tr	0
sections	1 cup	103	1	tr	0
Chiquita					
Tangerine	1 med (3.5 oz)	50	1	0	–
River Pride					
Sweet	1 (3.8 oz)	50	1	0	0
Sunkist					
Fresh	1 (3.8 oz)	50	1	0	–
TANGERINE JUICE					
canned sweetened	1 cup	124	1	tr	0
fresh	1 cup	106	tr	tr	0
Italian Volcano					
Organic	1 serv (6.75 oz)	94	1	–	0
Naked Juice					
Tangerine Scream	8 oz	110	0	0	0
Odwalla					
100% Juice	8 oz	110	0	0	0
SSips					
Drink	1 box (7 oz)	120	0	0	0
TAPIOCA					
pearl dry	¼ cup (1.3 oz)	136	tr	tr	0
starch	1 oz	98	tr	–	–
Let's Do Organic					
Granulated	1 tbsp	35	0	0	0
Starch	1 tbsp	0	0	0	0
TARO					
chips	10 (0.8 oz)	115	6	1	–
leaves cooked	½ cup	18	tr	tr	–
raw sliced	½ cup	56	tr	tr	–
shoots sliced cooked	½ cup	10	tr	tr	–
sliced cooked	½ cup (2.3 oz)	94	tr	tr	–
tahitian sliced cooked	½ cup	30	tr	tr	–
Frieda's					
Taro Root	⅔ cup (3 oz)	90	0	0	0

FOOD	PORTION	CALS	FAT	SAT FAT	TRANS FAT
TARPON					
fresh	3 oz	87	2	–	–
TARRAGON					
dried crumbled	1 tsp	2	tr	tr	0
ground	1 tsp	5	tr	tr	0
TEA/HERBAL TEA (see also ICED TEA)					
HERBAL					
chamomile brewed	1 cup	2	tr	tr	–
Celestial Seasonings					
Chamomile	1 cup	0	0	0	0
Dessert Tea English Toffee	1 cup	0	0	0	0
Moroccan Pomegranate Red	1 cup	0	0	0	0
Peppermint	1 cup	0	0	0	0
Red Safari Spice	1 cup	0	0	0	0
Roastaroma Herb	1 cup	0	0	0	0
Wellness Tea Ginseng Energy	1 tea bag	0	0	0	0
Zinger Acai Mango	1 cup	0	0	0	0
Zinger Lemon	1 cup	0	0	0	0
Eden					
Organic Genmaicha Tea	1 tea bag	0	0	0	0
Organic Kukicha Tea	1 tea bag	0	0	0	0
Guayaki					
Organic Yerba Mate Rooiboost	1 tea bag	5	0	0	0
Organic Yerba Mate Traditional	1 tea bag	5	0	0	0
Yerba Mate Magical Mint	1 tea bag	5	0	0	0
Lipton					
Cinnamon Apple	1 tea bag	0	0	0	0
Ginger Twist	1 tea bag	0	0	0	0
Honey Lemon	1 tea bag	0	0	0	0
Lemon	1 tea bag	0	0	0	0
Mango	1 tea bag	0	0	0	0
Orange	1 tea bag	0	0	0	0
Peach	1 tea bag	0	0	0	0
Peppermint	1 tea bag	0	0	0	0
Quietly Chamomile	1 tea bag	0	0	0	0
Raspberry	1 tea bag	0	0	0	0
Silk					
Chai	1 cup	140	4	0	–

FOOD	PORTION	CALS	FAT	SAT FAT	TRANS FAT
Tetley					
Chamomile	1 cup	0	0	0	0
Orange & Peach	1 cup	0	0	0	0
Peppermint	1 cup	0	0	0	0
REGULAR					
brewed tea	6 oz	2	0	0	0
Activitea					
Green Tea	1 cup	36	0	0	0
Celestial Seasonings					
Black Fast Lane	1 cup	0	0	0	0
Black Decaf Victorian Earl Grey	1 cup	0	0	0	0
Chai White Honey Vanilla	1 tea bag	0	0	0	0
Green Antioxidant	1 cup	0	0	0	0
Green Tropical Acai	1 cup	0	0	0	0
Green Tea	1 cup	0	0	0	0
Morning Thunder	1 cup	0	0	0	0
TeaHouse Chai Cinnamon Spice as prep	1 serv	110	0	0	0
White Tea Antioxidant Plum	1 tea bag	0	0	0	0
Daily Detox					
Original	1 teabag	0	0	0	0
DaVinci Gourmet					
Sugar Free Tea Concentrate Green	2 tbsp	0	0	0	0
Sugar Free Tea Concentrate Lemon	2 tbsp	0	0	0	0
Sugar Free Tea Concentrate Spiced Chai	1.5 tbsp	0	0	0	0
Eden					
Organic Bancha Green Tea	1 tea bag	0	0	0	0
Organic Hojicha Tea	1 tea bag	0	0	0	0
General Foods					
International Tea Chai Latte	1 serv	70	2	2	0
Guayaki					
Organic Yerba Mate Greener Green Tea	1 tea bag	5	0	0	0
Lipton					
Black Tea as prep	1 teabag	0	0	0	0
Black Tea French Vanilla	1 tea bag	0	0	0	0
Black Tea Honey & Lemon	1 tea bag	0	0	0	0

FOOD	PORTION	CALS	FAT	SAT FAT	TRANS FAT
Black Tea Mint	1 tea bag	0	0	0	0
Black Tea Orange & Spice	1 tea bag	0	0	0	0
Black Tea Spiced Chai	1 tea bag	0	0	0	0
Decaffeinated Black Tea as prep	1 serv	0	0	0	0
Earl Grey	1 tea bag	0	0	0	0
English Breakfast	1 tea bag	0	0	0	0
English Estate	1 tea bag	0	0	0	0
Green Tea as prep	1 tea bag	0	0	0	0
Green Tea Citrus Blossom	1 tea bag	5	0	0	0
Green Tea Decaffeinated	1 tea bag	0	0	0	0
Green Tea Lemon Ginseng	1 tea bag	0	0	0	0
Green Tea Mint	1 tea bag	0	0	0	0
Raspberry Truffle	1 tea bag	0	0	0	0
Vanilla Hazelnut	1 tea bag	0	0	0	0
Low Carb Creations					
Chai as prep	1 cup	25	2	0	–
Oregon Chai					
Chai Tea Latte Original Caffeine Free Concentrate	½ cup	78	0	0	0
Chai Tea Latte Original Concentrate	½ cup	78	0	0	0
Chai Tea Latte Spiced Original Mix	1 pkg	100	1	1	–
Chai Tea Latte Vanilla Mix	1 pkg	120	2	1	–
Organic Chai Cider Concentrate	½ cup	110	0	0	0
Oregon Chai					
Organic Chai Nog Concentrate	½ cup	90	0	0	0
Pacific Chai					
All Flavors as prep	1 serv	93	1	1	–
Red Rose					
Black Tea Tea Bag	1	0	0	0	0
Decaffeinated	1 cup	0	0	0	0
English Breakfast Tea Bag	1 cup	0	0	0	0
Salada					
Original Blend Black Tea	1 tea bag	0	0	0	0
Tea Tech					
Instant Green Tea All Flavors	1 tube	0	0	0	0
XtraGreen Tea Mix All Flavors	1 tube	0	0	0	0

FOOD	PORTION	CALS	FAT	SAT FAT	TRANS FAT
Tetley					
British Blend Round Tea Bags	1 cup	0	0	0	0
Chai Black Tea	1 cup	0	0	0	0
Decaffeinated Tea Bag as prep	1	0	0	0	0
Earl Grey	1 cup	0	0	0	0
English Breakfast	1 cup	0	0	0	0
Honey Lemon Green Tea	1 cup	0	0	0	0
TAKE-OUT					
chai spiced latte decaf	1 cup	130	3	1	–

TEMPEH

FOOD	PORTION	CALS	FAT	SAT FAT	TRANS FAT
tempeh	½ cup	165	6	1	–
Lightlife					
Garden Veggie	1 serv (4 oz)	230	10	2	–
Organic Flax	1 serv (4 oz)	230	10	2	–
Organic Grilles Lemon	1 patty (2.7 oz)	140	6	2	–
Organic Grilles Tamari	1 patty (2.7 oz)	130	5	2	–
Organic Soy	1 serv (4 oz)	210	9	1	–
Organic Three Grain	1 serv (4 oz)	240	9	2	–
Organic Wild Rice	1 serv (4 oz)	280	11	2	–
Tofurky					
Edamame Veggie	3 oz	145	4	1	0
Five Grain	3 oz	190	6	1	0
Soy	3 oz	160	4	1	0
White Wave					
Five Grain	⅓ block	140	4	1	–
Organic Original Soy	⅓ block	150	6	1	–
Organic Sea Veggie	⅓ block	120	3	0	–
Soy Rice	⅓ block	140	5	1	–
WildWood					
Organic Nori Seaweed	3 oz	170	7	1	0

TESTICLES (see SWEETBREAD)

THYME

FOOD	PORTION	CALS	FAT	SAT FAT	TRANS FAT
dried crumbled	1 tsp	3	tr	tr	0
fresh	1 tsp	1	tr	tr	0
ground	1 tsp	4	tr	tr	0

TILAPIA

FOOD	PORTION	CALS	FAT	SAT FAT	TRANS FAT
Beacon Light					
Farm Raised Fillets	3 oz	85	1	0	–

FOOD	PORTION	CALS	FAT	SAT FAT	TRANS FAT
Van de Kamp's					
Lightly Breaded Fillets	1 (4 oz)	240	11	3	0
TAKE-OUT					
battered & fried	1 filet (4 oz)	206	9	2	–
breaded & fried	1 filet (4 oz)	300	14	3	0
broiled w/o fat	1 filet (3.5 oz)	128	3	1	0
TILEFISH					
cooked	½ fillet (5.3 oz)	220	7	1	–
cooked	3 oz	125	4	1	–
raw	3 oz	81	2	tr	–
TOFU					
firm	½ cup	183	11	2	–
firm	¼ block (3 oz)	118	7	1	–
fresh fried	1 piece (0.5 oz)	35	3	tr	–
fuyu salted & fermented	1 block (0.3 oz)	13	1	tr	–
koyadofu dried frozen	1 piece (0.5 oz)	82	5	1	–
okara	½ cup	47	1	tr	–
regular	½ cup	94	6	1	–
regular	¼ block (4 oz)	88	6	1	–
Azumaya					
Extra Firm	1 serv (2.8 oz)	70	4	0	–
Firm	1 serv (2.8 oz)	70	4	1	–
Lite Silken	1 serv (3.2 oz)	40	1	0	–
Lite Extra Firm	1 serv (2.8 oz)	60	2	0	–
Seasoned Oriental Spice	1 serv (3 oz)	90	5	1	–
Seasoned Zesty Garlic & Onion	1 serv (3 oz)	90	5	1	–
Silken	1 serv (3.2 oz)	40	2	0	–
Eden					
Dried	1 piece (0.4 oz)	50	3	0	0
Nasoya					
Chinese Spice	¼ pkg (3 oz)	90	5	1	–
Extra Firm	⅕ pkg (2.8 oz)	80	4	1	–
Firm	⅕ pkg (2.8 oz)	70	3	0	–
Garlic & Onion	¼ pkg (3 oz)	90	5	1	–
Lite Firm	⅕ pkg (2.8 oz)	40	2	0	–
Lite Silken	⅕ pkg (3.2 oz)	30	1	tr	–
Seasoned Ginger Sesame	½ pkg (5.5 oz)	210	6	1	–
Seasoned Sweet & Sour	½ pkg (5.5 oz)	190	4	1	–
Seasoned Teriyaki	½ pkg (5.5 oz)	190	4	0	–

FOOD	PORTION	CALS	FAT	SAT FAT	TRANS FAT
Seasoned Thai Peanut	½ pkg (5.5 oz)	240	9	2	–
Silken	⅕ pkg (3.2 oz)	45	3	1	–
Soft	⅕ pkg (2.8 oz)	60	3	1	–
TofuMate Breakfast Scramble	¼ pkg	15	0	0	0
TofuMate Eggless Salad	¼ pkg	15	0	0	0
TofuMate Mandarin Stirfry	¼ pkg	25	0	0	0
TofuMate Mediterranean Herb	¼ pkg	15	0	0	0
TofuMate Szechwan StirFry	¼ pkg	25	0	0	0
TofuMate Texas Taco	¼ pkg	15	0	0	0
Pete's Tofu					
Dessert Peach Mango	1 serv (6 oz)	120	3	0	–
Medium Firm	3 oz	70	4	1	–
Soft	3 oz	56	3	1	–
Super Firm	3 oz	130	8	2	–
Super Firm Italian Herb	3 oz	120	7	1	–
Tofu 2 Go Lemon Pepper	2 pieces + sauce	160	9	1	–
Tofu 2 Go Santa Fe	2 pieces + sauce	150	9	1	–
Tofu 2 Go Sesame Ginger	2 pieces + sauce	160	10	2	–
Tofu 2 Go Thai Tango	2 pieces + sauce	165	10	2	–
Soyafarm					
Baked Tofu	10 pieces (3.5 oz)	147	10	–	–
Nuggets	4 (3.5 oz)	162	8	–	–
Tofu & Yuba Patties	1 (3.5 oz)	243	14	–	–
Tree Of Life					
30% Reduced Fat Firm	⅕ block (3.2 oz)	90	4	0	–
Organic Baked	⅓ block (2.7 oz)	150	8	1	–
Organic Baked Island Spice	⅓ pkg (2.7 oz)	130	7	1	–
Organic Baked Oriental	⅓ pkg (2.7 oz)	130	7	1	–
Organic Baked Savory	⅓ block (2.7 oz)	140	7	1	–
Organic Firm	⅕ block (3.2 oz)	100	5	0	–
Raw Firm	⅕ block (3.2 oz)	100	5	0	–
White Wave					
Baked Garlic Herb Italian	1 piece	120	6	1	–
Baked Hickory Smoke BBQ	1 piece	75	3	1	–
Baked Roma Italian Basil	1 piece	100	6	1	–
Baked Teriyaki Oriental	1 piece	120	6	1	–
Baked Thai Style	1 piece	120	6	1	–
Baked Zesty Lemon Pepper	1 piece	120	8	1	–
Extra Firm	¼ block	80	5	1	–
Organic Extra Firm	⅕ block	90	6	1	–

FOOD	PORTION	CALS	FAT	SAT FAT	TRANS FAT
Organic Soft	⅕ block	90	6	1	–
Reduced Fat	⅕ block	90	4	0	–
WildWood					
Organic Baked Aloha	1 piece (3.5 oz)	180	5	1	0
Organic Calcium Rich Medium	3 oz	70	4	1	0
Organic Golden Pineapple Teriyaki	3 oz	160	12	2	0
Organic High Protein Super Firm	3 oz	100	4	1	0
Organic Smoked Mild Szechuan	3 oz	150	6	1	0
TAKE-OUT					
breaded deep fried w/ soy sauce japanese style	1 piece (0.4 oz)	15	1	tr	–
soy sauce marinated & grilled	1 serv (4 oz)	181	11	2	–
TOMATILLO					
fresh	1 (1.2 oz)	11	tr	–	–
fresh chopped	½ cup	21	1	–	–
Las Palmas					
Tomatillos Crushed	½ cup	45	2	0	0
TOMATO					
CANNED					
paste	½ cup	110	1	tr	–
puree	1 cup	102	tr	tr	–
puree w/o salt	1 cup	102	tr	tr	–
red whole	½ cup	24	tr	tr	–
sauce	½ cup	37	tr	tr	–
sauce spanish style	½ cup	40	tr	tr	–
sauce w/ mushrooms	½ cup	42	tr	tr	–
sauce w/ onion	½ cup	52	tr	tr	–
stewed	½ cup	34	tr	tr	–
w/ green chiles	½ cup	18	tr	tr	–
wedges in tomato juice	½ cup	34	tr	tr	–
Cento					
Crushed	¼ cup	35	0	0	0
Paste	2 tbsp	30	0	0	0
Puree	¼ cup	25	0	0	0
Contadina					
Crushed w/ Italian Herbs	¼ cup	20	0	0	0

FOOD	PORTION	CALS	FAT	SAT FAT	TRANS FAT
Italian Paste Roasted Garlic	2 tbsp	35	1	–	–
Paste	2 tbsp (1.2 oz)	30	0	0	0
Paste Italian Herbs	2 tbsp	35	1	0	0
Petite Cut Diced	½ cup	25	0	0	0
Puree	¼ cup (2.2 oz)	20	0	0	0
Stewed	½ cup	35	0	0	0
Stewed w/ Celery & Green Peppers	½ cup	35	0	0	0
Del Monte					
Chunky Pasta Style	½ cup	45	0	0	0
Diced No Salt Added	½ cup	25	0	0	0
Diced w/ Garlic & Onion	½ cup	40	1	0	0
Diced w/ Green Pepper & Onion	½ cup	40	0	0	0
Diced Zesty Chili Style	½ cup	30	0	0	0
Diced Zesty w/ Mild Green Chilies	½ cup	30	0	0	0
Garden Select Petite Diced	½ cup	15	0	0	0
Organic Diced	½ cup	25	0	0	0
Organic Diced w/ Basil Garlic & Oregano	½ cup	50	0	0	0
Organic Tomato Paste	2 tbsp	30	0	0	0
Petite Cut	½ cup	25	0	0	0
Petite Cut Garlic & Olive Oil	½ cup	45	1	0	–
Sauce	¼ cup	20	0	0	0
Stewed Cajun Recipe	½ cup	35	0	0	0
Stewed Italian Recipe	½ cup	30	0	0	0
Stewed Mexican Recipe	½ cup	35	0	0	0
Stewed No Salt Added	½ cup	35	0	0	0
Stewed Original	½ cup	35	0	0	0
Wedges	½ cup	35	0	0	0
Eden					
Organic Crushed	¼ cup	20	0	0	0
Organic Diced	½ cup	30	0	0	0
Organic Whole Roma	½ cup	30	0	0	0
Hunt's					
Crushed	½ cup	30	0	0	0
Diced In Tomato Sauce	½ cup	30	0	0	0
Diced Original	½ cup	20	0	0	0

FOOD	PORTION	CALS	FAT	SAT FAT	TRANS FAT
Diced w/ Basil Garlic & Oregano	½ cup	25	0	0	0
Diced w/ Green Pepper Celery & Onions	½ cup	45	0	0	0
Diced w/ Mild Green Chilies	½ cup	30	0	0	0
Diced w/ Roasted Garlic	½ cup	30	0	0	0
Diced w/ Sweet Onion	½ cup	45	0	0	0
Family Favorites Meatloaf	¼ cup	30	0	0	0
Paste	2 tbsp	25	0	0	0
Paste No Salt Added	2 tbsp	30	0	0	0
Paste w/ Basil Garlic & Oregano	2 tbsp	25	0	0	0
Petite Diced	½ cup	20	0	0	0
Petite Diced w/ Mushrooms	½ cup	40	1	0	0
Puree	½ cup	30	0	0	0
Sauce	¼ cup	15	0	0	0
Sauce Garlic & Herb	½ cup	40	1	0	0
Sauce No Salt Added	2 tbsp	30	0	0	0
Sauce Roasted Garlic	¼ cup	15	0	0	0
Stewed	½ cup	35	0	0	0
Stewed No Salt Added	½ cup	40	0	0	0
Whole No Salt Added	¼ cup (4 oz)	20	0	0	0
Muir Glen					
Organic Chunky Tomato & Herb	½ cup	60	1	0	0
Organic Diced Fire Roasted	½ cup	30	0	0	0
Organic Diced w/ Basil & Garlic	½ cup	30	0	0	0
Pomi					
Chopped	½ cup	20	0	0	0
Progresso					
Crushed w/ Added Puree	¼ cup (2.1 oz)	20	0	0	0
Redpack					
Crushed In Puree	¼ cup	20	0	0	0
Diced In Juice	½ cup	25	0	0	0
Paste	2 tbsp	0	0	0	0
Petite Diced Onion Celery & Green Pepper	½ cup	45	0	0	0
Rienzi					
Paste	2 tbsp	25	0	0	0

FOOD	PORTION	CALS	FAT	SAT FAT	TRANS FAT
Ro-Tel					
Diced In Sauce	½ cup	40	0	0	0
Mexican Festival	½ cup	30	0	0	0
Original	½ cup	20	0	0	0
Tillen Farms					
Sunnyside Tomatoes	3 pieces (1 oz)	40	3	1	–
Tuttorosso					
Puree	¼ cup	20	0	0	0
DRIED					
sun dried	1 piece	5	tr	tr	–
sun dried	1 cup	140	2	tr	–
sun dried in oil	1 cup (4 oz)	235	15	2	–
sun dried in oil	1 piece (3 g)	6	tr	tr	–
Frieda's					
Red Chopped	⅓ cup (1.1 oz)	100	1	0	0
FRESH					
bruschetta	¼ cup	50	3	0	–
cooked	½ cup	32	1	tr	–
grape tomatoes	20	30	0	0	0
green	1	30	tr	tr	–
red	1 (4.5 oz)	26	tr	tr	–
red chopped	1 cup	35	tr	tr	–
Chiquita					
Tomato	1 med (5.2 oz)	35	1	0	–
Earthbound Farm					
Organic Roma	1 med (5.2 oz)	35	1	0	0
Eurofresh					
Tomatoes On The Vine	1 med (5.2 oz)	35	1	0	–
Foxy					
Roma	1 med (5 oz)	35	1	0	0
Frieda's					
Baby Roma	⅔ cup (3 oz)	120	0	0	0
Tear Drop	⅔ cup (3 oz)	20	0	0	0
TAKE-OUT					
bruschetta on toasted italian bread	1 slice	106	3	0	–
stewed	1 cup	80	3	1	–
TOMATO JUICE					
beef broth & tomato	1 can (5.5 oz)	62	tr	tr	–

FOOD	PORTION	CALS	FAT	SAT FAT	TRANS FAT
clam & tomato	1 can (5.5 oz)	77	tr	tr	–
tomato juice	½ cup	21	tr	tr	–
tomato juice	6 oz	32	tr	tr	–
Campbell's					
Healthy Request	8 oz	50	0	0	0
Low Sodium	8 oz	50	0	0	0
Organic	8 oz	50	0	0	0
Del Monte					
Juice	8 oz	50	0	0	0
Kagome					
Sweet Summer	8 oz	50	0	0	0
Lakewood					
Organic	8 oz	35	0	0	0
Luvli Juices					
Smashing Tomato	1 bottle (10 oz)	125	1	–	–
Spicy Tomato	1 bottle (10 oz)	125	1	–	–
TONGUE					
beef simmered	3 oz	241	19	7	0
lamb braised	3 oz	234	17	7	0
pork braised	3 oz	230	16	5	0
veal braised	3 oz	172	9	4	0
TORTILLA					
corn	1 (6 in)	56	1	tr	–
corn w/o salt	1 (6 in)	56	1	tr	–
flour w/o salt	1 (8 in)	114	3	tr	–
Alvarado Street Bakery					
Sprouted Wheat Burrito Size	1 (2.2 oz)	170	4	0	0
CarbOle					
Low-Carb	1 (2 oz)	100	4	0	–
Food For Life					
Sprouted Corn	2 (1.7 oz)	120	1	0	0
French Meadow Bakery					
Organic Fat Flush	1 (1 oz)	100	1	0	0
La Tortilla Factory					
Carb Cutting Original	1 (1.3 oz)	60	2	0	0
Organic Yellow Corn	2 (2.4 oz)	120	2	0	0
Smart & Delicious Low Fat Low Sodium	1 (2.5 oz)	150	2	1	0

FOOD	PORTION	CALS	FAT	SAT FAT	TRANS FAT
Manny's					
Burrito Tortilla	1 (2.1 oz)	180	5	1	1
Fajita Tortilla	1 (2 oz)	170	5	1	1
Fat Free	1 (1 oz)	65	0	0	0
Low Carb	1 (1.7 oz)	140	7	2	1
Soft Taco Tortilla	1 (1 oz)	80	2	1	0
Tortilla Wrap Tomato Basil	1 (1.4 oz)	100	2	1	–
White Corn Gluten Free	1 (2 oz)	60	1	0	0
Whole Wheat	1 (2 oz)	170	4	1	1
Rudi's Organic Bakery					
Spelt	1 (2 oz)	140	3	0	0
Super Bakery					
Organic	1 (2.5 oz)	210	5	0	0
Tumaro's					
Honey Wheat	1 (8 in)	110	2	0	–
Low In Carbs Garden Vegetable	1 (8 in)	100	3	0	0
Low In Carbs Green Onion	1 (8 in)	100	3	0	0
Low In Carbs Multi Grain	1 (8 in)	100	3	0	0
Low In Carbs Salsa	1 (8 in)	100	3	0	0
Pesto & Garlic	1 (8 in)	110	1	0	–
Premium White	1 (8 in)	120	2	0	–
Soy-full Heart 8 Grain 'N Soy	1 (1.4 oz)	100	0	0	0
Soy-full Heart Apple 'N Cinnamon	1 (1.4 oz)	90	3	0	0
Soy-full Heart Wheat Soy & Flax	1 (1.4 oz)	90	3	0	0
Spinach & Vegetables	1 (8 in)	110	2	0	–

TORTILLA CHIPS (see CHIPS)

TRAIL MIX
FOOD	PORTION	CALS	FAT	SAT FAT	TRANS FAT
Bowlby's					
Mix-Ups	½ cup	165	12	2	–
Mix-Ups Country	½ cup	170	14	2	–
Mix-Ups Nuttyest-Of-All	½ cup	160	13	2	–
Enjoy Life					
Gluten Free Not Nuts! Beach Bash	1 oz	130	7	1	0
Gluten Free Not Nuts! Mountain Mambo	1 oz	140	8	2	0

FOOD	PORTION	CALS	FAT	SAT FAT	TRANS FAT
Good Sense					
Dietary Snack Mix	¼ cup	130	6	2	0
Organic Tropical	⅓ cup	160	10	2	–
Maranatha					
Deluxe	¼ cup	150	11	1	–
High Energy Mix	¼ cup	120	7	1	–
Navajo	¼ cup	140	9	1	–
Olympic w/ Chocolate	¼ cup	140	8	2	–
Organic Harvest Mix	¼ cup	150	9	1	–
Organic Nature Mix	¼ cup	150	9	2	–
Organic Raw	¼ cup	140	9	2	–
Snack Attack Mix	¼ cup	140	8	3	–
Mauna Loa					
Tropical Nut & Fruit	¼ cup	180	8	2	–
Mrs. May's					
Coconut Almond Crunch	1 oz	183	15	1	0
Navitas Naturals					
3 Berry Cacao Nibs & Cashews	1 oz	110	5	2	0
Goji Cacao Nibs & Cashews	1 oz	120	6	2	0
Goji Golden Berry & Mulberry	1 oz	90	0	0	0
Organic Trails					
Summit Blend	¼ cup	150	8	2	0
Planters					
Berry Nut & Chocolate	3 tbsp (1 oz)	120	5	1	0
SunRise					
w/ Fruit	3 tbsp (1 oz)	130	6	1	0
TREE FERN					
chopped cooked	½ cup	28	tr	–	–
TRIPE					
beef simmered	3 oz	80	3	1	tr
TAKE-OUT					
mondongo w/ potatoes	1 cup	300	11	3	–
TRITICALE					
dry	½ cup (3.4 oz)	323	2	tr	–
TROUT					
baked	3 oz	162	7	1	–
rainbow cooked	3 oz	129	4	1	–
seatrout baked	3 oz	113	4	1	–

FOOD	PORTION	CALS	FAT	SAT FAT	TRANS FAT
TRUFFLES					
fresh	0.5 oz	4	tr	–	–
TUNA (see also TUNA DISHES)					
CANNED					
light in oil	1 can (6 oz)	399	14	3	–
light in oil	3 oz	169	7	1	–
light in water	1 can (5.8 oz)	192	1	tr	–
light in water	3 oz	99	1	tr	–
white in oil	1 can (6.2 oz)	331	14	–	–
white in oil	3 oz	158	7	–	–
white in water	1 can (6 oz)	234	4	1	–
white in water	3 oz	116	2	1	–
Bumble Bee					
Chunk Light In Oil	¼ cup	110	6	1	–
Chunk Light In Water	2 oz	60	1	0	0
Chunk Light Touch Of Lemon In Water	¼ cup	60	1	0	–
Chunk White In Oil	¼ cup	100	5	1	–
Chunk White In Water	¼ cup	60	1	0	–
Chunk White In Water Very Low Sodium	¼ cup	70	1	0	–
Light In Oil	¼ cup	110	6	1	–
Sensations Lemon & Pepper w/ Crackers	1 pkg (3.6 oz)	200	8	4	0
Solid White In Oil	¼ cup	90	3	1	–
Solid White In Water	2 oz	70	1	0	0
Tonno In Olive Oil	¼ cup	120	6	2	0
Chicken Of The Sea					
Albacore Solid In Water	2 oz	70	1	0	0
Chunk Light In Oil	2 oz	110	6	1	–
Chunk Light In Water	¼ cup (2 oz)	60	1	0	–
Chunk White In Spring Water	½ can	60	1	0	–
Chunk White Low Sodium In Spring Water	1 can (3 oz)	80	1	0	–
Premium Albacore Pouch	2 oz	60	1	0	–
Coral					
Light In Water	¼ cup	60	1	0	–

FOOD	PORTION	CALS	FAT	SAT FAT	TRANS FAT
StarKist					
Chunk Light In Water	¼ cup (2 oz)	60	1	0	–
Solid White Albacore In Water	¼ cup	70	1	0	0
FRESH					
bluefin cooked	3 oz	157	5	1	–
bluefin raw	3 oz	122	4	1	–
skipjack baked	3 oz	112	1	tr	–
yellowfin baked	3 oz	118	1	tr	–
MIX					
Chicken Of The Sea					
Salad Kit	1 serv (3.5 oz)	380	24	6	–
Tuna Salad Kit Single Mayo & Onion	1 pkg	380	24	6	–
SHELF-STABLE					
Bumble Bee					
Steak Entrees Ginger & Soy	1 pkg (4 oz)	170	3	0	0
Steak Entrees Lemon & Cracked Pepper	1 pkg (4 oz)	160	1	0	–
Steak Entrees Mesquite Grilled	1 pkg (4 oz)	150	2	0	–
TAKE-OUT					
tuna salad	1 cup	383	19	3	–
TURBOT					
european baked	3 oz	104	3	–	–
TURKEY (see also MEAT STICKS, TURKEY DISHES, TURKEY SUBSTITUTES)					
CANNED					
in broth	1 can (5 oz)	231	10	3	–
w/ broth	1 cup	220	9	3	–
Valley Fresh					
Chunk White	2 oz	80	2	1	–
FRESH					
breast pre-basted w/ skin roasted	3.5 oz	126	3	1	–
breast roasted w/ skin	4 oz	212	8	2	–
dark meat w/o skin roasted	1 cup (5 oz)	262	10	3	–
dark meat w/o skin roasted	3 oz	170	7	2	–
ground cooked	3 oz	193	11	3	–
leg w/ skin roasted	1 (19 oz)	1136	54	17	–
light meat w/ skin roasted half turkey	2.3 lbs	2069	87	25	–

FOOD	PORTION	CALS	FAT	SAT FAT	TRANS FAT
light meat w/o skin roasted	4 oz	183	4	1	–
neck simmered	1 (5.3 oz)	274	11	4	–
skin roasted	1 oz	141	13	3	–
skin roasted from half turkey	8.7 oz	1096	98	26	–
tail cooked	1 (2 oz)	197	16	5	–
w/ skin roasted	½ turkey (4 lbs)	3857	181	53	–
w/ skin roasted	8.4 oz	498	23	7	–
w/o skin roasted	1 cup (5 oz)	238	7	2	–
w/o skin roasted	7.3 oz	354	10	3	–
wing w/ skin roasted	1 (6.5 oz)	426	23	6	–
wing w/o skin roasted	1	237	5	2	–
Honeysuckle White					
85% Lean Ground	4 oz	240	17	5	0
93% Lean Patties	1 (4 oz)	160	8	3	0
97% Lean Ground White	4 oz	130	2	1	0
99% Fat Free Breast Tenderloin	4 oz	120	1	0	0
99% Fat Free Breast Cutlets	4 oz	120	1	0	0
Drumettes	4 oz	180	8	2	0
Marinated Strips Asian Grill	4 oz	160	7	2	–
Necks	4 oz	150	6	2	0
Tenderloins Creamy Dijon Mustard	4 oz	140	4	0	–
Tenderloins Homestyle	4 oz	130	4	0	–
Tenderloins Teriyaki	4 oz	140	4	0	–
Thighs	4 oz	190	11	4	0
Whole Honey Roasted	4 oz	180	9	3	–
Wings	4 oz	220	14	4	0
Jennie-O					
Ground	4 oz	160	8	3	–
Perdue					
Burger Cooked	1 (4 oz)	160	9	3	–
Dark Cooked	3 oz	180	11	4	–
Ground Cooked	3 oz	160	9	3	–
Shady Brook					
Breast Tenderloin	4 oz	130	1	0	–
Breast Tenderloin Creamy Dijon Mustard	4 oz	140	4	0	–
Breast Tenderloin Teriyaki	4 oz	140	4	0	–

FOOD	PORTION	CALS	FAT	SAT FAT	TRANS FAT
Breast Cutlets	4 oz	110	1	0	–
Ground 85% Lean	4 oz	220	17	5	–
Ground 93% Lean	4 oz	160	8	3	–
Ground 99% Lean	4 oz	120	1	0	–
Marinated Strips Asian Grill	4 oz	160	7	2	–
Marinated Strips Mild Herb	4 oz	130	4	2	–
Necks	4 oz	150	6	2	–
Tenderloins Turkey Breast Homestyle	4 oz	130	1	0	–
Thigh	4 oz	145	7	2	–
Whole Turkey	4 oz	180	9	3	–
Wing	4 oz	210	12	4	–
FROZEN					
roast boneless seasoned light & dark meat roasted	3.5 oz	155	6	2	–
sticks breaded fried	1 (2.2 oz)	179	11	3	–
Honeysuckle White					
Breast Boneless Roast	4 oz	170	7	3	–
Jennie-O					
Burger	1 (4 oz)	160	9	2	–
Organic Prairie					
Whole Young	4 oz	190	10	3	0
READY-TO-EAT					
bologna	1 slice (1 oz)	59	4	1	–
breast	1 slice (0.7 oz)	22	tr	tr	0
ham	1 slice (1 oz)	35	1	tr	–
pastrami	2 oz	70	2	1	–
salami	1 slice (1 oz)	48	3	1	0
Boar's Head					
Breast 50% Lower Sodium Skin On	2 oz	60	2	0	–
Breast Cracked Pepper Smoked	2 oz	60	1	0	–
Breast Hickory Smoked Black Forest	2 oz	60	1	0	–
Breast Maple Glazed Honey Coat	2 oz	70	1	0	–
Breast Ovengold	2 oz	60	2	0	–
Breast Ovengold Skinless	2 oz	60	1	0	–

FOOD	PORTION	CALS	FAT	SAT FAT	TRANS FAT
Breast Roasted Mesquite Smoked Skinless	2 oz	60	1	0	–
Breast Roasted Salsalito	2 oz	60	1	0	–
Healthy Choice					
Smoked Breast	4 slices (1.8 oz)	60	2	1	–
Healthy Ones					
Oven Roasted 97% Fat Free	7 slices (2 oz)	60	2	1	0
Hebrew National					
98% Fat Free Oven Roasted	5 slices (2 oz)	50	1	0	–
98% Fat Free Smoked Breast	5 slices (2 oz)	60	1	1	–
Honeysuckle White					
Simply Done Whole Breast	4 oz	160	7	2	–
Jennie-O					
Turkey Breast Golden Roast	3 oz	100	3	1	–
Jordan's					
Fat Free Turkey Breast	1 slice (1 oz)	25	0	0	0
Organic Prairie					
Roasted Breast Slices	2 oz	60	1	0	–
Oscar Mayer					
Breast Smoked Shaved	2 oz	50	1	0	0
Turkey Cotto Salami	3 slices (3 oz)	130	8	3	–
Perdue					
Breast Sliced Honey Smoked	2 oz	50	0	–	0
Breast Sliced Pan Roasted	2 oz	70	2	1	–
Ham Hickory Smoked	2 oz	60	3	1	–
Pastrami Hickory Smoked	2 oz	70	3	1	–
Sara Lee					
Breast Hardwood Smoked	4 slices (1.8 oz)	50	1	0	0
Breast Cracked Pepper	2 oz	50	1	0	–
Shady Brook					
Breast Bone-In Oven Roasted	3 oz	160	7	2	–
Hickory Smoked Breast Fat Free	2 oz	50	0	0	0
Turkey Ham Smoked	2 oz	60	2	1	–
Whole Oven Roasted	3 oz	160	8	2	–
Tyson					
Breast Oven Roasted	2 slices (1.6 oz)	40	1	0	0

FOOD	PORTION	CALS	FAT	SAT FAT	TRANS FAT
TURKEY DISHES					
FROZEN					
gravy & turkey	1 cup (8.4 oz)	160	6	2	–
Banquet					
Homestyle Gravy & Sliced Turkey	2 slices + gravy	130	9	3	–
READY-TO-EAT					
Jennie-O					
Stuffed Breast Cheddar Cheese & Broccoli	1 serv (6 oz)	240	9	5	–
Stuffed Turkey Breast Pepper Cheese & Rice	1 piece (6 oz)	250	7	4	–
Turkey Breast Roast In Homestyle Gravy	1 serv (5 oz)	110	1	0	–
Perdue					
Meal Time Starters Turkey Breast Roast w/ Homestyle Gravy	½ cup (4.6 oz)	144	5	2	0
TAKE-OUT					
boneless breast w/ cranberry apple stuffing	1 serv (5 oz)	260	9	2	–
fricassee	1 cup	322	18	5	–
salad	1 cup	417	32	6	–
tetrazzini	1 cup	369	18	6	–
turkey creole w/o rice	1 cup	189	4	1	–
turkey croquette	1 (2 oz)	158	9	2	–
turkey divan	1 cup	321	14	6	–
turkey meatloaf	1 lg slice (5 oz)	243	9	3	–
TURKEY SUBSTITUTES					
Lightlife					
Smart Deli Roast Turkey	4 slices (2 oz)	80	0	0	0
Tofurky					
Deli Slices Cranberry	3 (1.8 oz)	98	3	0	0
Deli Slices Hickory Smoked	3 (1.8 oz)	100	3	0	0
Deli Slices Italian	3 (1.8 oz)	103	4	1	0
Deli Slices Original	3 (1.8 oz)	103	3	0	0
Deli Slices Peppered	3 (1.8 oz)	103	3	0	0
Deli Slices Philly Steak	3 (1.8 oz)	110	3	0	0
Roast	1 serv (4 oz)	190	5	0	0

FOOD	PORTION	CALS	FAT	SAT FAT	TRANS FAT
Worthington					
Turkee Slices	3 (3.3 oz)	180	12	2	0
Yves					
Meatless Ground Turkey	⅓ cup	60	1	0	0
Meatless Deli Turkey Slices	4 slices	100	2	0	0
TURMERIC					
ground	1 tsp	8	tr	tr	0
TURNIPS					
canned greens	½ cup	17	tr	tr	–
cooked mashed	½ cup (4.2 oz)	47	tr	tr	–
cubed cooked	½ cup (3 oz)	33	tr	tr	–
frzn greens cooked	½ cup	24	tr	tr	–
greens chopped cooked	½ cup	15	tr	tr	–
greens raw chopped	½ cup	7	tr	tr	–
raw cubed	½ cup (2.4 oz)	25	tr	tr	–
Allens					
Green Seasoned Southern Style	½ cup	30	0	0	0
Glory					
Greens Fresh	2 cups	20	0	0	0
Greens Seasoned Canned	½ cup	35	0	0	0
Root Cut Fresh	½ cup	20	0	0	0
Sensibly Seasoned Greens	½ cup	20	0	0	0
TURTLE					
raw	3.5 oz	85	1	–	–
TUSK FISH					
raw	3.5 oz	79	tr	–	–
VANILLA					
vanilla extract	1 tsp	12	0	0	0
Bob's Red Mill					
Organic Extract	1 tsp	0	0	0	0
Steel's					
Sugar Free	1 tbsp	24	0	0	0
Virginia Dare					
Extract	1 tsp	10	0	0	0

FOOD	PORTION	CALS	FAT	SAT FAT	TRANS FAT
VEAL (see also VEAL DISHES)					
breast braised	3 oz	226	14	6	0
chop cooked	1 med (6.5 oz)	230	13	6	0
chop breaded fried	1 med (6.5 oz)	290	12	4	0
cubed braised	3 oz	160	4	1	0
cutlet cooked	3 oz	141	4	1	0
ground broiled	3 oz	146	6	3	0
leg roasted	3 oz	136	4	2	0
loin roasted	3 oz	184	10	4	0
patty breaded fried	1 (2.8 oz)	211	13	4	0
shank braised	3 oz	162	5	2	0
VEAL DISHES					
TAKE-OUT					
cordon bleu	1 serv (8 oz)	490	35	19	0
parmigiana	1 serv (6.4 oz)	362	21	8	0
scallopini	1 slice + sauce (3.4 oz)	238	17	5	0
stew	1 serv (8.8 oz)	192	6	3	0
veal marengo	1 serv (8.8 oz)	274	9	3	0
veal marsala	1 slice + sauce (3.4 oz)	268	19	9	0
veal paprikash	1 serv (8.6 oz)	280	12	5	0
veal picatta	1 piece + sauce (3.5 oz)	154	9	5	0
VEGETABLE JUICE					
low sodium tomato & vegetable juice	1 cup	53	tr	tr	0
vegetable juice cocktail	8 oz	46	tr	tr	0
Bolthouse Farms					
Vedge Tomato Carrot Celery	8 oz	60	0	0	0
Lakewood					
Super Veggie	6 oz	40	0	0	0
V8					
100% Vegetable Essential Antioxidants	8 oz	50	0	0	0
Acai Berry Blend	8 oz	110	0	0	0
Calcium Enriched	8 oz	50	0	0	0
High Fiber	8 oz	60	0	0	0

FOOD	PORTION	CALS	FAT	SAT FAT	TRANS FAT
Low Sodium	8 oz	50	0	0	0
Organic	8 oz	50	0	0	0
Walnut Acres					
Organic Incredible Vegetable	8 oz	50	0	0	0

VEGETABLES MIXED
CANNED

FOOD	PORTION	CALS	FAT	SAT FAT	TRANS FAT
mixed vegetables	½ cup	39	tr	tr	–
peas & carrots	½ cup	48	tr	tr	–
peas & carrots low sodium	½ cup	48	tr	tr	–
peas & onions	½ cup	30	tr	tr	–
succotash	½ cup	102	1	tr	–
Del Monte					
Mixed	½ cup	40	0	0	0
Mixed Vegetables w/ Potatoes	½ cup	45	0	0	0
Peas And Carrots	½ cup	60	0	0	0
Savory Sides Homestyle Vegetable Medley	½ cup	70	3	0	–
Savory Sides Rio Grande Vegetables	½ cup	70	0	0	0
S&W					
Mixed	½ cup (4.4 oz)	35	0	0	0
Peas & Carrots	½ cup (4.5 oz)	60	0	0	0
Peas & Onions	½ cup (4.3 oz)	40	0	0	0
Veg-All					
Original Mixed	½ cup	40	0	0	0
FRESH					
Mann's					
California Stir Fry	1 serv (3 oz)	30	0	0	0
River Ranch					
Broccoli & Carrots	1 cup	25	0	0	0
Broccoli & Cauliflower	1 cup	25	0	0	0
Stir Fry Blend	1 cup	30	0	0	0
Vegetable Medley	1 cup	25	0	0	0
FROZEN					
mixed vegetables cooked	½ cup	54	tr	tr	–
peas & carrots cooked	½ cup	38	tr	tr	–
peas & onions cooked	½ cup	40	tr	tr	–
succotash cooked	½ cup	79	1	tr	–

FOOD	PORTION	CALS	FAT	SAT FAT	TRANS FAT
Birds Eye					
Broccoli & Cauliflower	1 cup	30	0	0	0
Italian Herb Harvest Vegetables	1¼ cups	90	6	4	0
Spring Vegetables In Citrus Sauce	1¼ cups	70	4	2	0
Steamfresh Asian Medley	1 cup	50	2	0	0
Steamfresh Broccoli Carrots Sugar Snap Peas & Water Chestnuts	¾ cup	35	0	0	0
Steamfresh Broccoli Cauliflower & Carrots	¾ cup	30	0	0	0
Steamfresh Mixed Vegetables	⅔ cup	40	0	0	0
C&W					
Early Harvest Peas & Baby Carrots	⅔ cup	60	0	0	0
Petite Peas & Pearl Onions	⅔ cup	60	0	0	0
Cascadian Farm					
Organic Peas & Carrots	⅔ cup	50	0	0	0
Organic Mixed Vegetables	⅔ cup	60	0	0	0
Europe's Best					
Zen Garden	¾ cup	60	1	0	0
Fresh Like					
California Blend	3.5 oz	31	tr	–	–
Midwestern Blend	3.5 oz	42	tr	–	–
Mixed	3.5 oz	69	tr	–	–
Oriental Blend	3.5 oz	26	tr	–	–
Winter Blend	3.5 oz	26	tr	–	–
Green Giant					
Broccoli & Carrots w/ Garlic & Herbs as prep	½ cup	40	1	0	0
Garden Vegetable Medley as prep	½ cup	70	1	0	0
Mixed Vegetables as prep	½ cup	50	0	0	0
Southwestern Style as prep	½ cups	90	1	0	0
Szechuan Vegetables as prep	½ cup	50	1	0	0
Lean Cuisine					
Cafe Classics Roasted Potatoes w/ Broccoli & Cheddar Cheese Sauce	1 pkg (10.25 oz)	230	5	3	0

FOOD	PORTION	CALS	FAT	SAT FAT	TRANS FAT
McKenzie's					
Gumbo Mixture	1 serv (2.9 oz)	35	0	0	0
Okra Tomatoes w/ Onions	1 serv (2.8 oz)	20	0	0	0
Melrose Made Gourmet					
Vegetable Souffle Fat Free	1 serv (4 oz)	70	0	0	0
Pictsweet					
Peas & Carrots	⅔ cup	50	0	0	0
Roast Works					
Flame Roasted Redskins & Vegetables	1 serv (3 oz)	90	3	0	0
TAKE-OUT					
buddha's delight	1 serv (16 oz)	174	5	1	–
caponata	¼ cup	28	1	–	–
pakoras	1 (2 oz)	108	5	–	–
ratatouille	1 serv (3.5 oz)	96	7	1	–
samosa	1 (2.4 oz)	206	11	5	tr
succotash	½ cup	111	1	tr	–
tapenade grilled vegetables	¼ cup	40	3	0	–

VENISON (see also MEAT STICKS)

FOOD	PORTION	CALS	FAT	SAT FAT	TRANS FAT
roasted	4 oz	215	4	2	–

VINEGAR

FOOD	PORTION	CALS	FAT	SAT FAT	TRANS FAT
balsamic	1 tbsp	14	0	0	0
cider	1 tbsp	3	0	0	0
red wine	1 tbsp	3	0	0	0
vinegar	1 tbsp	3	0	0	0
white	1 tbsp	3	0	0	0
Carapelli					
Balsamic	1 tbsp	15	0	0	0
Red Wine	1 tbsp	5	0	0	0
White Wine	1 tbsp	5	0	0	0
Eden					
Organic Apple Cider	1 tbsp	0	0	0	0
Organic Brown Rice	1 tbsp	2	0	0	0
Red Wine	1 tbsp	0	0	0	0
Ume Plum	1 tsp	0	0	0	0
Heinz					
White	2 tbsp	2	0	0	0
Latino Chef					
Lulo	1 tbsp	35	3	–	–

FOOD	PORTION	CALS	FAT	SAT FAT	TRANS FAT
Passion Fruit	1 tbsp	40	3	–	–
Newman's Own					
Organic Balsamic	1 tbsp	20	0	0	0
Pacifica Culinaria					
Balsamic Dark Sweet Cherry	1 tbsp	15	0	0	0
Pear Pomegranate	1 tbsp	10	0	0	0
Regina					
Red Wine	1 tbsp	0	0	0	0
Spectrum					
Apple Cider Organic	1 tbsp	7	0	0	0
Balsamic Organic	1 tbsp	6	0	0	0
Brown Rice Organic	1 tbsp	10	0	0	0
Golden Balsamic Organic	1 tbsp	6	0	0	0
Red Wine Organic	1 tbsp	0	0	0	0
White Organic	1 tbsp	2	0	0	0
White Wine Organic	1 tbsp	0	0	0	0

WAFFLES
FROZEN

FOOD	PORTION	CALS	FAT	SAT FAT	TRANS FAT
Aunt Jemima					
Blueberry	2 (2.5 oz)	190	5	1	0
Low Fat	2 (2.5 oz)	160	3	1	0
Eggo					
Buttermilk	2	180	6	2	2
Homestyle	2	190	6	2	2
Homestyle Minis	12	250	9	2	3
Nutri-Grain Low Fat Whole Wheat	2	140	3	1	0
Special K	3	190	1	0	0
Waf-Fulls Strawberry	1	150	5	2	2
EnviroKidz					
Organic Gorilla Banana	2 (2.7 oz)	230	8	2	0
Kashi					
Heart To Heart Honey Oat	2 (3 oz)	160	3	0	0
Lifestream					
Organic Fig + Flax	2 (2.8 oz)	210	0	2	0
Organic Pomegran Plus	2 (2.8 oz)	190	5	1	0
Van's					
Belgian 7 Grain	2	230	4	1	0
Belgian Blueberry	2	184	4	0	0

FOOD	PORTION	CALS	FAT	SAT FAT	TRANS FAT
Belgian Original	2	172	4	0	0
Carb Manager Flax	2	200	13	3	0
Carb Manager Homestyle	2	200	12	3	0
Gourmet 97% Fat Free	2	230	8	1	0
Gourmet Blueberry	2	190	6	1	0
Gourmet Buckwheat	2	145	4	0	0
Gourmet Flax	2	157	4	0	0
Gourmet Multi Grain	2	260	11	1	0
Gourmet Original	2	180	2	1	0
Hearty Oat Berry Boost	2	200	8	1	0
Hearty Oat Maple Fusion	2	210	9	2	0
Hearty Oat Oats 'N Honey	2	200	8	1	0
Mini Blueberry	4	110	5	0	0
Mini Chocolate Chip	4	119	4	0	0
Mini Homestyle	4	116	4	0	0
Organic Blueberry	2	240	10	2	0
Organic Original	2	190	5	0	–
Organic Soy Flax	2	230	11	2	0
Wheat Free Blueberry	2	201	5	1	0
Wheat Free Cinnamon Apple	2	189	5	1	0
Wheat Free Flax	2	230	6	1	0
Wheat Free Mini	4	160	5	0	0
Wheat Free Original	2	189	5	1	0
MIX					
plain as prep (7 in diam)	1 (2.6 oz)	218	11	2	0
READY-TO-EAT					
Gol D Lite					
Low Carb Belgian	1 (0.9 oz)	100	5	0	–
Low Carb Belgian Chocolate Covered	1 (1.1 oz)	130	8	0	–
Kashi					
GoLean Blueberry	2 (3 oz)	170	3	0	0
GoLean Original	2 (3 oz)	170	3	0	0
Thomas'					
Homestyle	1 (1.6 oz)	140	5	1	–
TAKE-OUT					
belgian	1 (4.7 oz)	412	13	3	0
blueberry (9 in sq)	1 (7 oz)	556	16	3	0
round (10 in diam)	1 (6.8 oz)	598	18	4	0

FOOD	PORTION	CALS	FAT	SAT FAT	TRANS FAT
square (9 in)	1 (7 oz)	620	19	4	0
whole wheat (9 in sq)	1 (7 oz)	534	22	6	0

WALNUTS
black chopped	¼ cup	193	18	1	–
english chopped	¼ cup	191	19	2	0
english ground	¼ cup	131	13	1	0
english halves	14 (1 oz)	185	18	2	–
english in shell	7 (1 oz)	183	18	2	0
honey roasted	¼ cup	172	16	2	0
Diamond					
Chopped	¼ cup	200	20	2	0
Emerald					
Glazed	¼ cup	140	10	1	0
Good Sense					
Organic Raw	¼ cup	210	20	2	0
Sweet Delights					
Walnut Roasters	⅓ pkg (1 oz)	210	20	2	–

WASABI (see HORSERADISH)

WATER
ice cubes	3	0	0	0	0
tap water	8 oz	0	0	0	0
Absopure					
Natural Spring	8 oz	0	0	0	0
Aloe Breeze					
Organic All Flavors	8 oz	0	0	0	0
Aloe Splash					
All Flavors	8 oz	0	0	0	0
Apple & Eve					
Water Fruits All Flavors	10 oz	90	0	0	0
Aquafina					
Alive Wellness Berry Pomegranate	8 oz	10	0	0	0
Essentials Daily C Citrus	8 oz	40	0	0	0
Essentials Multi-V Watermelon	8 oz	40	0	0	0
Sparkling Citrus Twist	8 oz	0	0	0	0
Water	8 oz	0	0	0	0
Aroma Water					
All Flavors	8 oz	0	0	0	0

FOOD	PORTION	CALS	FAT	SAT FAT	TRANS FAT
Ayala's					
Herbal All Flavors	1 bottle	0	0	0	0
Base Energy + Water					
All Flavors	8 oz	28	0	0	0
Blu Italy					
Sparkling Lemon	8 oz	0	0	0	0
Bot					
Fortified All Flavors	12 oz	40	0	0	0
Calabria					
Mineral	8 oz	0	0	0	0
Carpe Diem					
Botanic Water All Flavors	8 oz	35	0	0	0
Clearly Canadian					
Sparkling Blackberry	8 oz	90	0	0	0
Sparkling Cherry	8 oz	85	0	0	0
Sparkling Raspberry	8 oz	75	0	0	0
Sparkling Strawberry	8 oz	85	0	0	0
Zero Sparkling All Flavors	8 oz	0	0	0	0
Crystal Geyser					
Spring Water	8 oz	0	0	0	0
Dasani					
Purfied Water	8 oz	0	0	0	0
w/ Lemon	8 oz	2	0	0	0
w/ Raspberry	8 oz	1	0	0	0
Eden					
Springs Artesian	8 oz	0	0	0	0
Evamor					
Artesian Water	8 oz	0	0	0	0
Evian					
Spring Water	1 bottle (11.5 oz)	0	0	0	0
Fiji					
Natural Artesian	1 bottle (16.9 oz)	0	0	0	0
FlavH2O					
All Flavors	1 can (12.3 oz)	80	0	0	0
Fruit2O					
Grape	8 oz	0	0	0	0
Natural Berry	8 oz	0	0	0	0
Watermelon Kiwi	8 oz	0	0	0	0
Fruit Refreshers					
Lemonade	8 oz	0	0	0	0

FOOD	PORTION	CALS	FAT	SAT FAT	TRANS FAT
Gerolsteiner					
Sparkling Mineral	8 oz	0	0	0	0
Glaceau Vitamin Water					
Balance Cran Grapefruit	8 oz	50	0	0	0
Defense	8 oz	50	0	0	0
Endurance Peach Mango	8 oz	50	0	0	0
Energy Tropical Citrus	8 oz	40	0	0	0
Essential Orange Orange	8 oz	40	0	0	0
Focus Kiwi Strawberry	8 oz	40	0	0	0
Formula 50	8 oz	50	0	0	0
Multi-V Lemonade	8 oz	40	0	0	0
Perform Lemon Lime	8 oz	50	0	0	0
Power-C Dragonfruit	8 oz	40	0	0	0
Rescue Green Tea	8 oz	40	0	0	0
Revive Fruit Punch	8 oz	50	0	0	0
Stress-B Lemon Lime	8 oz	40	0	0	0
H2Odwalla					
Enhanced Tropical Orange	20 oz	120	0	0	0
Organic Enhanced Blueberry Tea	20 oz	120	0	0	0
Organic Enhanced Jasmine Lime	20 oz	120	0	0	0
Hint					
All Flavors	15 oz	0	0	0	0
Flavored Water All Flavors	15 oz	0	0	0	0
Iceland Spring					
Spring Water	1 liter	0	0	0	0
IQ					
H2O Orange Mango	8 oz	40	0	0	0
Jones Soda					
24C Multi Vitamin Enhanced All Flavors	1 bottle	100	0	0	0
Liquid Salvation					
Ultra Hydrating	1 bottle	0	0	0	0
Metromint					
Peppermint or Spearmint Water	8 oz	0	0	0	0
Multi Vitamin Enhanced Water					
All Flavors	8 oz	50	0	0	0
No Carb All Flavors	8 oz	0	0	0	0

FOOD	PORTION	CALS	FAT	SAT FAT	TRANS FAT
Nestle					
Pure Life Splash All Flavors	8 oz	0	0	0	0
Nui					
All Natural Kid Water	10 oz	90	0	0	0
O Water					
Hydrate Black Raspberry	8 oz	25	0	0	0
Replenish Lemon Lime	8 oz	25	0	0	0
Vitalize Peach Mango	8 oz	25	0	0	0
Paradiso					
Slightly Sparkling	8 oz	0	0	0	0
Pellegrino					
Mineral Water	8 oz	0	0	0	0
Pink2O					
Fortified	20 oz	0	0	0	0
Propel					
Fitness Water All Flavors	23.7 oz	30	0	0	0
Rapid					
Hydra-Cell Water	16.9 oz	0	0	0	0
Replenish					
Elements Enhanced Water Orange	8 oz	40	0	0	0
San Benedetto					
Natural Mineral Water	1 liter	0	0	0	0
Sanfaustino					
Mineral	8 oz	0	0	0	0
SoBe					
All Flavors	8 oz	50	0	0	0
Spa					
Mineral Water Reine	1 bottle (17.5 oz)	0	0	0	0
Special K2O					
Protein Water All Flavors	1 bottle (16.6 oz)	50	0	0	0
Speedo Sportswater					
All Flavors	8 oz	10	0	0	0
Splash					
All Flavors	8 oz	0	0	0	0
Stacker 2					
Protein Water All Flavors	1 bottle (19.44 oz)	80	0	0	0
Sulinka					
Sparkling Mineral	8 oz	0	0	0	0

FOOD	PORTION	CALS	FAT	SAT FAT	TRANS FAT
TalkingRain					
Ice All Flavors	8 oz	5	0	0	0
Tao Tea					
Lychee Water	8 oz	67	0	0	0
Thorpedo					
Ultra Low GI Energy Water	8 oz	45	0	0	0
Tipperary					
Mineral Water	1 liter	0	0	0	0
Trinity					
Energize	8 oz	50	0	0	0
Multi-Essential	8 oz	50	0	0	0
Revive	8 oz	50	0	0	0
Strength	8 oz	50	0	0	0
Think	8 oz	50	0	0	0
Twist					
Organics All Flavors	8 oz	10	0	0	0
Ty Nant					
Mineral Water	1 liter	0	0	0	0
Vasa					
Natural Spring	8 oz	0	0	0	0
Veryfine					
Fruit 2 O Lemon	8 oz	0	0	0	0
Vittel					
Mineral Water	18 oz	0	0	0	0
Volvic					
Mineral Water	1 liter	0	0	0	0
Natural Lemon	8 oz	0	0	0	0
Natural Orange	8 oz	30	0	0	0
Voss					
Artesian	8 oz	0	0	0	0
W20 For Women					
All Flavors	8 oz	40	0	0	0
Wateroos					
All Flavors	1 box (8 oz)	0	0	0	0
WaterPlus					
Antioxidants Acai Berry	8 oz	50	0	0	0
Electrolytes Fruit Punch	8 oz	50	0	0	0
Extra-C Orange Tangerine	8 oz	50	0	0	0
Vitamins Dragonfruit Kiwi	8 oz	50	0	0	0

FOOD	PORTION	CALS	FAT	SAT FAT	TRANS FAT
Wild Waters					
All Flavors	8 oz	50	0	0	0
WATER CHESTNUTS					
chinese sliced canned	½ cup	35	tr	–	–
fresh sliced	½ cup	66	tr	–	–
WATERCRESS					
cooked w/o fat	1 cup	15	tr	tr	0
raw chopped	1 cup	4	tr	tr	0
Frieda's					
Watercress	1 cup	10	0	0	0
WATERMELON					
cut up	1 cup	46	tr	tr	0
seeds dried	¼ cup	150	13	3	0
wedge	1 sm (2.5 oz)	21	tr	tr	0
wedge	1 med (10 oz)	86	tr	tr	0
wedge	1 lg (20 oz)	172	1	tr	0
whole melon	1 (9 lb)	1227	6	1	0
Dulcinea					
Fresh Mini Seedless	2 cups	88	0	0	0
Frieda's					
Yellow Seedless	½ cup (3 oz)	25	0	0	0
Sundia					
Fresh	2 cups	80	0	0	0
WATERMELON JUICE					
juice	8 oz	71	tr	tr	0
Snapple					
What-A-Melon	8 oz	90	0	0	0
Sundia					
100% Natural	8 oz	110	1	0	–
Tang					
Watermelon Wallop	1 box (7 oz)	90	0	0	0
WHALE					
alaskan	3.5 oz	97	5	–	–
beluga dried	1 oz	92	2	tr	–
WHEAT					
sprouted	1 cup (3.8 oz)	214	1	tr	–
starch	3.5 oz	348	tr	–	–

FOOD	PORTION	CALS	FAT	SAT FAT	TRANS FAT
Arrowhead Mills					
Whole Grain Wheat	¼ cup (1.6 oz)	150	1	0	0
Bob's Red Mill					
Vital Wheat Gluten	¼ cup	120	1	0	0
Hodgson Mill					
Vital Wheat Gluten	4 tsp	40	0	0	0
Near East					
Pilaf Mix Wheat as prep	1 cup	220	5	2	–
Taboule Salad Mix as prep	⅔ cup	110	3	tr	–
NOW					
Wheat Gluten Flour	¼ cup	125	0	0	0
WHEAT GERM					
plain	¼ cup	108	3	1	0
Bob's Red Mill					
Wheat Germ	2 tbsp	59	2	0	0
Hodgson Mill					
Untoasted	2 tbsp	55	1	0	–
Kretschmer					
Original Toasted	2 tbsp	50	1	0	0
Mother's					
Toasted	2 tbsp	50	1	0	–
WHEY					
acid dry	1 tbsp	10	tr	tr	0
sweet dry	1 tbsp	26	tr	tr	0
sweet fluid	½ cup	33	tr	tr	0
whey cheese	1 oz	126	8	5	–
Bob's Red Mill					
Protein Concentrate	¼ cup	80	1	1	0
Sweet Dairy	1 tbsp	30	0	0	0
Wellements					
Whey Protein Chocolate	1 scoop (1 oz)	120	2	1	0
Whey Protein Vanilla	1 scoop (1 oz)	120	2	1	0
WHIPPED TOPPINGS					
cream pressurized	1 tbsp (3 g)	8	tr	tr	–
cream pressurized	1 cup (2.1 oz)	154	13	8	–
nondairy frzn	1 tbsp	13	1	1	–
nondairy powdered as prep w/ whole milk	1 cup	151	10	9	–

FOOD	PORTION	CALS	FAT	SAT FAT	TRANS FAT
nondairy pressurized	1 cup	184	16	13	–
nondairy pressurized	1 tbsp (4 g)	11	1	1	–
Cabot					
Whipped Cream	2 tbsp	15	2	1	0
Estee					
Whipped Topping as prep	1 serv	10	1	0	–
Hood					
Light Sugar Free Whipped Cream	2 tbsp	10	1	0	0
Whipped Light Cream	2 tbsp	20	2	1	0
Reddiwip					
Chocolate	2 tbsp	15	1	0	–
Extra Creamy	2 tbsp	15	2	1	–
Fat Free	2 tbsp	5	0	0	0
Original	2 tbsp	15	1	1	–
Soyatoo					
Soy Whip	2 tbsp	10	1	1	0

WHITE BEANS

FOOD	PORTION	CALS	FAT	SAT FAT	TRANS FAT
canned	1 cup	306	1	tr	–
dried regular cooked	1 cup	249	1	tr	–
dried small cooked	1 cup	253	1	tr	–

WHITEFISH

FOOD	PORTION	CALS	FAT	SAT FAT	TRANS FAT
baked	3 oz	146	6	1	–
smoked	1 oz	39	tr	tr	–
smoked	3 oz	92	1	tr	–

WHITING

FOOD	PORTION	CALS	FAT	SAT FAT	TRANS FAT
cooked	3 oz	98	1	tr	–
hake raw	3.5 oz	84	1	–	–
raw	3 oz	77	1	tr	–

WILD RICE

FOOD	PORTION	CALS	FAT	SAT FAT	TRANS FAT
cooked	1 cup (5.7 oz)	166	1	tr	–
Gourmet House					
Cracked not prep	¼ cup	170	0	0	0
Hand Harvested not prep	¼ cup	170	0	0	0
Quick Cooking not prep	½ cup	170	0	0	0
White & Wild not prep	¼ cup	170	0	0	0
Wild & Rice Garden Blend not prep	¼ cup	190	1	0	–

FOOD	PORTION	CALS	FAT	SAT FAT	TRANS FAT
Lundberg					
Organic Quick not prep	¼ cup	150	1	0	0
WINE					
chinese cooking	15 oz	559	0	0	0
cooking	1 oz	15	0	0	0
dessert dry	1 serv (4 oz)	179	0	0	0
haiku	1 serv	93	0	0	0
japanese plum	3 oz	139	tr	–	–
japanese sake	1 oz	33	0	0	0
kir	1 serv	78	0	0	0
madeira	3.5 oz	169	0	–	0
port	3.5 oz	156	0	–	0
red	1 serv (4 oz)	85	0	0	0
rosé	1 serv (4 oz)	84	0	0	0
sake screwdriver	1 serv	175	tr	tr	–
sangria	1 serv	88	tr	0	–
sangria blanco	1 serv	155	tr	tr	–
sherry	2 oz	84	0	0	0
sweet dessert	1 serv (4 oz)	189	0	0	0
vermouth dry	3.5 oz	105	0	0	0
vermouth sweet	3.5 oz	167	0	0	0
wassail wine	1 serv	142	tr	tr	–
white	1 serv (4 oz)	80	0	0	0
wine cooler	1 (7 oz)	118	tr	tr	0
Eden					
Mirin Rice Cooking Wine	1 tbsp	25	0	0	0
WINGED BEANS					
dried cooked	1 cup	252	10	1	–
WRAPS (see BREAD, SANDWICHES)					
YACON					
Navitas Naturals					
Slices Dried	1 oz	90	0	0	0
YAM (see also SWEET POTATO)					
CANNED					
Bruce's					
In Syrup	⅔ cup	150	1	0	0

FOOD	PORTION	CALS	FAT	SAT FAT	TRANS FAT
Glory					
Candied	½ cup	210	0	0	0
S&W					
Candied	½ cup (4.9 oz)	170	0	0	0
FRESH					
mountain yam hawaii cooked w/o salt	1 cup	119	tr	tr	0
yam cooked w/o salt	1 cup	158	tr	tr	0
Earthbound Farm					
Organic	1 med (4.6 oz)	130	0	0	0
Frieda's					
Name	¾ cup	100	0	0	0

YARDLONG BEANS

sliced cooked w/o salt	1 cup	49	tr	tr	0

YAUTIA (see MALANGA)

YEAST

baker's compressed	1 cake (0.6 oz)	18	tr	tr	0
baker's dry	1 pkg (7 g)	21	tr	tr	0
baker's dry	1 tbsp	35	1	tr	0
brewer's dry	1 tbsp	35	1	tr	0
Bob's Red Mill					
Active Dry	1 tbsp	25	1	0	0
Hodgson Mill					
Active Dry	1 tsp	30	0	0	0
Fast Rise	1 tsp (9 g)	25	0	0	0

YELLOW BEANS

fresh cooked w/o salt	1 cup	44	tr	tr	0
fresh raw	1 cup	34	tr	tr	0
Del Monte					
Wax Beans	½ cup	20	0	0	0
S&W					
Wax Beans Cut	½ cup (4.2 oz)	20	0	0	0

YELLOWTAIL

baked	4 oz	199	7	–	0

YOGURT (see also YOGURT DRINKS, YOGURT FROZEN)

plain low fat	8 oz	143	4	2	0
plain nonfat	8 oz	127	tr	tr	0

FOOD	PORTION	CALS	FAT	SAT FAT	TRANS FAT
plain whole milk	8 oz	138	7	5	0
tofu yogurt	1 cup	246	5	1	–
Axelrod					
Fat Free Lemon	1 pkg (6 oz)	90	0	0	0
Fat Free Raspberry	6 oz	90	0	0	0
Fat Free Vanilla	1 pkg (6 oz)	90	0	0	0
Breyers					
Creme Savers Orange & Creme	1 pkg (8 oz)	240	4	2	0
Creme Savers Raspberries & Creme	1 pkg (8 oz)	240	4	2	0
Light! Probiotic Plus Apple Cinnamon	1 pkg (8 oz)	100	2	1	0
Light! Probiotic Plus Blueberies 'N Cream	1 pkg (8 oz)	110	2	1	0
Light! Probiotic Plus Lemon Chiffon	1 pkg (8 oz)	100	2	1	0
Light! Probiotic Plus Peaches 'N Cream	1 pkg (8 oz)	100	2	1	0
Light! Probiotic Plus Strawberry Banana	1 pkg (8 oz)	110	2	1	0
Light! Probiotic Plus Strawberry Cheesecake	1 pkg (8 oz)	110	2	1	0
Smart! w/ DHA Mixed Berry	1 pkg (6 oz)	170	2	1	0
Smart! w/ DHA Strawberry	1 pkg (6 oz)	170	2	1	0
Smart! w/ DHA Strawberry Banana	1 pkg (6 oz)	170	2	1	0
Smart! w/DHA Black Cherry	1 pkg (6 oz)	170	2	1	0
Smart! w/DHA Peach	6 oz	170	2	1	0
Smart! w/DHA Pineapple	1 pkg (6 oz)	170	2	1	0
Smooth & Creamy Peaches 'N Cream	1 pkg (8 oz)	240	2	1	0
Smooth & Creamy Strawberry	1 pkg (8 oz)	230	2	1	0
Smooth & Creamy Vanilla Cream	1 pkg (8 oz)	240	2	1	0
Cabot					
Non Fat Berry Banana	8 oz	130	0	0	0
Non Fat Blueberry	8 oz	130	0	0	0
Non Fat French Vanilla	8 oz	130	0	0	0
Non Fat Lemon	8 oz	130	0	0	0
Non Fat Plain	8 oz	100	0	0	0

FOOD	PORTION	CALS	FAT	SAT FAT	TRANS FAT
Non Fat Raspberry	8 oz	130	0	0	0
Non Fat Very Berry	8 oz	130	0	0	0
Colombo					
Fat Free Plain	8 oz	100	0	0	0
Fat Free Vanilla	8 oz	160	0	0	0
French Vanilla	8 oz	180	2	2	–
Fruit On The Bottom Strawberry Banana	8 oz	230	2	2	–
Lowfat Plain	8 oz	130	3	2	–
Multipack Blended All Flavors	4 oz	110	1	1	–
Strawberry	8 oz	190	3	2	–
Dannon					
Activia Blueberry	1 pkg (4 oz)	110	2	1	0
Activia Mixed Berry	1 pkg (4 oz)	110	2	1	0
Activia Peach	1 pkg (4 oz)	110	2	1	0
Activia Prune	1 pkg (4 oz)	110	2	1	0
Activia Strawberry	1 pkg (4 oz)	110	2	1	0
Activia Vanilla	1 pkg (4 oz)	110	2	2	0
Activia Vanilla Light Fat Free	4 oz	70	0	0	0
All Natural Blended Mini Blueberry	1 (3.3 oz)	110	1	1	0
All Natural Blended Mini Strawberry	1 (3.3 oz)	110	1	1	0
Creamy Fruit Blends Raspberry	6 oz	170	2	1	0
Fruit On The Bottom Apple Cinnamon	6 oz	150	2	1	0
Fruit On The Bottom Peach	6 oz	150	2	1	0
Fruit On The Bottom Pineapple	6 oz	150	2	1	0
Fruit On The Bottom Raspberry	6 oz	150	2	1	0
La Creme Mousse French Vanilla	1 (2.6 oz)	110	5	4	0
La Creme Vanilla	4 oz	140	5	3	0
Light & Fit Carb & Sugar Control Blueberries 'N Cream	4 oz	60	3	2	0
Light & Fit Carb & Sugar Control Vanilla	4 oz	60	3	2	0
Light & Fit Nonfat Cherry Vanilla	6 oz	60	0	0	0
Light & Fit Nonfat Lemon Chiffon	6 oz	60	0	0	0

FOOD	PORTION	CALS	FAT	SAT FAT	TRANS FAT
Light & Fit Nonfat Raspberry	6 oz	60	0	0	0
Light & Fit Nonfat White Chocolate Raspberry	6 oz	90	0	0	0
Fage					
Sheep & Goat's Milk	1 pkg (7 oz)	190	12	8	0
Horizon Organic					
Fat Free Peach	1 pkg (6 oz)	140	0	0	0
Fat Free Vanilla	1 cup	180	0	0	0
Kids Strawberry	1 pkg (4 oz)	110	1	1	0
Lowfat Blended Blueberry	1 pkg (6 oz)	160	2	1	0
Tube Lowfat Blueberry	1 (2 oz)	70	1	1	0
Whole Milk Plain	1 cup	160	7	5	0
La Yogurt					
Lowfat Blueberries 'N' Cream	1 pkg (6 oz)	200	2	1	0
Lowfat Fruit On The Bottom Cherry	1 pkg (8 oz)	230	3	2	0
Lowfat Fruit On The Bottom Probiotic Peach	1 pkg (6 oz)	160	2	1	0
Lowfat Fruit On The Bottom Strawberry	1 pkg (8 oz)	220	2	2	0
Lowfat Peaches 'N' Cream	1 pkg (6 oz)	200	2	1	0
Lowfat Pina Colada	1 pkg (6 oz)	160	2	1	0
Lowfat Probiotic Pina Colada	1 pkg (6 oz)	160	2	2	0
Lowfat Probiotic Plain	1 pkg (6 oz)	100	2	2	0
Lowfat Probiotic Vanilla	1 pkg (6 oz)	150	2	2	0
Lowfat Vanilla 'N' Cream	1 pkg (6 oz)	200	2	1	0
Nonfat Banana Cream	1 pkg (6 oz)	100	0	0	0
Nonfat Probiotic Cherry	1 pkg (6 oz)	100	0	0	0
Nonfat Probiotic Peach	1 pkg (6 oz)	90	0	0	0
Nonfat Probiotic Raspberry	1 pkg (6 oz)	90	0	0	0
Nonfat Probiotic Vanilla	1 pkg (6 oz)	90	0	0	0
Sabor Latino Lowfat Dulce De Leche	1 pkg (6 oz)	190	2	1	0
Sabor Latino Lowfat Guava	1 pkg (6 oz)	190	2	1	0
Sabor Latino Lowfat Horchata	1 pkg (6 oz)	210	2	1	0
Sabor Latino Lowfat Papaya	1 pkg (6 oz)	190	2	1	0
LeCarb					
YoCarb Plain	1 pkg (4 oz)	50	3	2	–
Rachel's					
Essence Berry Jasmine w/ Zinc	1 pkg (6 oz)	160	3	2	0

FOOD	PORTION	CALS	FAT	SAT FAT	TRANS FAT
Essence Plum Honey Lavender	1 pkg (6 oz)	160	3	2	0
Essence Pomegrante Acai	1 pkg (6 oz)	170	3	2	0
Exotic Kiwi Passion Fruit Lime	1 pkg (6 oz)	160	3	2	0
Exotic Orange Strawberry Mango	1 pkg (6 oz)	160	3	2	0
Exotic Pomegranate Blueberry	1 pkg (6 oz)	170	3	2	0
Redwood Hill Farm					
Goat Milk Apricot Mango	1 cup	180	5	3	0
Goat Milk Cranberry Orange	1 cup	180	5	3	0
Goat Milk Plain	1 cup	130	6	4	0
Goat Milk Strawberry	1 cup	180	5	3	0
Goat Milk Vanilla	1 cup	190	5	4	0
Silk					
Soy Apricot Mango	1 pkg	160	2	0	–
Soy Banana Strawberry	1 pkg	160	2	0	–
Soy Black Cherry	1 pkg	160	2	0	–
Soy Blueberry	1 pkg	160	2	0	–
Soy Key Lime	1 pkg	170	2	0	–
Soy Lemon	1 pkg	160	2	0	–
Soy Lemon Kiwi	1 pkg	150	2	0	–
Soy Peach	1 pkg	170	2	0	–
Soy Plain	8 oz	120	3	0	–
Soy Raspberry	1 pkg	160	2	0	–
Soy Vanilla	1 pkg (8 oz)	120	2	0	–
Spega					
La Natura Low Fat	1 pkg (5.2 oz)	80	1	1	–
Stonyfield Farm					
Kids' Lowfat BaNilla	1 pkg (4 oz)	110	1	1	0
Light Black Cherry	1 pkg (6 oz)	100	0	0	0
Light Blueberry	1 pkg (4 oz)	100	0	0	0
Light Peach	1 pkg (6 oz)	100	0	0	0
Light Strawberry	1 pkg (4 oz)	100	0	0	0
Nonfat French Vanilla	1 pkg	90	0	0	0
Nonfat Strawberry	1 pkg	140	0	0	0
O'Soy Chocolate	1 pkg (6 oz)	160	3	0	0
O'Soy Peach	1 pkg (4 oz)	100	2	0	0
Squeezers Lowfat Strawberry	1 tube (2 oz)	60	1	1	0
Whole Milk French Vanilla	1 pkg (6 oz)	190	6	4	0
Total					
Greek Yogurt 0% Fat	1 pkg (5.3 oz)	80	0	0	0

FOOD	PORTION	CALS	FAT	SAT FAT	TRANS FAT
Greek Yogurt 2% Fat	1 pkg (7 oz)	130	4	3	0
Greek Yogurt Classic	1 pkg (7 oz)	180	20	16	0
Greek Yogurt Light	1 pkg (5.3 oz)	130	8	5	0
Honey	1 pkg (3.5 oz)	250	12	9	0
Wallaby					
Organic Banana Vanilla	1 pkg (6 oz)	150	3	2	0
Organic Lemon	1 pkg (6 oz)	150	3	2	0
Organic Maple	1 pkg (6 oz)	150	3	2	0
Organic Plain	1 cup	150	5	3	0
Organic Raspberry	1 pkg (6 oz)	150	3	2	0
Organic Vanilla	1 pkg (6 oz)	150	3	2	0
Organic Nonfat Mango Lime	1 pkg (6 oz)	140	0	0	0
Organic Nonfat Plain	1 cup	130	0	0	0
Organic Nonfat Vanilla Bean	1 pkg (6 oz)	140	0	0	0
WholeSoy & Co.					
Organic Soy Apricot Mango	1 pkg (6 oz)	160	3	0	0
Organic Soy Lemon	1 pkg (6 oz)	160	3	0	0
Organic Soy Plain	1 pkg (6 oz)	150	3	0	0
Organic Soy Raspberry	1 pkg (6 oz)	170	3	0	0
Organic Soy Vanilla	1 pkg (6 oz)	150	3	0	0
WildWood					
Organic Soyogurt Low Fat Peach	1 pkg (6 oz)	160	3	0	0
Organic Soyogurt Low Fat Vanilla	1 pkg (6 oz)	160	3	0	0
Organic Soyogurt Plain Unsweetened	1 pkg (6 oz)	110	4	1	0
Yoplait					
Go-Gurt All Fruit Flavors	1 pkg (2.25 oz)	80	2	1	0
Grande 99% Fat Free All Flavors	1 cup	250	3	2	0
Grande Fat Free Plain	1 cup	90	0	0	0
Kids Banana Vanilla	1 pkg (4 oz)	100	2	2	0
Kids Strawberry Vanilla	1 pkg (4 oz)	100	2	2	0
Light All Fruit Flavors	1 pkg (6 oz)	180	0	0	0
Light Indulgent All Flavors	1 pkg (6 oz)	110	0	0	0
Light Thick & Creamy All Fruit Flavors	1 pkg (6 oz)	100	0	0	0
Original All Fruit Flavors	1 pkg (6 oz)	170	2	1	0
Original Coconut Cream	1 pkg (6 oz)	190	3	2	0

FOOD	PORTION	CALS	FAT	SAT FAT	TRANS FAT
Original Lemon Burst	1 pkg (6 oz)	180	2	1	0
Original Pina Colada	1 pkg (6 oz)	170	2	2	0
Trix All Fruit Flavors	1 pkg (4 oz)	120	2	1	0
Yo Plus All Flavors	1 pkg (4 oz)	110	2	1	0

YOGURT DRINKS (see also SMOOTHIES)

FOOD	PORTION	CALS	FAT	SAT FAT	TRANS FAT
lassi	7 oz	78	5	3	–
Dannon					
DanActive Plain	1 bottle (3.3 oz)	90	2	2	0
DanActive Vanilla	1 bottle (3.3. oz)	90	2	1	0
Danimals Rockin' Raspberry	1 bottle (3.1 oz)	70	1	0	0
Danimals Strawberry Explosion	1 bottle (3.1 oz)	70	1	0	0
Danimals Strikin' Strawberry Kiwi	1 bottle (3.1 oz)	70	1	0	0
Frusion Cherry Berry Blend	1 bottle (10 oz)	260	4	2	0
Frusion Pina Colada	1 bottle (10 oz)	260	4	2	0
Frusion Strawberry Blend	1 bottle (10 oz)	260	4	2	0
Light & Fit Carb & Sugar Control Berries 'N Cream	1 bottle (7 oz)	60	3	2	0
Light & Fit Smoothie Peach Passion	1 bottle (7 oz)	70	0	0	0
Light & Fit Smoothie Strawberry Banana	1 bottle (7 oz)	70	0	0	0
Lifeway					
Lassi Lowfat All Flavors	8 oz	174	2	2	–
Promise					
Activ All Flavors	1 bottle (3.5 oz)	75	4	0	0
Stonyfield Farm					
Kids' Juice Smoothie Orange Strawberry Banana Wave	1 bottle (6 oz)	160	2	1	0
Smoothie Light Strawberry	1 bottle (10 oz)	130	0	0	0
Smoothie Lowfat Strawberry	1 bottle (10 oz)	250	3	2	0
Yo-Goat					
Blueberry	8 oz	150	8	5	–
Yoplait					
Nouriche All Fruit Flavors	1 bottle (11 oz)	260	0	0	0

YOGURT FROZEN

FOOD	PORTION	CALS	FAT	SAT FAT	TRANS FAT
chocolate soft serve	1 cup	230	9	5	0
vanilla soft serve	1 cup	236	8	5	0

FOOD	PORTION	CALS	FAT	SAT FAT	TRANS FAT
Breyers					
Chocolate	½ cup	150	5	3	–
Vanilla	½ cup	140	5	3	–
Vanilla No Sugar Added	½ cup	100	5	3	–
Edy's					
Black Cherry Vanilla Swirl	½ cup	90	0	0	0
Caramel Praline Crunch	½ cup	100	0	0	0
Chocolate	½ cup	90	0	0	0
Strawberry	½ cup	100	0	0	0
Vanilla	½ cup	90	0	0	0
Vanilla Chocolate Swirl	½ cup	90	0	0	0
Haagen-Dazs					
Lowfat Dulce De Leche	½ cup	190	3	2	–
Nonfat Chocolate	½ cup	140	0	0	0
Nonfat Coffee	½ cup	140	0	0	0
Nonfat Strawberry	½ cup	140	0	0	0
Nonfat Vanilla	½ cup	140	0	0	0
Nonfat Vanilla Raspberry Swirl	½ cup	130	0	0	0
Nonfat Vanilla Fudge	½ cup	160	0	0	0
Hood					
Fat Free Old Fashioned Vanilla	½ cup	110	0	0	0
Fat Free Strawberry	½ cup	100	0	0	0
Vanilla Swiss Almond	½ cup	150	5	2	0
Turkey Hill					
Black Raspberry	½ cup	110	3	–	–
Caramel Cashew Crunch	½ cup	160	9	–	–
Chocolate Chip Cookie Dough	½ cup	140	5	3	–
Clark Bar	½ cup	140	5	–	–
Fat Free Chocolate Cherry Cordial	½ cup	100	0	0	0
Fat Free Chocolate Marshmallow	½ cup	130	0	0	0
Fat Free Mint Cookie 'N Cream	½ cup	110	0	0	0
Fat Free Neapolitan	½ cup	100	0	0	0
Fat Free Orange Swirl	½ cup	100	0	0	0
Fat Free Vanilla Fudge	½ cup	110	0	0	0
Peach Raspberry	½ cup	110	2	2	–
Tin Roof Sundae	½ cup	140	5	3	–
Vanilla & Chocolate	½ cup	110	3	2	–
Vanilla Bean	½ cup	110	3	2	–

FOOD	PORTION	CALS	FAT	SAT FAT	TRANS FAT
WholeSoy & Co.					
Organic All Flavors	½ cup	120	1	0	0
ZUCCHINI					
baby raw	1 (0.5 oz)	3	tr	tr	0
canned italian style	1 cup	66	tr	tr	0
fresh	1 sm (4.1 oz)	19	tr	tr	0
pickled	¼ cup	16	tr	tr	0
raw sliced	1 cup	19	tr	tr	0
sliced cooked w/o salt	1 cup	29	tr	tr	0
C&W					
Yellow & Green	⅔ cup	20	0	0	0
Frieda's					
Baby	⅔ cup (3 oz)	20	0	0	0
TAKE-OUT					
breaded & fried	6 slices (3 oz)	141	11	1	0
indian pakora	1 serv	46	2	tr	–
sticks breaded & fried	6 (2 oz)	90	7	1	0

PART TWO

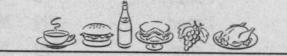

Restaurant Chains

FAT FACT

Go easy on the overindulging.

*A single high-fat meal
can increase your short-term risk for a heart attack
and chest pains.*

FOOD	PORTION	CALS	FAT	SAT FAT	TRANS FAT
A&W					
BEVERAGES					
Coke	1 sm (11 oz)	145	0	0	0
Diet Coke	1 sm (11 oz)	0	0	0	0
Diet Root Beer	1 sm (15 oz)	0	0	0	0
Float Diet Root Beer	1 sm (14 oz)	170	5	3	0
Float Root Beer	1 sm (14 oz)	330	5	3	0
Milkshake Chocolate	1 med	700	29	18	1
Milkshake Strawberry	1 med	670	29	18	1
Milkshake Vanilla	1 med	720	31	19	1
Root Beer	1 sm (15 oz)	220	0	0	0
DESSERTS					
Cone Vanilla	1 med	260	7	4	0
Freeze A&W Root Beer	1 med	480	10	6	1
Polar Swirl M&M's	1 med	710	25	16	1
Polar Swirl Oreo	1 med	690	24	11	1
Polar Swirl Reese's	1 med	740	31	14	1
Sundae Caramel	1 med	340	9	4	0
Sundae Chocolate	1 med	320	8	4	0
Sundae Hot Fudge	1 med	350	11	8	0
Sundae Strawberry	1 med	300	8	4	0
Sundae Vanilla	1 med	310	8	4	0
MAIN MENU SELECTIONS					
Cheese Curds	1 serv	570	40	21	1
Cheese Dog	1	320	20	7	1
Cheeseburger Original Bacon	1	570	33	10	4
Cheeseburger Original Bacon Double	1	800	48	17	4
Cheeseburger Original Double	1	720	42	15	4
Chicken Strips	3	500	29	5	2
Chili Bowl	1 serv	190	6	2	0
Coney Chili Dog	1	310	18	7	1
Coney Chili Dog Cheese	1	350	21	8	1
Fries	1 lg	430	18	5	6
Fries Cheese	1 serv	380	19	5	4
Fries Chili	1 serv	370	16	5	4
Fries Chili & Cheese	1 serv	400	19	8	4
Hot Dog Plain	1	280	17	6	1
Onion Rings	1 serv	350	18	4	5
Papa Burger	1	720	42	15	4

FOOD	PORTION	CALS	FAT	SAT FAT	TRANS FAT
Sandwich Crispy Chicken	1	590	29	5	5
Sandwich Grilled Chicken	1	440	19	4	3
SAUCES					
Dipping Sauce BBQ	1 serv (1 oz)	40	0	0	0
Dipping Sauce Honey Mustard	1 serv (1 oz)	100	6	2	0
Dipping Sauce Ranch	1 serv (1 oz)	160	17	3	0
Dipping Sauce Sweet & Sour	1 serv (1 oz)	45	0	0	0

ARBY'S
BEVERAGES

FOOD	PORTION	CALS	FAT	SAT FAT	TRANS FAT
Dr Pepper	1 (16 oz)	180	0	0	0
Pepsi	1 (16 oz)	130	0	0	0
Shake Chocolate	1 reg	507	13	8	0
Shake Jamocha	1 reg	498	13	8	0
Shake Orange Cream	1 (17 oz)	637	17	10	1
Shake Strawberry	1 reg	498	13	8	0
Shake Strawberry Banana Swirl	1 (17 oz)	567	16	9	1
Shake Vanilla	1 reg	437	13	8	0
Sierra Mist	1 (16 oz)	100	0	0	0
BREAKFAST SELECTIONS					
Biscuit	1	273	15	4	0
Biscuit Bacon Egg & Cheese	1	461	28	8	0
Biscuit Chicken	1	417	23	5	0
Biscuit Ham Egg & Cheese	1	437	23	6	0
Biscuit Sausage Egg & Cheese	1	557	38	11	0
Biscuit Sausage Gravy	1	961	68	14	0
Biscuit w/ Bacon	1	340	21	6	0
Biscuit w/ Ham	1	316	17	4	0
Biscuit w/ Sausage	1	436	31	9	0
Breakfast Syrup	1 serv (1 oz)	78	0	0	0
Cinnamon Roll Original Gourmet	1	507	10	4	0
Croissant	1	190	10	6	0
Croissant Bacon & Egg	1	337	22	10	0
Croissant Bacon Egg & Cheese	1	378	22	10	0
Croissant Ham & Cheese	1	274	12	7	0
Croissant Ham Egg & Cheese	1	434	24	10	0
Croissant Sausage & Egg	1	433	32	13	0
Croissant Sausage Egg & Cheese	1	475	32	13	0

FOOD	PORTION	CALS	FAT	SAT FAT	TRANS FAT
French Toastix	1 serv	312	13	2	0
Muffin Blueberry	1	320	12	2	0
Pecan Sticky Bun	1	688	22	5	0
Sourdough Bacon Egg & Cheese	1	437	16	5	0
Sourdough Egg & Cheese	1	392	12	3	0
Sourdough Ham Egg & Cheese	1	679	35	11	0
Sourdough Sausage Egg & Cheese	1	514	27	8	0
Twist Chocolate	1	250	12	4	0
Twist Cinnamon	1	260	14	5	4
Wrap Bacon Egg & Cheese	1	515	29	8	1
Wrap Ham Egg & Cheese	1	568	31	10	1
Wrap Sausage Egg & Cheese	1	689	45	15	1
CHILDREN'S MENU SELECTIONS					
Kids Meal Chicken Tenders	1 serv	289	14	2	0
Kids Meal Junior Roast Beef Sandwich	1	272	10	4	0
Market Fresh Mini Ham & Cheese Sandwich	1	228	5	1	0
Market Fresh Mini Turkey & Cheese Sandwich	1	235	4	1	0
DESSERTS					
Cookie Chocolate Chip	1 (1.6 oz)	202	10	4	2
Turnover Apple	1	377	16	5	7
Turnover Cherry	1	377	15	5	6
SALAD DRESSINGS AND SAUCES					
Arby's Sauce	1 serv (0.5 oz)	15	0	0	0
Dipping Sauce BBQ	1 pkg (1 oz)	40	0	0	0
Dipping Sauce Bronco Berry	1 serv (2 oz)	122	0	0	0
Dipping Sauce Buffalo	1 serv (1 oz)	10	1	0	0
Dipping Sauce Cool Ranch Sour Cream	1 serv (1.5 oz)	158	16	4	0
Dipping Sauce Honey Mustard	1 serv (1 oz)	129	12	2	0
Dressing Buttermilk Ranch	1 serv (2.2 oz)	325	34	5	1
Dressing Buttermilk Ranch Light	1 serv (2 oz)	112	6	1	0
Dressing Sante Fe Ranch	1 pkg (2.2 oz)	296	31	5	0
Horsey Sauce	1 pkg (0.5 oz)	62	5	1	0
Ketchup	1 pkg	13	0	0	0

FOOD	PORTION	CALS	FAT	SAT FAT	TRANS FAT
Sauce Cheddar Cheese	1 serv (0.7 oz)	30	2	1	1
Sauce Spicy Three Pepper	1 serv (0.5 oz)	22	1	0	0
Sauce Tangy Southwest	1 serv (2 oz)	333	35	5	1
SALADS					
Chicken Club	1 serv	487	25	8	1
Martha's Vineyard	1 serv	277	8	4	0
Santa Fe	1 serv	477	21	6	1
SANDWICHES					
Arby's Melt	1	302	12	4	1
Beef 'n Cheddar	1	445	21	6	2
Chicken Bacon & Swiss Crispy	1	624	29	7	0
Chicken Bacon & Swiss Grilled	1	462	17	4	0
Chicken Cordon Bleu Crispy	1	650	31	6	1
Chicken Cordon Bleu Grilled	1	488	19	4	0
Chicken Fillet Crispy	1	576	30	5	0
Chicken Fillet Grilled	1	414	17	3	0
Chicken Salad w/ Pecans	1	769	39	10	0
Corned Beef Reuben	1	606	33	9	1
Fish	1	543	25	6	0
French Dip	1	391	16	6	1
French Dip & Swiss	1	473	18	7	1
Ham & Swiss Melt	1	275	6	2	0
Roast Beef Regular	1	320	14	5	1
Roast Beef Super	1	398	19	6	1
Roast Beef & Swiss	1	777	41	13	2
Roast Beef 'N Cheddar	1	521	27	9	2
Roast Ham & Swiss	1	705	31	8	1
Roast Turkey Ranch & Bacon	1	834	38	11	1
Roast Turkey Reuben	1	611	30	8	1
Roast Turkey & Swiss	1	725	30	8	1
Sourdough Melt Beef	1	355	14	5	1
Sourdough Melt Ham	1	380	13	3	0
Spicy Cajun Fish	1	603	32	7	0
Sub Toasted Classic Italian	1	828	46	13	1
Sub Toasted French Dip & Swiss	1	622	20	7	2
Sub Toasted Philly Beef	1	739	37	9	1
Sub Toasted Turkey Bacon Club	1	619	18	4	0
Swiss Melt	1	303	12	4	1
Ultimate BLT	1	779	45	11	1

FOOD	PORTION	CALS	FAT	SAT FAT	TRANS FAT
Wrap Chicken Salad w/ Pecans	1	638	38	10	1
Wrap Corned Beef Reuben	1	577	29	8	1
Wrap Roast Turkey Ranch & Bacon	1	700	37	11	1
Wrap Roast Turkey Reuben	1	581	27	6	0
Wrap Southwest Chicken	1	567	29	9	1
Wrap Ultimate BLT	1	648	44	11	1
SIDES					
Bites Jalapeno	5	305	21	9	1
Bites Loaded Potato	5	353	22	7	1
Cheddar Fries	1 med	465	28	6	2
Chicken Tenders	3 pieces	379	18	3	0
Croutons Cheese & Garlic	1 pkg	77	5	1	0
Curly Fries	1 sm	338	20	4	0
Curly Fries	1 lg	631	37	7	1
Fruit Cup	1 serv	35	0	0	0
Homestyle Fries	1 sm	302	20	4	1
Homestyle Fries	1 lg	566	37	7	1
Mozzarella Sticks	8 pieces	849	56	26	2
Onion Petals	1 reg	331	23	4	0
Popcorn Chicken	1 reg	365	18	1	1
Potato Cakes	2	246	18	4	1
Seasoned Tortilla Strips	1 serv	71	3	0	0

AU BON PAIN
BAKED SELECTIONS

FOOD	PORTION	CALS	FAT	SAT FAT	TRANS FAT
Bagel Asiago Cheese	1	360	4	3	0
Bagel Cinnamon Raisin	1	320	1	0	0
Bagel Everything	1	350	5	0	0
Bagel Honey 9 Grain	1	330	2	0	0
Bagel Jalapeno Double Cheddar	1	350	10	6	0
Bagel Onion Dill	1	350	1	0	0
Bagel Plain	1	290	1	0	0
Bagel Poppy Seed	1	290	1	0	0
Bagel Sesame Seed	1	330	5	1	0
Baguette Artisan Salad Size	1 (3.5 oz)	210	1	0	0
Baguette Artisan Sandwich Size	1 (4.7 oz)	290	1	0	0
Baguette Artisan Honey Multigrain Salad Size	1 (3.5 oz)	240	3	0	0

FOOD	PORTION	CALS	FAT	SAT FAT	TRANS FAT
Baguette Artisan Honey Multigrain Sandwich Size	1 (4.7 oz	310	3	0	0
Blondie	1	330	19	6	0
Bread Artisan Multigrain	1 serv (4 oz)	260	3	0	0
Bread Artisan Sundried Tomato	1 serv (4 oz)	240	1	0	0
Bread Cheese	1 serv (4.8 oz)	290	8	4	0
Bread Country White	1 serv (4 oz)	240	1	0	0
Bread Bowl	1 (9.24 oz)	640	3	0	0
Breadstick Rosemary Garlic	1 (2.3 oz)	200	5	1	0
Brownie Chocolate Chip	1	380	17	5	0
Brownie Hazelnut Mocha	1	430	21	5	0
Brownie Rocky Road	1	410	17	5	0
Ciabatta	1 sm	180	1	0	0
Cinnamon Roll	1	350	12	7	0
Cookie Chocolate Chip	1 (2 oz)	260	12	6	0
Cookie Confetti	1 (2.4 oz)	310	14	5	0
Cookie Gingerbread	1 (2.7 oz)	300	9	4	0
Cookie Hazelnut Fudge	1 (2.25 oz)	290	16	6	0
Cookie Oatmeal Raisin	1 (2 oz)	230	8	4	0
Cookie Shortbread	1 (2.3 oz)	310	9	0	0
Cookie English Toffee	1 (2 oz)	210	11	4	0
Creme De Fleur	1 serv	550	26	15	0
Croissant Almond	1	560	36	13	0
Croissant Apple	1	230	10	6	0
Croissant Chocolate	1	330	17	10	0
Croissant Plain	1 (2.8 oz)	260	15	8	0
Croissant Raspberry Cheese	1	330	16	10	0
Croissant Sweet Cheese	1	320	16	10	0
Danish Cherry	1	370	19	9	0
Danish Sweet Cheese	1	380	20	10	0
Focaccia	1 piece (4.4 oz)	310	4	1	0
Lahvash	1 (4 oz)	320	1	0	0
Macaroon Chocolate Dipped Cranberry Almond	1	320	16	8	0
Mini Loaf Bacon & Cheese	1 (4.8 oz)	540	31	8	0
Muffin Banana Walnut	1 (5.4 oz)	430	21	4	–
Muffin Blueberry	1	510	19	2	0
Muffin Carrot Walnut	1	520	25	5	0
Muffin Corn	1	460	16	3	0
Muffin Cranberry Walnut	1	500	24	2	0

FOOD	PORTION	CALS	FAT	SAT FAT	TRANS FAT
Muffin Double Chocolate Chunk	1	590	20	6	0
Muffin Pumpkin	1	490	17	3	0
Muffin Raisin Bran	1	410	9	2	0
Muffin Low Fat Triple Berry	1	290	2	1	0
Pastry Hazelnut Creme	1	540	34	16	0
Pound Cake Cappuccino	1 slice (5.2 oz)	530	26	5	0
Pound Cake Chocolate	1 slice (4.7 oz)	500	29	6	0
Pound Cake Lemon	1 slice (4.9 oz)	520	27	6	0
Pound Cake Marble	1 slice (4.7 oz)	490	27	5	0
Roll Soft	1 (4.7 oz)	410	11	4	0
Roll Pecan	1	630	32	11	0
Scone Cinnamon	1	430	24	14	0
Scone Orange	1	410	20	11	0
Shortbread Chocolate Dipped	1	350	20	9	0
Toasts Basil Pesto Cheese	3 pieces (2 oz)	140	2	0	0
Tulip Blueberry	1	370	20	4	0
Tulip Chocolate Raspberry	1	430	21	5	0
Tulip Key Lime	1	440	22	5	0
BEVERAGES					
Blast Caramel	1 med (16 oz)	540	17	12	0
Blast Coffee	1 med (16 oz)	440	21	15	0
Blast Mocha	1 med (16 oz)	440	17	12	0
Blast Vanilla	1 med (12 oz)	540	17	12	0
Caffe Americano	1 sm (12 oz)	5	0	0	0
Caffe Latte	1 sm (12 oz)	200	11	7	0
Cappuccino	1 sm (12 oz)	120	7	4	0
Caramel Macchiato	1 sm (12 oz)	350	10	6	0
Chai Latte	1 sm (12 oz)	290	11	7	0
Chocolate Milk	1 (12 oz)	320	9	5	0
Hot Chocolate	1 sm (12 oz)	350	11	7	0
Iced Carfe Latte	1 sm (12 oz)	110	6	4	0
Iced Caramel Macchiato	1 sm (12 oz)	290	7	5	0
Iced Chai Latte	1 sm (12 oz)	190	5	4	0
Iced Mocha Latte	1 sm (12 oz)	210	11	7	0
Iced Tea Peach	1 med (22 oz)	120	0	0	0
Iced Vanilla Latte	1 sm (12 oz)	240	5	3	0
Iced White Chocolate Latte	1 sm (12 oz)	250	11	7	0
Lemonade	1 med (22 oz)	300	0	0	0
Mocha Latte	1 sm (12 oz)	300	16	10	0

FOOD	PORTION	CALS	FAT	SAT FAT	TRANS FAT
Orange Juice	1 (8 oz)	110	0	0	0
Smoothie Peach	1 med (16 oz)	310	1	0	0
Smoothie Strawberry	1 med (16 oz)	310	1	0	0
Vanilla Latte	1 sm (12 oz)	320	9	6	0
White Chocolate Latte	1 sm (12 oz)	310	14	9	0
MAIN MENU SELECTIONS					
Fruit Cup	1 sm (6 oz)	70	0	0	0
Harvest Rice Bowl Cajun Shrimp	1 (20 oz)	520	17	8	0
Harvest Rice Bowl Cajun Shrimp w/ Brown Rice	1 (20 oz)	560	20	7	0
Harvest Rice Bowl Mayan Chicken	1 (19.25 oz)	490	14	3	0
Harvest Rice Bowl Mayan Chicken w/ Brown Rice	1 (19.25 oz)	540	16	3	0
Harvest Rice Bowl Steak Teriyaki	1 (19.25 oz)	530	15	3	0
Harvest Rice Bowl Steak Teriyaki w/ Brown Rice	1 (19.25 oz)	570	18	3	0
Macaroni & Cheese	1 med (12 oz)	440	26	17	0
Stew Beef	1 med (12 oz)	300	16	3	0
Stew Chicken Vegetable	1 med (12 oz)	290	17	5	0
SALAD DRESSINGS AND SPREADS					
Artichoke Aioli	1 serv (1 oz)	130	14	2	0
Basil Pesto	1 serv (1 oz)	140	15	3	0
Chili Dijon	1 serv (1 oz)	120	12	2	0
Cream Cheese Honey Pecan	1 serv (2 oz)	120	10	7	0
Cream Cheese Honey Walnut	1 serv (2 oz)	140	9	6	0
Cream Cheese Lite	1 serv (2 oz)	120	9	6	0
Cream Cheese Plain	1 serv (2 oz)	170	16	11	1
Cream Cheese Strawberry	1 serv (2 oz)	180	15	10	1
Cream Cheese Sundried Tomato	1 serv (2 oz)	120	10	7	0
Cream Cheese Vegetable	1 serv (2 oz)	170	16	10	1
Dressing Balsamic Vinaigrette	1 serv (2.25 oz)	190	16	3	0
Dressing Blue Cheese	1 serv (1.75 oz)	230	24	5	0
Dressing Caesar	1 serv (2 oz)	280	28	5	0
Dressing Fat Free Raspberry Vinaigrette	1 serv (2.25 oz)	70	0	0	0
Dressing Light Honey Mustard	1 serv (2.25 oz)	180	11	2	0

FOOD	PORTION	CALS	FAT	SAT FAT	TRANS FAT
Dressing Light Olive Oil Vinaigrette	1 serv (2.25 oz)	130	10	2	0
Dressing Light Ranch	1 serv (2.25 oz)	150	15	3	0
Dressing Thai Peanut	1 serv (2.25 oz)	230	13	2	0
Guacomole	1 serv (1 oz)	60	6	1	0
Honey Mustard	1 serv (2.5 oz)	210	13	2	0
Hummus Roasted Red Pepper	1 serv (2 oz)	80	5	0	0
Mayonnaise	1 serv (1 oz)	200	22	3	0
Mayonnaise Herb	1 serv (1 oz)	210	23	4	0
Mayonnaise Jalapeno	1 serv (1 oz)	140	15	2	0
Mayonnaise Tarragon Sauce	1 serv (2 oz)	420	45	7	0
Mustard	1 tsp	0	0	0	0
Spread Herb Bagel	1 serv (2 oz)	130	11	7	0
Spread Sundried Tomato	1 serv (0.53 oz)	70	6	1	0
SALADS					
Caesar Asiago	1 serv	210	12	6	0
Caesar Asiago Grilled Chicken	1 (8.5 oz)	340	13	6	0
Caesar Asiago Side	1 (3.2 oz)	120	6	3	0
Chef's	1 serv	230	14	7	0
Garden	1 (7 oz)	80	2	0	0
Garden Side	1 (3.6 oz)	50	1	0	0
Mediterranean Chicken	1 (9.75 oz)	330	16	5	0
Riviera	1 (9.5 oz)	260	7	3	0
Thai Peanut Chicken	1 (11 oz)	250	8	0	0
Tuna Garden	1 (10.5 oz)	350	25	4	0
Turkey Medallion Cobb	1 (11 oz)	340	19	8	0
Turkey Spinach Sonoma	1 (12.3 oz)	310	13	7	0
SANDWICHES					
Arizona Chicken	1 (12 oz)	750	29	9	0
Baguette Turkey & Swiss	1 (12.3 oz)	770	38	10	0
Baja Turkey	1 (13 oz)	700	32	9	0
Breakfast Asiago Bagel Prosciutto & Egg	1 (9.6 oz)	660	25	8	0
Breakfast Asiago Bagel Sausage Egg & Cheddar	1 (10.2 oz)	770	45	21	0
Breakfast Bagel & Bacon	1 (4.2 oz)	340	6	2	0
Breakfast Egg On A Bagel	1 (6.8 oz)	370	4	1	0
Breakfast Egg On A Bagel w/ Bacon	1 (7.2 oz)	410	8	3	0

FOOD	PORTION	CALS	FAT	SAT FAT	TRANS FAT
Breakfast Egg On A Bagel w/ Bacon & Cheese	1 (7.9 oz)	500	15	6	0
Breakfast Egg On A Bagel w/ Cheese	1 (7.6 oz)	450	10	5	0
Breakfast Onion Dill Bagel Smoked Salmon & Wasabi	1 (7.1 oz)	490	11	4	0
Caprese	1 (11.8 oz)	700	35	15	0
Chicken Mozzarella	1 (14.5 oz)	800	27	8	0
Chicken Pesto	1 (12.5 oz)	700	23	5	0
Chicken Tarragon	1 (11 oz)	720	29	4	0
Ciabatta Bacon & Egg Melt	1 (7 oz)	400	15	6	0
Ciabatta Ham & Cheddar	1 (12 oz)	650	20	9	0
Club Smoked Turkey	1 (11.6 oz)	780	43	13	0
Croissant Ham & Cheese	1 (4.2 oz)	350	18	10	0
Croissant Spinach & Cheese	1	250	14	8	0
Hot BBQ Chicken On Farmhouse Roll	1 (14.3 oz)	970	44	12	0
Hot Eggplant & Mozzarella	1 (12.4 oz)	710	37	13	0
Hot Steakhouse On Ciabatta	1 (13 oz)	800	41	11	0
Melt Tuna	1 (12.5 oz)	760	41	10	0
Melt Turkey	1 (12.2 oz)	890	47	15	0
Portobello & Goat Cheese	1 (10 oz)	610	33	10	0
Portobello Egg & Cheddar	1 (8.5 oz)	590	37	21	0
Prosciutto Mozzarella	1 (12.7 oz)	880	49	17	0
Spicy Tuna	1 (10.3 oz)	640	34	5	0
The Montana	1 (12.5 oz)	560	23	12	0
Turkey & Cranberry Chutney	1 (10.9 oz)	680	24	4	0
Wrap Chicken Caesar Asiago	1	700	25	8	0
Wrap Chopped Turkey Cobb	1 (12 oz)	660	27	8	0
Wrap Mediterranean	1 (12.8 oz)	670	28	6	0
Wrap Southwest Tuna	1 (14 oz)	900	51	12	0
Wrap Thai Peanut Chicken	1 (14.5 oz)	660	19	2	0
Wrap Turkey Spinach Sonoma	1 (12 oz)	630	19	6	0
Wrap Hot Cajun Shrimp	1 (14.9 oz)	700	24	8	0
Wrap Hot Mayan Chicken	1 (13.5 oz)	630	19	3	0
Wrap Hot Steak Teriyaki	1 (13.5 oz)	660	19	4	0
SOUPS					
Baked Stuffed Potato	1 med (12 oz)	350	21	10	0
Broccoli Cheddar	1 med (12 oz)	310	21	10	0
Carrot Ginger	1 med (12 oz)	130	5	0	0

FOOD	PORTION	CALS	FAT	SAT FAT	TRANS FAT
Chicken Florentine	1 med (12 oz)	240	13	6	0
Chicken & Dumplings	1 med (12 oz)	210	7	3	0
Chicken Noodle	1 med (12 oz)	130	3	1	0
Clam Chowder	1 med (12 oz)	320	18	7	0
Corn & Green Chili Bisque	1 med (12 oz)	250	14	7	0
Corn Chowder	1 med (12 oz)	350	18	8	0
Curried Rice & Lentil	1 med (12 oz)	150	2	0	0
French Moroccan Tomato Lentil	1 med (12 oz)	180	2	0	0
French Onion	1 med (12 oz)	130	5	3	0
Garden Vegetable	1 med (12 oz)	80	2	0	0
Harvest Pumpkin	1 med (12 oz)	190	10	5	0
Hearty Cabbage	1 med (12 oz)	110	5	1	0
Italian Wedding	1 med (12 oz)	170	7	3	0
Jamaican Black Bean	1 med (12 oz)	180	1	0	0
Mediterranean Pepper	1 med (12 oz)	100	3	0	0
Old Fashioned Tomato Rice	1 med (12 oz)	120	1	0	0
Pasta E Fagioli	1 med (12 oz)	240	8	2	0
Portuguese Kale	1 med (12 oz)	120	5	1	0
Potato Cheese	1 med (12 oz)	250	14	8	0
Potato Leek	1 med (12 oz)	300	20	11	0
Red Beans Italian Sausage & Rice	1 med (12 oz)	200	5	2	0
Southern Black-Eyed Pea	1 med (12 oz)	180	2	0	0
Southwest Tortilla	1 med (12 oz)	200	11	3	0
Southwest Vegetable	1 med (12 oz)	160	3	0	0
Split Pea	1 med (12 oz)	210	2	0	0
Thai Coconut Curry	1 med (12 oz)	150	7	2	0
Tomato Florentine	1 med (12 oz)	120	3	1	0
Tomato Basil Bisque	1 med (12 oz)	210	8	5	0
Tomato Cheddar	1 med (12 oz)	240	15	6	0
Tuscan Vegetable	1 med (12 oz)	170	5	2	0
Vegetable Beef Barley	1 med (12 oz)	140	3	2	0
Vegetarian Lentil	1 med (12 oz)	140	2	0	0
Vegetarian Minestrone	1 med (12 oz)	120	2	0	0
Vegetarian Chili	1 med (12 oz)	230	3	0	0
Wild Mushroom Bisque	1 med (12 oz)	190	9	2	0
YOGURT					
Blueberry w/ Fruit	1 sm (7.5 oz)	220	2	2	0

FOOD	PORTION	CALS	FAT	SAT FAT	TRANS FAT
Blueberry w/ Granola & Fruit	1 sm (8.5 oz)	310	6	2	0
Strawberry w/ Blueberries	1 sm (7.5 oz)	220	2	2	0
Strawberry w/ Granola & Blueberries	1 sm (8.5 oz)	310	6	2	0
Vanilla w/ Blueberries	1 sm (7.5 oz)	190	2	1	0
Vanilla w/ Granola & Blueberries	1 sm (8.5 oz)	310	6	2	0

AUNTIE ANNE'S
BEVERAGES

FOOD	PORTION	CALS	FAT	SAT FAT	TRANS FAT
Dutch Ice Blue Raspberry	1 (14 oz)	165	0	0	0
Dutch Ice Grape	1 (14 oz)	180	0	0	0
Dutch Ice Kiwi Banana	1 (14 oz)	190	0	0	0
Dutch Ice Lemonade	1 (14 oz)	315	0	0	0
Dutch Ice Lemonade Strawberry	1 (14 oz)	330	0	0	0
Dutch Ice Mocha	1 (14 oz)	400	10	9	0
Dutch Ice Orange Creme	1 (14 oz)	280	0	0	0
Dutch Ice Pina Colada	1 (14 oz)	220	0	0	0
Dutch Ice Strawberry	1 (14 oz)	220	0	0	0
Dutch Ice Watermelon	1 (14 oz)	200	0	0	0
Dutch Ice Wild Cherry	1 (14 oz)	210	0	0	0
Dutch Latte Caramel	1 (14 oz)	350	15	11	0
Dutch Latte Coffee	1 (14 oz)	290	14	9	0
Dutch Latte Mocha	1 (14 oz)	160	17	11	0
Dutch Shake Chocolate	1 (14 oz)	580	27	18	0
Dutch Shake Coffee	1 (14 oz)	590	27	18	0
Dutch Shake Strawberry	1 (14 oz)	610	27	18	0
Dutch Shake Vanilla	1 (14 oz)	510	27	17	0
Dutch Smoothie Blue Raspberry	1 (14 oz)	230	8	5	0
Dutch Smoothie Grape	1 (14 oz)	230	8	5	0
Dutch Smoothie Kiwi Banana	1 (14 oz)	240	8	5	0
Dutch Smoothie Lemonade	1 (14 oz)	300	8	5	0
Dutch Smoothie Mocha	1 (14 oz)	330	13	9	0
Dutch Smoothie Orange Creme	1 (14 oz)	280	8	5	0
Dutch Smoothie Pina Colada	1 (14 oz)	260	8	5	0
Dutch Smoothie Strawberry	1 (14 oz)	250	8	5	0
Dutch Smoothie Wild Cherry	1 (14 oz)	250	8	5	0

FOOD	PORTION	CALS	FAT	SAT FAT	TRANS FAT
Lemonade	1 (22 oz)	180	0	0	0
Lemonade Strawberry	1 (22 oz)	190	0	0	0
DIPPING SAUCES					
Caramel Dip	1 serv (1.5 oz)	135	3	2	0
Cheese Sauce	1 serv (1.25 oz)	100	8	4	0
Cream Cheese Light	1 serv (1.25 oz)	70	6	4	0
Hot Salsa Cheese	1 serv (1.25 oz)	100	8	4	0
Marinara Sauce	1 serv (1.25 oz)	10	0	0	0
Sweet	1 serv (1.4 oz)	40	0	0	0
Sweet Mustard	1 serv (1.25 oz)	60	2	1	0
PRETZELS					
Almond	1	400	8	5	0
Almond w/o Butter	1	350	2	1	0
Cinnamon Raisin w/o Butter	1	350	2	0	0
Cinnamon Sugar	1	450	9	5	0
Garlic	1	350	5	3	0
Garlic w/o Butter	1	320	1	0	0
Glazin' Raisin	1	510	4	2	0
Glazin' Raisin w/o Butter	1	470	1	0	0
Jalapeno	1	310	5	3	0
Jalapeno w/o Butter	1	270	1	0	0
Original	1	370	4	2	0
Original w/o Butter	1	340	1	0	0
Pretzel Dog	1	290	16	7	1
Sesame	1	410	12	4	0
Sesame w/o Butter	1	350	6	1	0
Sour Cream & Onion	1	340	5	3	0
Sour Cream & Onion w/o Butter	1	310	1	0	0
Stix	6	370	4	2	0
Stix w/o Butter	6	340	1	0	0
Whole Wheat	1	370	5	2	0
Whole Wheat w/o Butter	1	350	2	0	0

BABS' DELI
BAGELS

FOOD	PORTION	CALS	FAT	SAT FAT	TRANS FAT
Apple Cinnamon	1	332	2	0	–
Banana Nut	1	340	2	0	–
Blueberry	1	330	2	0	–
Blueberry Cobbler	1	392	8	4	–

FOOD	PORTION	CALS	FAT	SAT FAT	TRANS FAT
Cheddar Herb	1	352	6	4	–
Cheddar Nacho	1	352	6	4	–
Chocolate Chip	1	348	2	2	–
Cinnamon Apple Pie	1	386	8	4	–
Cinnamon Bun	1	400	8	4	–
Cinnamon Danish	1	396	8	4	–
Cinnamon Raisin	1	336	2	0	–
Cinnamon Sugar	1	350	2	0	–
Cranberry Walnut	1	352	2	0	–
Egg	1	328	2	0	–
Everything	1	336	2	0	–
French Toast	1	372	4	4	–
Garlic	1	330	2	0	–
Honey Oat	1	320	2	0	–
Jalapeno	1	350	6	4	–
Onion	1	336	2	0	–
Pizzaah Cheese	1 piece	189	7	4	–
Plain	1	334	2	0	–
Poppy	1	344	2	0	–
Pumpernickel	1	332	2	0	–
Quiche Lorraine	1	354	8	4	–
Salt	1	324	2	0	–
Sesame	1	358	4	0	–
Spinach	1	356	2	0	–
Strawberry	1	342	2	0	–
Strawberry White Chocolate	1	364	4	2	–
Swiss Melt	1	368	8	4	–
Tomato Basil	1	322	2	0	–
Vegetable	1	318	2	0	–
Wheat	1	330	2	0	–
White Chocolate Swirl	1	396	8	4	–
BEVERAGES					
Americano	1 (16 oz)	12	0	0	0
Cafe Caramella	1 (16 oz)	212	8	5	–
Cappuccino 2% Milk	1 (16 oz)	195	7	4	–
Cappuccino Fat Free Milk	1 (16 oz)	133	1	1	–
Coffee Black Forest	1 (16 oz)	198	5	3	–
Icepresso Caramel Decadence	1 (16 oz)	300	12	12	–
Icepresso Classic	1 (16 oz)	300	5	1	–
Icepresso Java Chip	1 (16 oz)	360	18	14	–

FOOD	PORTION	CALS	FAT	SAT FAT	TRANS FAT
Icepresso Latte	1 (16 oz)	300	12	12	–
Icepresso Mocha	1 (16 oz)	300	12	12	–
Icepresso Strawberry	1 (16 oz)	340	12	12	–
Italiano 2% Milk	1 (16 oz)	131	5	3	–
Italiano Fat Free Milk	1 (16 oz)	89	1	0	–
Jittery Monkey 2% Milk	1 (16 oz)	482	11	7	–
Jittery Monkey Fat Free Milk	1 (16 oz)	429	6	4	–
Latte 2% Milk	1 (16 oz)	212	7	5	–
Latte Cinnamon Toast 2% Milk	1 (16 oz)	299	7	4	–
Latte Cinnamon Toast Fat Free Milk	1 (16 oz)	240	1	1	–
Latte Creme Caramel 2% Milk	1 (16 oz)	303	7	4	–
Latte Creme Caramel Fat Free Milk	1 (16 oz)	244	1	1	–
Latte Fat Free Milk	1 (16 oz)	145	1	1	–
Latte Oregon Chai Tea 2% Milk	1 (16 oz)	274	5	3	–
Latte Oregon Chai Tea Fat Free Milk	1 (16 oz)	231	1	0	–
Latte Raspberry Cheesecake 2% Milk	1 (16 oz)	319	7	4	–
Latte Raspberry Cheesecake Fat Free Milk	1 (16 oz)	259	1	1	–
Latte Vanilla Creme 2% Milk	1 (16 oz)	275	7	4	–
Mocha Whipped Cream 2% Milk	1 (16 oz)	454	12	7	–
Mocha Whipped Cream Fat Free Milk	1 (16 oz)	392	6	4	–
Turtle Mocha Fat Free Milk	1 (16 oz)	522	12	7	–
MUFFINS					
My Favorite Banana Nut	2 mini	195	11	2	–
My Favorite Blueberry	2 mini	168	8	2	–
My Favorite Blueberry Cheesecake	2 mini	199	12	5	–
My Favorite Boston Cream Pie	2 mini	176	7	2	–
My Favorite Cherry Cheesecake	2 mini	170	10	4	–
My Favorite Chocolate Cheesecake	2 mini	202	12	5	–
My Favorite Chocolate Chip	2 mini	211	11	3	–

FOOD	PORTION	CALS	FAT	SAT FAT	TRANS FAT
My Favorite Cinnamon Crumb Cake	2 mini	212	13	5	–
My Favorite Cinnamon Swirl Cheesecake	2 mini	214	11	3	–
My Favorite Deep Dish Apple	2 mini	177	8	2	–
My Favorite Double Chocolate	2 mini	210	9	3	–
My Favorite Fat Free Blueberry	2 mini	108	0	0	0
My Favorite Fat Free Cherry Pie	2 mini	109	0	0	0
My Favorite Fat Free Chocolate Marble	2 mini	125	0	0	0
My Favorite Fat Free Cinnamon Bun	2 mini	168	0	0	0
My Favorite Fat Free Raspberry Amaretto	2 mini	127	0	0	0
My Favorite Golden Corn Bread	2 mini	197	9	2	–
My Favorite Lemon Poppyseed	2 mini	201	10	3	–
My Favorite Pumpkin Spice	2 mini	181	8	3	–
SALADS					
Calypso Chicken	1 (13.6 oz)	637	49	8	–
Calypso Chicken w/ Lite Italian	1 (13.6 oz)	317	17	2	–
Chicken Caesar	1 (11.5 oz)	524	41	9	–
Chicken Caesar w/ Lite Italian	1 (11.5 oz)	268	12	3	–
Classic Caesar	1 (8.4 oz)	414	36	7	–
Classic Caesar Cafe	1 (4.3 oz)	225	19	4	–
Classic Caesar w/ Lite Italian	1 (8.4 oz)	158	8	2	–
Garden Mix	1 (12.4 oz)	197	9	2	–
Garden Mix Cafe	1 (6.5 oz)	100	5	1	–
Grilled Chicken Club	1 (17.9 oz)	820	69	21	–
Grilled Chicken Club w/ Lite Italian	1 (17.9 oz)	500	31	14	–
Low Carb Tuna Salad Plate	1 serv (8.9 oz)	356	25	4	–
Mediterranean Bread	1 (18.8 oz)	973	73	22	–
Mediterranean Bread w/ Lite Italian	1 (18.8 oz)	626	32	15	–
SANDWICHES					
Breakfast BLT	1	704	31	14	–
Breakfast Lox & Cream Cheese	1	602	21	14	–
Breakfast Morning Classic	1	486	11	5	–
Breakfast Northern Omelette	1	699	31	12	–

FOOD	PORTION	CALS	FAT	SAT FAT	TRANS FAT
Breakfast Southern Tradition w/ Bacon	1	566	18	8	–
Breakfast Southern Tradition w/ Ham	1	547	15	6	–
Breakfast Southern Tradition w/ Sausage	1	696	31	12	–
Build Your Own Ham	1	495	9	3	–
Build Your Own Roast Beef	1	480	6	2	–
Build Your Own Tuna	1	547	14	2	–
Build Your Own Turkey	1	465	3	0	–
Enchilada Bagellata	1	522	11	7	–
Gourmet Classic Turkey	1	552	14	2	–
Gourmet Holey Guacamole	1	476	5	1	–
Gourmet Kick-N Roast Beef	1	579	15	2	–
Gourmet Mediterranean Veg-Out	1	506	9	1	–
Overstuffed Classic Reuben	1	962	43	17	–
Overstuffed Corned Beef	1	661	19	6	–
Overstuffed Ham & Cheese	1	889	36	16	–
Overstuffed Manhattan Club	1	1122	40	15	–
Overstuffed Pastrami	1	661	19	6	–
Overstuffed TD Classic California	1	759	12	6	–
Overstuffed TD Classic Club	1	1110	43	13	–
Overstuffed TD Clubhouse	1	1079	37	14	–
Pizzaah Bruschetta	1 piece	162	12	7	–
Pizzaah Grilled Chicken Bruschetta	1 piece	343	21	12	–
Pizzaah Sausage	1 piece	211	17	7	–
Pizzaah Veggie	1 piece	238	10	4	–
Specialty All American Duo	1	752	28	13	–
Specialty Big Apple Club	1	797	37	13	–
Specialty Chicken Caesar	1	611	19	5	–
Specialty Roma Italian	1	764	34	14	–
Specialty Turkey Club	1	782	34	12	–
Toasted Cafe Chicken Melt	1	815	32	14	–
Toasted Deli Style Turkey	1	732	25	11	–
Toasted Roast Beef Parmesan Grinder	1	583	15	7	–

FOOD	PORTION	CALS	FAT	SAT FAT	TRANS FAT
Toasted Spicy Italian Sub	1	770	34	14	–
Toasted Tuna Melt	1	641	23	8	–
SOUPS					
Beef Barley Mushroom	1 serv (8 oz)	100	3	–	–
Boston Clam Chowder	1 serv (8 oz)	210	13	–	–
Chicken & Wild Rice	1 serv (8 oz)	190	9	–	–
Chicken Gumbo	1 serv (8 oz)	130	3	–	–
Cream Of Potato	1 serv (8 oz)	240	14	–	–
Hearty Vegetable Beef	1 serv (8 oz)	100	1	–	–
New England Clam Chowder	1 serv (8 oz)	220	13	–	–
Split Pea w/ Ham	1 serv (8 oz)	90	2	–	–
Wisconsin Cheese	1 serv (8 oz)	210	11	–	–
TOPPINGS					
Cream Cheese	2 tbsp	90	9	6	0
Cream Cheese Cheddar Jalapeno	2 tbsp	90	8	5	0
Cream Cheese Garden Vegetable	2 tbsp	90	9	6	0
Cream Cheese Lite	2 tbsp	60	5	3	0
Cream Cheese Onion Chive	2 tbsp	80	8	5	–
Cream Cheese Strawberry	2 tbsp	90	5	0	0
Cream Cheese Whipped	2 tbsp	70	7	5	0
Cream Cheese Whipped Brown Sugar Cinnamon	2 tbsp	70	5	4	0
Cream Cheese Whipped Reduced Fat Spring Veggie	2 tbsp	60	5	4	0

BAJA FRESH
CHILDREN'S MENU SELECTIONS

Kid's Mini Burrito Bean & Cheese	1 serv	540	14	7	0
Kid's Mini Burrito Bean & Cheese w/ Chicken	1 serv	590	15	7	0
Kid's Mini Quesadilla Cheese	1 serv	610	26	13	1
Kid's Mini Quesadilla Cheese w/ Chicken	1 serv	650	27	13	1
Kid's Taquitos Chicken	1 serv	630	33	7	1
MAIN MENU SELECTIONS					
Black Beans	1 serv	360	3	1	0

FOOD	PORTION	CALS	FAT	SAT FAT	TRANS FAT
Burrito Baja Breaded Fish	1 serv	850	44	16	2
Burrito Baja Carnitas	1 serv	830	45	18	1
Burrito Baja Chicken	1 serv	790	38	15	1
Burrito Baja Mahi Mahi	1 serv	780	38	15	1
Burrito Baja Shrimp	1 serv	760	37	15	1
Burrito Baja Steak	1 serv	850	46	18	1
Burrito Bare Carnitas	1 serv	600	14	4	0
Burrito Bare Chicken	1 serv	640	7	1	0
Burrito Bare Steak	1 serv	700	15	5	0
Burrito Bare Veggie & Cheese	1 serv	580	10	4	0
Burrito Bean & Cheese Breaded Fish	1 serv	1030	41	18	2
Burrito Bean & Cheese Carnitas	1 serv	1010	42	20	1
Burrito Bean & Cheese Chicken	1 serv	970	35	18	1
Burrito Bean & Cheese Mahi Mahi	1 serv	960	35	18	1
Burrito Bean & Cheese No Meat	1 serv	840	33	17	1
Burrito Bean & Cheese Shrimp	1 serv	950	34	17	1
Burrito Bean & Cheese Steak	1 serv	1030	43	21	2
Burrito Dos Manos Breaded Fish	1 serv	890	33	13	1
Burrito Dos Manos Carnitas	1 serv	780	30	14	1
Burrito Dos Manos Chicken	½ serv	760	26	12	1
Burrito Dos Manos Mahi Mahi	1 serv	780	26	12	1
Burrito Dos Manos Shrimp	1 serv	780	26	12	1
Burrito Dos Manos Steak	½ serv	795	30	14	1
Burrito Grilled Veggie	1 serv	506	33	17	1
Burrito Mexicano Breaded Fish	1 serv	850	19	4	1
Burrito Mexicano Carnitas	1 serv	830	20	6	0
Burrito Mexicano Chicken	1 serv	790	13	4	0
Burrito Mexicano Mahi Mahi	1 serv	790	13	4	0
Burrito Mexicano Shrimp	1 serv	770	13	4	0
Burrito Mexicano Steak	1 serv	860	21	7	1
Burrito Ultimo Breaded Fish	1 serv	940	42	19	2
Burrito Ultimo Carnitas	1 serv	920	44	21	1
Burrito Ultimo Chicken	1 serv	880	36	18	1
Burrito Ultimo Mahi Mahi	1 serv	880	36	18	1
Burrito Ultimo Shrimp	1 serv	860	36	18	1
Burrito Ultimo Steak	1 serv	950	44	21	2

FOOD	PORTION	CALS	FAT	SAT FAT	TRANS FAT
Chips & Guacamole	1 serv	1340	83	8	3
Chips & Salsa Baja	1 serv	810	37	4	2
Fajitas Corn Tortillas Breaded Fish	1 serv	1060	37	9	2
Fajitas Corn Tortillas Carnitas	1 serv	920	34	11	0
Fajitas Corn Tortillas Chicken	1 serv	860	24	7	0
Fajitas Corn Tortillas Mahi Mahi	1 serv	840	23	7	0
Fajitas Corn Tortillas Shrimp	1 serv	840	23	7	0
Fajitas Corn Tortillas Steak	1 serv	960	36	12	1
Fajitas Flour Tortillas Breaded Fish	1 serv	1340	46	12	2
Fajitas Flour Tortillas Carnitas	1 serv	1190	43	14	0
Fajitas Flour Tortillas Chicken	1 serv	1140	33	10	0
Fajitas Flour Tortillas Mahi Mahi	1 serv	1120	32	10	0
Fajitas Flour Tortillas Shrimp	1 serv	1120	32	10	0
Fajitas Flour Tortillas Steak	1 serv	960	36	12	1
Guacamole Side	1 (3 oz)	110	13	1	0
Nachos Breaded Fish	1 serv	2090	116	41	5
Nachos Carnitas	1 serv	2060	117	43	4
Nachos Cheese	1 serv	1890	108	40	4
Nachos Chicken	1 serv	2020	110	41	4
Nachos Mahi Mahi	1 serv	2020	110	41	4
Nachos Shrimp	1 serv	2000	110	41	0
Nachos Steak	1 serv	2120	118	44	5
Pico De Gallo Side	1 serv (8 oz)	50	1	0	0
Pinto Beans	1 serv	320	1	0	0
Pronto Guacamole Side	1 serv (6 oz)	560	34	3	1
Quesadilla Breaded Frish	1 serv	1400	86	38	3
Quesadilla Carnitas	1 serv	1370	87	40	3
Quesadilla Cheese	1 serv	1200	78	37	3
Quesadilla Chicken	1 serv	1330	80	37	3
Quesadilla Mahi Mahi	1 serv	1330	79	37	3
Quesadilla Shrimp	1 serv	1310	79	37	3
Quesadilla Steak	1 serv	1430	87	41	3
Quesadilla Veggie	1 serv	1260	78	37	3
Rice	1 serv	280	4	1	0
Rice & Beans Plate	1 serv	420	5	2	0
Salsa Baja Side	1 serv (8 oz)	70	3	0	0
Salsa Roja Side	1 serv (8 oz)	70	1	0	0

FOOD	PORTION	CALS	FAT	SAT FAT	TRANS FAT
Salsa Verde Side	1 serv (8 oz)	50	0	0	0
Soup Tortilla w/ Chicken	1 serv (13.6 oz)	320	14	4	0
Soup Tortilla w/o Chicken	1 serv (12.4 oz)	270	14	4	0
Taco Grilled Mahi Mahi	1 serv	230	9	2	0
Taco Baja Breaded Fish	1 serv	250	13	2	0
Taco Baja Chicken	1 serv	210	5	1	0
Taco Baja Shrimp	1 serv	200	5	1	0
Taco Baja Steak	1 serv	230	8	2	0
Taco Soft Breaded Fish	1 serv	240	11	5	0
Taco Soft Carnitas	1 serv	250	12	5	0
Taco Soft Chicken	1 serv	230	10	5	0
Taco Soft Mahi Mahi	1 serv	240	10	5	0
Taco Soft Shrimp	1 serv	230	10	5	0
Taco Soft Steak	1 serv	260	13	6	0
Taquitos Chicken w/ Beans	3	780	40	12	1
Taquitos Chicken w/ Rice	3	740	40	11	1
Veggie Mix	1 serv	110	0	0	0
SALAD DRESSINGS					
Chipotle Vinaigrette	1 serv (2.5 oz)	110	9	1	0
Fat Free Salsa Verde	1 serv (2.5 oz)	15	0	0	0
Olive Oil Vinaigrette	1 serv (2.5 oz)	290	31	5	0
Ranch	1 serv (2.5 oz)	260	26	6	1
SALADS					
Baja Ensalada w/ Chicken	1 serv	370	18	6	0
Baja Ensalada w/o Chicken	1 serv	310	7	2	0
Baja Ensalada Fish	1 serv	360	15	4	–
Baja Ensalada Shrimp	1 serv	230	6	2	0
Baja Ensalada Steak	1 serv	450	18	7	1
Chipotle w/ Carnitas	1 serv	640	30	10	2
Chipotle w/ Chicken	1 serv	590	22	6	1
Chipotle w/ Steak	1 serv	700	31	11	2
Side By Side Carnitas	1 serv	570	40	13	0
Side By Side Chicken	1 serv	500	27	8	0
Side By Side Steak	1 serv	620	42	14	1
Side Salad	1 (6.5 oz)	130	6	2	0
Tostada Breaded Fish	1 serv	1200	61	15	2
Tostada Carnitas	1 serv	1180	62	17	1
Tostada Chicken	1 serv	1140	55	14	1
Tostada Mahi Mahi	1 serv	1130	55	14	1
Tostada No Meat	1 serv	1010	53	13	1

FOOD	PORTION	CALS	FAT	SAT FAT	TRANS FAT
Tostada Shrimp	1 serv	1120	55	14	1
Tostada Steak	1 serv	1230	63	17	2

BASKIN-ROBBINS
FROZEN YOGURT

FOOD	PORTION	CALS	FAT	SAT FAT	TRANS FAT
Cafe Mocha Truly Free Soft Serve	1 reg	140	1	1	–
Chocolate Nonfat Soft Serve	1 reg	190	1	0	–
Lowfat Maui Brownie Madness	1 reg	250	9	4	–

ICE CREAM

FOOD	PORTION	CALS	FAT	SAT FAT	TRANS FAT
Cappuccino Blast w/ Whipped Cream	1 reg	340	16	10	–
Chocolate	1 reg	270	16	10	–
Chocolate Chip	1 reg	270	17	11	–
Espresso'n Cream Lowfat	1 reg	180	3	2	–
Jamoca Almond Fudge	1 reg	280	16	8	–
Peach Crumb Pie No Sugar Added	1 reg	180	5	3	–
Pralines'n Cream	1 reg	280	15	8	–
Shake Chocolate	16 oz	750	43	21	–
Shake Vanilla	16 oz	630	35	22	–
Smoothie Very Strawberry w/ Soft Serve Ice Cream	1 reg	320	1	1	–
Thin Mint No Sugar Added	1 reg	160	4	3	–
Vanilla	1 reg	270	16	10	–

ICES

FOOD	PORTION	CALS	FAT	SAT FAT	TRANS FAT
Daiquiri Ice	1 reg	130	0	0	0
Sherbet Rainbow	1 reg	160	2	2	–
Sorbet Peachy Keen	1 reg	110	0	0	0

BEAR ROCK CAFE
SANDWICHES

FOOD	PORTION	CALS	FAT	SAT FAT	TRANS FAT
Colorado Turkey Club	1	855	37	17	–
Coop's Chicken Salad Croissant	1	439	31	6	–
Garden Grill Ciabatta	1	406	25	7	–
Giant Panda Wrap	1	556	23	4	–
Hoot Owl	1	641	42	12	–
Rising Sunflower	1	596	35	9	–
Roast Turkey & Bacon	1	522	30	6	–
Rockslide Focaccia	1	958	62	17	–
The Moose	1	976	54	18	–

FOOD	PORTION	CALS	FAT	SAT FAT	TRANS FAT
BEN & JERRY'S					
FROZEN YOGURT					
Low Fat Cherry Garcia	½ cup	170	3	2	–
Low Fat Chocolate Fudge Brownie	½ cup	190	3	2	–
Low Fat Half Baked	½ cup	190	3	2	–
Phish Food	½ cup	220	5	4	–
ICE CREAM					
Bar Cherry Garcia	1	270	19	12	–
Bar Half Baked	1	340	16	10	–
Bar Vanilla	1	300	20	13	–
Bar Vanilla Almond	1	340	23	13	–
Black & Tan	½ cup	230	13	9	–
Brownie Batter	½ cup	310	18	10	–
Butter Pecan	½ cup	280	21	10	–
Cherry Garcia	½ cup	250	14	10	–
Chocolate	½ cup	260	16	11	–
Chocolate Chip Cookie Dough	½ cup	270	15	10	–
Chocolate Fudge Brownie	½ cup	260	13	9	–
Chubby Hubby	½ cup	330	20	11	–
Chunky Monkey	½ cup	300	18	10	–
Coffee	½ cup	240	15	10	–
Coffee Heath Bar Crunch	½ cup	290	18	11	–
Dave Matthews Band Magic Brownies	½ cup	250	13	8	–
Dublin Mudslide	½ cup	270	16	10	–
Everything But The	½ cup	310	19	12	–
Fossil Fuel	½ cup	280	17	11	–
Fudge Central	½ cup	300	18	12	–
Half Baked	½ cup	280	14	9	–
In A Crunch	½ cup	350	23	10	–
Karamel Sutra	½ cup	280	15	10	–
Marsha Marsha Marshmallow	½ cup	300	17	10	–
Mint Chocolate Cookie	½ cup	260	16	9	–
Neapolitan Dynamite	½ cup	250	13	9	–
New York Super Fudge Chunk	½ cup	310	20	11	–
Oatmeal Cookie Chunk	½ cup	270	15	9	–
Organic Chocolate Fudge Brownie	½ cup	270	13	9	–
Organic Strawberry	½ cup	210	12	8	–

FOOD	PORTION	CALS	FAT	SAT FAT	TRANS FAT
Organic Sweet Cream & Cookies	½ cup	250	15	9	–
Organic Vanilla	½ cup	240	16	11	–
Peanut Butter Cup	½ cup	360	26	13	–
Phish Food	½ cup	280	13	9	–
Pistachio Pistachio	½ cup	260	17	10	–
Sandwich 'Wich Ice Cream Cookie	1	350	18	13	–
Strawberry	½ cup	230	13	9	–
The Godfather	½ cup	270	14	9	–
Turtle Soup	½ cup	280	15	10	–
Uncanny Cashew	½ cup	290	19	13	–
Vanilla Caramel Fudge	½ cup	280	15	10	–
Vanilla Heath Bar Crunch	½ cup	290	18	11	–
Vermonty Python	½ cup	310	19	11	–
SORBETS					
Berried Treasure	½ cup	110	0	0	0
Jamaican Me Crazy	½ cup	130	0	0	0
Strawberry Kiwi Swirl	½ cup	110	0	0	0

BILLY'S BURGER HUT

BEVERAGES

FOOD	PORTION	CALS	FAT	SAT FAT	TRANS FAT
Shake Chocolate	1 (20 oz)	420	10	4	0
Shake Vanilla	1 (20 oz)	320	10	4	0
MAIN MENU SELECTIONS					
Big Billy's Roast Beef Sub	1	843	54	27	0
Billyburger	1	426	22	12	1
Billyburger w/ Cheese	1	498	35	19	1
Billy's Best Red Potato Salad	1 serv	190	9	2	0
Billy's Biggest Burger ½ Pounder w/ Everything	1	852	58	–	2
Billy's Famous 7 Layer Salad	1 serv	558	49	11	0
Billy's Seafood Sandwich	1	399	18	10	0
Caesar Side Salad	1 serv	360	28	4	0
Chili w/ Cheese & Onion	1 serv	380	12	6	0
Cowboy Cobb Salad	1 serv	735	45	14	0
Cowboy Coleslaw	1 serv	180	9	2	0
French Fries	1 reg	230	12	4	1
Onion Rings	1 serv	250	10	6	2
Super Billy Burger w/ Bacon	1	663	41	21	1

FOOD	PORTION	CALS	FAT	SAT FAT	TRANS FAT
BLIMPIE					
COOKIES					
Chocolate Chunk	1	200	10	6	–
Macadamia White Chunk	1	210	10	5	–
Oatmeal Raisin	1	190	8	2	–
Peanut Butter	1	220	12	5	–
Sugar	1	330	17	5	–
SALAD DRESSINGS AND TOPPINGS					
Caesar Dressing	1 serv (1.5 oz)	208	22	4	–
Cracked Peppercorn Dressing	1 serv (1.5 oz)	237	25	1	–
Frank's Red Hot Buffalo Sauce	1 serv (1 oz)	13	tr	tr	–
French's Honey Mustard	1 tbsp	5	0	0	0
GourMayo Chipotle Chili	1 tbsp	50	5	1	–
GourMayo Sun Dried Tomato	1 tbsp	50	5	1	–
GourMayo Wasabi Horseradish	1 tbsp	50	5	1	–
Guacamole	1 serv (1.5 oz)	194	18	3	–
Oil & Vinegar	1 serv	36	4	1	–
Pesto Dressing	1 serv (1 oz)	132	13	2	–
SALADS					
Antipasto	1 reg serv	244	13	6	–
Chef	1 reg serv	212	9	5	–
Chili Ole	1 reg serv	480	27	11	–
Grilled Chicken w/ Caesar Dressing	1 reg serv	347	27	5	–
Grilled Chicken w/o Dressing	1 serv	139	5	2	–
Roast Beef 'N Blue	1 reg serv	390	16	10	–
Seafood	1 reg serv	122	4	1	–
Tuna	1 reg serv	261	20	3	–
Zesto Pesto Turkey	1 reg serv	370	19	8	–
SANDWICHES					
6 Inch Hot Sub BLT	1	588	32	10	–
6 Inch Hot Sub Buffalo Chicken	1	400	13	7	–
6 Inch Hot Sub Buffalo Chicken w/o Cheese	1	320	7	3	–
6 Inch Hot Sub ChiliMax	1	511	13	2	–
6 Inch Hot Sub Grilled Chicken	1	373	9	3	–
6 Inch Hot Sub Meatball	1	572	27	10	–
6 Inch Hot Sub MexiMelt	1	425	9	2	–
6 Inch Hot Sub Pastrami	1	507	17	7	–

FOOD	PORTION	CALS	FAT	SAT FAT	TRANS FAT
6 Inch Hot Sub Steak & Onion Melt	1	440	16	6	–
6 Inch Hot Sub VegiMax	1	395	7	2	–
6 Inch Sub Blimpie Best	1	476	16	7	–
6 Inch Sub Club	1	440	12	6	–
6 Inch Sub Ham & Cheese	1	436	13	6	–
6 Inch Sub Roast Beef	1	468	14	6	–
6 Inch Sub Roast Beef w/o Cheese	1	388	8	2	–
6 Inch Sub Seafood	1	355	8	2	–
6 Inch Sub Tuna	1	493	23	4	–
6 Inch Sub Turkey	1	424	11	5	–
6 Inch Sub Turkey w/o Cheese	1	344	5	1	–
Cheddar	1 slice	52	5	3	
Grilled Subs Beef Turkey & Cheddar	1	600	31	10	–
Grilled Subs Cuban	1	462	12	6	–
Grilled Subs Pastrami	1	462	14	6	–
Grilled Subs Reuben	1	630	33	5	–
Provolone	1 slice	80	6	4	–
Swiss	1 slice	80	6	4	–
Wraps Beef & Cheddar	1	714	37	11	–
Wraps Chicken Caesar	1	646	35	7	–
Wraps Southwestern	1	674	35	8	–
Wraps Steak & Onions	1	716	37	10	–
Wraps Ultimate BLT	1	831	50	15	–
Wraps Zesty Italian	1	638	33	10	–
SIDE ORDERS					
Cole Slaw	1 serv (5 oz)	180	13	2	–
Macaroni Salad	1 serv (5 oz)	360	25	4	–
Mustard Potato Salad	1 serv (5 oz)	160	5	1	–
Potato Chips Cheddar & Sour Cream	1 bag	210	11	2	–
Potato Chips Jalapeno	1 bag	210	11	2	–
Potato Chips Lea & Perrins Barbecue	1 bag	210	10	2	–
Potato Chips Regular	1 bag	210	11	2	–
Potato Chips Romano & Garlic	1 bag	210	11	2	–

FOOD	PORTION	CALS	FAT	SAT FAT	TRANS FAT
Potato Chips Sour Cream & Onion	1 bag	210	11	2	–
Potato Salad	1 serv (5 oz)	270	19	3	–
SOUPS					
Chicken w/ White & Wild Rice	1 serv (8 oz)	230	12	2	–
Cream Of Broccoli & Cheese	1 serv (8 oz)	190	12	5	–
Cream Of Potato	1 serv (8 oz)	190	9	3	–
Garden Vegetable	1 serv (8 oz)	80	1	0	–
Grande Chili w/ Beans & Beef	1 serv (8 oz)	250	7	4	–
Homestyle Chicken Noodle	1 serv (8 oz)	120	3	1	–
Tomato Basil w/ Raviolini	1 serv (8 oz)	110	1	0	–
Vegetable Beef	1 serv (8 oz)	80	2	1	–

BOB EVANS
BAKED SELECTIONS

FOOD	PORTION	CALS	FAT	SAT FAT	TRANS FAT
Biscuit	1	277	12	3	–
Bread Apple Walnut	1 slice	142	6	1	–
Bread Banana Nut	1 slice	186	7	1	–
Bread Garlic	1 slice	218	16	3	–
Bread Sourdough	1	130	1	0	–
Bun Kaiser	1	167	2	0	–
Bun Mini	1	105	1	0	–
English Muffin	1	139	1	0	–
Roll Cinnamon Swirl Frosted	1	607	26	6	–
Roll Cinnamon Swirl Unfrosted	1	510	23	5	–
Roll Dinner	1	201	5	1	–
Texas Toast	1 slice	120	1	0	–
BEVERAGES					
Coca-Cola	12.5 oz	145	0	0	0
Coffee Decaf	7 oz	5	0	0	0
Coffee Regular	7 oz	2	0	0	0
Creamer Half & Half	0.5 oz	40	3	0	–
Creamer Non-Dairy	0.5 oz	19	1	0	–
Diet Coke	12.5 oz	4	0	0	0
Dr Pepper	12.5 oz	145	0	0	0
Hot Chocolate	1 serv (8.8 oz)	142	3	5	–
Hot Tea	7 oz	2	0	0	0
Iced Tea	9.4 oz	3	0	0	0
Iced Tea Blackberry	9.4 oz	92	0	0	0
Iced Tea Strawberry	9.4 oz	120	0	0	0

FOOD	PORTION	CALS	FAT	SAT FAT	TRANS FAT
Kool-Aid Ice Blue Raspberry Lemonade	1 kids cup (8 oz)	70	0	0	0
Lemonade	12 oz	136	0	0	0
Lemonade Blackberry	12 oz	214	0	0	0
Lemonade Strawberry	12 oz	242	0	0	0
Root Beer	12.5 oz	145	0	0	0
Sprite	12.5 oz	142	0	0	0
Strawberry Splash	12.5 oz	218	0	0	0
BREAKFAST SELECTIONS					
Bacon	1 piece	36	4	2	0
Benedict Ham & Cheese	1 serv	826	52	19	5
Country Benedict Sausage	1 serv	936	66	24	5
Country Benedict Spinach Bacon & Tomato	1 serv	729	48	16	5
Country Biscuit Breakfast	1 serv	659	45	16	6
Egg Hardcooked	1	60	4	2	0
Egg Over Easy	1	101	8	2	0
Egg Beaters	1 serv	173	12	2	0
Eggs Scrambled	1 serv	255	17	5	0
French Toast	1 slice	131	2	0	0
French Toast Stuffed Plain	1 serv	599	20	12	0
Fruit & Yogurt Plate	1 serv	403	2	1	0
Grits	1 serv	178	7	2	1
Ham Smoked	1 slice	87	2	1	0
Hotcake Blueberry	1	328	9	2	3
Hotcake Buttermilk	1	318	9	2	3
Hotcake Cinnamon	1	417	15	4	5
Hotcake Multigrain	1	322	10	3	1
Mush	1 serv	79	3	1	0
Oatmeal	1 serv	172	3	0	0
Omelette Bacon & Cheese	1 serv	825	66	25	0
Omelette Border Scramble	1	756	58	20	0
Omelette Egg Beaters Bacon & Cheese	1 serv	615	47	20	0
Omelette Egg Beaters Border Scramble	1 serv	517	37	14	0
Omelette Egg Beaters Farmer's Market	1 serv	569	41	19	1
Omelette Egg Beaters Garden Harvest	1 serv	444	31	14	1

FOOD	PORTION	CALS	FAT	SAT FAT	TRANS FAT
Omelette Egg Beaters Ham & Cheddar	1 serv	426	29	12	0
Omelette Egg Beaters Sausage & Cheddar	1 serv	502	40	15	0
Omelette Egg Beaters Three Cheese	1 serv	435	34	16	0
Omelette Farmer's Market	1	778	60	24	1
Omelette Garden Harvest	1 serv	654	50	20	1
Omelette Ham & Cheddar	1 serv	634	48	17	0
Omelette Sausage & Cheddar	1 serv	741	61	21	0
Omelette Three Cheese	1 serv	645	52	21	0
Omelette Western	1 serv	654	48	17	0
Pot Roast Hash	1 serv	652	39	14	1
Sausage Gravy Bowl	1 serv	268	17	11	0
Sausage Link	1	125	11	3	0
Skillet Sunshine	1 serv	842	60	18	3
Waffles Sweet Cream	1 serv	598	12	7	3
CHILDREN'S MENU SELECTIONS					
Fruit & Yogurt Dippers	1 serv	275	2	1	0
Hotcakes	1 serv	501	17	6	4
Kids Macaroni & Cheese	1 serv	320	11	3	0
Kids Pasta	1 serv	113	5	1	0
Mini Cheeseburgers	1 serv	306	19	7	0
Smiley Face Potatoes	1 serv	524	31	6	0
Sundae Fudge Blast	1 serv	244	11	8	1
Sundae Reese's I'm Smiling	1 serv	330	17	9	1
DESSERTS					
A La Mode Vanilla Ice Cream	1 serv	159	8	6	–
Cake Hershey's Hot Fudge	1 slice	688	25	20	–
Cake Pineapple Upside Down	1 slice	500	25	8	–
Oreo Cheesecake	1 slice	625	38	19	–
Peach Cobbler	1 serv	499	25	6	–
Pie Apple Dumpling	1 slice	682	30	8	–
Pie Banana Cream	1 slice	456	25	17	–
Pie Coconut Cream	1 slice	461	23	16	–
Pie French Silk	1 slice	653	44	23	–
Pie Lemon Meringue	1 slice	536	18	5	–
Pie Reese's Peanut Butter Cup	1 slice	1130	60	33	–
Pie Strawberry Supreme	1 slice	589	39	20	–
Pie No Sugar Added Apple	1 slice	483	28	7	–

FOOD	PORTION	CALS	FAT	SAT FAT	TRANS FAT
Sundae Fudge	1	501	19	13	–
Sundae Reese's	1 serv	769	35	19	–
MAIN MENU SELECTIONS					
Applesauce	1 serv	101	0	0	0
Baked Potato Loaded	1	427	18	10	–
Baked Potato Plain	1	207	0	0	0
Broccoli Florets	1 serv	156	1	0	–
Broccoli Florets Cheddar	1 serv	230	9	4	–
Carrots Glazed	1 serv	188	8	3	–
Catfish Grilled New Orleans	1 piece	255	19	3	–
Cheeseburger Bacon Plain	1	1005	76	34	–
Cheeseburger Plain	1	691	46	19	–
Chicken Quesadilla	1 serv	502	36	16	–
Chicken & Broccoli Alfredo	1 serv	826	29	7	–
Chicken Fried	1 piece	291	30	6	–
Chicken Grilled	1 piece	229	10	2	–
Chicken Pot Pie	1 serv	758	49	22	–
Chicken Tenders Grilled	1 piece	103	7	1	–
Chicken-N-Noodle	1 serv	407	22	5	–
Coleslaw	1 serv	198	13	2	–
Corn Buttered	1 serv	225	14	5	–
Cottage Cheese	1 serv	122	5	3	–
Country Fried Steak w/ Gravy	1 serv	535	37	13	–
Country Fried Steak w/o Gravy	1 serv	481	33	12	–
Dressing Bread & Celery	1 serv	362	20	0	–
Fish Market Halibut	1 piece	209	12	2	–
French Fries	1 serv	217	7	2	–
Green Beans w/ Ham	1 serv	83	3	1	–
Grilled Garden Vegetables	1 serv	290	23	4	–
Hamburger Patty	1	388	30	13	–
Hamburger Plain	1	585	36	14	–
Hamburger Shroomin' Onion Plain	1	695	44	19	–
Home Fries	1 serv	193	7	1	–
Mashed Potatoes	1 serv	171	6	4	–
Meat Loaf	1 serv	626	44	19	–
Mushrooms Grilled	1 serv	152	12	2	–
Onion Rings	1 serv	460	27	5	–
Open Faced Roast Beef Dinner	1 serv	633	29	10	–
Pork Chop Dinner	1 serv	466	28	9	–

FOOD	PORTION	CALS	FAT	SAT FAT	TRANS FAT
Pork Chop Dinner w/ Garlic Herb Butter	1 serv	624	39	11	–
Pork Chop Dinner w/ Wildfire Barbecue Sauce	1 serv	645	35	10	–
Rice Pilaf	1 serv	163	3	1	–
Salmon	1 serv	334	18	4	–
Salmon w/ Garlic Herb Butter	1 serv	491	29	6	–
Salmon w/ Wildfire Barbecue Sauce	1 serv	512	25	5	–
Sandwich Bob's BLT	1	795	54	21	–
Sandwich Chicken Salad	1	694	43	7	–
Sandwich Fish Market Haddock	1	570	25	4	–
Sandwich Fried Chicken	1	508	23	4	–
Sandwich Fried Chicken Club	1	994	70	26	–
Sandwich Grilled Cheese	1	391	17	7	–
Sandwich Grilled Chicken	1	447	18	3	–
Sandwich Grilled Chicken Club	1	993	70	29	–
Sandwich Pot Roast	1	728	35	15	–
Sandwich Turkey Bacon Melt	1	872	52	23	–
Seniors Chicken Parmesan	1 serv	522	26	9	0
Seniors Garden Vegetable Alfredo	1 serv	363	23	9	1
Seniors Garden Vegetable Alfredo Chicken	1 serv	452	26	10	1
Seniors Steak Tips & Noodles	1 serv	422	22	6	0
Seniors Stir-Fry Chicken	1 serv	368	13	2	0
Spaghetti & Marinara Sauce	1 serv	619	7	3	–
Spaghetti w/ Meatballs	1 serv	1087	45	17	–
Steak Monterey	1 serv	584	41	17	–
Steak Tips & Noodles	1 serv	985	37	10	–
Stir-Fry Grilled Chicken	1 serv	728	28	6	–
Stir-Fry Grilled Shrimp	1 serv	713	17	3	–
Stir-Fry Vegetable	1 serv	497	7	1	–
T-Bone Steak Plain	1 serv	1335	92	35	–
T-Bone Steak w/ Garlic Herb Butter	1 serv	1492	102	37	–
Turkey & Dressing	1 serv	542	24	7	–
SALAD DRESSINGS AND TOPPINGS					
Dressing Blue Cheese	1 serv (1.5 oz)	220	23	4	–

FOOD	PORTION	CALS	FAT	SAT FAT	TRANS FAT
Dressing Colonial	1 serv (1.5 oz)	232	21	3	–
Dressing French	1 serv (1.5 oz)	219	21	3	–
Dressing Honey Mustard	1 serv (1.5 oz)	192	18	3	–
Dressing Hot Bacon	1 serv (1.5 oz)	106	3	1	–
Dressing Lite Italian	1 serv (1.5 oz)	82	7	1	–
Dressing Oriental	1 serv (1.5 oz)	194	16	2	–
Dressing Ranch	1 serv (1.5 oz)	156	16	3	–
Dressing Ranch Lite	1 serv (1.5 oz)	103	10	2	–
Dressing Raspberry Vinaigrette	1 serv (1.5 oz)	155	13	2	–
Dressing Thousand Island	1 serv (1.5 oz)	212	20	3	–
Dressing Wildfire Ranch	1 serv (1.5 oz)	212	9	1	–
Gravy Chicken	1 serv (3 oz)	29	1	1	–
Gravy Country	1 serv (3 oz)	54	4	1	–
Gravy Sausage	1 serv (7 oz)	244	12	8	–
Syrup	1 serv (3 oz)	213	0	0	0
Syrup Sugar Free	1 serv (3 oz)	47	0	0	0
Topping Oregon Berry	1 serv (3 oz)	49	0	0	0
Topping Strawberry	1 serv (3 oz)	50	0	0	0
Whipped Topping	1 serv	69	5	5	–
SALADS					
Chicken Salad Plate	1 serv	789	46	7	–
Cobb Salad w/ Grilled Chicken	1 serv	778	54	22	–
Country Spinach w/ Grilled Chicken	1 serv	532	38	10	–
Frisco Salad w/ Fried Chicken	1 serv	672	40	14	–
Frisco Salad w/ Grilled Chicken	1 serv	599	40	14	–
Fruit & Yogurt	1 serv	414	2	1	–
Raspberry Grilled Chicken	1 serv	637	42	16	–
Speciality Side	1 serv	174	9	4	–
Wildfire Fried Chicken Salad	1 serv	806	31	9	–
Wildfire Grilled Chicken Salad	1 serv	733	30	9	–
SOUPS					
Bean	1 cup	144	3	1	0
Cheddar Baked Potato	1 cup	294	20	8	3
Sausage Chili	1 cup	268	17	6	0
Vegetable Beef	1 cup	135	5	2	0

BOJANGLES

FOOD	PORTION	CALS	FAT	SAT FAT	TRANS FAT
Biscuit	1	243	12	3	–
Biscuit Sandwich Bacon	1	290	17	5	–

FOOD	PORTION	CALS	FAT	SAT FAT	TRANS FAT
Biscuit Sandwich Bacon Egg Cheese	1	550	42	14	–
Biscuit Sandwich Cajun Filet	1	454	21	6	–
Biscuit Sandwich Country Ham	1	270	15	4	–
Biscuit Sandwich Egg	1	400	30	6	–
Biscuit Sandwich Sausage	1	350	23	7	–
Biscuit Sandwich Smoked Sausage	1	380	26	9	–
Biscuit Sandwich Steak	1	649	49	13	–
Botato Rounds	1 serv	235	11	4	–
Buffalo Bites	1 serv	180	5	2	–
Cajun Pintos	1 serv	110	0	0	0
Cajun Spiced Breast	1 serv	278	17	–	–
Cajun Spiced Leg	1 serv	264	16	–	–
Cajun Spiced Thigh	1 serv	310	23	–	–
Cajun Spiced Wing	1 serv	355	25	–	–
Chicken Supremes	1 serv	337	16	6	–
Corn On The Cob	1 serv	140	2	0	–
Dirty Rice	1 serv	166	6	2	–
Green Beans	1 serv	25	0	0	0
Macaroni & Cheese	1 serv	198	14	5	–
Marinated Cole Slaw	1 serv	136	3	0	–
Potatoes w/o Gravy	1 serv	80	1	0	–
Sandwich Cajun Filet w/o Mayo	1	337	11	5	–
Sandwich Cajun Filet w/ Mayo	1	437	22	7	–
Sandwich Grilled Filet w/ Mayo	1 serv	335	16	5	–
Sandwich Grilled Filet w/o Mayo	1	235	5	3	–
Seasoned Fries	1 serv	344	19	5	–
Southern Style Breast	1 serv	261	16	–	–
Southern Style Leg	1 serv	254	15	–	–
Southern Style Thigh	1 serv	308	21	–	–
Southern Style Wing	1 serv	337	21	–	–
Sweet Biscuit Bo Berry	1	320	18	4	–
Sweet Biscuit Cinnamon	1	320	18	4	–

BOSTON MARKET
DESSERTS

FOOD	PORTION	CALS	FAT	SAT FAT	TRANS FAT
Apple Pie	1 slice	420	20	4	5

FOOD	PORTION	CALS	FAT	SAT FAT	TRANS FAT
Brownie Chocolate Chip Fudge	1	580	23	5	0
Chocolate Cake	1 serv	600	32	7	5
Cookie Chocolate Chip	1	370	19	9	0
Cornbread	1 piece	180	5	2	2
MAIN MENU SELECTIONS					
Broccoli w/ Garlic Butter	1 serv	80	6	2	0
Butternut Squash	1 serv	140	5	3	0
Carver Boston Chicken	1	700	29	7	0
Carver Boston Meatloaf	1	940	45	18	0
Carver Boston Sirloin Dip	1	1000	51	15	2
Carver Boston Turkey	1	770	27	8	0
Carver Boston Turkey Dip	1	770	27	8	0
Carver Half Boston Chicken	1	340	15	4	0
Carver Half Boston Sirloin Dip	1	500	25	8	1
Carver Half Boston Turkey	1	390	14	4	0
Cinnamon Apples	1 serv	210	3	0	0
Cranberry Walnut Relish	1 serv	140	2	0	–
Creamed Spinach	1 serv	280	23	15	0
Dip Spinach Artichoke	1 serv	100	8	4	0
Family Meals Boneless Turkey Breast	1 serv (5 oz)	180	3	1	0
Family Meals Raosted Turkey	1 serv (5 oz)	180	3	1	0
Family Meals Rotisserie Chicken	1 serv (6 oz)	290	14	4	0
Family Meals Spiral Sliced Ham	1 serv (8 oz)	450	26	10	0
Family Meals Whole Turkey	1 serv (6.7 oz)	310	18	5	0
Fresh Vegetable Stuffing	1 serv	190	8	1	0
Garden Fresh Coleslaw	1 serv	170	9	2	0
Garlic Dill New Potatoes	1 serv	140	3	1	0
Green Bean Casserole	1 serv	60	2	1	0
Green Beans	1 serv	60	4	2	0
Individual Meal ¼ White Rotisserie Chicken	1 serv	290	11	4	0
Individual Meal Award Winning Roasted Sirloin	1 serv	290	15	6	1
Individual Meal Meatloaf	1	480	33	13	0
Individual Meals 1 Thigh & 1 Drumstick	1 serv	300	17	5	0

FOOD	PORTION	CALS	FAT	SAT FAT	TRANS FAT
Individual Meals ¼ White Rotisserie Chicken No Skin	1 serv	210	2	1	0
Individual Meals 3 Piece Dark	1 serv	380	19	6	0
Individual Meals 3 Piece Dark Skinless	1 serv	240	8	3	0
Individual Meals Roasted Turkey	1 serv	180	3	1	0
Macaroni & Cheese	1 serv	330	12	7	1
Mashed Potatoes	1 serv	210	9	6	0
Pot Pie Pastry Topped Chicken	1	780	47	17	7
Poultry Gravy	1 serv (4 oz)	15	1	0	0
Seasonal Fresh Fruit Salad	1 serv	60	0	0	0
Spinach w/ Garlic Butter Sauce	1 serv	130	9	6	0
Squash Casserole	1 serv	320	24	11	1
Steamed Fresh Vegetables	1 serv	60	2	0	0
Sweet Corn	1 serv	170	4	1	0
Sweet Potato Casserole	1 serv	460	17	6	0
SALADS					
Entree Caesar	1	500	45	11	0
Entree Caesar w/o Dressing	1 serv	140	8	5	0
Entree Market Chopped	1 serv	580	48	9	1
Entree Market Chopped w/o Dressing	1 serv	210	9	4	0
Side Caesar	1 serv	400	40	8	1
Side Caesar w/o Dressing	1 serv	40	2	2	0
Side Market Chopped	1 serv	440	43	7	1
Side Market Chopped w/o Dressing	1 serv	80	4	1	0
SOUPS					
Chicken Noodle	1 serv	170	5	2	0
Chicken Tortilla w/ Toppings	1 serv	340	22	7	0
Tortilla Soup w/o Toppings	1 serv	980	5	1	0

BOSTON PIZZA
CHILDREN'S MENU SELECTIONS

FOOD	PORTION	CALS	FAT	SAT FAT	TRANS FAT
Baked Salmon w/ Ceasar Salad	1 serv	330	14	–	–
Bugs 'N Cheese	1 serv	500	13	–	–
Chicken Fingers w/ Fries	1 serv	390	19	–	–
Pizza Pint Size	1	390	7	–	–

FOOD	PORTION	CALS	FAT	SAT FAT	TRANS FAT
Quesadilla Bacon Double Cheeseburger w/ Caesar Salad	1 serv	540	27	–	–
Reduced Size Fruit Cup	1 serv	80	0	0	0
Sandwich Grilled Chicken w/ Garden Greens	1 serv	600	38	–	–
Sandwich Grilled Chicken w/ Garden Greens	1 serv	780	52	–	–
Super Spaghetti	1 serv	440	13	–	–
Wrap Ham & Cheese w/ Fries	1 serv	550	28	–	–
DESSERTS					
Blondie Maple	1	850	43	–	–
Blondie Maple Bite Size	1	430	21	–	–
Brownie Chocolate Addiction	1	490	13	–	–
Brownie Chocolate Addiction Bite Size	1	200	7	–	–
Cheesecake New York	1 slice	620	33	–	–
Cheesecake Vanilla Bean	1 slice	770	52	–	–
Chocolate Explosion	1 serv	890	50	–	–
Tarte Au Sucre	1 serv	310	21	–	–
MAIN MENU SELECTIONS					
Angus Beef Sirloin Steak w/ Spaghetti	1 serv	1260	70	–	–
Baked 3 Cheese Penne	1 half order	460	14	–	–
Baked Seven Cheese Ravioli	1 half order	310	14	–	–
Baked Shrimp & Feta Penne	1 half order	480	19	–	–
Boston's Lasagne	1 half order	340	10	–	–
Boston's Smokey Mountain Spaghetti	1 order	1290	47	–	–
Chicken & Mushroom Fettuccini	1 half order	710	38	–	–
Chicken Parmesan w/ Seasonal Vegetables	1 serv	1060	74	–	–
Fries	1 serv	430	25	–	–
Garlic Mashed Potatoes	1 serv	730	60	–	–
Garlic Toast	1 slice	150	6	–	–
Homestyle Lasagna	1 order	590	33	–	–
Jambalaya Fettuccini	1 half order	860	51	–	–
Lemon Baked Salmon w/ Fries	1 serv	1150	74	–	–
Mama Meata Penne	1 half order	940	62	–	–

FOOD	PORTION	CALS	FAT	SAT FAT	TRANS FAT
Mushroom Chicken w/ Garlic Mashed Potatoes	1 serv	1030	62	–	–
Pad Thai w/ Chicken	1 serv	2110	47	–	–
Pad Thai w/ Shrimp	1 serv	2090	45	–	–
Pollo Pomodoro Spaghetti	1 serv	520	14	–	–
Salmon Filet Lemon Baked	1 serv	430	13	–	–
Scallop & Prawn Fettuccini	1 half order	710	41	–	–
Seasoned Vegetables	1 serv	70	0	–	0
Shrimp Skewers Lime & Parmesan	1 serv	190	7	–	–
Sicilan Penne	1 half order	720	48	–	–
Sirloin Steak w/ Prawns & Fries	1 serv	1480	104	–	–
Slow Roasted Pork Back Ribs w/ Fries	1 serv	1680	123	–	–
Spaghetti w/ Alfredo Sauce	1 half order	440	11	–	–
Spaghetti w/ Bolognese Sauce	1 half order	400	5	–	–
Spaghetti w/ Creamy Tomato Sauce	1 half order	410	11	–	–
Spaghetti w/ Pomodoro Sauce	1 half order	450	14	–	–
Spicy Italian Penne	1 half order	980	61	–	–
Starter Baked Raviolo Bites	1 serv	450	22	–	–
Starter Basket Garlic Twist	1 serv	1140	39	–	–
Starter Basket Three Cheese Toast	1 serv	730	34	–	–
Starter Boston's Poutine	1 serv	740	45	–	–
Starter Bruschetta Sun Dried Tomato	1 serv	470	21	–	–
Starter Cactus Cuts Potatoes & Dip	1 serv	1150	89	–	–
Starter Chicken Fingers	1 serv	360	14	–	–
Starter Chicken Fingers Buffalo Style	1 serv	370	14	–	–
Starter Cracked Pepper Dry Ribs	1 serv	380	41	–	–
Starter Nachos Cactus w/ Cactus Dip	1 serv	1830	128	–	–
Starter Nachos Spicy Chicken w/ Sour Cream & Salsa	1 serv	1430	72	–	–
Starter Nachos Taco Beef w/ Sour Cream & Salsa	1 serv	1560	86	–	–

FOOD	PORTION	CALS	FAT	SAT FAT	TRANS FAT
Starter Nachos w/ Sour Cream & Salsa	1 serv	1320	71	–	–
Starter Panzerotti Roll	1	820	32	–	–
Starter Pizza Bread Bandera w/ Santa Fe Ranch Dip	1 serv	960	54	–	–
Starter Pizza Bread w/o Sauce	1 serv	500	12	–	–
Starter Potato Skins	1 serv	650	46	–	–
Starter Quesadilla Southwest w/ Sour Cream & Salsa	1 serv	770	27	–	–
Starter Quesadilla Oven Roasted Chicken	1 serv	900	39	–	–
Starter Shrimp Stuffed Mushroom Caps	1 serv	490	41	–	–
Starter Team Platter w/ Dips & Sauces	1 serv	3030	205	–	–
Starter Thai Chicken Bites	1 serv	540	15	–	–
Starter Wings Breaded BBQ	1 serv	930	52	–	–
Starter Wings Breaded Honey Garlic	1 serv	940	52	–	–
Starter Wings Breaded Mild	1 serv	880	52	–	–
Starter Wings Breaded Teriyaki	1 serv	940	52	–	–
Starter Wings Breaded Thai	1 serv	1110	52	–	–
Starter Wings Oven Roasted BBQ	1 serv	670	42	–	–
Starter Wings Oven Roasted Honey Garlic	1 serv	700	42	–	–
Starter Wings Oven Roasted Hot	1 serv	620	42	–	–
Starter Wings Oven Roasted Teriyaki	1 serv	670	42	–	–
Starter Wings Oven Roasted Thai Chili	1 serv	770	40	–	–
The Ribber w/ Spaghetti	1 serv	970	43	–	–
Tortellini w/ Alfredo Sauce	1 half order	340	15	–	–
Tortellini w/ Bolognese Sauce	1 half order	300	9	–	–
Tortellini w/ Creamy Tomato Sauce	1 half order	310	14	–	–
Tortellini w/ Pomodoro Sauce	1 half order	340	18	–	–
Veal Parmesan w/ Spaghetti	1 serv	1020	72	–	–

FOOD	PORTION	CALS	FAT	SAT FAT	TRANS FAT
PIZZA					
Bacon Double Cheeseburger Individual	1 pie	1140	54	–	–
Bacon Double Cheeseburger Slice	1 med	280	12	–	–
BBQ Chicken Individual	1 pie	730	24	–	–
BBQ Chicken Slice	1 med	190	6	–	–
Boston Royal Individual	1 pie	840	27	–	–
Boston Royal Slice	1 med	210	6	–	–
Californian Slice	1 med	280	15	–	–
Clubhouse Individual	1 pie	1040	56	–	–
Deluxe Individual	1 pie	850	29	–	–
Deluxe Slice	1 med	220	7	–	–
Great White North Individual	1 pie	960	39	–	–
Great White North Slice	1 med	240	9	–	–
Hawaiian Individual	1 pie	780	20	–	–
Hawaiian Slice	1 med	210	5	–	–
Indy California	1 (11.3 oz)	440	12	–	–
La Quebecoise Individual	1 pie	770	27	–	–
La Quebecoise Slice	1 med	200	7	–	–
Meateor Individual	1 pie	950	37	–	–
Meateor Slice	1 med	260	10	–	–
Pepperoni Individual	1 pie	750	27	–	–
Pepperoni Slice	1 med	200	7	–	–
Pepperoni & Mushroom Individual	1 pie	750	27	–	–
Pepperoni & Mushroom Slice	1 med	200	7	–	–
Popeye Individual	1 pie	720	22	–	–
Popeye Slice	1 med	200	7	–	–
Rustic Italian Individual	1 pie	950	39	–	–
Rustic Italian Slice	1 med	260	10	–	–
Spicy Perogy Individual	1 pie	980	45	–	–
Spicy Perogy Slice	1 med	280	13	–	–
Szechuan Individual	1 pie	750	17	–	–
Szechuan Slice	1 med	200	4	–	–
Tandoori Individual	1 med	730	24	–	–
Tandoori Slice	1 med	200	6	–	–
Thai Chicken Individual	1 pie	840	28	–	–
Thai Chicken Slice	1 med	240	8	–	–
The Basic Individual	1 pie	620	16	–	–

FOOD	PORTION	CALS	FAT	SAT FAT	TRANS FAT
The Basic Slice	1 med	160	4	–	–
Tropical Chicken Individual	1 pie	970	39	–	–
Tropical Chicken Slice	1 med	260	10	–	–
Tuscan Individual	1 pie	940	37	–	–
Tuscan Slice	1 med	250	10	–	–
Ultimate Pepperoni Individual	1 pie	870	37	–	–
Ultimate Pepperoni Slice	1 med	230	9	–	–
Vegetarian Individual	1 pie	680	16	–	–
Vegetarian Slice	1 med	180	4	–	–
Zorba The Greek Individual	1 pie	800	29	–	–
Zorba The Greek Slice	1 med	210	8	–	–
SALAD DRESSINGS AND TOPPINGS					
House Dressing	1 serv (2 oz)	270	28	–	–
Ketchup	1 serv (2 oz)	60	1	–	–
Salsa	1 serv (2 oz)	20	1	–	–
Sour Cream	1 serv (2 oz)	100	9	–	–
SALADS					
Chipotle Chicken & Bacon	1 serv	630	41	–	–
Crispy Chicken Pecan	1 serv	1100	86	–	–
Entree Caesar	1 serv	500	38	–	–
Entree Spinach	1 serv	450	41	–	–
Garden Greens w/ House Dressing	1 serv	310	29	–	–
Garden Greens w/ Low Fat Raspberry Vinagrette	1 serv	130	6	–	–
Side Caesar	1 serv	170	11	–	–
Starter Spinach	1 serv	250	22	–	–
Taco Salad Beef w/o Sour Cream & Salsa	1 serv	610	33	–	–
Taco Salad Chicken w/o Sour Cream & Salsa	1 serv	480	19	–	–
Thai Chicken Salad	1 serv	1060	40	–	–
SANDWICHES					
Beef Dip w/ Fries & Au Jus	1 serv	1340	62	–	–
Boston Brute w/ Caesar Salad & Au Jus	1 serv	820	30	–	–
Boston Cheesesteak w/ Caesar Salad & Au Jus	1 serv	1300	66	–	–
Buffalo Chicken w/ Fries	1 serv	1220	53	–	–
Chicken Parmesan w/ Fries	1 serv	1370	81	–	–

FOOD	PORTION	CALS	FAT	SAT FAT	TRANS FAT
Ciabatta Chicken w/ Caesar Salad	1 serv	920	53	–	–
New York Steak w/ Garden Greens & Au Jus	1 serv	660	39	–	–
Stromboli Bacon Double Cheeseburger w/ Caesar Salad	1 serv	910	38	–	–
Stromboli Chicken Santa Fe w/ Caesar Salad	1 serv	750	22	–	–
Stromboli Smoked Ham & Chicken w/ Caesar Salad	1 serv	880	31	–	–
Wrap Thai Chicken	1	570	9	–	–
SOUPS					
Baked French Onion	1 serv	330	14	–	–
Clam Chowder	1 serv	260	14	–	–

BROWN'S CHICKEN & PASTA

FOOD	PORTION	CALS	FAT	SAT FAT	TRANS FAT
Breadsticks Garlic	1	50	1	–	–
Breast	3 oz	284	15	–	–
Cheezy Potatoes	1 serv (12 oz)	188	11	6	–
Coleslaw	3 oz	131	10	–	–
Corn Fritters	3 oz	415	25	–	–
Corn On Cob	1 ear (3 inch)	126	3	–	–
French Fries	3 oz	503	22	–	–
Gizzard	3 oz	387	20	–	–
Leg	3 oz	287	16	–	–
Liver	3 oz	341	19	–	–
Mostaccioli w/ Meat Sauce	1 serv (12 oz)	835	14	2	–
Mostaccioli w/ Meatless Sauce	1 serv (12 oz)	792	10	2	–
Mushrooms	3 oz	289	16	–	–
Potato Salad	3 oz	94	4	–	–
Ravioli w/ Meat Sauce	1 serv (12 oz)	865	20	–	–
Ravioli w/ Meatless Sauce	1 serv (12 oz)	822	16	–	–
Shrimp	3 oz	277	10	–	–
Spaghetti w/ Meat Sauce	1 serv (12 oz)	835	14	2	–
Spaghetti w/ Meatless Sauce	1 serv (12 oz)	792	10	2	–
Thigh	3 oz	355	24	–	–
Wing	3 oz	385	25	–	–

BRUEGGER'S BAGELS
BAGELS

FOOD	PORTION	CALS	FAT	SAT FAT	TRANS FAT
Asiago Parmesan	1	330	4	2	0

FOOD	PORTION	CALS	FAT	SAT FAT	TRANS FAT
Baked Apple	1	370	3	0	–
BAGELS					
Blueberry	1	330	2	0	0
Chocolate Chip	1	350	5	2	0
Cinnamon Sugar	1	330	2	0	0
Cranberry Orange	1	330	2	0	0
Everything	1	320	2	0	0
Garlic	1	320	2	0	0
Honey Grain	1	330	3	0	0
Jalapeno	1	320	2	0	0
Multi-Grain	1	350	4	0	0
Onion	1	320	2	0	0
Plain	1	320	2	0	0
Poppy	1	320	3	0	0
Pumpernickel	1	330	3	0	0
Pumpkin	1	330	2	0	–
Rosemary Olive Oil	1	350	7	1	0
Salt	1	320	2	0	0
Sesame	1	360	3	0	0
Sourdough	1	340	2	0	0
Square Asiago Parmesan	1	360	5	2	0
Square Everything	1	320	2	0	0
Square Plain	1	350	3	0	0
Square Sesame	1	360	3	0	0
Sun Dried Tomato	1	320	2	0	0
Whole Wheat	1	390	6	1	0
DESSERTS					
Brownie Chocolate Chunk	1	330	18	7	0
Cake Lemon Pound	1 slice	320	13	7	0
Cookie Chocolate Chip	1	500	22	12	0
Cookie Oatmeal Raisin	1	460	19	9	0
Cookie Peanut Butter	1	480	23	9	0
Cookie Triple Chocolate Chunk	1	560	28	16	0
Cookie White Chocolate Macadamia	1	580	31	16	0
Luscious Lemon Bar	1	300	16	9	0
Marshmallow Chew	1	280	6	3	0
Muffin Blueberry	1	450	19	4	0
Muffin Chocolate	1	460	24	6	0
Oreo Dream Bar	1	470	28	14	0

FOOD	PORTION	CALS	FAT	SAT FAT	TRANS FAT
Pecan Chocolate Chunk	1 slice	310	19	6	0
Raspberry Sammies	1 slice	340	16	10	0
Seven Layer Bar	1	650	43	23	0
Toffee Almond Bar	1	400	19	8	0
SALADS					
Caesar w/ Dressing	1 serv	270	17	5	0
Tossed Chicken Caesar w/ Dressing	1 serv	370	20	5	0
Tossed Mandarin Medley	1 serv	340	17	5	0
Tossed Sesame Chicken	1 serv	480	28	3	0
SANDWICHES					
BLT w/ Mayo	1	570	23	5	0
Chicken Breast	1	660	11	3	0
Chicken Fajita	1	530	11	5	0
Chicken Salad w/ Mayo	1	630	26	4	0
Cranberry Gobbler	1	620	21	6	0
Cuban Chicken	1	680	25	7	0
Denver Egg	1	460	18	6	0
Egg Cheese	1	420	18	6	0
Egg Cheese Sausage	1	640	38	13	0
Egg Cheese Bacon	1	460	23	8	0
Egg Cheese Ham	1	460	18	6	0
Ham	1	460	7	1	0
Herby Turkey	1	560	14	7	0
Leonardo Da Veggie	1	480	12	6	0
Radishy Roast Beef	1	560	18	6	0
Roadhouse Chicken	1	710	19	8	0
Roast Beef	1	730	36	5	0
Santa Fe Turkey	1	490	9	4	0
Smoked Salmon	1	490	10	5	0
Softwich BLT w/ Mayo	1	600	25	6	0
Softwich Chicken Breast	1	630	11	3	0
Softwich Chicken Fajita	1	570	10	4	0
Softwich Chicken Salad	1	670	27	4	0
Softwich Cranberry Gobbler	1	730	28	10	0
Softwich Cuban Chicken	1	810	32	10	0
Softwich Garden Veggie	1	380	3	0	0
Softwich Ham	1	510	6	2	0
Softwich Herby Turkey	1	580	14	7	0
Softwich Hummus	1	540	13	2	0

FOOD	PORTION	CALS	FAT	SAT FAT	TRANS FAT
Softwich Leonardo Da Veggie	1	550	15	8	0
Softwich Mediterranean	1	790	33	15	0
Softwich Peanut Chicken	1	590	12	3	0
Softwich Radishy Roast Beef	1	670	26	10	0
Softwich Roadhouse Chicken	1	670	19	8	0
Softwich Roast Beef	1	750	40	6	0
Softwich Roasted Turkey	1	550	15	2	0
Softwich Smoked Salmon	1	520	11	5	0
Softwich Supreme Club w/o Mayo	1	880	39	14	0
Softwich Tuna Salad	1	720	34	5	0
Softwich Western Wheat	1	820	58	13	0
Supreme Club w/o Mayo	1	470	9	2	0
Tuna Salad	1	620	27	4	0
Turkey	1	510	14	2	0
Wrap Classic w/ Bacon	1	520	45	15	0
Wrap Classic w/ Ham	1	510	41	14	0
Wrap Classic w/ Sausage	1	660	60	21	1
Wrap Rio Grande Bacon	1	560	49	16	0
Wrap Rio Grande Ham	1	630	34	10	0
Wrap Rio Grande Sausage	1	510	47	15	0
Wrap Sesame Chicken Salad	1	770	36	5	0
Wrap Tossed Chicken Caesar	1	660	28	7	0
Wrap Tossed Mandarin Medley Salad	1	630	25	7	0
SOUPS					
Chicken Pot Pie	1 cup	250	19	10	0
Chicken Spaeztle	1 cup	120	5	2	0
Chicken Wild Rice	1 cup	260	19	11	0
Creamy Tomato	1 cup	150	9	4	0
Hearty Mushroom Barley	1 cup	110	2	0	0
Italian Wedding	1 cup	160	8	4	0
Minestrone	1 cup	120	2	1	0
Moroccan Stew	1 cup	140	3	0	0
New England Clam	1 cup	300	18	8	0
Sweet Potato Cheddar	1 cup	200	11	5	0
TOPPINGS					
Cream Cheese Bacon Scallion	1 scoop (1.5 oz)	140	12	7	0
Cream Cheese Cucumber Dill	1 scoop (1.5 oz)	140	13	6	0
Cream Cheese Garden Veggie	1 scoop (1.5 oz)	130	11	6	0

FOOD	PORTION	CALS	FAT	SAT FAT	TRANS FAT
Cream Cheese Honey Walnut	1 scoop (1.5 oz)	150	12	6	0
Cream Cheese Jalapeno	1 scoop (1.5 oz)	140	13	8	0
Cream Cheese Light Garden Veggie	1 scoop (1.5 oz)	90	6	4	0
Cream Cheese Light Herb Garlic	1 scoop (1.5 oz)	100	6	4	0
Cream Cheese Light Plain	1 scoop (1.5 oz)	100	6	3	0
Cream Cheese Olive Pimento	1 scoop (1.5 oz)	140	13	6	0
Cream Cheese Onion & Chive	1 scoop (1.5 oz)	140	13	8	0
Cream Cheese Plain	1 scoop (1.5 oz)	130	11	7	0
Cream Cheese Pumpkin	1 scoop (1.5 oz)	120	11	7	0
Cream Cheese Strawberry	1 scoop (1.5 oz)	140	13	7	0
Cream Cheese Wildberry	1 scoop (1.5 oz)	140	12	7	0
Hummus	1 scoop (2 oz)	110	6	1	0

BURGER KING
BEVERAGES

FOOD	PORTION	CALS	FAT	SAT FAT	TRANS FAT
Apple Juice	1 (6.67 oz)	90	0	0	0
BK Joe Regular	1 sm	5	0	0	0
BK Joe Turbo	1 sm (12 oz)	10	0	0	0
Chocolate Milk 1% Low Fat	1 (9 oz)	180	3	2	0
Coke Classic	1 sm (16 oz)	140	0	0	0
Diet Coke	1 sm (16 oz)	0	0	0	0
Dr Pepper	1 sm (16 oz)	140	0	0	0
Iced Coffee Mocha BK Joe	1 (16 oz)	380	10	6	0
Icee Coca-Cola	1 sm (16 oz)	110	0	0	0
Icee Minute Maid Cherry	1 sm (16 oz)	110	0	0	0
Milk 1% Low Fat	1	110	3	2	0
Minute Maid Orange Juice	8 oz	140	0	0	0
Shake Chocolate	1 sm (16 oz)	470	14	9	0
Shake Oreo Sundae Chocolate	1 sm (16 oz)	680	24	15	1
Shake Oreo Sundae Strawberry	1 sm (16 oz)	660	23	15	1
Shake Oreo Sundae Vanilla	1 sm (16 oz)	610	24	16	1
Shake Strawberry	1 sm (16 oz)	460	14	9	0
Shake Vanilla	1 sm (16 oz)	400	15	9	0
Sprite	1 sm (16 oz)	140	0	0	0
Water Nestle Pure Life	1 bottle (16 oz)	0	0	0	0

BREAKFAST SELECTIONS

FOOD	PORTION	CALS	FAT	SAT FAT	TRANS FAT
Biscuit Bacon Egg & Cheese	1	410	25	8	5
Biscuit Ham Egg & Cheese	1	390	22	7	5

FOOD	PORTION	CALS	FAT	SAT FAT	TRANS FAT
Biscuit Sausage	1	390	26	8	5
Biscuit Sausage Egg & Cheese	1	530	37	12	6
Croissan'wich Bacon Egg & Cheese	1	340	20	7	2
Croissan'wich Double w/ Bacon Egg & Cheese	1	430	27	10	2
Croissan'wich Double w/ Sausage Bacon Egg & Cheese	1	550	39	14	3
Croissan'wich Double w/ Sausage Egg & Cheese	1	680	51	18	3
Croissan'wich Double w/ Ham Bacon Egg & Cheese	1	420	24	9	2
Croissan'wich Double w/ Ham Egg & Cheese	1	420	23	9	2
Croissan'wich Double w/ Ham Sausage Egg & Cheese	1	550	37	14	0
Croissan'wich Egg & Cheese	1	300	17	6	2
Croissan'wich Ham Egg & Cheese	1	340	18	6	2
Croissan'wich Sausage & Cheese	1	370	25	9	2
Croissan'wich Sausage Egg & Cheese	1	470	32	11	3
French Toast Sticks	3 pieces	240	13	3	2
Hash Browns	1 lg	620	40	11	13
Hash Browns	1 sm	260	17	5	5
Omelet Sandwich Enormous	1	730	45	16	1
Omelet Sandwich Ham	1	290	13	5	0
DESSERTS					
Cini-minis	1 serv	390	18	5	4
Dutch Apple Pie	1 serv	300	13	3	3
Hershey Sundae Pie	1	310	19	12	0
MAIN MENU SELECTIONS					
BK Chicken Fries	6 pieces	260	15	4	3
BK Stacker Double	1	610	39	16	2
BK Stacker Quad	1	1000	68	30	3
BK Stacker Triple	1	800	54	23	2
BK Veggie Burger	1	420	16	3	0

FOOD	PORTION	CALS	FAT	SAT FAT	TRANS FAT
Cheeseburger	1	330	16	7	1
Cheeseburger Double	1	500	29	14	2
Chicken Sandwich Original	1	660	40	8	3
Chicken Sandwich Tendercrisp	1	790	44	8	4
Chicken Sandwich Tendergrill	1	510	19	4	1
Chicken Tenders	5 pieces	210	12	3	2
Chick'n Crisp Spicy Sandwich	1	480	31	5	2
Double Cheeseburger	1	410	21	9	1
French Fries No Salt Added	1 sm	230	13	3	3
French Fries No Salt Added	1 lg	500	28	6	6
French Fries Salted	1 sm	230	13	3	3
French Fries Salted	1 lg	500	28	6	6
Hamburger	1	290	12	5	0
Onion Rings	1 sm	140	7	2	1
Onion Rings	1 lg	440	22	5	4
Sandwich BK Big Fish	1	640	32	6	3
The Angus Steak Burger	1	640	33	10	2
Whopper	1	670	39	11	2
Whopper Double	1	900	57	19	2
Whopper Double w/ Cheese	1	990	64	25	3
Whopper Jr.	1	370	21	6	1
Whopper Jr. w/ Cheese	1	410	24	8	1
Whopper Triple	1	1130	74	27	3
Whopper Triple w/ Cheese	1	1230	82	32	4
Whopper w/ Cheese	1	760	47	16	2
SALAD DRESSINGS & TOPPINGS					
Breakfast Syrup	1 serv (1 oz)	80	0	0	0
Croutons Garlic Parmesan	1 serv	60	2	0	0
Dipping Sauce Barbecue	1 serv (1 oz)	40	0	0	0
Dipping Sauce Honey Mustard	1 serv (1 oz)	90	6	1	0
Dipping Sauce Ranch	1 serv (1 oz)	140	15	3	0
Dipping Sauce Sweet & Sour	1 serv (1 oz)	40	0	0	0
Dressing Ken's Creamy Caesar	1 serv (2 oz)	210	21	4	0
Dressing Ken's Fat Free Ranch	1 serv (2 oz)	60	0	0	0
Dressing Ken's Honey Mustard	1 serv (2 oz)	270	23	3	0
Dressing Ken's Ranch	1 serv (2 oz)	190	20	3	0
Jam Grape	1 serv	30	0	0	0
Jam Strawberry	1 serv	30	0	0	0
Ketchup	1 pkg	10	0	0	0
Mayonnaise	1 pkg	80	9	1	0

FOOD	PORTION	CALS	FAT	SAT FAT	TRANS FAT
SALADS					
Chicken Garden Tendercrisp	1	410	22	6	4
Chicken Garden Tendergrill w/o Dressing or Croutons	1	240	9	4	0
Side Garden w/o Dressing	1	15	0	0	0
BURGERVILLE					
BEVERAGES					
Milkshake Black Forest	1 (16 oz)	600	20	–	–
Milkshake Blackberry	1 (16 oz)	610	25	–	–
Milkshake Caramel Apple	1 (16 oz)	540	26	–	–
Milkshake Chocolate	1 (16 oz)	520	23	–	–
Milkshake Fresh Strawberry	1 (16 oz)	560	21	–	–
Milkshake Mocha Perk	1 (16 oz)	590	25	–	–
Milkshake Pumpkin	1 (16 oz)	460	22	–	–
Milkshake Vanilla	1 (16 oz)	500	20	–	–
Smoothies Chocolate Monkey	1 (16 oz)	470	1	–	–
Smoothies Fresh Blackberry	1 (16 oz)	420	0	0	0
Smoothies Fresh Raspberry	1 (16 oz)	470	0	0	0
Smoothies Fresh Strawberry	1 (16 oz)	390	0	0	0
Smoothies Strawberry Splash	1 (16 oz)	310	1	–	–
Smoothies Triple Berry Blast	1 (16 oz)	360	0	0	0
BREAKFAST SELECTIONS					
American Cheese	2 slices	90	7	–	–
Bagel Bacon Egg	1	450	11	–	–
Bagel Cheese	1	290	6	–	–
Bagel Ham Egg	1	450	8	–	–
Bagel Plain	1	310	1	–	–
Bagel Sausage Egg	1	640	29	–	–
Biscuit Bacon Egg	1	400	23	–	–
Biscuit Ham Egg	1	400	20	–	–
Biscuit Sausage Egg	1	590	41	–	–
Tillamook Cheese	1 slice	120	10	–	–
MAIN MENU SELECTIONS					
Cheeseburger	1	370	20	–	–
Cheeseburger Double Beef	1	470	27	–	–
Cheeseburger Pepper Bacon	1	680	45	–	–
Cheeseburger Tillamook	1	630	40	–	–
Cheeseburger Walla Walla Onion	1	679	44	–	–

FOOD	PORTION	CALS	FAT	SAT FAT	TRANS FAT
Chicken Strips	5 pieces	550	30	–	–
Colossal	1	530	30	–	–
French Fries	1 kid size	220	12	–	–
French Fries	1 reg	390	22	–	–
Gardenburger	1	460	19	–	–
Gardenburger Spicy Black Bean	1	550	32	–	–
Halibut	3 pieces	230	14	–	–
Hamburger	1	320	16	–	–
Onion Rings Walla Walla	3 pieces	485	29	–	–
Roasted Turkey Salad w/o Hazelnuts	1 serv	375	19	–	–
Rogue River Blue Cheese Bacon Burger	1	510	56	–	–
Sandwich Crispy Chicken	1	450	18	–	–
Sandwich Deluxe Crispy Chicken	1	610	30	–	–
Sandwich Grilled Chicken	1	350	3	–	–
Sandwich Halibut	1	490	30	–	–
Sandwich Turkey Club	1	490	32	–	–
Side Salad w/o Dressing	1 serv	70	4	–	–
Smoked Salmon Salad w/o Hazelnuts	1 serv	370	18	–	–
Sweet Potato Fries	1 serv	530	29	–	–
Turkey Burger	1	470	21	–	–

CAPTAIN D'S SEAFOOD

FOOD	PORTION	CALS	FAT	SAT FAT	TRANS FAT
Baked Chicken Dinner	1 serv	350	5	1	–
Baked Fish Dinner	1 serv	390	5	0	–
Baked Potato	1 serv	190	0	0	0
Baked Salmon Dinner	1 serv	470	8	0	–
Carb Counter Chicken Dinner	1 serv	320	15	3	–
Carb Counter Fish Dinner	1 serv	350	15	3	–
Cole Slaw	1 serv	150	6	2	–
Corn On The Cob	1 serv	150	3	0	–
Fresh Steamed Broccoli	1 serv	25	1	0	–
Green Beans	1 serv	90	3	1	–
Rice Pilaf	1 serv	160	1	0	–
Shrimp Scampi Dinner	1 serv	370	5	1	–

FOOD	PORTION	CALS	FAT	SAT FAT	TRANS FAT
Side Salad w/o Dressing	1	30	1	0	–
Tuscan Style Vegetables	1 serv	30	0	0	0

CARIBOU COFFEE

FOOD	PORTION	CALS	FAT	SAT FAT	TRANS FAT
Black Forest Mocha	1 med	553	19	–	–
Black Forest Wild Drink	1 med	553	19	–	–
Cappuccino	1 med (16 oz)	113	1	–	–
Cappuccino 2%	1 med (16 oz)	162	7	–	–
Caramel High Rise	1 med (16 oz)	414	13	–	–
Chai Latte 2%	1 med (16 oz)	286	5	–	–
Cooler Caramel	1 med (12 oz)	450	10	–	–
Cooler Chocolate	1 med (12 oz)	257	3	–	–
Cooler Coffee	1 med (16 oz)	230	3	–	–
Cooler Espresso	1 med (16 oz)	193	2	–	–
Cooler Mint Oreo	1 med (12 oz)	614	19	–	–
Cooler Vanilla	1 med (16 oz)	257	4	–	–
Glacier Gum	2 pieces	5	0	0	0
Hot Apple Blast	1 med	379	8	–	–
Latte 2%	1 med (16 oz)	171	6	–	–
Latte Skim	1 med (16 oz)	121	1	–	–
Latte Skinny Bou Low Cal	1 med	120	1	–	–
Lite White Berry	1 med (16 oz)	311	5	–	–
Mint Condition	1 med (16 oz)	520	19	–	–
Mints All Flavors	3 pieces	5	0	0	0
Mocha 2%	1 med (16 oz)	347	16	–	–
Mocha Skim	1 med (16 oz)	302	12	–	–
Mocha Turtle	1 med (16 oz)	559	19	–	–
Smoothie Passion Green Tea	1 med (16 oz)	252	tr	–	–
Smoothie Raspberry	1 med (12 oz)	293	tr	–	–
Smoothie Strawberry Banana	1 med (16 oz)	253	tr	–	–
Smoothie Wild Berry	1 med (16 oz)	235	tr	–	–

CARL'S JR.
BAKED SELECTIONS

FOOD	PORTION	CALS	FAT	SAT FAT	TRANS FAT
Cheese Danish	1	400	23	6	–
Cheesecake Strawberry Swirl	1 serv	290	17	9	–
Chocolate Cake	1 serv	300	12	3	–
Chocolate Chip Cookie	1	350	18	7	–
Muffin Blueberry	1	340	14	2	–
Muffin Bran Raisin	1	370	13	2	–

FOOD	PORTION	CALS	FAT	SAT FAT	TRANS FAT
BEVERAGES					
Coca-Cola Classic	1 reg (21 oz)	220	0	0	0
Coffee	1 reg (12 oz)	2	tr	0	–
Diet Coke	1 reg (21 oz)	tr	0	0	0
Dr Pepper	1 reg (21 oz)	200	0	0	0
Hot Chocolate	1 serv (12 oz)	120	2	2	–
Iced Tea	1 reg (12 oz)	5	0	0	0
Lemonade Minute Maid	1 reg (21 oz)	200	0	0	0
Milk 1%	1 (10 fl oz)	150	3	2	–
Minute Maid Orange Soda	1 reg (21 oz)	200	0	0	0
Nestea Raspberry	1 reg (21 oz)	160	0	0	0
Orange Juice	1 (10 oz)	150	0	0	0
Ramblin' Root Beer	1 reg (21 oz)	220	0	0	0
Shake Chocolate	1 reg (32 oz)	770	15	10	–
Shake Strawberry	1 reg (32 oz)	750	15	10	–
Shake Vanilla	1 reg (32 oz)	700	16	11	–
Sprite	1 reg (21 oz)	200	0	0	0
BREAKFAST SELECTIONS					
Bacon	2 strips	45	4	2	–
Breakfast Burrito	1	560	32	11	–
Breakfast Quesadilla	1	370	17	5	–
English Muffin w/ Margarine	1	210	9	2	–
French Toast Dips w/o Syrup	1 serv	370	20	3	–
Grape Jelly	1 serv (0.5 oz)	40	0	0	0
Hash Brown Nuggets	1 serv	330	21	5	–
Sausage	1 patty	190	18	6	–
Scrambled Eggs	1 serv	180	14	3	–
Sourdough Breakfast	1 serv	410	20	10	–
Strawberry Jam	1 serv (0.5 oz)	40	0	0	0
Sunrise Sandwich w/o Meat	1	360	21	8	–
Table Syrup	1 serv (1 oz)	90	0	0	0
MAIN MENU SELECTIONS					
American Cheese	1 sm	50	4	3	–
BBQ Sauce	1 serv (1.1 oz)	50	0	0	0
Breadstick	1 (0.3 oz)	35	1	0	–
Carl's Famous Star	1	590	32	9	–
Chicken Stars	6 pieces	260	16	5	–
CrissCut Fries	1 serv	410	24	5	–
Croutons	1 serv (0.5 oz)	30	1	0	–

FOOD	PORTION	CALS	FAT	SAT FAT	TRANS FAT
Double Sourdough Bacon Cheeseburger	1	880	59	24	–
Double Western Bacon Cheeseburger	1	920	50	21	–
Famous Bacon Cheeseburger	1	700	41	13	–
French Fries	1 kid size	250	12	3	–
French Fries	1 med	460	22	5	–
Hamburger	1	280	9	4	–
Honey Sauce	1 serv (1 oz)	90	0	0	0
Mustard Sauce	1 serv (1 oz)	50	0	0	0
Onion Rings	1 serv	430	22	5	–
Potato Bacon & Cheese	1	640	29	9	–
Potato Broccoli & Cheese	1 serv	530	21	5	–
Potato Plain w/o Margarine	1	290	0	0	0
Potato Sour Cream & Chives	1	430	14	4	–
Salsa	1 serv (0.9 oz)	10	0	0	0
Sandwich Bacon Swiss Crispy Chicken	1	760	38	11	–
Sandwich Carl's Catch Fish	1	530	28	7	–
Sandwich Charbroiled Sirloin Steak	1	550	24	5	–
Sandwich Chargrilled BBQ Chicken	1	290	4	1	–
Sandwich Chargrilled Chicken Club	1	470	23	7	–
Sandwich Chargrilled Santa Fe Chicken	1	540	31	8	–
Sandwich Ranch Crispy Chicken	1	660	31	7	–
Sandwich Southwest Spicy Chicken	1	620	41	10	–
Sandwich Spicy Chicken	1	480	26	5	–
Sandwich Western Bacon Crispy Chicken	1	750	28	11	–
Sourdough Bacon Cheeseburger	1	640	41	15	–
Sourdough Ranch Bacon Cheeseburger	1	720	46	16	–
Super Star	1	790	47	15	–
Sweet N' Sour Sauce	1 serv (1 oz)	50	0	0	0

FOOD	PORTION	CALS	FAT	SAT FAT	TRANS FAT
Swiss Cheese	1 serv	50	4	3	–
Western Bacon Cheeseburger	1	660	30	12	–
Zucchini	1 serv	320	19	5	–
SALAD DRESSINGS					
1000 Island	1 serv (2 oz)	230	23	4	–
Blue Cheese	1 serv (2 oz)	320	35	7	–
French Fat Free	1 serv (2 oz)	60	0	0	0
House	1 serv (2 oz)	220	22	4	–
Italian Fat Free	1 serv (2 oz)	15	0	0	0
SALADS					
Salad-To-Go Charbroiled Chicken	1 serv	200	7	3	–
Salad-To-Go Garden	1	50	3	2	–
CARVEL					
Cake 6 Inch	1 piece (3 oz)	210	11	8	0
Cone Cake Chocolate	1 sm	260	13	8	0
Cone Cake Chocolate	1 lg	600	30	18	0
Cone Cake Vanilla	1 sm	280	16	10	0
Cone Cake Vanilla	1 lg	650	36	24	0
Cone Sugar Chocolate	1 sm	300	13	35	0
Cone Sugar Vanilla	1 sm	320	15	10	0
Cone Waffle Chocolate	1 sm	330	13	35	0
Cone Waffle Chocolate	1 lg	660	30	18	0
Cone Waffle Vanilla	1 sm	350	16	11	0
Cone Waffle Vanilla	1 lg	710	36	25	0
Flying Saucer 98% Fat Free Chocolate	1	180	3	1	0
Flying Saucers 98% Fat Free Vanilla	1	180	3	0	0
Thinny Thin Classic Sundae No Fat Strawberry	1 reg	320	0	0	0
Thinny Thin Classic Sundae No Fat Fudge	1 reg	380	2	0	0
Thinny Thin Minature Sundae No Fat	1	190	0	0	0
Thinny Thin Minature Sundae No Sugar Added	1	200	3	2	0
Thinny Thin No Fat Carvelanche Strawberry	1 (16 oz)	430	0	0	0

FOOD	PORTION	CALS	FAT	SAT FAT	TRANS FAT
Thinny Thin No Fat Chocolate	1 sm	160	0	0	0
Thinny Thin No Fat Vanilla	1 sm	160	0	0	0
Thinny Thin No Sugar Added Vanilla	1 sm	180	3	0	0
Thinny Thin Parfait No Fat	1	190	0	0	0
Thinny Thin Shake No Fat Chocolate	1 (16 oz)	440	0	0	0
Thinny Thin Shake No Fat Mocha	1 (16 oz)	440	0	0	0
Thinny Thin Shake No Fat Vanilla	1 (16 oz)	300	0	0	0

CHEVYS

FOOD	PORTION	CALS	FAT	SAT FAT	TRANS FAT
Black Beans	1 serv	59	0	–	0
Catch Of The Day w/ San Antonio Vegetables Salsa & Tamalito	1 serv	428	16	–	–
Chicken Fajitas w/ San Antonio Vegetables & Tamalito	1 serv	285	6	–	–
Fish Tacos w/ Taco Dressing Lettuce & Pico De Gallo	1 serv	483	18	–	–
Grilled Chicken Salad w/ Salsa Vinaigrette	1 serv	533	18	–	–
Guacamole	1 serv (2 oz)	103	10	–	–
Mexican Rice	1 serv	211	3	–	–
Mixed Green Salad w/ Salsa Vinaigrette	1 serv	358	16	–	–
Salsa	1 serv (5 oz)	40	0	0	0
Shrimp Fajitas w/ San Antonio Vegetables & Tamalito	1 serv	286	7	–	–
Sour Cream	1 serv	121	12	–	–
Tortilla Corn	1	80	1	–	–
Tortilla El Machino	1	167	4	–	–
Veggie Burrito w/ San Antonio Vegetables Pico De Gallo & Ranchero Sauce	1 serv	430	19	–	–
Veggie Fajitas w/ San Antonio Vegetables & Tamalito	1 serv	345	28	–	–

FOOD	PORTION	CALS	FAT	SAT FAT	TRANS FAT
CHICKEN OUT ROTISSERIE					
MAIN MENU SELECTIONS					
Apple Cornbread Stuffing	1 serv (6 oz)	215	2	–	–
Baked Potato Wedges	1 serv (6 oz)	110	tr	–	–
Biscuit	1	150	4	–	–
Chicken Breast Skinless	1 serv (6 oz)	210	4	–	–
Chicken Burger w/o Cheese	1	285	7	–	–
Chunky Cinnamon Applesauce	1 serv (6 oz)	60	0	–	0
Creamed Spinach w/ Artichokes	1 serv (6 oz)	160	6	–	–
Farm Fresh Cole Slaw	1 serv (6 oz)	55	0	–	0
French Baguette	1	80	1	–	–
Fresh Fruit Salad	1 serv (6 oz)	77	tr	–	–
Mandarin Walnut Cranberry Relish	1 serv (6 oz)	240	1	–	–
Mashed Sweet Potatoes	1 serv (6 oz)	120	tr	–	–
Oriental Green Beans	1 serv (6 oz)	34	0	–	0
Pulled White Meat	1 serv (6 oz)	180	4	–	–
Real Cheese & Macaroni	1 serv (6 oz)	311	12	–	–
Red Skin Mashed Potatoes	1 serv (6 oz)	181	6	–	–
Rice Pilaf	1 serv (6 oz)	140	1	–	–
Roasted Peas Corn & Carrots	1 serv (6 oz)	120	tr	–	–
Rotisserie Chicken Quarter Dark No Skin	1 serv	232	6	–	–
Rotisserie Chicken Quarter White No Skin	1 serv	196	4	–	–
Sandwich BBQ Pulled Chicken	1	406	8	–	–
Sandwich Grilled Chicken Breast	1	350	6	–	–
Sandwich Open Faced Pulled Chicken	1	682	18	–	–
Sandwich Pulled Chicken	1	320	6	–	–
Sandwich Signature Chicken Salad	1	370	5	–	–
Steamed Broccoli & Carrots	1 serv (6 oz)	30	0	–	0
Vegetarian Baked Beans	1 serv (6 oz)	150	1	–	–
Wrap Chinese Chicken Salad w/o Dressing	1	330	9	–	–
Wrap Fajita	1	360	10	–	–

FOOD	PORTION	CALS	FAT	SAT FAT	TRANS FAT
Wrap Fresh Vegetable Salad w/o Dressing	1	170	4	–	–
Wrap Grilled Chicken Caesar	1	355	11	–	–
Wrap Pesto Chicken	1	405	11	–	–
Wrap Pulled Chicken	1	300	7	–	–
Wrap Skinless Grilled Chicken	1	330	7	–	–
SALAD DRESSINGS					
Balsamic Vinaigrette	1 oz	18	0	–	0
Caesar	1 oz	55	5	–	–
Chinese	1 oz	72	7	–	–
Low Fat Honey Mustard	1 oz	23	1	–	–
Ranch	1 oz	90	6	–	–
Southwestern	1 oz	85	7	–	–
SALADS					
Caesar w/ Grilled Chicken w/o Dressing	½ serv	235	8	–	–
Caesar w/o Dressing	½ serv	140	4	–	–
Chicken Salad Apricot	1 serv (6 oz)	300	8	–	–
Chicken Salad BBQ Pulled	1 serv (6 oz)	263	5	–	–
Chicken Salad Chinese w/o Dressing	½ serv	210	6	–	–
Chicken Salad Pesto	1 serv (6 oz)	285	8	–	–
Chicken Salad Pulled w/o Dressing	½ serv	204	4	–	–
Chicken Salad Santa Fe w/o Dressing	½ serv	240	7	–	–
Chicken Salad Signature	1 serv (6 oz)	230	5	–	–
Garden w/ Grilled Chicken w/o Dressing	½ serv	200	4	–	–
Garden w/o Dressing	½ serv	25	1	–	–
Young Spinach w/ Grilled Chicken w/o Dressing	½ serv	270	4	–	–
Young Spinach w/o Dressing	½ serv	180	2	–	–
SOUPS					
Chicken Noodle	1 serv (6 oz)	130	3	–	–
Vegetable Minestrone	1 serv (6 oz)	96	2	–	–

CHICK-FIL-A

BEVERAGES

Coca-Cola Classic	1 sm	110	0	0	0

FOOD	PORTION	CALS	FAT	SAT FAT	TRANS FAT
Diet Coke	1 sm	0	0	0	0
Diet Lemonade	1 sm	25	0	0	0
Ice Tea Sweetened	1 sm	80	0	0	0
Iced Tea Unsweetened	1 sm	0	0	0	0
Lemonade	1 sm	170	1	0	0
BREAKFAST SELECTIONS					
Bagel Chicken Egg & Cheese	1	500	20	7	0
Bagel Wheat	1	220	3	0	0
Biscuit Bacon	1	300	14	4	3
Biscuit Bacon & Egg	1	390	20	5	3
Biscuit Bacon Egg Cheese	1	440	24	8	3
Biscuit Buttered	1	270	12	3	3
Biscuit Chicken	1	420	19	5	3
Biscuit Chicken w/ Cheese	1	470	23	8	3
Biscuit Egg	1	350	16	5	3
Biscuit Egg Cheese	1	400	21	7	3
Biscuit Sausage	1	410	23	9	3
Biscuit Sausage Egg	1	500	29	10	3
Biscuit Sausage Egg Cheese	1	550	33	13	3
Biscuit w/ Gravy	1	330	15	4	4
Burrito Chicken	1	420	19	6	2
Burrito Sausage	1	460	24	10	2
Chick-N-Minis	1 serv	270	11	4	1
Hashbrowns	1 serv	260	17	4	1
DESSERTS					
Cheesecake	1 slice	340	21	12	1
Fudge Nut Brownie	1	330	15	4	3
Icedream Cone	1 sm	160	4	2	0
Lemon Pie	1 slice	390	13	5	2
MAIN MENU SELECTIONS					
Carrot & Raisin Salad	1 sm	170	6	1	0
Chicken Filet	1	230	11	3	0
Chicken Filet Chargrilled	1	100	2	0	0
Chick-N-Strips	4	290	13	3	0
Cole Slaw	1 sm	260	21	4	0
Cool Wrap Chargrilled Chicken	1	390	7	3	0
Cool Wrap Chicken Caesar	1	460	10	6	0
Cool Wrap Spicy Chicken	1	380	6	3	0
Fruit Cup	1 serv	60	0	0	0
Hearty Breast of Chicken Soup	1 cup	140	4	1	0

FOOD	PORTION	CALS	FAT	SAT FAT	TRANS FAT
Nuggets	8	260	12	3	0
Polynesian Sauce	1 pkg	110	6	1	0
Sandwich Chargrilled Chicken	1	270	4	1	0
Sandwich Chicken	1	410	16	4	0
Sandwich Chicken Deluxe	1	420	16	4	0
Sandwich Chicken Salad On Wheat Bread	1	350	15	3	0
Waffle Fries w/o Salt	1 sm	280	14	5	–
Waffle Potato Fries	1 sm	270	13	3	2
SALAD DRESSINGS AND SAUCES					
Barbecue Sauce	1 pkg	45	0	0	0
Blue Cheese	2 tbsp	150	16	3	0
Buffalo Sauce	1 pkg	15	2	0	0
Buttermilk Ranch	2 tbsp	160	16	3	0
Buttermilk Ranch Sauce	1 pkg	110	12	2	0
Caesar	2 tbsp	160	17	3	0
Fat Free Honey Mustard	2 tbsp	60	0	0	0
Honey Mustard	1 pkg	45	0	0	0
Honey Roasted BBQ Sauce	1 pkg	60	6	1	0
Light Italian	2 tbsp	15	1	0	0
Raspberry Vinaigrette Reduced Fat	2 tbsp	80	2	0	0
Spicy	2 tbsp	140	14	2	0
Thousand Island	2 tbsp	150	14	2	0
SALADS					
Chargrilled Chicken Garden Salad	1 serv	180	6	3	0
Chick-N-Strips Salad	1 serv	390	18	5	0
Croutons Garlic & Butter	1 pkg	50	3	0	0
Honey Roasted Sunflower Kernels	1 pkg	80	7	1	0
Side Salad	1 serv	60	3	2	0
Southwest Chargrilled Salad	1 serv	240	8	4	0
Tortilla Strips	1 pkg	70	4	1	0

CHILI'S
CHILDREN'S MENU SELECTIONS

FOOD	PORTION	CALS	FAT	SAT FAT	TRANS FAT
Corn Dog	1	250	17	4	–
Grilled Chicken Platter	1 serv	140	3	1	–
Little Chicken Crispers	1 serv	590	42	8	–

FOOD	PORTION	CALS	FAT	SAT FAT	TRANS FAT
Little Mouth Burger	1 serv	280	15	5	–
Little Mouth Cheeseburger	1 serv	350	21	9	–
Macaroni & Cheese	1 serv	510	18	6	–
Pepper Pal Pasta w/ Alfredo	1 serv	410	19	9	–
Pepper Pal Pasta w/ Marinara	1 serv	290	5	1	–
Pizza	1	570	24	10	–
Rib Basket	1 serv	370	24	9	–
Sandwich Grilled Cheese	1 serv	420	27	16	–
Sandwich Grilled Chicken	1 serv	140	3	1	–
DESSERTS					
Cheesecake	1 serv	760	44	25	–
Chocolate Chip Paradise Pie w/ Vanilla Ice Cream	1 serv	1600	78	35	–
Frosty Chocolate Shake w/ Chocolate Sprinkles	1 serv	850	36	22	–
Molten Chocolate Cake w/ Vanilla Ice Cream	1 serv	1270	62	31	–
MAIN MENU SELECTIONS					
Awesome Blossom	1 serv	2710	203	36	–
Baby Back Ribs & Chicken	1 serv	1460	67	26	–
Black Bean Burger	1 serv	650	12	2	–
Boneless Buffalo Wings	1 serv	1250	80	15	–
Boneless Shanghai Wings	1 serv	1260	71	12	–
Bottomless Tostada Chips	1 basket	400	36	6	–
Burger Bacon	1 serv	1080	71	22	–
Burger BBQ Ranch	1 serv	1110	71	22	–
Burger Chipotle Bleu Cheese Bacon	1 serv	1090	71	21	–
Burger Ground Peppercorn	1 serv	1050	68	17	–
Burger Mushroom Swiss	1 serv	1100	71	21	–
Burger Oldtimer	1 serv	800	44	13	–
Chicken Crispers	1 serv	1870	129	25	–
Chicken Tacos	1 serv	1200	41	19	–
Cinnamon Apples	1 serv	210	8	2	–
Citrus Fire Chicken & Shrimp	1 serv	760	27	5	–
Classic Nachos	1 serv	1570	115	58	–
Country Fried Steak	1 serv	1890	107	29	–
Fried Cheese w/ Marinara Sauce	1 serv	1210	89	28	–
Garlic Toast	1 piece	200	12	3	–

FOOD	PORTION	CALS	FAT	SAT FAT	TRANS FAT
Grilled Baby Back Ribs	1 serv	1370	82	24	–
Grilled Salmon w/ Garlic & Herbs	1 serv	700	33	8	–
Guiltless Grill Chicken Pita	1 serv	550	9	3	–
Guiltless Grill Chicken Platter	1 serv	580	9	3	–
Guiltless Grill Chicken Sandwich	1 serv	490	8	2	–
Guiltless Grill Salmon	1 serv	480	14	3	–
Guiltless Grill Tomato Basil Pasta	1 serv	650	14	3	–
Homestyle Fries	1 serv	520	31	4	–
Kettle Black Beans	1 serv	140	1	0	–
Loaded Mashed Potatoes	1 serv	560	37	13	–
Margarita Grilled Chicken	1 serv	690	14	3	–
Monterey Chicken	1 serv	1170	71	29	–
Pasta Cajun Chicken	1 serv	1460	75	38	–
Pasta Grilled Shrimp Alfredo	1 serv	1340	72	37	–
Pasta Tomato Basil Chicken	1 serv	860	26	5	–
Pita Chicken Caesar	1 serv	650	41	7	–
Pita Chicken Fajita	1 serv	450	17	3	–
Pita Steak Fajita	1 serv	580	33	10	–
Quesadillas Fajita Chicken	1 serv	1720	82	44	–
Quesadillas Fajita Combo	1 serv	1840	94	48	–
Quesadillas Fajita Steak	1 serv	1970	106	53	–
Ribeye Cajun	1 serv	870	76	28	–
Ribeye Flame Grilled	1 serv	960	87	30	–
Rice	1 serv	210	2	0	–
Sandwich Cajun Chicken	1 serv	820	43	11	–
Sandwich Chicken Ranch	1 serv	1150	70	11	–
Sandwich Chili's Cheesesteak	1 serv	1010	55	24	–
Sandwich Grilled Chicken	1 serv	840	47	12	–
Sandwich Smoked Turkey	1 serv	930	57	15	–
Sauteed Mushrooms Onions & Bell Peppers	1 serv	120	10	2	–
Seasonal Grilled Veggies	1 serv	90	6	1	–
Seasonal Steamed Veggies w/ Parmesan Cheese	1 serv	60	1	1	–
Sirloin Chili's Classic	1 serv	530	41	14	–
Sirloin Honey BBQ	1 serv	800	56	21	–
Skillet Queso	1 serv	670	53	30	–

FOOD	PORTION	CALS	FAT	SAT FAT	TRANS FAT
Southwestern Eggrolls	1 serv	810	51	10	–
Steamed Broccoli	1 serv	80	6	1	–
Sweet Corn On The Cob	1 serv	180	2	0	–
Triple Play	1 serv	2330	177	31	–
Wings Over Buffalo	1 serv	1140	100	22	–
SALAD DRESSINGS AND SAUCES					
Dressing Asian Sesame Ginger	1 serv (2 oz)	250	22	3	–
Dressing Avocado Ranch	1 serv (2 oz)	150	15	2	–
Dressing Bleu Cheese	1 serv (2 oz)	330	35	6	–
Dressing Caesar	1 serv (2 oz)	350	37	6	–
Dressing Chipotle Ranch	1 serv (2 oz)	170	18	3	–
Dressing Citrus Balsamic Vinaigrette	1 serv (2 oz)	350	35	5	–
Dressing Creamy Cilantro	1 serv (2 oz)	300	32	5	–
Dressing Honey Lime	1 serv (2 oz)	270	22	3	–
Dressing Honey Mustard	1 serv (2 oz)	260	28	4	–
Dressing Ranch	1 serv (2 oz)	240	25	4	–
Dressing Thousand Island	1 serv (2 oz)	270	26	4	–
Dressing Low Fat Ranch	1 serv (2 oz)	110	6	1	–
Dressing No Fat Balsamic Vinaigrette	1 serv (2 oz)	50	0	0	0
Dressing No Fat Honey Mustard	1 serv (2 oz)	90	1	0	–
Sauce Peanut Dipping	1 serv (2 oz)	190	13	2	–
Sauce Picante Salsa	1 serv (2 oz)	40	0	0	0
Sauce Sesame Dipping	1 serv (2 oz)	70	0	0	0
SALADS					
Boneless Buffalo Chicken	1 serv	870	55	13	–
Chicken Caesar w/ Dressing	1 serv	1010	76	13	–
Crispy Chicken	1 serv	810	47	7	–
Dinner Caesar w/ Dressing	1 serv	430	34	6	–
Dinner House	1 serv	140	7	3	–
Grilled Caribbean	1 serv	440	10	2	–
Lettuce Wraps	1 serv	330	21	3	–
Lime Grilled Shrimp Caesar w/ Dressing	1 serv	980	77	13	–
Quesadilla Explosion	1 serv	850	45	21	–
Southwestern Cobb	1 serv	650	32	10	–
SOUPS					
Broccoli Cheese	1 cup	160	9	5	–

FOOD	PORTION	CALS	FAT	SAT FAT	TRANS FAT
Chicken Enchilada	1 cup	220	14	5	–
Chicken Noodle	1 cup	50	1	0	–
Chicken Tortilla	1 cup	140	7	3	–
Chili w/ Cheese	1 cup	500	35	15	–
New England Clam Chowder	1 cup	470	33	17	–
Potato	1 cup	220	16	10	–
Southwestern Vegetable	1 cup	110	5	2	–

CHIPOTLE

FOOD	PORTION	CALS	FAT	SAT FAT	TRANS FAT
Barbacoa	1 serv (5 oz)	285	16	4	–
Black Beans	1 serv (4 oz)	130	1	tr	–
Carnitas	1 serv (4 oz)	227	12	3	–
Cheese	1 serv (1 oz)	110	9	6	–
Chicken	1 serv (4 oz)	219	11	2	–
Chips	1 serv (4 oz)	490	19	4	–
Crispy Taco Shells	4	240	9	2	–
Fajita Vegetables	1 serv (3 oz)	100	8	1	–
Flour Tortilla	1 (6 inch)	300	8	2	–
Flour Tortilla	1 (13 inch)	340	9	2	–
Guacamole	1 serv (4 oz)	170	15	3	–
Lettuce	1 serv (1 oz)	5	0	0	0
Pinto Beans	1 serv (4 oz)	138	1	tr	–
Rice	1 serv (5 oz)	240	7	1	–
Salsa Corn	1 serv (4 oz)	100	1	0	–
Salsa Tomato	1 serv (4 oz)	25	0	0	0
Sour Cream	1 serv (2 oz)	120	10	7	–
Steak	1 serv (4 oz)	230	12	4	–
Tomatillo Green	1 serv (2 oz)	15	tr	0	–
Tomatillo Red	1 serv (2 oz)	28	1	0	–

CHURCH'S CHICKEN
DESSERTS

FOOD	PORTION	CALS	FAT	SAT FAT	TRANS FAT
Pie Apple	1 pie (3 oz)	280	11	4	2
Pie Edward's Double Lemon	1 pie (3 oz)	300	14	6	–
Pie Edward's Strawberry Cream Cheese	1 pie (2.8 oz)	280	15	8	–

MAIN MENU SELECTIONS

FOOD	PORTION	CALS	FAT	SAT FAT	TRANS FAT
Biscuit Honey Butter	1	240	12	3	2
Cajun Rice	1 reg	130	7	3	0
Chicken Fried Steak w/ White Gravy	1 serv (7.5 oz)	610	43	13	4

FOOD	PORTION	CALS	FAT	SAT FAT	TRANS FAT
Cole Slaw	1 reg	150	10	2	0
Corn On The Cob	1 ear	140	3	0	0
Country Fried Steak w/ White Gravy	1 serv (5.8 oz)	470	28	7	2
Crunchy Tenders	1 (2 oz)	120	6	2	1
French Fries	1 reg	290	14	3	3
Jalapeno Cheese Bombers	4 (4 oz)	240	10	6	–
Macaroni & Cheese	1 reg	210	11	4	–
Mashed Potatoes & Gravy	1 reg	70	2	0	0
Okra	1 reg	350	22	7	1
Original Breast	1	200	11	3	2
Original Leg	1	110	6	2	1
Original Thigh	1	330	23	6	3
Original Wing	1	300	19	5	3
Sandwich Bigger Better Chicken w/ Cheese	1	510	27	7	2
Sandwich Country Fried Steak	1	490	32	8	2
Sandwich Spicy Fish	1	320	20	4	3
Spicy Breast	1	320	20	5	4
Spicy Crunchy Tenders	1 (2 oz)	135	7	2	2
Spicy Fish Fillet	1 piece (2.3 oz)	160	9	2	3
Spicy Leg	1	180	11	3	2
Spicy Thigh	1	480	35	9	5
Spicy Wing	1	430	27	7	4
Sweet Corn Nuggets	1 reg	600	29	2	–
Whole Jalapeno Peppers	2	10	0	0	0
SAUCES					
BBQ	1 pkg	30	0	0	0
Creamy Jalapeno	1 pkg	100	11	2	–
Honey	1 pkg	27	0	0	0
Honey Mustard	1 pkg	110	11	2	–
Hot Sauce	1 pkg	0	0	0	0
Ketchup	1 pkg	18	0	0	0
Purple Pepper	1 pkg	45	0	0	0
Ranch	1 pkg	130	13	2	0
Sweet & Sour	1 pkg	30	0	0	0

CICI'S
EXTRAS

FOOD	PORTION	CALS	FAT	SAT FAT	TRANS FAT
Apple Pizza	1 slice	149	4	1	0

FOOD	PORTION	CALS	FAT	SAT FAT	TRANS FAT
Brownie	1	143	6	1	0
Cinnamon Roll	1	139	6	1	0
Garlic Bread	1 slice	99	5	1	0
PIZZA					
Buffet 12 Inch Alfredo	1 slice	139	5	3	0
Buffet 12 Inch Bacon Cheddar	1 slice	145	5	2	0
Buffet 12 Inch Bar-B-Que	1 slice	172	6	4	0
Buffet 12 Inch Beef	1 slice	170	7	4	0
Buffet 12 Inch Cheese	1 slice	152	5	3	0
Buffet 12 Inch Ham & Pineapple	1 slice	141	4	3	0
Buffet 12 Inch Olé	1 slice	108	4	2	0
Buffet 12 Inch Pepperoni	1 slice	175	7	2	0
Buffet 12 Inch Pepperoni & Jalapeno	1 slice	163	6	4	0
Buffet 12 Inch Sausage	1 slice	197	7	4	0
Buffet 12 Inch Spinach Alfredo	1 slice	151	5	3	0
Buffet 12 Inch Zesty Ham & Cheese	1 slice	153	6	3	0
Buffet 12 Inch Zesty Pepperoni	1 slice	157	7	3	0
Buffet 12 Inch Zesty Tomato Alfredo	1 slice	136	5	3	0
Buffet 12 Inch Zesty Veggie	1 slice	124	4	2	0
To-Go 15 Inch Bar-B-Que	1 slice	289	10	7	0
To-Go 15 Inch Cheese	1 slice	223	8	5	0
To-Go 15 Inch Ham & Pineapple	1 slice	225	8	5	0
To-Go 15 Inch Olé	1 slice	169	4	2	0
To-Go 15 Inch Pepperoni	1 slice	240	10	6	0
To-Go 15 Inch Spinach Alfredo	1 slice	243	8	5	0
To-Go 15 Inch Zesty Pepperoni	1 slice	246	12	5	0
To-Go 15 Inch Zesty Veggie	1 slice	213	9	4	0

CINNABON
BAKED SELECTIONS

FOOD	PORTION	CALS	FAT	SAT FAT	TRANS FAT
Caramel Pecanbon	1	1100	56	10	–
Cinnabon Bites	6	520	16	4	5
Cinnabon Classic	1	813	32	8	–
Cinnabon Stix	1	379	21	6	–
Cinnamon Filled Churro	1	281	11	2	0

FOOD	PORTION	CALS	FAT	SAT FAT	TRANS FAT
Minibon	1	339	13	3	–
BEVERAGES					
CarameLatta Chill	1 (16 oz)	520	19	12	0
Chillatta Cappuccino	1 (16 oz)	330	11	7	0
Chillatta Caramel	1 (16 oz)	480	18	11	–
Chillatta Chocolate Mocha	1 (16 oz)	460	14	8	–
Chillatta Mango	1 (16 oz)	340	11	7	0
Chillatta Strawberry	1 (16 oz)	330	11	7	0
Chillatta Strawberry Banana	1 (16 oz)	350	11	7	0
Chillatta Tropical Blast	1 (16 oz)	330	7	4	0
MochaLatta Chill	1 (16 oz)	450	18	11	–

COLD STONE CREAMERY

FOOD	PORTION	CALS	FAT	SAT FAT	TRANS FAT
Waffle Cone Dipped	1	310	15	7	–
Waffle Cone Dipped w/ Candy	1	390	20	7	–
Waffle Cone or Bowl	1	160	4	1	–
FROZEN YOGURT					
Cheesecake	1 serv (6 oz)	170	0	0	0
Low Fat Chocolate	1 serv (6 oz)	230	2	1	0
Nonfat Coffee	1 serv (6 oz)	220	0	0	0
Nonfat Sweet Cream	1 serv (6 oz)	220	0	0	0
ICE CREAM					
Amaretto	1 serv (6 oz)	390	24	15	1
Banana	1 serv (6 oz)	370	22	14	1
Black Cherry	1 serv (6 oz)	390	22	14	1
Butter Pecan	1 serv (6 oz)	390	24	15	1
Cake A Cheesecake Named Desire	1 slice (5 oz)	410	19	17	–
Cake Batter	1 serv (6 oz)	410	23	14	1
Cake Butterfinger Bonanza	1 slice (5 oz)	450	22	13	–
Cake Celebration Sensation	1 slice (4.5 oz)	350	17	11	–
Cake Chocolate Chipper	1 slice (4.6 oz)	450	28	11	–
Cake Coffeehouse Crunch	1 slice (5 oz)	530	31	10	–
Cake Cookie Dough Delirium	1 slice (4.8 oz)	420	21	11	–
Cake Cookies & Creamery	1 slice (4.5 oz)	390	20	11	–
Cake Midnight Delight	1 slice (5.3 oz)	510	28	12	–
Cake MMMMMM Chip	1 slice (4.5 oz)	380	20	12	–
Cake Peanut Butter Playground	1 slice (5 oz)	490	29	11	–
Cake Raspberry Truffle Temptation	1 slice (5 oz)	480	27	18	–

FOOD	PORTION	CALS	FAT	SAT FAT	TRANS FAT
Cake Snickers Supreme	1 slice (5 oz)	510	29	11	–
Cake Strawberry Passion	1 slice (5 oz)	380	19	10	–
Cake Zebra Stripes	1 slice (4.8 oz)	400	22	15	–
Candy Cane	1 serv (6 oz)	420	24	14	2
Caramel Latte	1 serv (6 oz)	400	22	14	1
Carrot Cake Batter	1 serv (6 oz)	450	24	13	1
Cheesecake	1 serv (6 oz)	390	22	14	1
Chocolate	1 serv (6 oz)	390	24	15	1
Cinnamon	1 serv (6 oz)	400	24	15	1
Coconut	1 serv (6 oz)	390	23	15	0
Coffee	1 serv (6 oz)	400	24	15	1
Cookie Batter	1 serv (6 oz)	450	24	13	1
Cotton Candy	1 serv (6 oz)	390	23	15	1
Dark Chocolate Peppermint	1 serv (6 oz)	410	23	15	1
Egg Nog	1 serv (6 oz)	400	22	14	1
Expresso	1 serv (6 oz)	350	21	13	1
French Vanilla	1 serv (6 oz)	400	23	16	1
Irish Cream	1 serv (6 oz)	390	24	15	1
Macadamia Nut	1 serv (6 oz)	390	24	15	1
Mango	1 serv (6 oz)	370	22	14	1
Mint	1 serv (6 oz)	400	23	15	1
Mocha	1 serv (6 oz)	390	24	15	1
Oatmeal Batter	1 serv (6 oz)	400	23	15	1
Orange Dreamsicle	1 serv (6 oz)	380	22	14	1
Peanut Butter	1 serv (6 oz)	440	29	15	1
Pecan Praline	1 serv (6 oz)	400	22	14	1
Pistachio	1 serv (6 oz)	390	24	15	1
Pumpkin	1 serv (6 oz)	390	22	14	1
Raspberry	1 serv	390	22	14	1
Sinless Sans Fat Sweet Cream	1 serv (6 oz)	160	0	0	0
Strawberry	1 serv (6 oz)	380	22	14	1
Sweet Cream	1 serv (6 oz)	390	24	15	1
Vanilla Bean	1 serv (6 oz)	400	23	15	1
White Chocolate	1 serv (6 oz)	390	23	15	1
MIX-INS AND TOPPINGS					
Almond Joy	1 piece	180	9	6	0
Apple Pie Filling	¾ oz	60	0	0	0
Banana	½	60	0	0	0
Black Cherries	¾ oz	80	0	0	0
Blackberries	¾ oz	10	0	0	0

FOOD	PORTION	CALS	FAT	SAT FAT	TRANS FAT
Blueberries	¾ oz	10	0	0	0
Brownies	1 piece	180	6	2	1
Butterfinger	½ bar	140	6	3	0
Butterscotch Fat Free	1 oz	80	0	0	0
Caramel	1 oz	100	0	0	0
Caramel Topping Fat Free	1 oz	110	0	0	0
Cashews	1 oz	170	14	3	0
Chocolate Chips	1 oz	130	7	5	0
Cinnamon	⅛ tsp	15	0	0	0
Coconut	1 oz	80	5	5	0
Cookie Dough	1 piece	180	8	3	2
Fudge	1 oz	100	3	3	0
Fudge Topping Fat Free	1 oz	80	0	0	0
Granola	1 oz	120	2	0	0
Gumballs	1 oz	120	0	0	0
Gummi Bears	1 oz	120	0	0	0
Heath Candy	1 bar	110	7	0	0
Honey	1 oz	90	0	0	0
Kit Kat	½ bar	100	5	4	0
M&M's	1 oz	170	7	5	0
M&M's Peanut	1 oz	150	8	4	0
Macadamia Nuts	1 oz	180	19	3	0
Maraschino Cherries	1	5	0	0	0
Marshmallo Creme	1 oz	100	0	0	0
Marshmallows	1 oz	100	0	0	0
Nestle Crunch	½ bar	130	7	4	0
Oreo Cookies	2	120	5	1	0
Peach Pie Filling	1 oz	60	0	0	0
Peanut Butter	¾ oz	150	13	3	0
Peanuts	1 oz	200	17	3	0
Pecan Pralines	1 oz	210	21	2	0
Pecans	1 oz	140	14	1	0
Pie Crust Graham Cracker	1 oz	110	3	0	0
Pie Crust Oreo	1 oz	180	8	2	0
Pistachios	1 oz	210	18	3	0
Raisins	1 oz	80	0	0	0
Raspberries	¾ oz	15	0	0	0
Reese's Peanut Butter Cup	1 piece	190	11	4	0
Reese's Pieces	1 oz	170	7	6	0
Roasted Almonds	1 oz	190	17	2	0

FOOD	PORTION	CALS	FAT	SAT FAT	TRANS FAT
Sliced Almonds	1 oz	210	20	2	0
Snickers	½ bar	170	9	3	0
Sprinkles Chocolate	1 oz	25	0	0	0
Sprinkles Rainbow	1 oz	25	0	0	0
Strawberries	¾ oz	20	0	0	0
Toasted Coconut	1 oz	180	14	13	0
Twix	1 cup	150	7	3	0
Vanilla Wafers	3	70	3	0	0
Walnuts	1 oz	130	12	1	0
Whipped Topping	1 serv	45	3	1	0
White Chocolate Chips	1 oz	160	9	8	0
Whoppers	1 oz	100	4	3	0
Yellow Sponge Cake	1 piece	70	1	0	0
York Peppermint Patties	2 pieces	120	2	2	0
SORBET					
Sinless Lemon	1 serv	180	0	0	0
Sinless Raspberry	1 serv (6 oz)	200	0	0	0
Sinless Tangerine	1 serv (6 oz)	200	0	0	0

COLOMBO FROZEN YOGURT

FOOD	PORTION	CALS	FAT	SAT FAT	TRANS FAT
Strawberry Lowfat	½ cup	110	2	1	–
Strawberry Nonfat	½ cup	100	0	0	0

COSÌ
BEVERAGES

FOOD	PORTION	CALS	FAT	SAT FAT	TRANS FAT
Arctic Double Chi	1 tall (12 oz)	621	25	–	–
Arctic Latte	1 tall (12 oz)	396	12	–	–
Arctic Mocha	1 tall (12 oz)	623	11	–	–
Arctic Raspberry Chai	1 tall (12 oz)	300	8	–	–
Arctic Thai	1 tall (12 oz)	432	9	–	–
Caramel Mocha	1 tall (9 oz)	344	20	–	–
Chai Tea Latte	1 tall (8 oz)	109	4	–	–
Hot Chocolate	1 tall (12 oz)	436	29	–	–
Kefir Blueberry	1 (12 oz)	278	3	–	–
Lemonade	1 (15 oz)	112	0	0	0
Lemonade Strawberry	1 tall (12 oz)	290	0	–	0
Smoothie Mango Mania	1 tall (12 oz)	186	0	–	0
Smoothie Peach	1 tall (12 oz)	186	0	–	0
Smoothie Strawberry Banana	1 tall (12 oz)	186	0	–	0
Smores Latte	1 tall (11 oz)	401	20	–	–
Wildberry Blast	1 tall (12 oz)	186	0	–	0

FOOD	PORTION	CALS	FAT	SAT FAT	TRANS FAT
BREAKFAST SELECTIONS					
Bagel Asiago Cheese	1 (6 oz)	327	1	–	–
Bagel Cinnamon Raisin	1 (6 oz)	438	1	–	–
Bagel Cranberry Orange	1 (6 oz)	372	1	–	–
Bagel Everything	1 (5.5 oz)	353	3	–	–
Bagel Plain	1 (5.5 oz)	326	1	–	–
Bagel Poppy Seed	1 (5.5 oz)	346	3	–	–
Cream Cheese Honey Pecan	1 serv (2 oz)	159	14	–	–
Cream Cheese Plain	1 serv (2 oz)	182	18	–	–
Cream Cheese Plain Low Fat	1 serv (2 oz)	121	12	–	–
Cream Cheese Veggie Low Fat	1 serv (2 oz)	113	9	–	–
Croissant Almond	1	340	16	–	–
Croissant Butter	1	330	17	–	–
Croissant Chocolate	1	370	18	–	–
Fruit Salad	1 serv	216	1	–	–
Granola Cereal	1 serv	564	12	–	–
Granola Parfait Peach	1 serv	389	6	–	–
Granola Parfait Strawberry	1 serv	426	6	–	–
Muffin Banana Nut	1	480	22	–	–
Muffin Blueberry	1	440	19	–	–
Muffin Carrot Raisin	1	470	22	–	–
Muffin Corn	1	450	25	–	–
Muffin Lowfat Bran	1	351	6	–	–
Scone Blueberry	1	410	17	–	–
DESSERTS					
Apple Tart	1 serv	396	6	–	–
Blondie Brownie	1	570	36	–	–
Cheesecake	1 serv	567	33	–	–
Cheesecake Brownie	1 serv	470	28	–	–
Cinnamon Apple Pie	1 serv	960	40	–	–
Cookie Chocolate Chunk	1	480	20	–	–
Cookie Oatmeal Raisin	1	440	14	–	–
Ice Cream Double Scoop	1 serv	225	14	–	–
Sundae	1 med	408	24	–	–
SALAD DRESSINGS					
Caesar	1 serv (2 oz)	301	32	–	–
Così Vinaigrette	1 serv (2 oz)	357	39	–	–
Fat Free Balsamic Vinaigrette	1 serv (2 oz)	45	0	0	0
Lowfat Ginger Soy	1 serv (2 oz)	74	2	–	–

FOOD	PORTION	CALS	FAT	SAT FAT	TRANS FAT
Pepperanch	1 serv (2 oz)	262	28	–	–
Reduced Fat Roasted Shallot Sherry Vinaigrette	1 serv (2 oz)	85	5	–	–
Roasted Shallot Sherry Vinaigrette	1 serv (2 oz)	308	31	–	–
SALADS					
Bombay Chicken No Dressing	1 serv	176	3	–	–
Caesar No Dressing	1 serv	182	8	–	–
Caesar w/ Grilled Chicken No Dressing	1 serv	340	10	–	–
Cosi Cobb No Dressing	1 serv	419	28	–	–
Greek No Dressing	1 serv	236	17	–	–
Mixed Greens No Dressing	1 serv	46	1	–	–
Shanghai Chicken No Dressing	1 serv	221	9	–	–
Signature No Dressing	1 serv	375	21	–	–
SANDWICHES					
Buffalo Blue	1	649	30	–	–
Così Club	1	729	35	–	–
Green Market	1	555	17	–	–
Grilled Chicken T.B.M.	1	791	43	–	–
Hummus & Fresh Veggies	1	432	8	–	–
Italiano	1	834	47	–	–
Melts Bacon Turkey Cheddar	1	682	25	–	–
Melts Chicken TBM	1	926	47	–	–
Melts Grilled Chicken Parmesan	1	701	27	–	–
Melts Pesto Chicken	1	809	39	–	–
Melts Tomato Basil & Mozzarella	1	666	34	–	–
Melts Tuna	1	1012	60	–	–
Polpette Rustica	1	553	23	–	–
Roasted Turkey & Brie	1	772	36	–	–
Sesame Ginger Chicken	1	508	11	–	–
Shrimp Salad	1	471	17	–	–
Smoked Ham & Brie	1	639	25	–	–
T.B.M.	1	729	42	–	–
Tandoori Chicken	1	633	26	–	–
Tuna Cheddar	1	956	55	–	–
Turkey Light	1	476	9	–	–
Turkey Rustica	1	619	27	–	–

FOOD	PORTION	CALS	FAT	SAT FAT	TRANS FAT
Tuscan Pesto Chicken	1	571	22	–	–
Vegi Muffaletta	1	824	51	–	–
Wasabi Roast Beef	1	626	28	–	–
SOUPS					
Cajun Gumbo	1 serv (10 oz)	251	18	–	–
Chicken Gumbo	1 serv (6 oz)	151	11	–	–
Chicken Noodle	1 serv (10 oz)	116	4	–	–
Grilled Chicken Corn Chowder	1 serv (10 oz)	305	16	–	–
Lentil	1 serv (10 oz)	199	3	–	–
Minestone	1 serv (10 oz)	174	3	–	–
New England Clam Chowder	1 serv (10 oz)	440	29	–	–
Three Bean Chili	1 serv (10 oz)	162	1	–	–

DAIRY QUEEN
FOOD SELECTIONS

FOOD	PORTION	CALS	FAT	SAT FAT	TRANS FAT
Chicken Strip Basket	4 pieces	520	49	9	12
Chili Cheese Dog	1	330	21	9	0
DQ Homestyle Bacon Double Cheeseburger	1	610	36	18	0
DQ Homestyle Burger	1	290	12	5	0
DQ Homestyle Cheeseburger	1	340	17	8	0
DQ Homestyle Double Cheeseburger	1	540	31	16	0
DQ Ultimate Burger	1	670	43	19	0
French Fries	1 sm	300	12	3	4
Grillburger ½ Lb	1	800	50	21	5
Grillburger ½ Lb w/ Cheese	1	930	60	27	5
Grillburger ¼ Lb FlameThrower	1	850	64	19	3
Grillburger Bacon Cheddar	1	710	45	19	4
Grillburger California	1	630	42	13	3
Grillburger Classic	1	540	30	11	3
Grillburger Classic w/ Cheese	1	610	36	15	4
Grillburger Mushroom Swiss	1	700	47	16	4
Hot Dog	1	240	14	5	0
Onion Rings	1 reg	470	30	6	7
Salad Crispy Chicken No Dressing	1 serv	350	20	6	3
Salad Grilled Chicken No Dressing	1 serv	240	10	5	0

FOOD	PORTION	CALS	FAT	SAT FAT	TRANS FAT
Sandwich Crispy Chicken	1	590	34	6	2
Sandwich Grilled Chicken	1	340	16	3	0
Side Salad	1 serv	60	3	2	0
ICE CREAM					
Banana Split	1	510	12	8	0
Blizzard Banana Split	1 sm	460	14	9	0
Blizzard Chocolate Chip Cookie Dough	1 sm	720	28	14	3
Blizzard Oreo Cookies	1 sm	570	21	10	1
Blizzard Reese's Peanut Butter Cup	1 sm	600	21	16	0
Blizzard Strawberry Cheesecake	1 sm	530	21	13	1
Brownie Earthquake	1	740	27	16	1
Buster Bar	1	500	28	15	1
Cake 8 Inch Round	1/8 cake	370	13	8	1
Cake Blizzard Oreo Cookie	1/8 cake	490	20	12	1
Cake Blizzard Reese's Peanut Butter Cup	1/8 cake	490	20	13	0
Cone Chocolate	1 sm	240	8	5	0
Cone Vanilla	1 sm	230	7	5	0
Cone Dipped	1 sm	340	17	9	1
Dilly Bar Chocolate	1	220	13	10	1
DQ Fudge Bar No Sugar Added	1	50	0	0	0
DQ Sandwich	1	200	6	3	1
DQ Soft Serve Chocolate	1/2 cup	150	5	4	0
DQ Soft Serve Vanilla	1/2 cup	140	5	3	0
DQ Vanilla Orange Bar No Sugar Added	1	60	0	0	0
Malt Chocolate	1 sm	640	16	11	1
MooLatte Cappuccino	1 (16 oz)	490	18	14	0
MooLatte Caramel	1 (16 oz)	630	20	15	1
MooLatte French Vanilla	1 (16 oz)	570	18	14	0
MooLatte Mocha	1 (16 oz)	590	23	15	0
Peanut Buster Parfait	1	730	31	17	0
Shake Chocolate	1 sm	560	15	10	1
Slush Arctic Rush	1 sm	220	0	0	0
Starkiss	1	80	0	0	0
Sundae Chocolate	1 sm	280	7	5	0
Sundae Strawberry	1 sm	240	7	5	0

FOOD	PORTION	CALS	FAT	SAT FAT	TRANS FAT
SALAD DRESSINGS					
Blue Cheese	1 serv (2 oz)	210	20	4	0
Honey Mustard	1 serv (2 oz)	260	21	4	0
Italian Fat Free	1 serv (2 oz)	10	0	0	0
Ranch	1 serv (2 oz)	310	33	5	0

D'ANGELO
CHILDREN'S MENU SELECTIONS

FOOD	PORTION	CALS	FAT	SAT FAT	TRANS FAT
D'Lite Turkey	1	217	3	0	0
Sub Cheeseburger	1	294	13	6	0
Sub Ham & Cheese	1	227	5	2	0
Sub Kidz Tuna	1	438	29	4	0
Sub Meatball	1	330	15	5	0
SALAD DRESSINGS					
Bleu Cheese	1 serv	152	15	3	0
Caesar	1 serv	397	43	7	0
Caesar Fat Free	1 serv	57	0	0	0
Creamy Italian	1 serv	340	37	6	0
Greek w/ Feta Cheese	1 serv	227	26	4	0
Honey Mustard	1 serv	150	142	2	0
Olive Oil Vinaigrette	1 serv	170	17	3	–
Ranch Lite	1 serv	240	19	3	0
SALADS					
Antipasto	1 serv	284	18	7	0
Caesar w/ Dressing	1 serv	474	39	7	0
Chicken Caesar w/ Dressing	1 serv	533	38	8	0
Chicken Stir Fry w/o Dressing	1 serv	168	3	1	0
Cobb w/o Dressing	1 serv	292	17	7	0
Greek	1 serv	290	23	9	0
Lobster w/o Dressing	1 serv	376	26	4	0
Roast Beef w/o Dressing	1 serv	131	3	1	0
Steak Tip Caesar	1 serv	661	50	13	0
Tossed Garden w/o Dressing	1 serv	49	1	tr	0
Turkey w/o Dressing	1 serv	157	2	tr	0
SANDWICHES					
D'Lite Chicken Caesar Salad	1	374	7	3	0
D'Lite Chicken Stir Fry	1	426	6	2	0
D'Lite Classic Veggie	1	362	7	3	0
D'Lite Fresh Veggie	1	348	7	3	0
D'Lite Grilled Chicken Breast	1	388	7	1	0

FOOD	PORTION	CALS	FAT	SAT FAT	TRANS FAT
D'Lite Roast Beef	1	338	5	1	0
D'Lite Turkey	1	347	4	0	0
D'Lite Turkey Cranberry	1	444	4	0	0
Pokket Big Papi	1	469	11	6	0
Pokket BLT & Cheese	1	397	17	8	0
Pokket Caesar Salad	1	616	39	7	0
Pokket Capacola & Cheese	1	362	13	7	0
Pokket Cheese	1	519	27	18	0
Pokket Cheeseburger	1	459	25	11	0
Pokket Chicken Caesar Salad	1	674	39	8	0
Pokket Chicken Club	1	526	28	6	0
Pokket Chicken Honey Dijon	1	508	20	7	0
Pokket Chicken Salad	1	623	42	7	0
Pokket Chicken Stir Fry	1	380	9	5	0
Pokket Classic Vegetable	1	368	13	8	0
Pokket Classic Vegetable No Cheese	1	212	1	tr	0
Pokket Greek	1	790	61	14	0
Pokket Grilled Chicken	1	303	5	1	0
Pokket Ham	1	229	3	1	0
Pokket Ham & Cheese	1	326	10	6	0
Pokket Ham & Salami	1	386	17	8	0
Pokket Hamburger	1	399	20	8	0
Pokket Italian	1	525	30	12	0
Pokket Lobster	1	530	31	5	0
Pokket Meatball	1	574	31	10	0
Pokket Mortadella & Cheese	1	410	21	9	0
Pokket Number 9	1	407	18	9	0
Pokket Pastrami	1	438	25	9	0
Pokket Pepperoni	1	407	20	9	0
Pokket Roast Beef	1	247	3	1	0
Pokket Salad	1	196	1	tr	0
Pokket Salami & Cheese	1	509	30	13	0
Pokket Seafood Salad	1	449	22	3	0
Pokket Steak	1	305	12	5	0
Pokket Steak & Cheese	1	377	17	9	0
Pokket Steak Bomb	1	631	32	14	0
Pokket Steak Tip	1	452	16	5	0
Pokket Tuna	1	664	49	8	0
Pokket Turkey	1	256	2	0	0

FOOD	PORTION	CALS	FAT	SAT FAT	TRANS FAT
Pokket Turkey Club	1	332	7	2	0
Sub Big Papi	1 sm	525	15	9	0
Sub BLT & Cheese	1 sm	463	19	8	0
Sub Capicola & Cheese	1 sm	408	13	6	0
Sub Cheese	1 sm	589	28	18	0
Sub Cheeseburger	1 sm	526	26	11	0
Sub Chicken Club	1 sm	593	29	6	0
Sub Chicken Honey Dijon	1 sm	575	22	7	0
Sub Chicken Salad	1 sm	692	44	7	0
Sub Chicken Stir Fry	1 sm	449	11	5	0
Sub Classic Veggie	1 sm	462	15	8	0
Sub Grilled Chicken	1 sm	369	7	1	0
Sub Ham	1 sm	302	5	1	0
Sub Ham & Cheese	1 sm	395	11	6	0
Sub Ham & Salami	1 sm	456	19	8	0
Sub Hamburger	1 sm	466	22	8	0
Sub Italian	1 sm	614	31	12	0
Sub Lobster	1 sm	598	33	5	0
Sub Meatball	1 sm	644	33	10	0
Sub Meatballs & Cheese	1 sm	750	41	15	0
Sub Mortadella & Cheese	1 sm	479	23	9	0
Sub Number 9	1 sm	450	19	9	0
Sub Pastrami	1 sm	613	34	14	0
Sub Pepperoni	1 sm	603	33	13	0
Sub Roast Beef	1 sm	320	5	1	0
Sub Salad	1 sm	281	3	tr	0
Sub Salami & Cheese	1 sm	579	32	13	0
Sub Seafood Salad	1 sm	498	23	3	0
Sub Steak	1 sm	373	14	5	0
Sub Steak & Cheese	1 sm	446	19	9	0
Sub Steak Bomb	1 sm	670	33	14	0
Sub Steak Tip	1 sm	545	18	5	0
Sub Tuna	1 sm	685	46	7	0
Sub Turkey Club	1 sm	401	9	2	0
Sub Toasted Italian Bistro	1 sm	585	31	12	0
Sub Toasted Pastrami Reuben	1 sm	750	47	14	1
Sub Toasted Roast Beef & Cheddar	1 sm	564	26	10	1
Sub Toasted Spicy Meatball	1 sm	933	57	20	2
Sub Toasted Tuna & Swiss	1 sm	796	54	12	0

FOOD	PORTION	CALS	FAT	SAT FAT	TRANS FAT
Sub Toasted Turkey Thanksgiving	1 sm	705	20	2	0
Sub Toasted Turkey & Ham	1 sm	532	24	5	0
Wrap Big Papi	1	593	23	11	0
Wrap BLT & Cheese	1	544	26	10	0
Wrap Buffalo Chicken Salad	1	823	44	7	0
Wrap Caesar Salad	1	711	44	9	0
Wrap Capicola & Cheese	1	494	20	8	0
Wrap Cheese	1	675	35	20	0
Wrap Cheeseburger	1	609	33	13	0
Wrap Chicken Caesar Salad	1	830	47	10	0
Wrap Chicken Cobb	1	931	55	14	0
Wrap Chicken Filet & Bacon	1	639	28	6	0
Wrap Chicken Honey Dijon	1	672	29	9	0
Wrap Chicken Salad	1	782	51	9	0
Wrap Chicken Stir Fry	1	535	17	7	0
Wrap Classic Veggie	1	486	13	8	0
Wrap Greek	1	765	61	14	0
Wrap Grilled Chicken	1	422	6	1	0
Wrap Ham & Cheese	1	435	10	6	0
Wrap Ham & Salami	1	513	18	9	0
Wrap Hamburger	1	509	21	8	0
Wrap Italian	1	631	29	12	0
Wrap Lobster	1	749	43	7	0
Wrap Meatball	1	687	31	10	0
Wrap Mortadella & Cheese	1	522	21	9	0
Wrap Number 9	1	517	24	10	0
Wrap Pastrami	1	550	25	9	0
Wrap Peppercorn Steak	1	702	40	14	0
Wrap Pepperoni	1	519	21	9	0
Wrap Roast Beef	1	448	13	3	0
Wrap Salad	1	324	2	tr	0
Wrap Salami & Cheese	1	605	29	12	0
Wrap Seafood Salad	1	541	22	3	0
Wrap Steak	1	392	13	5	0
Wrap Steak & Cheese	1	464	18	9	0
Wrap Steak Bomb	1	670	33	14	0
Wrap Steak Tip	1	432	16	5	0
Wrap Tuna	1	731	44	7	0

FOOD	PORTION	CALS	FAT	SAT FAT	TRANS FAT
Wrap Turkey	1	369	3	0	0
Wrap Turkey Club	1	415	8	2	0
SOUPS					
Beef Stew	1 sm	220	8	4	0
Broccoli & Cheddar Cheese	1 sm	270	21	11	0
Chicken Noodle	1 sm	110	3	1	0
Hearty Vegetable	1 sm	40	0	0	0
Italian Wedding	1 sm	120	6	2	0
Lobster Bisque	1 sm	360	29	18	0
New England Clam Chowder	1 sm	320	18	10	0
Portuguese Kale	1 sm	130	4	2	0
Thanksgiving Everyday	1 sm	250	17	9	–

DEL TACO
BEVERAGES

FOOD	PORTION	CALS	FAT	SAT FAT	TRANS FAT
Barq's Root Beer	1 sm	278	0	0	0
Classic Coke	1 sm	248	0	0	0
Diet Coke	1 sm	2	0	0	0
Iced Tea	1 sm	0	0	0	0
Light Lemonade Minute Maid	1 sm	13	0	0	0
Milk 2% Low Fat	1 serv	152	6	3	–
Pibb Xtra	1 sm	243	0	0	0
Orange Juice	1 serv	140	0	0	0
Shake Chocolate	1 (15 oz)	680	18	12	–
Shake Strawberry	1 (15 oz)	540	8	6	–
Shake Vanilla	1 (15 oz)	550	10	6	–
Sprite	1 sm	243	0	0	0
BREAKFAST SELECTIONS					
Burrito Breakfast	1	250	11	6	–
Burrito Egg & Cheese	1	450	24	13	–
Burrito Macho Bacon & Egg	1	1030	60	20	–
Burrito Steak & Egg	1	580	34	16	–
Hash Brown Sticks	5 pieces	250	19	1	–
Quesadilla Bacon & Egg	1	450	23	12	–
Side of Bacon	2 strips	50	4	2	–
MAIN MENU SELECTIONS					
Beans 'n Cheese Cup	1 serv	260	3	2	–
Bun Taco	1	440	21	12	–
Burrito Crispy Fish	1	497	21	5	–
Burrito Del Beef	1	550	30	17	–

FOOD	PORTION	CALS	FAT	SAT FAT	TRANS FAT
Burrito Del Classic Chicken	1	560	36	13	–
Burrito Del Combo	1	530	22	13	–
Burrito Deluxe Combo	1	570	26	15	–
Burrito Deluxe Del Beef	1	590	33	19	–
Burrito Green Bean & Cheese	1	280	8	5	–
Burrito Green Half Pound	1	430	12	9	–
Burrito Macho Beef	1	1170	62	29	–
Burrito Macho Chicken	1	930	33	15	–
Burrito Macho Combo	1	1050	44	21	–
Burrito Red Bean & Cheese	1	270	8	5	–
Burrito Red Half Pound	1	430	12	9	–
Burrito Spicy Chicken	1	480	16	10	–
Burrito Works Chicken	1	520	23	12	–
Burrito Works Steak	1	590	31	16	–
Burrito Works Veggie	1	490	18	11	–
Cheeseburger	1	330	13	6	–
Cheeseburger Double Del	1	560	35	12	–
Cheeseburger Double Del Bacon	1	610	39	14	–
Chips & Salsa	1 sm	156	7	3	–
Del Cheeseburger	1	430	25	7	–
Fries	1 sm	350	23	4	–
Fries Chili Cheese	1 serv	670	46	15	–
Fries Deluxe Chili Cheese	1 serv	710	49	16	–
Hamburger	1	280	9	3	–
Nachos	1 serv	380	24	8	–
Nachos Macho	1 serv	1100	63	24	–
Quesadilla Cheddar	1	500	27	20	–
Quesadilla Spicy Jack	1	490	28	17	–
Quesadilla Spicy Jack Chicken	1	570	30	16	–
Quesadillas Chicken Cheddar	1	580	31	21	–
Rice Cup	1 serv	140	2	1	–
Taco	1	160	10	4	–
Taco Big Fat	1	320	11	5	–
Taco Big Fat Chicken	1	340	13	4	–
Taco Big Fat Steak	1	390	19	6	–
Taco Carne Asada	1	237	8	5	–
Taco Crispy Fish	1	290	16	3	–
Taco Del Carbon Chicken	1	170	5	1	–
Taco Del Carbon Steak	1	220	11	4	–

FOOD	PORTION	CALS	FAT	SAT FAT	TRANS FAT
Taco Macho	1	504	37	18	–
Taco Soft	1	160	8	4	–
Taco Soft Chicken	1	210	12	4	–
SALADS					
Deluxe Chicken Salad	1 serv	740	34	15	–
Taco Salad	1 serv	350	30	10	–
Taco Salad Deluxe	1	780	40	18	–

DENNY'S
BEVERAGES

FOOD	PORTION	CALS	FAT	SAT FAT	TRANS FAT
2% Milk	10 oz	151	6	4	–
Apple Juice	1 reg	126	0	0	0
Cappuccino French Vanilla	8 oz	100	2	2	–
Cappuccino Original	8 oz	100	3	3	–
Chocolate Milk	10 oz	235	9	6	–
Grapefruit	1 serv (10 oz)	162	0	0	0
Hot Chocolate	8 oz	100	2	2	–
Lemonade	16 oz	150	0	0	0
Malted Milk Shake Chocolate Or Vanilla	12 oz	583	26	16	–
Orange Juice	10 oz	126	0	0	0
Raspberry Ice Tea	16 oz	78	0	0	0
Tomato Juice	1 serv (10 oz)	56	0	0	0

BREAKFAST SELECTIONS

FOOD	PORTION	CALS	FAT	SAT FAT	TRANS FAT
All American Slam	1 serv	816	67	24	–
Applesauce	1 serv	60	0	0	0
Bacon	4 strips	162	18	5	–
Bagel Dry	1	235	1	0	–
Banana	1	110	0	0	0
Belgian Waffle	1	619	45	22	–
Breakfast Dagwood	1 serv	1446	90	35	–
Buttermilk Hotcakes	3	466	23	7	–
Cantaloup	¼	32	0	0	0
Chicken Fajita Skillet	1 serv	855	49	15	–
Corned Beef Hash Slam	1 serv	668	55	19	–
Country Fried Potatoes	1 serv	394	20	6	–
Egg	1	120	10	3	–
English Muffin Dry	1	125	1	0	–
Fabulous French Toast	1 serv	1146	71	24	–
Farmer's Slam	1 serv	1200	80	24	–

FOOD	PORTION	CALS	FAT	SAT FAT	TRANS FAT
French Slam	1 serv	1119	77	25	–
Fruit Mix	1 serv	36	0	0	0
Grand Slam Slugger	1 serv	927	55	15	–
Grapefruit	½	60	0	0	0
Grapes	1 serv	55	1	0	–
Grits	1 serv	80	0	0	0
Ham & Cheddar Omelette	1 serv	595	47	16	–
Ham & Cheese Omelette w/ Egg Beaters	1 serv	468	32	11	–
Ham Slice	1	94	3	1	–
Hashed Browns	1 serv	197	12	2	–
Hashed Browns Covered	1 serv	280	19	6	–
Hashed Browns Covered & Smothered	1 serv	493	25	9	–
Honeydew	¼	31	0	0	0
Lumberjack Slam w/ Hash Browns	1 serv	1035	58	17	–
Meat Lover's Skillet	1 serv	1031	74	24	–
Moon Over My Hammy	1 serv	841	51	22	–
Oatmeal	1 serv	100	2	0	–
Oatmeal Deluxe	1 serv	460	6	3	–
Original Grand Slam	1 serv	665	49	15	–
Ready To Eat Cereal	1 serv	100	0	0	0
Sausage	4 links	354	32	2	–
Scram Slam	1 serv	827	68	21	–
Senior Belgian Waffle Slam	1 serv	399	33	8	–
Senior Omelette	1 serv	429	20	12	–
Sirloin Steak & Eggs	1 serv	675	45	16	–
Slim Slam	1 serv	438	6	3	–
T-Bone Steak & Eggs	1 serv	991	77	31	–
Toast Dry	1 slice	92	1	0	–
Two Egg Breakfast w/ Hash Browns	1 serv	825	67	17	–
Ultimate Omelette	1 serv	611	50	17	–
Veggie Cheese Omelette	1 serv	494	39	12	–
CHILDREN'S MENU SELECTIONS					
Burgerlicious	1 serv	296	17	6	–
Burgerlicious w/ Cheese	1 serv	341	20	6	–
Dennysaur Chicken Nuggets	1 serv	190	13	4	–
Frenchtastic Slam	1 serv	452	33	9	–

FOOD	PORTION	CALS	FAT	SAT FAT	TRANS FAT
Junior Fish & Chips	1 serv	698	45	8	–
Junior Grand Slam	1 serv	397	25	7	–
Junior Shrimps Ahoy!	1 serv	411	18	4	–
Oreo Blender Blaster	1 serv	580	29	15	–
Pizza Party	1 serv	400	15	3	–
Smiley-Face Hotcakes w/ Meat	1 serv	463	22	7	–
Smiley-Face Hotcakes w/o Meat	1 serv	344	9	3	–
The Big Cheese	1 serv	334	20	2	–
DESSERTS					
Apple Pie	1 serv	470	24	6	–
Banana Split	1	894	43	19	–
Carrot Cake	1 serv	799	45	13	–
Cheesecake	1 serv	580	38	24	–
Chocolate Topping	1 serv	317	25	0	–
Chocolate Peanut Butter Pie	1 serv	653	39	19	–
Double Scoop Sundae	1 serv	375	27	12	–
Float Rootbeer or Coke	12 oz	280	10	6	–
Hot Fudge Brownie A La Mode	1 serv	997	42	6	–
Milkshake Vanilla Or Chocolate	12 oz	560	26	16	–
Oreo Blender Blaster	1 serv	895	46	23	–
Single Scoop Sundae	1 serv	188	14	6	–
MAIN MENU SELECTIONS					
Albacore Tuna Melt	1 serv	640	39	13	–
Applesauce	1 serv	60	0	0	0
Bacon Lettuce & Tomato	1	610	38	9	–
Baked Potato Plain	1	220	0	0	0
BBQ Chicken Sandwich	1 serv	1089	62	14	–
Bread Stuffing Plain	1 serv	100	1	0	–
Buffalo Chicken Sandwich	1 serv	708	28	6	–
Buffalo Chicken Strips	5 pieces	734	42	4	–
Buffalo Wings	12 pieces	856	54	17	–
Burger Bacon Cheddar	1	875	52	19	–
Burger BBQ	1 serv	953	52	21	–
Burger Boca	1 serv	601	27	6	–
Burger Classic	1	694	35	12	–
Burger Classic w/ Cheese	1	852	48	20	–
Burger Mushroom Swiss	1 serv	880	49	19	–
Carrots In Honey Glaze	1 serv	80	3	1	–
Chicken Strips	5 pieces	720	33	4	–

FOOD	PORTION	CALS	FAT	SAT FAT	TRANS FAT
Chicken Ranch Melt	1 serv	758	45	14	–
Chicken Strips	1 serv	635	25	1	–
Club Sandwich	1	718	38	7	–
Coleslaw	1 serv	274	30	24	–
Corn In Butter Sauce	1 serv	120	4	2	–
Cottage Cheese	1 serv	72	3	2	–
Country Fried Steak	1 serv	644	48	10	–
Fish & Chips Dinner	1 serv	955	57	37	–
French Fries Unsalted	1 serv	423	20	5	–
Fried Shrimp Dinner	1 serv	219	10	2	–
Fried Shrimp & Shrimp Scampi	1 serv	346	20	4	–
Green Beans w/ Bacon	1 serv	60	4	2	–
Grilled Cheese Sandwich	1	510	30	14	–
Grilled Chicken Dinner	1 serv	130	4	1	–
Grilled Chicken Sandwich	1	469	14	3	–
Ham & Swiss On Rye	1	417	16	8	–
Herb Toast	1 serv	170	11	2	–
Hoagie Chicken Melt	1	751	44	12	–
Hoagie Philly Melt	1 serv	874	50	16	–
Mashed Potatoes Plain	1 serv	168	7	3	–
Mozzarella Sticks	8 pieces	710	41	24	–
Onion Rings	1 serv	381	23	6	–
Patty Melt	1	798	51	21	–
Pot Roast Dinner w/ Gravy	1 serv	292	11	5	–
Roast Turkey & Stuffing w/ Gravy	1 serv	388	3	1	–
Sampler	1 serv	1405	80	24	–
Seasoned Fries	1 serv	261	12	3	–
Senior Chicken Strip Dinner	1 serv	285	10	0	–
Senior Club	1 serv	540	31	5	–
Senior Country Fried Steak	1 serv	341	23	5	–
Senior Fish & Chips	1 serv	756	47	35	–
Senior French Slam	1 serv	820	65	22	–
Senior Fried Shrimp Dinner	1 serv	129	5	1	–
Senior Grilled Chicken Breast	1 serv	200	5	1	–
Senior Pot Roast	1 serv	160	6	3	–
Senior Starter	1 serv	544	42	11	–
Senior Turkey & Stuffing	1 serv	220	2	0	–
Shrimp Scampi Skillet Dinner	1 serv	289	19	4	–
Sirloin Steak Dinner	1 serv	337	28	8	–

FOOD	PORTION	CALS	FAT	SAT FAT	TRANS FAT
Sliced Tomatoes	3 slices	13	0	0	0
Smothered Cheese Fries	1 serv	767	48	17	–
Steak & Shrimp Dinner	1 serv	645	42	14	–
T-Bone Steak Dinner	1 serv	860	65	29	–
The Super Bird Sandwich	1	620	32	5	–
Turkey Breast On Multigrain w/o Mayo	1	277	4	tr	–
SALAD DRESSINGS AND TOPPINGS					
BBQ Sauce	1.5 oz	47	1	0	–
Bleu Cheese	1 oz	163	18	3	–
Blueberry Topping	1 serv	71	0	0	0
Caesar	1 oz	133	14	2	–
Cherry Topping	1 serv	57	0	0	0
Cream Cheese	1 oz	100	10	6	–
French	1 oz	106	10	2	–
Fudge Topping	1 serv	201	10	7	–
Gravy Brown	1 serv	13	0	0	0
Gravy Chicken	1 serv	14	1	0	–
Gravy Country	1 serv	17	1	0	–
Honey Mustard	1 serv	160	15	8	–
Low Calorie Italian	1 oz	15	1	0	–
Marinara Sauce	1 serv	48	2	1	–
Ranch	1 oz	129	14	2	–
Ranch Fat Free	1 serv	25	tr	0	–
Sour Cream	1.5 oz	91	9	6	–
Strawberry Topping	1 serv	77	1	0	–
Syrup	3 tbsp	143	0	0	0
Syrup Sugar Free	1 serv	23	0	0	0
Tartar Sauce	1 serv	225	23	4	–
Thousand Island	1 oz	118	11	2	–
Thousand Island	2 tbsp	170	18	3	–
Whipped Margarine	1 serv	87	10	2	–
Whipped Cream	2 tbsp	23	2	0	–
SALADS					
Garden Salad w/ Albacore Tuna	1 serv	444	29	8	–
Garden Salad w/ Fried Chicken Strips	1 serv	438	26	6	–
Garden Salad w/ Grilled Chicken Breast	1 serv	264	11	5	–

FOOD	PORTION	CALS	FAT	SAT FAT	TRANS FAT
Grilled Chicken Caesar Salad w/ Dressing	1 serv	600	41	10	–
Side Caesar w/ Dressing	1 serv	362	26	7	–
Side Garden Salad w/o Dressing	1 serv	113	4	1	–
SOUPS					
Chicken Noodle	1 serv	60	2	0	–
Clam Chowder	1 serv	624	42	34	–
Cream Of Broccoli	1 serv	574	43	34	–
Vegetable Beef	1 serv	79	1	1	–

DESERT MOON CAFE
CHILDREN'S MENU SELECTIONS

FOOD	PORTION	CALS	FAT	SAT FAT	TRANS FAT
Burrito Bean & Cheese	1 serv	650	26	11	–
Kids Nachos	1 serv	500	23	9	–
Kids Taco w/ Chicken	1	280	7	3	–
Kids Taco w/ Steak	1	290	8	3	–
Kidsadilla	1 serv	630	30	15	–
MAIN MENU SELECTIONS					
Alamo Burger	1	810	51	18	–
Burrito Adobe Moon w/ Chicken	1	730	28	8	–
Burrito Adobe Moon w/ Steak	1	750	31	10	–
Burrito Black Bean w/ Chicken	1	770	25	10	–
Burrito Black Bean w/ Steak	1	790	27	12	–
Burrito Full Moon w/ Chicken	1	620	24	9	–
Burrito Full Moon w/ Steak	1	640	26	10	–
Burrito Get It Smothered	1	120	9	5	–
Burrito Harvest Wrap w/ Chicken	1	620	30	9	–
Burrito Harvest Wrap w/ Steak	1	300	33	10	–
Enchilada Mesa	1	710	27	13	–
Enchilada Queso	1	730	26	13	–
Enchilada Shrimp	1	830	28	13	–
Fajita Platter w/ Chicken	1 serv	1160	51	22	–
Fajita Platter w/ Shrimp	1 serv	1060	49	21	–
Fajita Platter w/ Steak	1 serv	1190	55	24	–
Hell Canyon Chili	1 serv	260	14	6	–
Mucho Nachos	1 serv	800	47	21	–
Mucho Nachos w/ Chicken	1 serv	900	49	21	–

FOOD	PORTION	CALS	FAT	SAT FAT	TRANS FAT
Mucho Nachos w/ Steak	1 serv	920	52	23	–
Pizza Texas BBQ	1	330	37	19	–
Quesadilla Baja Chicken	1	650	32	16	–
Quesadilla Coyote w/ Chicken	1	660	32	16	–
Quesadilla Coyote w/ Steak	1	680	35	17	–
Quesadilla Sonoran	1	660	39	17	–
Rice Bowl Black Bean w/ Chicken	1 serv	790	14	5	–
Rice Bowl Black Bean w/ Steak	1 serv	820	17	7	–
Rice Bowl Chili w/ Chicken	1 serv	760	17	7	–
Rice Bowl Chili w/ Steak	1 serv	790	20	9	–
Rice Bowl Shrimp Creole	1 serv	910	19	5	–
Shrimp Dippers	1 serv	430	15	7	–
Soup Black Bean	1 serv	360	7	3	–
Soup Tortilla	1 serv	330	13	4	–
Taco Acapulco Shrimp	1	230	9	1	–
Taco Classic w/ Chicken	1	190	6	3	–
Taco Classic w/ Steak	1	200	7	3	–
Taco Fajita w/ Chicken	1	200	6	3	–
Taco Fajita w/ Steak	1	210	8	3	–
SALAD DRESSINGS AND SAUCES					
BBQ Sauce	1 serv (1 oz)	50	1	0	–
Buffalo Wing Sauce	1 serv (1 oz)	45	5	1	–
Dressing Bleu Cheese	1 serv (2 oz)	300	32	7	–
Dressing Creamy Caesar	1 serv (2 oz)	320	36	3	–
Dressing Honey Dijon Fat Free	1 serv (2 oz)	80	0	0	0
Dressing Lite Ranch	1 serv (2 oz)	150	13	2	–
Dressing Lite Raspberry Vinaigrette	1 serv (2 oz)	150	11	2	–
Dressing Poblano	1 serv (1 oz)	150	16	3	–
Guacamole	1 serv (2 oz)	100	9	2	–
Pepper Cream Sauce	1 serv (2 oz)	100	9	5	–
Pico De Gallo	1 serv (2 oz)	15	0	0	0
Salsa Black Bean	1 serv (2 oz)	20	0	0	0
Salsa Fruit	1 serv (2 oz)	60	2	0	–
Salsa Mild Tomato	1 serv (2 oz)	15	0	0	0
Salsa Rattlesnake	1 serv (2 oz)	15	0	0	0
SALADS W/O TORTILLA BOWL					
Caesar	1 serv	530	47	9	–
Caesar w/ Chicken	1 serv	640	49	9	–

FOOD	PORTION	CALS	FAT	SAT FAT	TRANS FAT
Caesar w/ Shrimp	1 serv	570	48	9	–
Chopped Chicken	1 serv	520	35	9	–
Taco w/ Chicken	1 serv	310	15	8	–
Taco w/ Steak	1 serv	340	17	10	–

DOMINO'S PIZZA
12 INCH MEDIUM PIZZAS

FOOD	PORTION	CALS	FAT	SAT FAT	TRANS FAT
Deep Dish Cheese Only	2 slices	482	22	8	–
Hand Tossed America's Favorite Feast	1 serv	508	22	9	–
Hand Tossed Bacon Cheeseburger Feast	2 slices	549	26	12	–
Hand Tossed Barbeque Feast	2 slices	506	20	9	–
Hand Tossed Cheese Only	2 slices	375	11	5	–
Hand Tossed Deluxe Feast	2 slices	465	18	8	–
Hand Tossed ExtravaganZZa Feast	2 slices	576	27	12	–
Hand Tossed Hawaiian Feast	2 slices	450	16	7	–
Hand Tossed MeatZZa Feast	2 slices	560	26	11	–
Hand Tossed Pepperoni Feast	2 slices	534	25	11	–
Hand Tossed Vegi Feast	2 slices	439	16	7	–
Thin Crust Cheese	¼ pie	273	12	4	–
Toppings Pineapple	1 serv	12	0	0	0

DESSERTS

FOOD	PORTION	CALS	FAT	SAT FAT	TRANS FAT
Cinna Stix	1 serv	111	5	1	–
Sweet Icing	1 serv	283	5	3	–

MAIN MENU SELECTIONS

FOOD	PORTION	CALS	FAT	SAT FAT	TRANS FAT
Breadstick	1	116	4	1	–
Buffalo Chicken Kickers	1 piece	47	2	tr	–
Buffalo Wings Barbeque	1 piece	50	2	1	–
Buffalo Wings Hot	1 piece	45	2	1	–
Cheesy Bread	1 piece	142	6	2	–

TOPPINGS

FOOD	PORTION	CALS	FAT	SAT FAT	TRANS FAT
Blue Cheese	1 serv	223	23	4	–
Hot Sauce	1 serv	14	tr	0	–
Medium Pizza Anchovies	1 serv	34	1	tr	–
Medium Pizza Bacon	1 serv	102	9	3	–
Medium Pizza Banana Peppers	1 serv	5	tr	0	–
Medium Pizza Beef	1 serv	78	7	3	–
Medium Pizza Cheddar Cheese	1 serv	57	5	3	–

FOOD	PORTION	CALS	FAT	SAT FAT	TRANS FAT
Medium Pizza Extra Cheese	1 serv	49	4	2	–
Medium Pizza Green Olives	1 serv	19	2	tr	–
Medium Pizza Green Peppers	1 serv	4	tr	0	–
Medium Pizza Ham	1 serv	23	1	tr	–
Medium Pizza Italian Sausage	1 serv	77	6	2	–
Medium Pizza Mushrooms	1 serv	6	tr	tr	–
Medium Pizza Onion	1 serv	5	tr	0	–
Medium Pizza Pepperoni	1 serv	74	7	3	–
Medium Pizza Ripe Olives	1 serv	21	2	tr	–
Ranch	1 serv	197	20	3	–

DONATOS PIZZA
PIZZA

FOOD	PORTION	CALS	FAT	SAT FAT	TRANS FAT
Dessert Apple	¼ pie	722	20	4	–
Dessert Cherry	¼ pie	818	20	4	–
Original	¼ pie	660	33	14	–
Original Chicken Vegy Medley	¼ pie	500	19	8	–
Original Chicken Vegy Medley No Cheese	¼ pie	392	10	3	–
Original Founders	¼ pie	737	42	17	–
Original Hawaiian	¼ pie	620	30	10	–
Original Hawaiian No Cheese	¼ pie	411	13	2	–
Original Mariachi Beef	¼ pie	613	30	14	–
Original Mariachi Chicken	¼ pie	580	25	12	–
Original Serious Cheese	¼ pie	640	28	20	–
Original Serious Meat	¼ pie	817	47	20	–
Original Vegy	¼ pie	564	24	10	–
Original Vegy No Cheese	¼ pie	370	9	2	–
Original Works	¼ pie	729	41	17	–
Traditional Chicken Vegy Medley	¼ pie	647	17	8	–
Traditional Founders	¼ pie	900	40	17	–
Traditional Hawaiian	¼ pie	794	30	12	–
Traditional Mariachi Beef	¼ pie	797	31	15	–
Traditional Mariachi Chicken	¼ pie	770	26	13	–
Traditional Original	¼ pie	928	39	28	–
Traditional Serious Cheese	¼ pie	830	36	30	–
Traditional Serious Meat	¼ pie	977	46	20	–
Traditional Vegy	¼ pie	752	26	12	–
Traditional Works	¼ pie	892	39	17	–

FOOD	PORTION	CALS	FAT	SAT FAT	TRANS FAT
SALAD DRESSINGS					
Italian	1 serv (1.5 oz)	230	24	4	–
Italian Lite	1 serv (1.5 oz)	20	1	0	–
SALADS					
Grilled Chicken w/o Dressing	1 serv	314	18	7	–
Italian Chef w/o Dressing	1 serv	338	23	9	–
Side w/o Dressing	1 serv	106	7	3	–
SIDE ORDERS					
Breadsticks	2	220	5	1	–
Chicken Wings Hot	5	449	29	–	–
Chicken Wings Mild	5	451	29	–	–
Three Cheese Garlic Bread	1 bun	605	28	8	–
SUBS					
Big Don Italian	1 serv	705	33	10	
Big Don Lite Italian	1 serv	631	25	9	–
Grilled Chicken	1 serv	786	43	12	–
Ham & Cheese Italian	1 serv	609	22	5	–
Ham & Cheese Lite Italian	1 serv	534	14	4	–
Southwest Turkey	1 serv	710	33	7	–
Steak & Cheese	1 serv	929	52	18	–
Vegy Italian	1 serv	730	36	9	–
Vegy Lite Italian	1 serv	661	28	8	–

DUNKIN' DONUTS
BAGELS AND CREAM CHEESE

FOOD	PORTION	CALS	FAT	SAT FAT	TRANS FAT
Bagel Blueberry	1	330	3	1	0
Bagel Cinnamon Raisin	1	330	3	1	0
Bagel Everything	1	370	6	1	0
Bagel Harvest	1	350	6	1	0
Bagel Onion	1	320	4	1	0
Bagel Plain	1	320	3	1	0
Bagel Poppyseed	1	370	7	1	0
Bagel Reduced Carb w/ Cheese	1	380	12	5	0
Bagel Salsa	1	310	3	1	0
Bagel Salt	1	370	3	1	0
Bagel Sesame	1	380	8	1	0
Bagel Wheat	1	330	4	1	0
Cream Cheese Chive	2 oz	170	17	11	0
Cream Cheese Garden Vegetable	2 oz	170	15	11	0

FOOD	PORTION	CALS	FAT	SAT FAT	TRANS FAT
Cream Cheese Lite	2 oz	110	9	7	0
Cream Cheese Plain	2 oz	190	17	13	0
Cream Cheese Salmon	2 oz	170	17	11	0
Cream Cheese Strawberry	2 oz	190	17	9	0
BAKED SELECTIONS					
Biscuit	1	250	13	4	8
Bismark Chocolate Iced	1	340	15	4	2
Coffee Roll	1	270	14	3	0
Coffee Roll Chocolate Frosted	1	290	15	3	1
Coffee Roll Maple Frosted	1	290	14	3	0
Coffee Roll Vanilla Frosted	1	290	14	3	0
Cookie Chocolate Chunk	2	220	11	7	0
Cookie Chocolate Chunk w/ Walnuts	2	230	12	6	0
Cookie Oatmeal Raisin Pecan	2	220	10	5	0
Cookie White Chocolate Chunk	2	230	12	7	0
Croissant Plain	1	330	18	5	7
Danish Apple	1	330	20	9	0
Danish Cheese	1	340	22	10	0
Danish Strawberry Cheese	1	320	20	9	0
Donut Apple Crumb	1	230	10	3	1
Donut Apple Crumb Cake	1	290	15	13	1
Donut Apple N' Spice	1	200	8	2	3
Donut Bavarian Kreme	1	210	9	2	3
Donut Black Raspberry	1	210	8	2	4
Donut Blueberry	1	290	16	4	3
Donut Blueberry Crumb	1	240	10	3	1
Donut Boston Kreme	1	240	9	2	4
Donut Bow Tie	1	300	17	4	5
Donut Chocolate Coconut	1	300	19	6	5
Donut Chocolate Frosted	1	360	20	5	5
Donut Chocolate Glazed	1	290	16	4	4
Donut Chocolate Kreme Filled	1	270	13	3	4
Donut Cinnamon	1	330	20	5	4
Donut Double Chocolate	1	310	17	4	5
Donut Frosted Lemon	1	240	14	4	3
Donut Glazed	1	180	8	2	4
Donut Glazed Gingerbread	1	260	11	3	4
Donut Glazed Lemon	1	240	14	4	3

FOOD	PORTION	CALS	FAT	SAT FAT	TRANS FAT
Donut Jelly Filled	1	210	8	2	4
Donut Lemon Burst	1	300	14	5	3
Donut Maple Frosted	1	210	9	2	3
Donut Marble Frosted	1	200	9	2	3
Donut Old Fashioned	1	300	19	5	4
Donut Powdered	1	330	19	5	4
Donut Strawberry	1	210	8	2	4
Donut Strawberry Frosted	1	210	9	2	3
Donut Sugar Raised	1	170	8	2	1
Donut Vanilla Kreme Filled	1	270	13	3	4
Donut Whole Wheat Glazed	1	310	19	4	4
Eclair	1	270	11	3	1
English Muffin	1	160	2	0	0
French Cruller	1	150	8	2	3
Fritter Apple	1	300	14	3	3
Fritter Glazed	1	260	14	3	3
Muffin Banana Walnut	1	540	25	4	0
Muffin Blueberry	1	470	17	3	0
Muffin Chocolate Chip	1	630	26	8	0
Muffin Coffee Cake	1	580	19	3	0
Muffin Corn	1	510	18	4	0
Muffin Cranberry Orange	1	440	17	3	0
Muffin Honey Bran Raisin	1	480	15	3	0
Muffin Reduced Fat Blueberry	1	400	5	2	0
Munchkins Chocolate Glazed	3	200	10	2	5
Munchkins Cinnamon	4	270	19	4	4
Munchkins Glazed	3	280	13	3	4
Munchkins Jelly Filled	5	210	9	2	3
Munchkins Lemon Filled	4	170	8	2	3
Munchkins Plain	4	270	16	4	4
Munchkins Powdered	4	270	14	4	4
Munchkins Sugar Raised	7	220	12	3	1
Stick Cinnamon	1	450	30	7	5
Stick Glazed	1	490	29	7	5
Stick Glazed Chocolate	1	470	29	7	5
Stick Jelly	1	530	29	7	5
Stick Plain	1	420	29	7	5
Stick Powdered	1	450	29	7	5
BEVERAGES					
Cappuccino	1 (10 oz)	60	5	3	0

FOOD	PORTION	CALS	FAT	SAT FAT	TRANS FAT
Cappuccino w/ Soy Milk	1 (10 oz)	70	3	0	0
Cappuccino w/ Soy Milk Sugar	1 (10 oz)	120	3	0	0
Cappuccino w/ Sugar	1 (10 oz)	130	4	3	0
Coffee Blueberry	1 (10 oz)	20	0	0	0
Coffee Caramel	1 (10 oz)	20	0	0	0
Coffee Chocolate	1 (10 oz)	20	0	0	0
Coffee Cinnamon	1 (10 oz)	20	0	0	0
Coffee Coconut	1 (10 oz)	20	0	0	0
Coffee French Vanilla	1 (10 oz)	20	0	0	0
Coffee Hazelnut	1 (10 oz)	20	0	0	0
Coffee Marshmallow	1 (10 oz)	20	0	0	0
Coffee Regular	1 (10 oz)	15	0	0	0
Coffee Toasted Almond	1 (10 oz)	20	0	0	0
Coffee w/ Cream	1 (10 oz)	70	6	4	0
Coffee w/ Cream Sugar	1 (10 oz)	120	6	4	0
Coffee w/ Milk	1 (10 oz)	35	1	1	0
Coffee w/ Milk Sugar	1 (10 oz)	80	1	1	0
Coffee w/ Skim Milk	1 (10 oz)	25	0	0	0
Coffee w/ Skim Milk Sugar	1 (10 oz)	70	0	0	0
Coffee w/ Sugar	1 (10 oz)	60	0	0	0
Coolatta Lemonade	1 (16 oz)	240	0	0	0
Coolatta Strawberry Fruit	1 (16 oz)	290	0	0	0
Coolatta Tropicana Orange	1 (16 oz)	370	0	0	0
Coolatta Vanilla Bean	1 (16 oz)	440	17	15	1
Coolatta Coffee w/ 2% Milk	1 (16 oz)	190	2	2	0
Coolatta Coffee w/ Cream	1 (16 oz)	350	22	14	0
Coolatta Coffee w/ Milk	1 (16 oz)	210	4	3	0
Coolatta Coffee w/ Skim Milk	1 (16 oz)	170	0	0	0
Dunkaccino	1 (10 oz)	230	10	3	5
Espresso	1 (2 oz)	0	0	0	0
Espresso w/ Sugar	1 (2 oz)	30	0	0	0
Hot Chocolate	1 (10 oz)	220	8	2	4
Ice Coffee w/ Milk	1 (16 oz)	35	1	1	0
Iced Coffee	1 (16 oz)	15	0	0	0
Iced Coffee w/ Cream	1 (16 oz)	70	6	4	0
Iced Coffee w/ Cream Sugar	1 (16 oz)	120	6	4	0
Iced Coffee w/ Milk Sugar	1 (16 oz)	80	1	1	0
Iced Coffee w/ Skim Milk	1 (16 oz)	25	0	0	0
Iced Coffee w/ Skim Milk Sugar	1 (16 oz)	70	0	0	0
Iced Coffee w/ Sugar	1 (16 oz)	60	0	0	0

FOOD	PORTION	CALS	FAT	SAT FAT	TRANS FAT
Iced Latte	1 (16 oz)	120	7	4	0
Iced Latte Caramel Creme	1 (16 oz)	260	9	6	0
Iced Latte Caramel Swirl	1 (16 oz)	240	7	4	0
Iced Latte Caramel Swirl w/ Skim Milk	1 (16 oz)	180	0	0	0
Iced Latte Lite	1 (16 oz)	80	0	0	0
Iced Latte Mocha Almond	1 (16 oz)	290	10	7	0
Iced Latte Mocha Swirl	1 (16 oz)	240	8	5	0
Iced Latte Mocha Swirl w/ Skim Milk	1 (16 oz)	180	1	1	0
Iced Latte w/ Skim Milk	1 (16 oz)	70	0	0	0
Iced Latte w/ Skim Milk Sugar	1 (16 oz)	120	0	0	0
Iced Latte w/ Sugar	1 (16 oz)	170	7	4	0
Latte	1 (10 oz)	120	6	4	0
Latte Caramel Creme	1 (10 oz)	260	9	6	0
Latte Caramel Swirl	1 (10 oz)	230	6	4	0
Latte Caramel Swirl w/ Soy Milk	1 (10 oz)	210	4	0	0
Latte Lite	1 (10 oz)	70	0	0	0
Latte Mocha Almond	1 (10 oz)	290	10	7	0
Latte Mocha Swirl	1 (10 oz)	230	7	4	0
Latte Mocha Swirl w/ Soy Milk	1 (10 oz)	210	5	1	0
Latte w/ Soy Milk	1 (10 oz)	90	4	0	0
Latte w/ Soy Milk Sugar	1 (10 oz)	150	4	1	0
Latte w/ Sugar	1 (10 oz)	160	6	4	0
Smoothie Mango Passion Fruits	1 (16 oz)	360	3	2	0
Smoothie Strawberry Banana	1 (16 oz)	360	3	2	0
Smoothie Wildberry	1 (16 oz)	360	3	2	0
Tea Regular Or Decaffeinated	1 (10 oz)	0	0	0	0
Tea w/ Milk	1 (10 oz)	25	1	1	0
Tea w/ Milk Sugar	1 (10 oz)	70	1	1	0
Tea w/ Skim Milk	1 (10 oz)	25	0	0	0
Tea w/ Skim Milk Sugar	1 (10 oz)	60	0	0	0
Tea w/ Sugar	1 (10 oz)	50	0	0	0
Turbo Ice	1 (16 oz)	120	7	4	0
Vanilla Chai	1 (10 oz)	230	8	6	0
SANDWICHES					
Bagel Bacon Egg Cheese	1	540	18	7	0
Bagel Egg Cheese	1	470	15	6	0

FOOD	PORTION	CALS	FAT	SAT FAT	TRANS FAT
Bagel Ham Egg Cheese	1	510	16	6	0
Bagel Sausage Egg Cheese	1	660	35	13	1
Biscuit Egg Cheese	1	410	25	9	7
Biscuit Sausage Egg Cheese	1	610	43	14	7
Croissant Bacon Egg Cheese	1	520	33	10	7
Croissant Egg Cheese	1	550	34	11	7
Croissant Ham Egg Cheese	1	520	32	10	7
Croissant Sausage Egg Cheese	1	490	51	17	7
English Muffin Bacon Egg Cheese	1	360	16	6	0
English Muffin Egg Cheese	1	280	9	5	0
English Muffin Ham Egg Cheese	1	310	10	5	0
English Muffin Sausage Egg Cheese	1	530	32	12	1
Panini Meatball	1	480	19	9	0
Panini Southwestern Chicken	1	420	10	5	0
Panini Steak	1	450	12	5	1

EDDIE'S PIZZA

Bar Pie	1 pie	350	11	–	–
Bar Pie No Fat Cheese	1 pie	270	1	–	–

EINSTEIN BROS BAGELS
BAGELS AND BREADS

Bagel Asiago Cheese	1	360	3	2	–
Bagel Cranberry Special	1	350	1	0	–
Bagel Egg	1	340	3	1	–
Bagel Honey Whole Wheat	1	320	1	0	–
Bagel Jalapeno	1	330	1	0	–
Bagel Lucky Green	1	320	1	0	–
Bagel Mango	1	360	1	0	–
Bagel Marble Rye	1	340	2	0	–
Bagel Potato	1	350	5	1	–
Bagel Power	1	410	5	1	–
Bagel Power w/ Peanut Butter	1	750	34	6	–
Bagel Pumpkin	1	330	2	0	–
Bagel Roasted Red Pepper & Pesto	1	410	7	4	–
Bagel Six Cheese	1	390	6	3	–
Bagel Spicy Nacho	1	450	9	5	–

FOOD	PORTION	CALS	FAT	SAT FAT	TRANS FAT
Bagel Spinach Florentine	1	410	7	4	–
Bagel Croutons	¼ cup	25	1	0	–
Bagel Twist	1	220	4	2	–
Bread Ciabatta	1 serv	320	3	1	–
Chocolate Chip	1	370	3	2	–
Chopped Garlic	1	380	3	1	–
Chopped Onion	1	330	1	0	–
Cinnamon Raisin Swirl	1	350	1	0	–
Cinnamon Sugar	1	330	1	0	–
Dark Pumpernickel	1	320	1	0	–
Everything	1	340	2	0	–
Focaccia Cheese Pizza	1 serv	500	11	7	–
Focaccia Margherita	1 serv	400	17	2	–
Focaccia Pepperoni Pizza	1 serv	590	19	10	–
Nutty Banana	1	360	3	1	–
Plain	1	320	1	0	–
Poppy Dip'd	1	350	2	0	–
Roll Challah	1	300	5	1	–
Salt	1	330	1	0	–
Sesame Dip'd	1	380	5	1	–
Sun Dried Tomato	1	320	1	0	–
Wild Blueberry	1	350	1	0	–
BEVERAGES					
Americano	1 reg	1	0	0	0
Cafe Latte	1 reg	140	5	4	–
Cafe Latte Nonfat	1 reg	100	0	0	0
Cappuccino	1 reg	90	4	2	–
Cappuccino Nonfat	1 reg	60	0	0	0
Chai 2% Milk	1 reg	210	2	2	–
Chai Skim Milk	1 reg	190	0	0	0
Coffee	1 reg	0	0	0	0
Espresso	1 reg	1	0	0	0
Half & Half	2 tbsp	40	3	2	–
Hot Chocolate	1 reg	290	11	8	–
Hot Chocolate Lower Fat	1 reg	260	7	6	–
Hot Tea All Flavors	1 cup	0	0	0	0
Iced Americano	1 serv	1	0	0	0
Iced Coffee	1 serv	0	0	0	0
Iced Latte	1 serv	120	5	3	–
Iced Latte Nonfat	1 serv	90	0	0	0

FOOD	PORTION	CALS	FAT	SAT FAT	TRANS FAT
Iced Mocha	1 serv	210	6	4	–
Iced Mocha Low Fat	1 serv	180	3	2	–
Mocha	1 reg	230	6	5	–
Mocha Low Fat	1 reg	190	3	2	–
DESSERTS					
Brownie Iced	1	550	24	6	–
Brownie Iced w/ Walnuts	1	600	29	6	–
Cherry Figure 8	1	400	18	6	–
Cinnamon Roll	1	810	32	9	–
Cookie Chocolate Chunk	1	640	31	10	–
Cookie Oatmeal Raisin	1	600	27	6	–
Cookie Peanut Butter	1	640	34	7	–
Muffin Banana Nut	1	640	32	4	–
Muffin Blueberry	1	540	22	4	–
Muffin Chocolate Chip	1	620	27	8	–
Pound Cake Lemon Iced	1 slice	540	25	13	–
Pound Cake Marble	1 slice	460	24	12	–
Rice Krispy Bar	1	420	8	2	–
Scone Blueberry w/ Icing	1	450	18	8	–
Scone Lemon Currant	1	430	15	5	–
Strudel Cinnamon Walnut	1 piece	550	31	11	–
Sweetie Pie	1	620	20	2	–
SALAD DRESSINGS					
Asian Sesame	2 tbsp	80	2	0	–
Caesar	2 tbsp	150	16	3	–
Chipotle Vinaigrette	2 tbsp	110	10	2	–
Horseradish Sauce	2 tbsp	170	18	3	–
Raspberry Vinaigrette	2 tbsp	160	14	2	–
Thousand Island	2 tbsp	110	9	20	–
SALADS					
Asian Chicken	1 serv (14.5 oz)	550	9	2	–
Bros Bistro	1 serv (9.5 oz)	520	43	10	–
Chicken Caesar	1 serv (12.5 oz)	750	53	11	–
Chicken Chipotle	1 serv	710	43	9	–
Chicken Salad On Greens	1 serv (10.5 oz)	210	9	2	–
Egg	1 serv (4 oz)	200	17	4	–
Fresh Fruit Cup	1 serv (8 oz)	110	1	0	–
Mixed Greens	1 serv (3.5 oz)	228	18	3	–
Potato	½ cup	290	21	3	–
Tuna Salad On Greens	1 serv (10.5 oz)	170	5	1	–

FOOD	PORTION	CALS	FAT	SAT FAT	TRANS FAT
SANDWICHES					
12 Grain Bread Deli Chicken Salad	1	440	13	2	–
12 Grain Bread Deli Egg Salad	1	490	21	4	–
12 Grain Bread Deli Ham	1	560	25	7	–
12 Grain Bread Deli Roast Beef	1	560	24	7	–
12 Grain Bread Deli Smoked Turkey	1	530	21	6	–
12 Grain Bread Deli Tuna Salad	1	440	13	2	–
12 Grain Bread Deli Turkey Pastrami	1	540	21	6	–
12 Grain Bread Ultimate Toasted Cheese w/ Tomato	1	870	50	25	–
Bagel Chicken Salad	1	500	10	2	–
Bagel Egg Bacon	1	580	19	7	–
Bagel Egg Ham	1	530	13	5	–
Bagel Egg Salad	1	560	18	5	–
Bagel Egg Sausage	1	550	14	5	–
Bagel Ham	1	450	6	2	–
Bagel Holey Cow	1	900	50	13	–
Bagel Hummus & Feta	1	540	13	4	–
Bagel New York Lox	1	660	27	19	–
Bagel Original	1	480	10	4	–
Bagel Roast Beef	1	460	4	2	–
Bagel Rueben Deli	1	660	19	6	–
Bagel Salmon & Shmear	1	650	22	12	–
Bagel Sante Fe	1	650	24	8	–
Bagel Smoked Turkey	1	420	2	0	–
Bagel Tasty Turkey	1	570	15	9	–
Bagel The Veg Out	1	490	13	7	–
Bagel Tuna Salad	1	470	6	2	–
Bagel Turkey Pastrami	1	440	2	0	–
Challah BBQ Chicken	1	380	8	2	–
Challah Club Mex	1	750	45	14	–
Challah Cobbie	1	630	33	12	–
Challah Deli Chicken Salad	1	480	14	3	–
Challah Deli Egg Salad	1	430	20	5	–
Challah Deli Pastrami	1	480	21	7	–
Challah Deli Roast Beef	1	500	23	8	–

FOOD	PORTION	CALS	FAT	SAT FAT	TRANS FAT
Challah Deli Smoked Turkey	1	470	21	7	–
Challah Deli Tuna Salad	1	370	10	3	–
Challah Deli Turkey Ham	1	500	25	8	–
Challah Roasted Chicken & Smoked Gouda	1	440	13	6	–
Chicago Bagel Dog Asiago	1	740	34	15	–
Chicago Bagel Dog Chili Cheese	1	810	38	17	–
Chicago Bagel Dog Everything	1	730	34	12	–
Chicago Bagel Dog Onion w/o Cheese	1	680	30	12	–
Country White Deli Chicken Salad	1	540	15	4	–
Country White Deli Egg Salad	1	590	23	6	–
Country White Deli Ham	1	660	27	9	–
Country White Deli Roast Beef	1	660	26	9	–
Country White Deli Smoked Turkey	1	630	23	8	–
Country White Deli Tuna Salad	1	510	11	3	–
Country White Deli Turkey Pastrami	1	640	23	8	–
Country White Ultimate Toasted Cheese w/ Tomato	1	870	51	26	–
Panini Cali Club	1	730	24	9	–
Panini Cuban Ham	1	700	31	11	–
Panini Denver Omelet Breakfast	1	740	33	13	–
Panini Italian Chicken	1	770	36	13	–
Panini Taos Turkey	1	740	25	9	–
Panini Ultimate Toasted Cheese	1	900	44	24	–
Roll Ups Albuquerque Turkey	1	790	39	15	–
Roll Ups Thai Vegetable	1	630	21	2	–
Roll Ups Thai Vegetable w/ Chicken	1	670	18	1	–
SOUPS					
Broccoli Sharp Cheddar	1 cup	230	15	8	–
Chicken & Wild Rice	1 cup	190	4	1	–
Chicken Noodle	1 cup	220	9	3	–
Clam Chowda	1 cup	160	11	6	–
Minestroni Low Fat	1 cup	180	3	1	–

FOOD	PORTION	CALS	FAT	SAT FAT	TRANS FAT
Tomato Bisque	1 cup	190	10	3	–
Tortilla	1 cup	90	3	0	–
Turkey Chili	1 cup	140	5	1	–
SPREADS					
Butter	1 tbsp	100	11	8	–
Butter & Margarine Blend	1 tbsp	60	7	2	–
Cream Cheese Blueberry	1 tbsp	70	5	4	–
Cream Cheese Cappuccino	2 tbsp	70	5	4	–
Cream Cheese Garden Vegetable	2 tbsp	60	5	4	–
Cream Cheese Honey Almond Reduced Fat	2 tbsp	70	5	3	–
Cream Cheese Jalapeno Salsa	1 tbsp	60	5	3	–
Cream Cheese Maple Walnut Raisin	2 tbsp	60	5	4	–
Cream Cheese Onion & Chive	2 tbsp	70	6	4	–
Cream Cheese Plain	2 tbsp	60	7	5	–
Cream Cheese Plain Reduced Fat	2 tbsp	60	5	4	–
Cream Cheese Pumpkin	2 tbsp	100	8	6	–
Cream Cheese Smoked Salmon	2 tbsp	60	5	4	–
Cream Cheese Strawberry	2 tbsp	70	5	4	–
Cream Cheese Sun Dried Tomato & Basil	2 tbsp	60	5	4	–
Fruit Spread Apricot	1 serv	75	0	0	0
Fruit Spread Grape	1 serv (1 oz)	75	0	0	0
Fruit Spread Strawberry	1 serv (1 oz)	75	0	0	0
Honey Butter	1 tbsp	90	8	4	–
Hummus	1 serv	110	7	1	–
Mayo Ancho Lime	1 tbsp	50	5	1	–
Mustard French Dijon	1 tsp	10	0	0	0
Mustard Grain Dijon	1 tsp	5	0	0	0
Mustard Honey	1 tsp	15	0	0	0
Mustard Raspberry	2 tbsp	50	2	0	–
Mustard Yellow	1 tbsp	5	0	0	0
Peanut Butter	2 tbsp	190	15	2	–
Salsa Ancho Lime	¼ cup	20	1	0	–

FOOD	PORTION	CALS	FAT	SAT FAT	TRANS FAT
EL POLLO LOCO					
DESSERTS					
Caramel Flan	1 serv (5.5 oz)	290	12	10	0
Churros	2	300	18	4	1
Cone Vanilla	1	330	8	5	0
Soft Serve Vanilla	1 cup (5 oz)	300	8	5	0
MAIN MENU SELECTIONS					
BBQ Black Beans	1 serv (6 oz)	200	3	0	0
Bowl The Original Pollo	1 serv	540	4	1	0
Burrito BRC	1 (7.5 oz)	390	10	5	0
Burrito Classic Chicken	1 (10.3 oz)	500	14	6	0
Burrito Twice Grilled	1 (15 oz)	830	37	18	0
Burrito Ultimate Grilled	1 (13.6 oz)	650	20	8	0
Chicken Breast	1 (4.3 oz)	220	9	3	0
Chicken Breast Skinless	1 (4 oz)	180	4	1	0
Chicken Leg	1 (1.8 oz)	90	4	1	0
Chicken Thigh	1 (3.1 oz)	220	15	5	0
Chicken Wing	1 (1.3 oz)	90	5	2	0
Cole Slaw	1 serv (6 oz)	120	9	2	0
Corn Cobbette	1 (5 oz)	90	1	0	0
French Fries	1 serv (5.5 oz)	440	21	4	0
Fresh Vegetables w/ Margarine	1 serv (4.1 oz)	60	3	0	0
Fresh Vegetables w/o Margarine	1 serv (4 oz)	35	0	0	0
Gravy	1 serv (1 oz)	10	0	0	0
Loco Nachos	1 serv	170	14	3	0
Macaroni & Cheese	1 serv (5.5 oz)	280	17	11	0
Mashed Potatoes	1 serv (5 oz)	100	1	0	0
Pinto Beans	1 serv (6 oz)	140	0	0	0
Quesadilla Cheese	1 (4.5 oz)	420	23	13	0
Refried Beans w/ Cheese	1 serv (6.3 oz)	270	7	2	0
Skinless Breast Meal	1 serv	310	12	5	0
Soup Chicken Tortilla w/o Tortilla Strips	1 serv (10 oz)	140	6	2	0
Spanish Rice	1 serv (4.5 oz)	160	1	0	0
Taco Al Carbon	1 (3.1 oz)	150	5	2	0
Taco Soft Chicken	1 (4.5 oz)	270	13	6	0
Taquito Chicken	1	190	9	2	0
Tortilla Chips	1 serv (1.5 oz)	210	10	2	0

FOOD	PORTION	CALS	FAT	SAT FAT	TRANS FAT
Tortilla Corn 6 Inches	2	120	2	0	0
Tortilla Flour 6.5 Inches	2	210	7	3	0
SALAD DRESSINGS AND TOPPINGS					
Creamy Cilantro	1 serv (1.5 oz)	220	23	4	0
Creamy Cilantro Light	1 pkg	70	5	1	0
Guacamole	1 serv (1 oz)	45	4	1	0
Hot Sauce Jalapeno	1 pkg	5	0	0	0
Jack & Poblano Queso	1 serv (1.8 oz)	100	8	5	0
Ketchup	1 pkg	10	0	0	0
Light Italian	1 pkg	20	1	0	0
Pico De Gallo Medium	1 serv (1 oz)	10	1	0	0
Ranch	1 pkg	230	24	4	0
Salsa Avocado Hot	1 serv (1 oz)	30	3	0	0
Salsa Chipotle Hot	1 serv (1 oz)	5	0	0	0
Salsa House Mild	1 serv (1 oz)	5	0	0	0
Sour Cream	1 serv (1 oz)	60	5	4	0
Thousand Island	1 pkg	220	21	3	0
SALADS					
Caesar Pollo	1 (11.4 oz)	520	38	7	0
Ceasar Pollo w/o Dressing	1 (9.4 oz)	220	7	2	0
Garden	1 (4.8 oz)	120	4	0	0
Tostada Chicken	1 (17.3 oz)	840	40	11	0
Tostada Chicken w/o Shell	1 (14.7 oz)	410	11	6	0

FAZOLI'S
BEVERAGES

FOOD	PORTION	CALS	FAT	SAT FAT	TRANS FAT
Lemon Ice All Flavors	1	360	0	0	0
Lemon Ice Original	1 reg	180	0	0	0
Lemon Ice Strawberry	1	320	0	0	0
CHILDREN'S MENU SELECTIONS					
Fettuccine Alfredo	1 serv	290	5	2	0
Meat Lasagna	1 serv	260	13	6	0
Ravioli w/ Marinara	1 serv	290	7	4	0
Spaghetti w/ Meat Sauce	1 serv	300	4	1	0
Spaghetti w/ Meatballs	1 serv	350	7	3	0
Ziti w/ Meat Sauce	1 serv	190	6	3	0
DESSERTS					
Cheesecake Original	1 slice	290	22	14	0
Cheesecake Turtle	1 slice	450	28	16	0
Cookie Chocolate Chunk	1	510	26	15	0

FOOD	PORTION	CALS	FAT	SAT FAT	TRANS FAT
MAIN MENU SELECTIONS					
Breadstick	1	100	2	0	0
Breadstick Garlic	1	150	7	2	0
Fettuccine Alfredo	1 sm	520	12	4	0
Fettuccine w/ Marinara	1 serv	450	3	0	0
Fettuccine w/ Meat Sauce	1 serv	500	7	2	0
Oven Baked Chicken Parmesan	1 serv	960	33	11	1
Oven Baked Meat Lasagna	1 serv	510	25	12	0
Oven Baked Rigatoni Romano	1 serv	1090	54	20	1
Oven Baked Spaghetti	1 serv	680	22	9	1
Oven Baked Spaghetti w/ Meatballs	1 serv	940	40	17	1
Panini Four Cheese & Tomato	1	510	22	12	1
Panini Grilled Chicken	1	540	18	5	0
Panini Smoked Turkey	1	620	29	11	0
Penne w/ Alfredo	1 serv	520	12	4	0
Penne w/ Marinara	1 serv	450	3	0	0
Penne w/ Meat Sauce	1 serv	500	7	2	0
Pizza Slice Cheese	1	270	11	4	1
Pizza Slice Pepperoni	1	310	14	5	1
Platter Classic Sampler	1	810	25	10	0
Platter Ultimate Sampler	1	980	29	12	0
Ravioli w/ Marinara	1 serv	500	15	8	0
Ravioli w/ Meat Sauce	1 serv	550	20	10	0
Spaghetti w/ Alfredo	1 serv	520	12	4	0
Spaghetti w/ Marinara	1 sm	450	3	0	0
Spaghetti w/ Meat Sauce	1 sm	500	7	2	0
Submarinos Club	half	973	34	10	0
Submarinos Ham n' Swiss	1	680	30	9	0
Submarinos Italian Beef	half	660	24	9	0
Submarinos Original	half	940	58	17	0
Topping Broccoli	1 serv	25	0	0	0
Topping Broccoli & Tomatoes	1 serv	30	0	0	0
Topping Garlic Shrimp	1 serv	160	12	3	0
Topping Italian Sausage	1 serv	240	21	7	0
Topping Meatballs	1 serv	160	18	8	0
Topping Peppery Chicken	1 serv	70	1	0	0
Ziti w/ Meat Sauce	1 serv	480	15	6	1
SALAD DRESSINGS					
Caesar	1 serv	220	25	4	0

FOOD	PORTION	CALS	FAT	SAT FAT	TRANS FAT
Fat Free Honey Mustard	1 serv	60	0	0	0
Fat Free Italian	1 serv	25	0	0	0
Honey French	1 serv	220	18	3	0
Italian	1 serv	160	14	2	0
Ranch	1 serv	220	24	4	0
Ranch Lite	1 serv	120	12	2	0
SALADS					
Chicken & Fruit	1	220	2	0	0
Chicken & Pasta Caesar	1	440	15	4	0
Chicken BLT Ranch	1	270	10	4	0
Parmesan Chicken	1	360	15	5	0
Side Caesar	1	40	2	1	0
Side Garden	1	25	0	0	0
Side Pasta	1 serv	320	12	3	0
FRESHENS					
PRETZELS					
Bites	1 serv (3 oz)	255	3	tr	–
Gourmet	1 (6 oz)	510	6	1	–
SMOOTHIES					
Berry Berry	1 serv (21 oz)	280	tr	–	–
Blueberry Breeze	1 serv (21 oz)	396	1	–	–
Caribbean Craze	1 serv (21 oz)	315	tr	–	–
Cayman Cooler	1 serv (21 oz)	320	tr	–	–
Club Trim	1 serv (21 oz)	291	0	0	0
Fitness Fuel	1 serv (21 oz)	521	5	–	–
Immune Support	1 serv (21 oz)	377	3	–	–
Jamaican Jammer	1 serv (21 oz)	378	1	–	–
Maui Mango	1 serv (21 oz)	354	tr	–	–
Mocha Coffee	1 serv (21 oz)	385	3	–	–
Mystic Mango	1 serv (21 oz)	407	3	–	–
Orange Shooter	1 serv (21 oz)	330	3	–	–
Orange Sunrise	1 serv (21 oz)	367	3	–	–
Peach Sunset	1 serv (21 oz)	388	tr	–	–
Peachy Pineapple	1 serv (21 oz)	415	1	–	–
Peanut Butter Chocolate	1 serv (21 oz)	312	20	–	–
Pina Colada	1 serv (21 oz)	451	4	–	–
Pineapple Passion	1 serv (21 oz)	389	4	–	–
Raspberry Royale	1 serv (21 oz)	346	tr	–	–
Rockin' Raspberry	1 serv (21 oz)	332	tr	–	–

FOOD	PORTION	CALS	FAT	SAT FAT	TRANS FAT
Strawberry Shooter	1 serv (21 oz)	251	tr	–	–
Strawberry Squeeze	1 serv (21 oz)	313	1	–	–
Vanilla Coffee	1 serv (21 oz)	438	3	–	–
Vanilla Fudge	1 serv (21 oz)	275	17	–	–

FRUITFULL
BREADS

FOOD	PORTION	CALS	FAT	SAT FAT	TRANS FAT
Almond Cherry	½ slice	226	11	2	–
Apple Spice	½ slice	186	7	1	–
Banana	½ slice	165	6	1	–
Cappuccino Chocolate Chip	½ slice	229	13	3	0
Carrot	½ slice	190	9	1	–
Chocolate	½ slice	120	0	0	0
Lemon Blueberry	½ slice	120	0	0	0
Old Fashion Pound Cake	½ slice	227	13	3	–
Orange Cranberry	½ slice	130	0	0	0
Pumpkin	½ slice	150	0	0	0
Sweet Potato	½ slice	176	6	1	–
Zucchini	½ slice	190	9	1	–

DIPS

FOOD	PORTION	CALS	FAT	SAT FAT	TRANS FAT
Banana Cream	1 serv (4.5 oz)	250	15	11	0
Banana Split	1 serv (4.5 oz)	290	16	12	0
Cherry Cream	1 serv (4.5 oz)	280	15	11	0
Coconut Cream	1 serv (4.5 oz)	300	15	7	0
Mud Pie	1 serv (4.5 oz)	380	24	17	0
Strawberry Cream	1 serv (4.5 oz)	270	16	12	0

FROZEN BARS

FOOD	PORTION	CALS	FAT	SAT FAT	TRANS FAT
Cream Banana	1	110	3	2	–
Cream Coconut	1	130	5	4	0
Cream Peaches 'n' Cream	1	150	5	4	0
Cream Pina Colada	1	90	3	2	0
Cream Raspberry Cream	1	110	3	2	0
Cream Strawberry Cream	1	110	3	1	0
Happy Indulgence Berry Cobbler	1	200	8	5	0
Happy Indulgence Key Lime Pie	1	220	8	5	0
Happy Indulgence Peach Cobbler	1	170	8	3	0
Juice Fuzzy Navel	1	70	0	0	0

FOOD	PORTION	CALS	FAT	SAT FAT	TRANS FAT
Juice Green Tea Melon	1	90	0	0	0
Juice Guava	1	70	0	0	0
Juice Lemon	1	90	0	0	0
Juice Lime	1	80	0	0	0
Juice Passionate Cherry	1	80	0	0	0
Juice Pineapple	1	80	0	0	0
Juice Raspberry	1	70	0	0	0
Juice Strawberry	1	70	0	0	0
Juice Tamarind	1	90	0	0	0
Juice Tropical Splash	1	80	0	0	0
Juice Watermelon	1	60	0	0	0
Yogurt Blueberry	1	120	0	0	0
Yogurt Chocolate	1	160	0	0	0
Yogurt Vanilla	1	140	0	0	0
SMOOTHIES					
Berry Berry Best	1 (4 oz)	160	2	1	–
Make Mine Mango	4 oz	160	0	0	0
Strawberry Ana Banana	4 oz	120	1	0	–
SNACKS					
All About Almonds	1 pkg (1 oz)	170	15	1	0
Buzzworthy Banana	1 pkg (1.1 oz)	140	8	3	0
Calypso Cashews	1 pkg (1.1 oz)	170	13	2	0
Chocolate Twisted Bliss	1 pkg (1.4 oz)	190	8	6	0
Debbie Loves Fruit	1 pkg (1 oz)	110	2	2	0
Got Nuts?	1 pkg (1.1 oz)	180	13	1	0
Hit The Road Jack	1 pkg (1.1 oz)	130	6	1	0
Honey I Ate The Peanuts	1 pkg (1 oz)	160	12	2	0
Jamaican Me Crazy Cranberry Mix	1 pkg (1.1 oz)	100	0	0	0
Judy's Apple Crisps	1 pkg (1 oz)	140	7	1	0
Nacho Chips They're Mine	1 pkg (1.1 oz)	120	2	1	0
Nature Lover's Choice	1 pkg (1.1 oz)	140	7	1	0
Power Pistachios	1 pkg (1.1 oz)	100	9	2	0
Reggae Rice Crackers	1 pkg (1.1 oz)	120	0	0	0
Rockin' Raisins	1 pkg (1.4 oz)	170	7	4	0
Rocky Mountain Munch	1 pkg (1.1 oz)	120	4	2	0
Sour Wiggle Giggle	1 pkg (1.5 oz)	150	0	0	0
Soy Glad You're Healthy	1 pkg (1.1 oz)	160	10	2	0
Survivor Snacks	1 pkg (1.1 oz)	140	8	1	0
Swinging Sesame Stix	1 pkg (1.1 oz)	180	13	2	0

FOOD	PORTION	CALS	FAT	SAT FAT	TRANS FAT
Tammy's Flax Snacks	1 pkg (1.1 oz)	170	13	2	0
Whassup Wasabi!	1 pkg (1.1 oz)	150	7	1	0
Yogurt Twisted Bliss	1 pkg (1.4 oz)	190	8	6	0
You've Got Trail	1 pkg (1.1 oz)	150	8	3	0
Yummy Gummy In My Tummy	1 pkg (1.4 oz)	150	0	0	0
Zydeco Cajun Mix	1 pkg (1.1 oz)	108	11	2	0

FRULLATI CAFE

Smoothie	1 (14 oz)	195	3	2	–

GODFATHER'S PIZZA

Breadstick	1	80	2	–	–
Golden All Meat Combo	1 med slice	300	14	–	–
Golden Apple Dessert	1/6 sm	202	5	–	–
Golden Bacon Cheeseburger	1 med slice	270	12	–	–
Golden Cheese	1 med slice	220	8	–	–
Golden Cherry Dessert	1/6 sm	206	5	–	–
Golden Cinnamon Streusel	1/6 sm	226	6	–	–
Golden Combo	1 med slice	290	13	–	–
Golden Hawaiian	1 med slice	240	8	–	–
Golden Hot Stuff	1 med slice	290	14	–	–
Golden Humble Pie	1 med slice	310	15	–	–
Golden M&M Streusel Dessert	1/6 sm	249	7	–	–
Golden Pepperoni	1 med slice	260	11	–	–
Golden Super Combo	1 med slice	320	15	–	–
Golden Super Hawaiian	1 med slice	250	10	–	–
Golden Super Taco	1 med slice	330	17	–	–
Golden Taco	1 med slice	300	14	–	–
Golden Veggie	1 med slice	230	8	–	–
Monkey Bread	1/6	120	2	–	–
Original All Meat Combo	1 med slice	370	16	–	–
Original Bacon Cheeseburger	1 med slice	330	13	–	–
Original Cheese	1 med slice	260	7	–	–
Original Combo	1 med slice	350	14	–	–
Original Hawaiian	1 med slice	280	8	–	–
Original Hot Stuff	1 med slice	360	6	–	–
Original Humble Pie	1 med slice	380	18	–	–
Original Pepperoni	1 med slice	290	10	–	–
Original Super Combo	1 med slice	390	17	–	–
Original Super Hawaiian	1 med slice	280	8	–	–
Original Super Taco	1 med slice	390	18	–	–

FOOD	PORTION	CALS	FAT	SAT FAT	TRANS FAT
Original Taco	1 med slice	360	16	–	–
Original Veggie	1 med slice	270	9	–	–
Potato Wedges	1 serv (4 oz)	192	9	–	–
Thin All Meat Combo	1 med slice	280	15	–	–
Thin Bacon Cheeseburger	1 med slice	250	13	–	–
Thin Cheese	1 med slice	180	8	–	–
Thin Combo	1 med slice	250	13	–	–
Thin Hawaiian	1 med slice	200	9	–	–
Thin Hot Stuff	1 med slice	270	15	–	–
Thin Humble Pie	1 med slice	270	16	–	–
Thin Pepperoni	1 med slice	220	11	–	–
Thin Super Combo	1 med slice	300	16	–	–
Thin Super Hawaiian	1 med slice	230	11	–	–
Thin Super Taco	1 med slice	310	18	–	–
Thin Taco	1 med slice	260	15	–	–
Thin Veggie	1 med slice	190	9	–	–

HÄAGEN-DAZS
FROZEN YOGURT

FOOD	PORTION	CALS	FAT	SAT FAT	TRANS FAT
Pinapple Coconut	½ cup	230	13	8	–
Soft Serve Nonfat Chocolate	½ cup	110	0	0	0
Soft Serve Nonfat Chocolate Mousse	½ cup	80	0	0	0
Soft Serve Nonfat Coffee	½ cup	110	0	0	0
Soft Serve Nonfat Strawberry	½ cup	110	0	0	0
Soft Serve Nonfat Vanilla	½ cup	110	0	0	0
Soft Serve Nonfat Vanilla Mousse	½ cup	70	0	0	0
Soft Serve Nonfat White Chocolate	½ cup	110	0	0	0
Vanilla Fudge	½ cup	160	0	0	–
Vanilla Raspberry Swirl	½ cup	130	0	0	0

ICE CREAM

FOOD	PORTION	CALS	FAT	SAT FAT	TRANS FAT
Bailey's Irish Cream	½ cup	270	17	10	–
Bar Chocolate	1 (2.7 oz)	200	12	8	–
Bar Chocolate & Dark Chocolate	1 (3.6 oz)	350	24	15	–
Bar Coffee	1 (2.7 oz)	190	13	8	–
Bar Coffee & Almond Crunch	1 (3.7 oz)	370	27	15	–
Bar Vanilla	1 (2.7 oz)	190	13	8	–

FOOD	PORTION	CALS	FAT	SAT FAT	TRANS FAT
Bar Vanilla & Almonds	1 (3.7 oz)	380	28	14	–
Bar Vanilla & Milk Chocolate	1 (3.5 oz)	340	24	14	–
Belgian Chocolate Chocolate	½ cup	330	21	12	–
Brownies A La Mode	½ cup	280	16	10	–
Butter Pecan	½ cup	300	22	10	–
Cappuccino Commotion	½ cup	310	21	12	–
Chocolate	½ cup	269	17	10	–
Chocolate Chocolate Chip	½ cup	300	19	11	–
Chocolate Chocolate Mint	½ cup	300	20	11	–
Chocolate Swiss Almond	½ cup	300	20	11	–
Coffee	½ cup	250	17	10	–
Coffee Mocha Chip	½ cup	270	19	12	–
Cookie Dough Dynamo	½ cup	310	20	12	–
Cookies & Cream	½ cup	270	17	10	–
Cookies & Fudge	½ cup	180	3	2	–
Deep Chocolate Peanut Butter	½ cup	350	24	11	–
Dulce De Leche Caramel	½ cup	270	16	10	–
Lowfat Coffee Fudge	½ cup	170	3	2	–
Macadamia Brittle	½ cup	280	19	11	–
Macadamia Nut	½ cup	320	24	12	–
Mint Chip	½ cup	280	18	12	–
Pistachio	½ cup	280	19	10	–
Pralines & Cream	½ cup	280	17	9	–
Rum Raisin	½ cup	260	17	10	–
Strawberry	½ cup	250	16	9	–
Vanilla	½ cup	250	17	10	–
Vanilla Chocolate Chip	½ cup	290	19	12	–
Vanilla Swiss Almond	½ cup	290	20	11	–
SORBET					
Bar Raspberry & Vanilla	1 (2.5 oz)	90	0	0	0
Mango	½ cup	120	0	0	0
Orange	½ cup	120	0	0	0
Raspberry	½ cup	120	0	0	0
Soft Serve Raspberry	½ cup	110	0	0	0
Strawberry	½ cup	120	0	0	0
Zesty Lemon	½ cup	120	0	0	0

HARDEE'S
BEVERAGES

FOOD	PORTION	CALS	FAT	SAT FAT	TRANS FAT
Barq's Root Beer	1 sm (20 oz)	290	0	0	0

FOOD	PORTION	CALS	FAT	SAT FAT	TRANS FAT
Cherry Coke	1 sm (20 oz)	260	0	0	0
Coca-Cola	1 sm (20 oz)	260	0	0	0
Coffee Black	1 sm (12 oz)	5	0	0	0
Diet Coke	1 sm (20 oz)	0	0	0	0
Dr Pepper	1 sm (20 oz)	260	0	0	0
Hi-C Fruit Punch	1 sm (20 oz)	260	0	0	0
Hi-C Orange	1 sm (20 oz)	280	0	0	0
Lemonade Minute Maid	1 sm (20 oz)	250	0	0	0
Mello Yellow	1 sm (20 oz)	265	0	0	0
Milk 2%	1 (10 oz)	150	3	2	–
Orange Juice	1 serv (10 oz)	150	0	0	0
Shake Chocolate	1 (16 oz)	700	34	24	–
Shake Strawberry	1 (16 oz)	700	33	23	–
Shake Vanilla	1 (16 oz)	710	33	23	–
Sprite	1 sm	260	0	0	0
BREAKFAST SELECTIONS					
Big Country Breakfast Platter Bacon	1 serv	980	56	13	–
Big Country Breakfast Platter Breaded Pork Chop	1 serv	1220	68	13	–
Big Country Breakfast Platter Chicken	1 serv	1140	61	13	–
Big Country Breakfast Platter Country Ham	1 serv	970	53	12	–
Big Country Breakfast Platter Country Steak	1 serv	1150	68	16	–
Big Country Breakfast Platter Grilled Pork Chop	1 serv	1130	61	15	–
Big Country Breakfast Platter Sausage	1 serv	1060	64	15	–
Biscuit Bacon	1 serv	430	28	7	–
Biscuit Bacon Egg Cheese	1	560	38	11	–
Biscuit Breaded Pork Chop	1 serv	690	42	8	–
Biscuit Chicken Fillet	1 serv	600	34	7	–
Biscuit Cinnamon 'N' Raisin	1	280	12	3	–
Biscuit Country Ham	1	440	26	6	–
Biscuit Country Steak	1 serv	620	41	11	–
Biscuit Country Steak & Egg	1 serv	690	47	11	–
Biscuit Egg	1 serv	450	29	6	–
Biscuit Ham Egg Cheese	1	560	35	10	–

FOOD	PORTION	CALS	FAT	SAT FAT	TRANS FAT
Biscuit Loaded Omelet	1 serv	640	44	14	–
Biscuit Made From Scratch	1	370	23	5	–
Biscuit 'N' Gravy	1	530	34	8	–
Biscuit Sausage	1	530	36	10	–
Biscuit Sausage Egg	1	610	44	11	–
Breakfast Bowl Loaded Biscuit 'N' Gravy	1 serv	770	54	14	–
Breakfast Bowl Low Carb	1 serv	620	50	21	–
Burrito Loaded Breakfast	1	780	51	20	–
Burrito Steak 'N' Egg Breakfast	1	470	22	8	–
Folded Egg	1 serv	80	6	2	–
Frisco Breakfast Sandwich	1	410	17	7	–
Grits	1 serv	110	5	1	–
Hash Rounds	1 sm	260	16	4	–
Loaded Omelet	1	270	21	9	–
Pancake Platter	1 serv	300	5	1	–
Scrambled Egg	1 serv	160	12	3	–
Sunrise Croissant	1	210	10	4	–
Sunrise Croissant w/ Bacon	1	450	29	12	–
Sunrise Croissant w/ Ham	1	430	26	10	–
Sunrise Croissant w/ Sausage	1	550	38	15	–
CHILDREN'S MENU SELECTIONS					
French Fries	1 serv	250	12	3	–
Kids Meal Cheeseburger	1 serv	600	27	6	–
Kids Meal Chicken Strips	1 serv	500	25	5	–
Kids Meal Hamburger	1 serv	560	24	6	–
DESSERTS					
Apple Turnover	1	290	15	5	–
Cone Single Scoop	1	285	13	8	–
Cookie Chocolate Chip	1	290	11	5	–
Ice Cream Bowl Single Scoop	1 serv	235	13	8	–
Peach Cobbler	1 serv	280	7	2	–
MAIN MENU SELECTIONS					
Burger Six Dollar	1	1060	72	30	–
Cheeseburger	1 sm	350	16	4	–
Cheeseburger	1 lg	680	39	19	–
Cheeseburger Double	1	510	26	5	–
Chicken Strips	3 pieces	380	21	4	–
Cole Slaw	1 serv	170	10	2	–
Crispy Curls	1 sm	340	17	4	–

FOOD	PORTION	CALS	FAT	SAT FAT	TRANS FAT
French Fries	1 sm	390	19	4	–
Fried Chicken Breast	1 piece	370	15	4	–
Fried Chicken Leg	1 piece	170	7	2	–
Fried Chicken Thigh	1 piece	330	15	4	–
Fried Chicken Wing	1 piece	200	8	2	–
Grilled Onions	1 serv	35	3	3	–
Hamburger	1	310	12	4	–
Hamburger Double	1	420	19	5	–
Hot Dog	1	420	30	12	–
Hot Ham 'N' Cheese	1	420	18	10	–
Hot Ham 'N' Cheese Big	1	520	24	13	–
Mashed Potatoes	1 sm	90	2	0	–
Roast Beef Big	1	470	23	10	–
Roast Beef Regular	1	330	16	7	–
Sandwich Big Chicken Fillet	1	850	42	9	–
Sandwich Charbroiled Chicken Club	1	560	30	8	–
Sandwich Fish Supreme	1	500	27	7	–
Thickburger	1	850	57	22	–
Thickburger Bacon Cheese	1	910	63	24	–
Thickburger Double	1	1240	90	38	–
Thickburger Double Bacon Cheese	1	1300	96	40	–
Thickburger Low Carb	1	420	32	12	–
Thickburger Monster	1	1410	107	45	–
Thickburger Mushroom 'N Swiss	1	720	42	21	–
SAUCES AND TOPPINGS					
Au Jus Sauce	1 serv (3 oz)	10	0	0	0
Chicken Gravy	1 serv (1.5 oz)	20	1	0	–
Dipping Sauce BBQ	1 serv (0.5 oz)	15	0	0	0
Dipping Sauce Honey Mustard	1 serv (1 oz)	110	9	2	–
Dipping Sauce Ranch Dressing	1 serv (1 oz)	160	16	3	–
Dipping Sauce Sweet N Sour	1 serv (1 oz)	45	0	0	0
Gravy Biscuit	1 serv (5 oz)	160	11	3	–
Horseradish Sauce	1 pkg	25	2	0	–
Hot Sauce	1 pkg	0	0	0	0
Jam Grape	1 serv	10	0	0	0
Jam Strawberry	1 serv	35	0	0	0
Ketchup	1 pkg	10	0	0	0

FOOD	PORTION	CALS	FAT	SAT FAT	TRANS FAT
Mayonnaise	1 pkg	90	9	2	–
Pancake Syrup	1 serv (1 oz)	90	0	0	0

HUNGRY HOWIE'S
PIZZA

FOOD	PORTION	CALS	FAT	SAT FAT	TRANS FAT
Medium Cheese	1 slice	153	5	2	–
Medium Cheese + Beef	1 slice	177	6	3	–
Medium Cheese + Green Peppers	1 slice	155	5	3	–
Medium Cheese + Ham	1 slice	159	6	2	–
Medium Cheese + Mushrooms	1 slice	155	5	2	–
Medium Cheese + Onions	1 slice	155	5	3	–
Medium Cheese + Pepperoni	1 slice	171	6	3	–
Medium Cheese + Sausage	1 slice	175	6	2	–
Small Cheese	1 slice	121	3	2	–
Small Cheese + Bacon	1 slice	138	3	2	–
Small Cheese + Beef	1 slice	137	4	2	–
Small Cheese + Black Olives	1 slice	125	3	2	–
Small Cheese + Green Olives	1 slice	125	3	2	–
Small Cheese + Green Peppers	1 slice	122	3	2	–
Small Cheese + Ham	1 slice	126	3	2	–
Small Cheese + Mushrooms	1 slice	123	3	2	–
Small Cheese + Onions	1 slice	122	3	2	–
Small Cheese + Pepperoni	1 slice	136	4	3	–
Small Cheese + Pineapple	1 slice	124	3	2	–
Small Cheese + Sausage	1 slice	136	3	2	–

IHOP

FOOD	PORTION	CALS	FAT	SAT FAT	TRANS FAT
Pancake Buckwheat	1 (1.7 oz)	110	4	1	–
Pancake Buttermilk	1 (1.7 oz)	110	3	1	–
Pancake Country Griddle	1 (2 oz)	120	4	1	–
Pancake Harvest Grain 'N Nut	1 (2.25 oz)	180	9	2	–

IN-N-OUT BURGER
BEVERAGES

FOOD	PORTION	CALS	FAT	SAT FAT	TRANS FAT
Coca-Cola	1 (16 oz)	198	0	0	0
Coffee Black	1 (10 oz)	5	0	0	0
Diet Coca-Cola	1 (16 oz)	0	0	0	0
Dr Pepper	1 (16 oz)	180	0	0	0
Iced Tea	1 (16 oz)	0	0	0	0
Lemonade	1 (16 oz)	180	0	0	0

FOOD	PORTION	CALS	FAT	SAT FAT	TRANS FAT
7Up	1 (16 oz)	200	0	0	0
Milk	1 (10 oz)	108	6	4	–
Root Beer	1 (16 oz)	222	0	0	0
Shake Chocolate	1 (15 oz)	690	36	24	–
Shake Strawberry	1 (15 oz)	690	33	22	–
Shake Vanilla	1 (15 oz)	680	37	25	–
MAIN MENU SELECTIONS					
Cheeseburger w/ Onions	1	480	27	10	–
Cheeseburger w/ Onions Lettuce Bun	1	330	25	9	–
Cheeseburger w/ Onions Mustard Ketchup No Spread	1	400	18	9	–
French Fries	1 serv (4.4 oz)	400	18	5	–
Hamburger Double Double w/ Onions	1	670	41	18	–
Hamburger Double Double w/ Onions Lettuce Bun	1	520	39	17	–
Hamburger Double Double w/ Onions Mustard Ketchup No Spread	1	590	32	17	–
Hamburger w/ Onions	1	390	19	5	–
Hamburger w/ Onions Lettuce Bun	1	240	17	4	–
Hamburger w/ Onions Mustard Ketchup No Spread	1	310	10	4	–

JACK IN THE BOX
BEVERAGES

FOOD	PORTION	CALS	FAT	SAT FAT	TRANS FAT
Barq's Root Beer	1 (20 oz)	180	0	0	0
Chocolate Milk Low Fat Chug	1 (3.5 oz)	200	3	2	–
Coca-Cola Classic	1 (20 oz)	170	0	0	0
Coffee Regular & Decaf	1 (11 oz)	5	0	0	0
Diet Coke	1 (20 oz)	0	0	0	0
Dr Pepper	1 (20 oz)	150	0	0	0
Fanta Orange	1 (20 oz)	150	0	0	0
Fanta Strawberry	1 (20 oz)	150	0	0	0
Iced Tea	1 (20 oz)	5	0	0	0
Lemonade	1 (20 oz)	160	0	0	0
Orange Juice	1 (10 oz)	140	0	0	0
Reduced Fat Milk Chug	1 (3.5 oz)	130	5	3	0

FOOD	PORTION	CALS	FAT	SAT FAT	TRANS FAT
Shake Chocolate	1 (16 oz)	880	45	31	2
Shake Oreo	1 (16 oz)	910	49	32	2
Shake Strawberry	1 (16 oz)	880	44	31	2
Shake Vanilla	1 (16 oz)	790	44	31	2
Sprite	1 (20 oz)	160	0	0	0
BREAKFAST SELECTIONS					
Biscuit Bacon Egg Cheese	1	430	25	8	5
Biscuit Chicken	1	450	24	6	6
Biscuit Sausage	1	440	29	8	5
Biscuit Sausage Egg Cheese	1	740	55	17	6
Biscuit Spicy Chicken	1	460	22	5	0
Breakfast Sandwich Ciabatta	1	710	30	10	1
Breakfast Sandwich Ultimate	1	570	27	10	1
Breakfast Jack	1	290	12	5	0
Breakfast Jack Bacon	1	300	14	5	1
Breakfast Jack Sausage	1	450	28	10	1
Burrito Hearty Breakfast	1	480	29	10	1
Burrito Sirloin Steak & Egg w/o Salsa	1	790	48	15	4
Croissant Sausage	1	580	39	13	4
Croissant Supreme	1	450	25	9	4
French Toast Sticks	4 (4.2 oz)	470	23	5	5
French Toast Sticks Blueberry	4	450	20	5	5
Hash Brown	1 serv	150	10	3	3
DESSERTS					
Cake Chocolate Overload	1 serv (3.2 oz)	300	7	2	0
Cheesecake	1 serv (3.6 oz)	310	16	9	1
MAIN MENU SELECTIONS					
Bacon Cheddar Potato Wedges	1 serv (9 oz)	720	48	15	12
Cheeseburger Bacon Ultimate	1	1090	77	30	3
Cheeseburger Junior Bacon	1	430	25	9	1
Cheeseburger Sourdough Ultimate	1	950	73	29	5
Cheeseburger Ultimate	1	1010	71	28	3
Chicken Fajita Pita	1	280	9	4	0
Chicken Sandwich	1	400	21	5	3
Chicken Strips Crispy	4	500	25	6	6
Chicken Strips Grilled	4 (5 oz)	180	2	1	0
Ciabatta Chipotle w/ Grilled Chicken	1	690	28	9	0

FOOD	PORTION	CALS	FAT	SAT FAT	TRANS FAT
Ciabatta Chipotle w/ Spicy Crispy Chicken	1	750	34	10	0
Ciabatta Sirloin Steak & Cheddar	1	770	38	8	0
Ciabatta Burger Bacon & Cheese	1	1120	76	28	3
Ciabatta Burger Single Bacon & Cheese	1	870	54	18	0
Club Sourdough Grilled Chicken	1	530	28	7	2
Curly Fries Seasoned	1 sm (3 oz)	270	15	3	5
Dipping Sauce Barbeque	1 serv (1 oz)	45	0	0	0
Egg Rolls	1	130	6	2	1
Fish & Chips	1 serv (7.6 oz)	570	30	7	9
Fries Natural Cut	1 sm	340	17	4	5
Fruit Cup	1 serv	90	0	0	0
Hamburger	1	310	14	6	1
Hamburger Deluxe	1	370	21	7	1
Hamburger Deluxe w/ Cheese	1	460	28	11	1
Hamburger w/ Cheese	1	350	17	8	1
Jack's Spicy Chicken	1 serv	620	31	6	3
Jack's Spicy Chicken w/ Cheese	1	700	37	10	3
Jumbo Jack	1	600	35	12	2
Jumbo Jack w/ Cheese	1	690	42	16	2
Mozzarella Cheese Sticks	3	240	12	5	2
Onion Rings	8 (4.2 oz)	500	30	6	10
Sampler Trio	1 serv	750	39	14	7
Sandwich Bacon Chicken	1	440	24	6	3
Sirloin Burger w/ American Cheese & Red Onion	1	1120	73	24	3
Sirloin Burger w/ Swiss & Grilled Onions	1	1070	71	25	2
Sirloin Steak Melt	1	640	40	13	2
Sourdough Jack	1	710	51	18	3
Spicy Chicken Bites	1 serv	290	14	3	3
Stuffed Jalapeno	3 (2.5 oz)	230	13	6	2
Taco Monster Beef	1	240	14	5	2
Taco Regular Beef	1	160	8	3	1
SALAD DRESSINGS AND TOPPINGS					
Asian Sesame	1 serv (2.5 oz)	230	17	3	0

FOOD	PORTION	CALS	FAT	SAT FAT	TRANS FAT
Dipping Sauce Buttermilk House	1 serv (0.9 oz)	130	13	2	0
Dipping Sauce Frank's Red Hot Buffalo	1 serv (1 oz)	10	0	0	0
Dipping Sauce Sweet & Sour	1 serv (1 oz)	45	0	0	0
Dipping Sauce Teriyaki	1 serv (1 oz)	60	0	0	0
Dipping Sauce Zesty Marinara	1 serv (0.8 oz)	15	0	0	0
Dressing Bacon Ranch	1 serv (2.5 oz)	320	33	5	1
Dressing Creamy Southwest	1 serv (2.5 oz)	270	27	5	1
Low Fat Balsamic	1 serv (2.5 oz)	40	2	0	0
Mayo Onion Sauce	1 serv (0.5 oz)	90	10	2	0
Ranch	1 serv (2.5 oz)	390	41	6	0
Ranch Lite	1 serv (2.5 oz)	190	18	3	0
Soy Sauce	1 serv (0.3 oz)	5	0	0	0
Syrup Log Cabin	1 serv (2 oz)	190	0	0	0
Taco Sauce	1 serv (0.3 oz)	0	0	0	0
Tartar Sauce	1 serv (1.5 oz)	210	22	4	0
SALADS					
Asian w/ Crispy Chicken w/o Dressing	1 (13.8 oz)	330	13	3	3
Asian w/ Grilled Chicken w/o Dressing	1 (12.8 oz)	160	2	0	0
Chicken Club w/ Crispy Chicken w/o Dressing	1 (14 oz)	480	27	7	0
Chicken Club w/ Grilled Chicken w/o Dressing	1 (13 oz)	320	16	6	0
Side w/o Dressing	1 (4.3 oz)	50	3	2	0
Southwest Chicken w/ Crispy Chicken w/o Dressing	1 (16 oz)	480	23	8	3
Southwest w/ Grilled Chicken w/o Dressing	1 (15 oz)	320	12	6	0
JAMBA JUICE					
Acai Supercharger Original	1 (24 oz)	420	5	1	0
Aloha Pineapple Original	1 (26 oz)	500	2	1	–
Banana Berry Original	1 (25 oz)	480	1	0	–
Berry Fulfilling Original	1 (24 oz)	290	1	0	–
Berry Lime Sublime Original	1 (26 oz)	460	2	1	–
Caribbean Passion Original	1 (26 oz)	440	2	1	–
Chocolate Moo'd Original	1 (24 oz)	680	8	5	–

FOOD	PORTION	CALS	FAT	SAT FAT	TRANS FAT
Citrus Squeeze Original	1 (26 oz)	470	2	1	–
Coldbuster Original	1 (25 oz)	430	3	1	–
Grape Escape Original	1 (24 oz)	300	0	0	0
Mango Mantra Original	1 (25 oz)	310	1	0	–
Mango-A-Go-Go Original	1 (24 oz)	440	2	1	0
Matcha Green Tea Blast Original	1 (24 oz)	440	1	0	0
Matcha Green Tea Mist Original	1 (24 oz)	280	0	0	0
Mega Mango Original	1 (24 oz)	330	1	0	0
Mighty Cherry Charger Original	1 (24 oz)	490	1	0	0
Orange Berry Blitz Original	1 (26 oz)	410	3	1	–
Orange Dream Machine Original	1 (24 oz)	540	3	1	–
Orange-A-Peel Original	1 (25 oz)	440	2	0	–
Passion Berry Breeze Original	1 (24 oz)	270	1	0	0
Peach Pleasure Original	1 (25 oz)	460	2	1	–
Peanut Butter Moo'd Original	1 (24 oz)	840	21	5	–
Peenya Kowlada Original	1 (26 oz)	690	5	4	–
Protein Berry Pizazz Original	1 (24 oz)	440	2	0	–
Raspberry Rainbow Original	1 (24 oz)	300	1	0	0
Razzmatazz Original	1 (26 oz)	480	2	1	–
Strawberries Wild Original	1 (25 oz)	450	1	0	–
Strawberry Nirvana Original	1 (25 oz)	280	1	0	–
Strawberry Surf Rider Original	1 (25 oz)	490	2	1	0
Strawberry Whirl Original	1 (24 oz)	310	1	0	0

JERSEY MIKE'S

FOOD	PORTION	CALS	FAT	SAT FAT	TRANS FAT
Ham On Wheat	1	240	4	2	–
Ham On White	1	240	5	2	–
Ham/Turkey Wheat	1	230	3	1	–
Ham/Turkey White	1	240	4	1	–
Roast Beef Wheat	1	290	5	2	–
Roast Beef White	1	280	5	2	–
Turkey On Wheat	1	230	2	1	–
Turkey On White	1	230	3	1	–
Veggie On Wheat	1	170	2	0	–
Veggie On White	1	170	2	1	–

FOOD	PORTION	CALS	FAT	SAT FAT	TRANS FAT

KENTUCKY FRIED CHICKEN
BEVERAGES

FOOD	PORTION	CALS	FAT	SAT FAT	TRANS FAT
Diet Pepsi	1 med (14 oz)	0	0	0	0
Mountain Dew	1 med (14 oz)	190	0	0	0
Pepsi	1 med (14 oz)	180	0	0	0

DESSERTS

FOOD	PORTION	CALS	FAT	SAT FAT	TRANS FAT
Cake Double Chocolate Chip	1 slice	330	16	4	1
Cookie Sweet Life Chocolate Chip	1 (1.2 oz)	160	7	4	0
Cookie Sweet Life Oatmeal Raisin	1 (1.2 oz)	150	5	3	0
Cookie Sweet Life Sugar	1 (1.2 oz)	160	6	3	0
Lil' Bucket Chocolate Cream	1	280	13	9	1
Lil' Bucket Lemon Creme	1 serv	410	15	7	2
Lil' Bucket Strawberry Short Cake	1 serv	210	7	5	0
Pie Mini's Apple	3 (4 oz)	370	20	6	0
Teddy Graham Cinnamon Snacks	1 serv	90	3	1	0

MAIN MENU SELECTIONS

FOOD	PORTION	CALS	FAT	SAT FAT	TRANS FAT
Baked Beans	1 serv	220	1	0	0
Biscuit	1 (2 oz)	220	11	3	4
Bowl Chicken & Biscuit	1	870	44	11	5
Bowl Mashed Potato w/ Gravy	1	740	36	9	2
Bowl Rice w/ Gravy	1	620	28	7	1
Chicken Pot Pie	1 (15 oz)	770	40	15	14
Cole Slaw	1 serv	180	10	2	0
Corn On The Cob	1 ear (3 inch)	70	2	2	0
Crispy Strips	2 (3.5 oz)	240	13	3	0
Extra Crispy Breast	1 (5.7 oz)	440	27	6	0
Extra Crispy Drumstick	1 (2 oz)	160	10	2	0
Extra Crispy Thigh	1 (4 oz)	370	28	6	0
Extra Crispy Whole Wing	1 (1.8 oz)	170	11	3	0
Green Beans	1 serv	50	2	0	0
KFC Snacker	1	290	13	3	0
KFC Snacker Buffalo	1	260	8	2	0
KFC Snacker Fish	1	330	15	3	0
KFC Snacker Fish w/o Sauce	1	290	12	3	0
KFC Snacker Honey BBQ	1	210	3	1	0
KFC Snacker Ultimate Cheese	1	280	11	3	1

FOOD	PORTION	CALS	FAT	SAT FAT	TRANS FAT
Macaroni & Cheese	1 serv	180	8	4	1
Mashed Potatoes w/ Gravy	1 serv	140	5	1	1
Mashed Potatoes w/o Gravy	1 serv	110	4	1	0
Original Recipe Breast	1 (5.6 oz)	360	21	5	0
Original Recipe Breast w/o Skin Or Breading	1 (3.8 oz)	140	2	0	0
Original Recipe Drumstick	1 (2 oz)	130	8	2	0
Original Recipe Thigh	1 (4.4 oz)	330	24	6	0
Original Recipe Whole Wing	1 (1.6 oz)	130	8	2	0
Popcorn Chicken	1 reg (4 oz)	400	26	5	0
Potato Salad	1 serv	180	9	2	0
Potato Wedges	1 serv	260	13	3	0
Sandwich Crispy Twister	1	550	28	6	0
Sandwich Double Crunch	1	470	23	5	0
Sandwich Honey BBQ	1	280	4	1	0
Sandwich Tender Roast	1	380	13	3	0
Sandwich Tender Roast w/o Sauce	1	300	5	2	0
Seasoned Rice	1 serv	180	1	0	0
Twister Oven Roasted	1	420	17	4	0
Twister Oven Roasted w/o Sauce	1	330	7	3	0
Wings Fiery Buffalo	5	380	24	5	0
Wings Honey BBQ	5	390	24	5	0
Wings Hot	5	350	24	5	0
Wings Hot & Spicy	5	400	24	5	0
Wings Teriyaki	5	480	25	5	0
Wings Boneless Fiery Buffalo	5	420	20	4	0
Wings Boneless Honey BBQ	5	450	20	4	0
Wings Boneless Sweet & Spicy	5	440	19	4	0
Wings Boneless Teriyaki	5	500	21	4	0
SALAD DRESSINGS					
Creamy Parmesan Caesar	1 serv (2 oz)	260	26	5	0
Golden Italian Light	1 serv (1.5 oz)	45	3	0	0
Ranch	1 serv (2 oz)	200	20	3	0
Ranch Fat Free	1 serv (1.5 oz)	35	0	0	0
SALADS					
Crispy BLT w/o Dressing	1 (12 oz)	330	17	4	0
Crispy Caesar w/o Dressing & Croutons	1 (11 oz)	350	19	6	0

FOOD	PORTION	CALS	FAT	SAT FAT	TRANS FAT
Croutons Parmesan Garlic	1 pkg	60	3	0	0
Roasted BLT w/o Dressing	1 (12 oz)	200	6	2	0
Roasted Caesar w/o Dressing & Croutons	1 (11 oz)	220	8	5	0
Side Caesar w/o Dressing & Croutons	1 (3 oz)	50	3	2	0
Side House w/o Dressing	1 (3 oz)	15	0	0	0

KOO-KOO-ROO

FOOD	PORTION	CALS	FAT	SAT FAT	TRANS FAT
Original Breast	1 piece	187	6	1	–
Original Chicken Dark	3 pieces	320	16	5	–
Rotisserie Chicken Breast & Wing	1 serv	355	16	4	–
Rotisserie Chicken Leg & Thigh	1 serv	300	18	5	–
Rotisserie Half Chicken	1 serv	655	34	9	–
Sandwich BBQ Chicken	1	562	12	4	–
Sandwich Chicken Caesar	1	781	36	11	–
Sandwich Original Chicken	1	661	29	5	–
Traditional Turkey Dinner	1 serv	692	29	10	–
Turkey Pot Pie	1 serv	883	44	12	–
Turkey Sandwich Hand Carved	1	599	32	8	–
Wrap Caesar Chicken	1	757	39	8	–
Wrap Chipotle Chicken	1	924	43	15	–

KRISPY KREME
BEVERAGES

FOOD	PORTION	CALS	FAT	SAT FAT	TRANS FAT
Chillers Fruity Orange You Glad	1 (12 oz)	180	0	0	0
Chillers Fruity Very Berry	1 (12 oz)	170	0	0	0
Chillers Kremey Berries & Kreme	1 (12 oz)	620	28	24	0
Chillers Kremey Chocolate Chocolate	1 (12 oz)	970	29	24	0
Chillers Kremey Lemon Sherbert	1 (12 oz)	630	28	24	0
Chillers Kremey Lotta Latte	1 (12 oz)	670	28	24	0
Chillers Kremey Mocha Dream	1 (12 oz)	670	28	24	0
Chillers Kremey Oranges & Kreme	1 (12 oz)	630	28	24	0

DOUGHNUTS

FOOD	PORTION	CALS	FAT	SAT FAT	TRANS FAT
Apple Fritter	1	380	20	10	0

FOOD	PORTION	CALS	FAT	SAT FAT	TRANS FAT
Caramel Kreme Crunch	1	380	19	9	0
Chocolate Iced Cake	1	280	14	6	0
Chocolate Iced Custard Filled	1	300	17	8	0
Chocolate Iced Glazed	1	250	12	6	0
Chocolate Iced Kreme Filled	1	350	20	11	0
Chocolate Iced w/ Sprinkles	1	270	12	6	0
Cinnamon Apple Filled	1	290	16	8	0
Cinnamon Bun	1	260	16	8	0
Cinnamon Twist	1	240	15	7	0
Dulce De Leche	1	300	18	9	0
Glazed Chocolate Cake	1	300	15	7	0
Glazed Cinnamon	1	210	12	6	0
Glazed Creme Filled	1	340	20	10	0
Glazed Cruller	1	240	14	7	0
Glazed Cruller Chocolate	1	290	15	7	0
Glazed Lemon Filled	1	290	16	8	0
Glazed Maple Iced	1	240	12	6	0
Glazed Original	1	200	12	6	0
Glazed Pumpkin Spice	1	300	14	7	0
Glazed Raspberry Filled	1	300	16	8	0
Glazed Sour Cream	1	300	13	7	0
Holes Glazed Blueberry	4	220	12	5	0
Holes Glazed Cake	4	210	10	5	0
Holes Glazed Chocolate Cake	4	210	10	5	0
Holes Glazed Original	4	200	11	5	0
Holes Glazed Pumpkin Spice	4	210	10	5	0
Maple Iced Glazed	1	240	12	6	0
New York Cheesecake	1	340	20	10	0
Powdered Cake	1	290	14	6	0
Powdered Strawberry Filled	1	290	16	8	0
Sugar	1	200	12	6	0
Traditional Cake	1	230	13	6	0

KRYSTAL
BEVERAGES

Coca-Cola Classic	1 sm (16 oz)	129	0	0	0
Coco-Cola Classic frzn	1 (16 oz)	130	0	0	0
Diet Coke	1 sm (16 oz)	tr	0	0	0
Sprite	1 sm (16 oz)	126	0	0	0

BREAKFAST SELECTIONS

Biscuit	1	270	13	3	–

FOOD	PORTION	CALS	FAT	SAT FAT	TRANS FAT
Biscuit & Gravy	1	280	14	3	–
Biscuit Bacon Egg & Cheese	1	390	23	7	–
Biscuit Chik	1	360	15	3	–
Biscuit Sausage	1	480	33	10	–
Country Breakfast	1 serv	660	42	14	–
Kryspers	1 serv	190	13	5	–
Krystal Sunriser	1	240	14	5	–
Scrambler	1 serv	440	26	11	–
DESSERTS					
Fried Apple Turnover	1	220	10	4	–
Lemon Icebox Pie	1 serv	260	9	2	–
MAIN MENU SELECTIONS					
Chik'n Bites	1 sm	310	19	8	–
Chik'n Bites Salad	1 serv	290	20	11	–
Fries	1 med	470	20	8	–
Fries Chili Cheese	1 serv	540	28	13	–
Krystal	1	160	7	3	–
Krystal Bacon Cheese	1	190	10	5	–
Krystal Cheese	1	180	9	4	–
Krystal Chik	1	240	11	4	–
Krystal Chili	1 serv	200	7	4	–
Krystal Double	1	260	13	6	–
Krystal Double Cheese	1	310	16	7	–
Pup	1	170	9	4	–
Pup Chili Cheese	1	210	12	5	–
Pup Corn	1	260	19	8	–

LITTLE CAESARS
MAIN MENU SELECTIONS

FOOD	PORTION	CALS	FAT	SAT FAT	TRANS FAT
Baby Pan! Pan!	1 piece	360	16	7	–
Crazy Bread	1 piece	90	3	tr	–
Crazy Bread Cinnamon	2 pieces	100	2	tr	–
Crazy Sauce	1 serv (4 oz)	45	0	0	0
Deli Sandwich Ham & Cheese	1	640	29	3	–
Deli Sandwich Italian	1	800	45	10	–
Deli Sandwich Veggie	1	600	28	3	–
Italian Cheese Bread	1 piece	130	6	3	–
PIZZA					
14 Inch Round Meatsa	1/10 pie	280	13	6	–
14 Inch Round Supreme	1/10 pie	270	10	5	–
14 Inch Round Veggie	1/10 pie	240	8	4	–

FOOD	PORTION	CALS	FAT	SAT FAT	TRANS FAT
14 Inch Thin Crust Cheese	¹⁄₁₀ pie	160	7	4	–
16 Inch Round Cheese	¹⁄₁₂ pie	220	7	4	–
18 Inch Round Cheese	¹⁄₁₄ pie	230	7	4	–
Deep Dish Large	⅛ pie	320	12	5	–
Deep Dish Medium	⅛ pie	230	9	4	–
SALAD DRESSINGS					
Caesar	1 serv (1.5 oz)	230	25	4	–
Greek	1 serv (1.5 oz)	270	29	5	–
Italian	1 serv (1.5 oz)	220	23	4	–
Italian Fat Free	1 serv (1.5 oz)	25	0	0	0
Ranch	1 serv (1.5 oz)	230	24	4	–
SALADS					
Antipasto	1 serv	140	8	2	–
Caesar	1 serv	90	3	1	–
Greek	1 serv	128	7	5	–
Tossed Salad	1 serv	100	3	1	–
TOPPINGS PER SLICE					
Bacon	1 serv	41	4	1	–
Beef	1 serv	20	2	1	–
Black Olives	1 serv	12	2	tr	–
Extra Cheese	1 serv	26	2	1	–
Green Peppers	1 serv	2	tr	–	–
Ham	1 serv	5	tr	tr	–
Italian Sausage	1 serv	22	2	1	–
Mushrooms	1 serv	2	tr	tr	–
Onion	1 serv	3	tr	–	–
Pepperoni	1 serv	26	2	1	–
Tomato	1 serv	2	tr	–	–

LONG JOHN SILVER'S
BEVERAGES

FOOD	PORTION	CALS	FAT	SAT FAT	TRANS FAT
Coca-Cola	1 sm	150	0	0	0
Diet Coke	1 sm	0	0	0	0
Sprite	1 sm	140	0	0	0
DESSERTS					
Pie Chocolate Cream	1 pie	310	44	14	–
Pie Pecan	1 pie	370	15	3	–
Pie Pineapple Cream	1 pie	290	13	7	–
MAIN MENU SELECTIONS					
Baked Cod	1 piece	120	5	1	–
Battered Chicken	1 piece	140	8	3	–

FOOD	PORTION	CALS	FAT	SAT FAT	TRANS FAT
Battered Fish	1 piece	230	13	4	–
Battered Shrimp	1 piece	45	3	1	–
Breaded Clams	1 serv	240	13	2	–
Cheesesticks	3 pieces	140	8	2	–
Clam Chowder	1 bowl	220	10	4	–
Corn Cobbette	1 piece	90	3	1	–
Crumblies	1 serv	170	12	3	–
Crunchy Shrimp	21 pieces	330	18	5	–
Fries	1 reg	230	10	3	–
Hushpuppy	1 piece	60	3	1	–
Rice	1 serv	180	4	1	–
Sandwich Chicken	1	360	15	4	–
Sandwich Fish	1	440	20	3	–
Sandwich Ultimate Fish	1	500	28	9	–
Slaw	1 serv	200	15	3	–

MAGGIE MOO'S

FOOD	PORTION	CALS	FAT	SAT FAT	TRANS FAT
Ice Cream Fat Free	½ cup	80	0	0	0
Ice Cream Low Carb Sugar Added	½ cup	100	6	4	–
Ice Cream Udderly Cream	½ cup	180	11	8	–
Sorbet	½ cup	90	0	0	0

MANHATTAN BAGEL

FOOD	PORTION	CALS	FAT	SAT FAT	TRANS FAT
Blueberry	1	260	tr	0	–
Cheddar Cheese	1	270	4	2	–
Chocolate Chip	1	290	3	2	–
Cinnamon Raisin	1	280	tr	0	–
Cranberry Orange	1	270	1	0	–
Egg	1	270	2	0	–
Everything	1	290	3	0	–
Garlic	1	270	tr	0	–
Jalapeno Cheddar	1	260	2	0	–
Marble	1	260	tr	0	–
Oat Bran	1	260	1	0	–
Oat Bran Raisin Walnut	1	270	3	0	–
Onion	1	270	tr	0	–
Plain	1	260	tr	0	–
Poppy	1	300	4	1	–
Pumpernickel	1	250	1	0	–
Rye	1	260	1	0	–

FOOD	PORTION	CALS	FAT	SAT FAT	TRANS FAT
Salt	1	260	tr	tr	–
Sesame	1	310	5	1	–
Spinach	1	270	tr	0	–
Sun-Dried Tomato	1	260	1	0	–
Whole Wheat	1	260	tr	0	–

MARBLE SLAB CREAMERY

FOOD	PORTION	CALS	FAT	SAT FAT	TRANS FAT
Cone Honey Wheat	1	130	3	0	–
Cone Sugar	1	130	3	0	–
Cone Vanilla Cinnamon	1	130	3	0	–
Frozen Yogurt Nonfat	½ cup	100	1	1	–
Frozen Yogurt Nonfat No Sugar Added	½ cup	90	1	1	–
Ice Cream Reduced Fat	1 serv (6.75 oz)	390	20	13	–
Ice Cream Superpremium	1 serv (6.75 oz)	450	28	18	–
Sorbet	½ cup	90	0	0	0

MAUI WOWI

FOOD	PORTION	CALS	FAT	SAT FAT	TRANS FAT
Smoothie Rip Sticks All Flavors	1	88	0	0	0

MAX & ERMA'S

FOOD	PORTION	CALS	FAT	SAT FAT	TRANS FAT
Black Bean Roll Up	1 serv	577	10	2	–
Caribbean Chicken Lunch Portion	1 serv	536	20	8	–
Fruit Smoothie	1	124	tr	tr	–
Garlic Breadstick	1	156	6	0	–
Hula Bowl w/ Fat Free Honey Mustard Dressing w/o Breadsticks	1 serv	823	7	1	–
Salad Baby Greens w/o Breadsticks	1 serv	119	11	1	–
Salad Shrimp Stack	1 serv	322	12	2	–
Salad Dressing Bleu Cheese	2 tbsp	201	21	4	–
Salad Dressing French Fat Free	2 tbsp	126	tr	0	–
Salad Dressing Honey Mustard Fat Free	2 tbsp	60	0	0	0
Salad Dressing Italian	2 tbsp	110	12	2	–
Salad Dressing Ranch	2 tbsp	120	13	2	–
Salad Dressing Tex Mex Low Fat	2 tbsp	23	tr	0	–

FOOD	PORTION	CALS	FAT	SAT FAT	TRANS FAT

MCALISTER'S DELI
CHILDREN'S MENU SELECTIONS

FOOD	PORTION	CALS	FAT	SAT FAT	TRANS FAT
Kid's Nacho	1 serv	734	43	9	0
Mac's Dog	1	307	19	0	0
Pita Pizza	1	503	21	10	0
Sandwich Ham & Cheese	1	455	22	11	0
Sandwich PB&J	1	714	32	5	0
Sandwich Toasted Cheese	1	620	38	0	0
Sandwich Turkey & Cheese	1	451	21	11	0

DESSERTS

FOOD	PORTION	CALS	FAT	SAT FAT	TRANS FAT
Brownie Chocolate	1 (3.5 oz)	424	18	4	0
Brownie Delight	1 (11 oz)	917	48	22	0
Chocolate Loving Spoon Cake	1 (4 oz)	538	35	9	0
Ice Cream Vanilla Bean	1 scoop (5 oz)	160	10	6	0
Kentucky Pie	1 slice (12 oz)	807	64	27	0
New York Cheesecake	1 slice (5 oz)	505	35	12	1
Sundae Topping Caramel	2 tbsp	100	0	0	0
Sundae Topping Chocolate	1 tbsp	110	0	0	0

MAIN MENU SELECTIONS

FOOD	PORTION	CALS	FAT	SAT FAT	TRANS FAT
Appetizers Chips & Salsa	1 serv (5 oz)	87	5	1	0
Appetizers Dip Cheese & Chili	1 serv (5 oz)	572	35	8	0
Appetizers Dip Cheese & Veggie Chili	1 serv (5 oz)	552	31	7	0
Appetizers Nacho Basket	1 serv (6 oz)	579	33	7	0
Appetizers Nacho Chili	1 serv (6 oz)	564	37	10	0
Appetizers Nacho Veggie Chili	1 serv (6 oz)	537	31	9	0
Chicken Cordon Bleu	1 serv	810	39	39	0
Chili Vegetarian	1 serv (8 oz)	133	1	0	0
Cole Slaw	1 serv (4 oz)	190	15	3	0
Fruit Cup	1 serv (4 oz)	98	0	0	0
Giant Spud Cheese	1 (27 oz)	930	48	6	0
Giant Spud Grilled Chicken	1 (27 oz)	839	25	–	0
Giant Spud Just A Spud	1 (26 oz)	604	4	0	0
Giant Spud Olé	1 (30 oz)	1252	60	28	0
Giant Spud Olé w/ Chili	1 (33 oz)	1512	78	29	0
Giant Spud Olé w/ Veggie Chili	1 (33 oz)	1457	67	27	0
Giant Spud Veggie	1 (28 oz)	668	18	0	0
Macaroni & Cheese	1 serv (4 oz)	200	7	4	1
Mashed Potatoes	1 serv (4 oz)	136	8	2	2
Meatloaf w/ Gravy	1 serv	340	37	11	0

FOOD	PORTION	CALS	FAT	SAT FAT	TRANS FAT
Open-Faced Roast Beef	1 serv	751	21	7	0
Pot Roast Spud	1 serv	906	30	10	0
Potato Salad	1 serv (4 oz)	200	11	2	0
Salmon Filet	1 serv	235	4	2	0
Steamed Vegetables	1 serv (4 oz)	43	0	0	0
SALAD DRESSINGS AND SAUCES					
Au Jus	1 serv (4 oz)	10	0	0	0
Comeback Gravy	1 serv (4 oz)	37	2	0	0
Dressing Blue Cheese	2 tbsp	140	15	2	0
Dressing Greek	2 tbsp	90	9	2	0
Dressing Parmesan Peppercorn	2 tbsp	150	16	3	0
Dressing Ranch	2 tbsp	100	11	2	0
Dressing Tomato Basil	2 tbsp	30	0	0	0
Dressing Lite Olive Oil Vinaigrette	2 tbsp	60	6	1	0
Dressing Lite Ranch	2 tbsp	100	10	2	0
Dressing Low Calorie Italian	2 tbsp	25	2	0	0
SALADS					
Caesar w/ Salmon	1 (17 oz)	800	53	8	0
Chicken Fiesta	1 (20 oz)	493	22	14	0
Chicken Grill	1 (21 oz)	840	15	0	0
Garden	1 (15 oz)	264	17	9	0
Garden w/ Chicken Salad	1 (18 oz)	537	45	4	0
Garden w/ Salmon	1 (17 oz)	315	10	1	0
Garden w/ Tuna Salad	1 (18 oz)	373	18	2	0
Greek Chicken	1 (19 oz)	584	32	3	0
Side Caesar	1 (6 oz)	328	24	3	0
Side Garden	1 (8 oz)	138	9	5	0
Taco	1 (26 oz)	641	40	15	0
Taco w/ Veggie Chili	1 (26 oz)	641	40	15	0
SANDWICHES					
BLT	1	654	38	9	0
Chicken Salad	1	677	43	10	0
Deli Corned Beef On Wheat	1	369	9	2	0
Deli Ham On Wheat	1	350	9	1	0
Deli Pastrami On Wheat	1	371	10	1	0
Deli Roast Beef On Wheat	1	398	12	1	0
Deli Salami On Wheat	1	565	32	14	0
Deli Turkey On Wheat	1	342	9	0	0

FOOD	PORTION	CALS	FAT	SAT FAT	TRANS FAT
French Dip	1	676	34	19	0
Grilled Chicken Breast	1	751	36	14	0
Grilled Chicken Club	1	1234	64	27	0
Ham Melt	1	700	34	16	0
McAlisters Club	1	1225	69	29	0
Meatloaf Parmesan	1	708	36	15	0
Memphian	1	585	26	12	0
Muffuletta	¼ (8 oz)	615	35	15	0
New Yorker	1	628	25	12	0
Orange Cranberry Club	1	954	52	26	0
Reuben On Rye	1	492	30	9	0
Roast Beef Melt	1	635	32	15	0
Salmon	1	608	21	3	0
Submarine	1	833	48	17	0
Sweetberry Chicken On Wheatberry	1	701	24	11	0
Tuna Salad On Wheat	1	452	19	2	0
Turkey Melt	1	700	35	16	0
Veggie On Pita	1	522	36	9	0
Wrap Greek Chicken	1	630	25	4	0
Wrap Grill Chicken Caesar	1	533	25	3	0
SOUPS					
Asiago Cheese Bisque	1 serv (8 oz)	240	17	8	0
Broccoli Cheddar	1 serv (8 oz)	213	15	8	0
Cheddar Potato	1 serv (8 oz)	213	13	8	0
Cheesy Chicken Tortilla	1 (8 oz)	150	6	3	0
Chicken & Sausage Gumbo	1 serv (8 oz)	150	5	2	0
Clam Chowder	1 serv (8 oz)	200	11	6	0
Country Potato	1 serv (8 oz)	173	8	4	0
Country Vegetable	1 serv (8 oz)	93	1	0	0
French Onion	1 serv (8 oz)	80	1	1	0
Red Beans & Rice	1 serv (8 oz)	107	3	1	0
Southwest Roasted Corn	1 serv (8 oz)	90	4	1	0

MCDONALD'S
BEVERAGES

FOOD	PORTION	CALS	FAT	SAT FAT	TRANS FAT
Apple Juice	1 box (6.8 oz)	90	0	0	0
Chocolate Milk 1% Low Fat	8 oz	170	3	2	0
Coca-Cola Classic	1 sm (16 oz)	150	0	0	0
Coffee	1 sm (12 oz)	0	0	0	0

FOOD	PORTION	CALS	FAT	SAT FAT	TRANS FAT
Diet Coke	1 sm (16 oz)	0	0	0	0
Half & Half Creamer	1 pkg	20	2	2	0
Hi-C Orange Lavaburst	1 sm (16 oz)	160	0	0	0
Iced Coffee Caramel	1 sm (16 oz)	130	5	4	0
Iced Coffee Hazelnut	1 sm (16 oz)	130	5	4	0
Iced Coffee Regular	1 sm (16 oz)	140	5	4	0
Iced Coffee Vanilla	1 sm (16 oz)	130	5	4	0
Iced Tea	1 sm (16 oz)	0	0	0	0
Milk Lowfat 1%	1 pkg	100	3	2	0
Orange Juice	1 sm (12 oz)	140	0	0	0
Powerade Mountain Blast	1 sm (16 oz)	100	0	0	0
Shake Triple Thick Chocolate	1 sm (12 oz)	440	10	6	1
Shake Triple Thick Strawberry	1 sm (12 oz)	420	10	6	1
Shake Triple Thick Vanilla	1 sm (16 oz)	420	10	6	1
Sprite	1 sm (16 oz)	150	0	0	0
BREAKFAST SELECTIONS					
Big Breakfast Regular Biscuit	1 serv	720	46	16	3
Biscuit	1 reg	250	11	5	0
Biscuit Regular Bacon Egg Cheese	1	450	25	11	0
Biscuit Regular Sausage	1	410	27	10	0
Biscuit Regular Sausage w/ Egg	1	500	32	12	0
Burrito Sausage	1	300	16	7	1
Deluxe Breakfast Regular Biscuit w/o Syrup & Margarine	1 serv	1070	55	18	3
English Muffin	1	160	3	1	0
Hash Browns	1 serv	140	8	2	2
Hotcake Syrup	1 pkg (2 oz)	180	0	0	0
Hotcakes & Sausage w/o Syrup & Margarine	1 serv	520	24	7	0
Hotcakes w/o Syrup & Margarine	1 serv	350	9	2	0
McGriddles Bacon Egg Cheese	1	460	21	9	0
McGriddles Sausage	1	420	22	8	0
McGriddles Sausage Egg & Cheese	1	560	32	12	0
McMuffin Sausage	1	370	22	8	0
McMuffin Sausage w/ Egg	1	250	27	10	0
McSkillet Burrito w/ Sausage	1	610	36	14	1
McSkillet Burrito w/ Steak	1	570	30	12	1

FOOD	PORTION	CALS	FAT	SAT FAT	TRANS FAT
Sausage Patty	1	170	15	5	0
Scrambled Eggs	2	170	11	4	0
DESSERTS					
Apple Dippers	1 pkg	35	0	0	0
Apple Pie Baked	1	270	12	4	5
Caramel Dip Low Fat	1 pkg	70	1	0	0
Cinnamon Melts	1 serv	460	19	9	0
Cookie Chocolate Chip	1	180	7	3	0
Cookie Oatmeal	1 (1.1 oz)	150	6	2	2
Cookie Sugar	1 (1.1 oz)	150	6	2	2
Cookies McDonaldland	1 pkg (2 oz)	250	8	2	3
Cookies McDonaldland Chocolate Chip	1 pkg	270	11	6	0
Fruit 'n Yogurt Parfait	1 serv	160	2	1	0
Ice Cream Cone Reduced Fat Vanilla	1	150	4	2	0
Kiddie Cone	1	45	1	1	0
McFlurry w/ M&M's	1 (12 oz)	620	20	12	1
McFlurry w/ Oreos	1 (12 oz)	560	16	9	2
Peanuts For Sundae	1 serv	45	4	1	0
Sundae Hot Caramel	1	340	7	5	0
Sundae Hot Fudge	1	330	10	7	0
Sundae Strawberry	1	280	6	4	0
MAIN MENU SELECTIONS					
Apple Sauce Strawberry	1 serv	90	0	0	0
Big Mac	1	540	29	10	2
Big N' Tasty	1	460	24	8	2
Big N' Tasty w/ Cheese	1	510	28	43	2
Cheeseburger	1	300	12	6	1
Cheeseburger Double	1	440	23	11	2
Cheesy Tots	6 pieces	210	12	5	2
Chicken McNuggets	4 pieces	170	10	2	1
Chicken Selects	3 pieces	380	20	4	3
Filet-O-Fish	1	380	18	4	1
French Fries	1 lg	570	30	6	0
French Fries	1 sm	250	13	3	0
Hamburger	1	250	9	4	1
McChicken	1	360	16	4	1
McRib	1	500	26	10	0
Onion Rings	1 sm	140	7	2	1

FOOD	PORTION	CALS	FAT	SAT FAT	TRANS FAT
Quarter Pounder	1	410	19	7	1
Quarter Pounder Double w/ Cheese	1	740	42	19	3
Quarter Pounder w/ Cheese	1	510	26	12	2
Sandwich Chicken Classic Crispy	1	500	17	4	2
Sandwich Chicken Classic Grilled	1	420	10	2	0
Sandwich Club Chicken Crispy	1	660	28	8	2
Sandwich Club Chicken Grilled	1	570	21	7	0
Sandwich Ranch BLT Chicken Crispy	1	600	23	5	2
Sandwich Ranch BLT Chicken Grilled	1	520	16	4	0
Snack Wrap w/ Chipotle BBQ	1	320	14	5	1
Snack Wrap w/ Honey Mustard	1	320	15	5	1
Snack Wrap w/ Ranch	1	140	16	5	1
Snack Wrap Grilled w/ Chipotle BBQ	1	260	8	4	0
Snack Wrap Grilled w/ Honey Mustard	1	260	9	4	0
Snack Wrap Grilled w/ Ranch	1	270	10	4	0
SALAD DRESSINGS AND SAUCES					
Dipping Sauce Buffalo	1 serv (1 oz)	80	8	2	0
Dipping Sauce Zesty Onion Ring	1 serv (1 oz)	150	15	3	0
Dressing Ken's Light Italian	1 pkg (2 oz)	120	11	2	0
Dressing Newman's Own Creamy Caesar	1 pkg (2 oz)	170	18	4	0
Dressing Newman's Own Creamy Southwest	1 pkg (1.5 oz)	100	6	1	0
Dressing Newman's Own Low Fat Balsamic Vinaigrette	1 pkg (1.5 oz)	40	3	0	0
Dressing Newman's Own Low Fat Family Recipe Italian	1 pkg (1.5 oz)	60	3	0	0
Dressing Newman's Own Low Fat Sesame Ginger	1 pkg (1.5 oz)	90	3	0	0
Dressing Newman's Own Ranch	1 pkg (2 oz)	170	15	3	0
Honey	1 pkg (0.5 oz)	50	0	0	0

FOOD	PORTION	CALS	FAT	SAT FAT	TRANS FAT
Ketchup	1 pkg	15	0	0	0
Sauce Barbecue	1 pkg (1 oz)	50	0	0	0
Sauce Creamy Ranch	1 pkg (1.5 oz)	200	22	4	0
Sauce Hot Mustard	1 pkg (1 oz)	60	3	0	0
Sauce Southwestern Chipotle Barbeque	1 pkg (1.5 oz)	70	0	0	0
Sauce Spicy Buffalo	1 pkg (1.5 oz)	60	7	1	0
Sauce Sweet'N Sour	1 pkg (1 oz)	50	0	0	0
Sauce Tangy Honey Mustard	1 pkg (1.5 oz)	70	3	0	0
SALADS					
Asian w/ Crispy Chicken w/o Dressing	1 serv	380	17	3	2
Asian w/ Grilled Chicken w/o Dressing	1 serv	300	10	1	0
Asian w/o Chicken & Dressing	1 serv	150	7	1	0
Bacon Ranch w/ Crispy Chicken	1 serv	350	16	5	2
Bacon Ranch w/ Grilled Chicken w/o Dressing	1 serv	260	9	4	0
Bacon Ranch w/o Chicken	1 serv	140	7	4	0
Caesar w/ Crispy Chicken	1 serv	300	13	4	2
Caesar w/ Grilled Chicken	1 serv	220	6	3	0
Caesar w/o Chicken	1 serv	90	4	3	0
Croutons Butter Garlic	1 pkg	60	2	0	0
Fruit & Walnut Snack Size	1 serv	210	8	2	0
Side Salad	1 serv	20	0	0	0
Southwest w/ Crispy Chicken w/o Dressing	1 serv	400	16	4	2
Southwest w/ Grilled Chicken	1 serv	320	9	3	0
Southwest w/o Chicken & Dressing	1 serv	140	5	2	0
MIAMI SUBS					
Burger Deluxe	1	784	59	17	–
Cheeseburger Deluxe	1	859	65	21	–
Cheeseburger Deluxe Bacon	1	919	70	23	–
Cheesesteak Classic	1 (6 in)	420	11	7	–
Cheesesteak Original	1 (6 in)	409	11	7	–
Cheesesteak Works	1 (6 in)	532	23	8	–
Chicken Philly Classic	1 (6 in)	551	27	8	–
Mozzarella Sticks	1 serv	757	57	16	–

FOOD	PORTION	CALS	FAT	SAT FAT	TRANS FAT
Onion Rings	1 serv	869	68	10	–
Pita Chicken	1	392	13	3	–
Pita Gyros	1	662	39	27	–
Platter Chicken Breast	1 serv	743	41	11	–
Platter Gyros	1 serv	1420	93	9	–
Salad Caesar w/ Dressing	1 serv	459	34	6	–
Salad Chicken Caesar w/ Dressing	1 serv	609	39	7	–
Salad Chicken Club	1 serv	490	25	10	–
Salad Garden	1 serv	310	18	7	–
Salad Greek	1 serv	284	15	5	–
Salad Greek Side w/ Dressing	1 serv	78	5	2	–
Spicy Fries	1 reg	532	39	10	–
Subs 6 Inch Ham & Cheese	1	452	18	5	–
Subs 6 Inch Italian Deli	1	516	25	8	–
Subs 6 Inch Meatball	1	491	22	9	–
Subs 6 Inch Tuna	1	468	18	2	–
Subs 6 Inch Turkey	1	484	18	5	–
Wings w/ Fries Celery & Blue Cheese	1 serv	1020	67	17	–

MR. HERO
MAIN MENU SELECTIONS

Breadsticks w/ Sauce	1 serv	291	9	2	–
Spaghetti Dinner	1 serv	606	8	2	–
Spaghetti w/ Meatballs	1 serv	846	26	2	–

SALAD DRESSINGS

Buttermilk	1 serv (2 oz)	290	29	–	–

SALADS

Garden Salad	1 serv	36	tr	0	–
Grilled Chicken	1 serv	225	10	3	–
Seafood Crab	1 serv	452	37	7	–
Side Salad	1 serv	27	tr	0	–
Tuna	1 serv	745	69	13	–

SANDWICHES

Cheesesteaks Grilled Steak	7 in	450	14	6	–
Cheesesteaks Hot Buttered Deluxe	7 in	566	33	18	–
Cold Subs Classic Italian	7 in	586	36	9	–
Cold Subs Tuna & Cheese	7 in	666	47	9	–

FOOD	PORTION	CALS	FAT	SAT FAT	TRANS FAT
Cold Subs Turkey & Cheese	7 in	453	21	5	–
Hot Subs Grilled Chicken Philly	7 in	438	14	5	–
Hot Subs Meatball	7 in	620	32	3	–
Hot Subs Romanburger	7 in	717	47	15	–
Round Chicken	1	420	23	5	–
Round Tuna	1	302	34	6	–

MR. PITA

FOOD	PORTION	CALS	FAT	SAT FAT	TRANS FAT
Cranberry Turkey	1 reg	424	1	tr	–
Grilled Raspberry Chicken	1 reg	342	3	1	–
Grilled Chicken & Broccoli	1 reg	373	4	1	–
Grilled Chicken Caesar	1 reg	353	4	1	–
Grilled Hawaiian Chicken	1 reg	375	4	1	–
Ultra Combo	1 reg	354	3	1	–
Ultra Grilled Chicken	1 reg	367	4	1	–
Ultra Supreme	1 reg	350	3	1	–
Ultra Turkey	1 reg	343	1	tr	–

MRS. FIELDS

FOOD	PORTION	CALS	FAT	SAT FAT	TRANS FAT
Brownie Double Fudge	1 (2.7 oz)	360	19	11	–
Brownie Frosted Fudge	1 (3.7 oz)	440	21	12	–
Brownie Pecan Fudge	1 (2.7 oz)	340	21	9	–
Brownie Pecan Pie	1 (2.7 oz)	340	20	9	–
Brownie Walnut Fudge	1 (2.7 oz)	380	23	10	–
Bundt Cake Banana Walnut	1 piece (2.9 oz)	350	21	5	–
Bundt Cake Banana Walnut w/ Chocolate Chips	1 piece (2.9 oz)	370	22	7	–
Bundt Cake Blueberry	1 piece (2.9 oz)	270	12	5	–
Bundt Cake Raspberry	1 piece (2.9 oz)	270	12	5	–
Bundt Cake White w/ Chocolate Chips	1 piece (2.9 oz)	350	17	8	–
Cookie Butter Toffee	1 (2.3 oz)	290	13	8	–
Cookie Cinnamon Sugar	1 (2.3 oz)	300	12	8	–
Cookie Coconut Macadamia	1 (2.3 oz)	280	13	5	–
Cookie Debra's Special	1 (2.3 oz)	280	12	6	–
Cookie Milk Chocolate	1 (2.3 oz)	280	13	8	–
Cookie Milk Chocolate & Walnuts	1 (2.3 oz)	320	17	9	–
Cookie Milk Chocolate Macadamia	1 (2.3 oz)	320	18	9	–

FOOD	PORTION	CALS	FAT	SAT FAT	TRANS FAT
Cookie Oatmeal Chocolate Chip	1 (2.3 oz)	280	13	8	–
Cookie Oatmeal Raisin & Walnuts	1 (2.3 oz)	280	12	6	–
Cookie Peanut Butter	1 (2.3 oz)	310	16	8	–
Cookie Peanut Butter w/ Milk Chocolate Chips	1 (2.3 oz)	300	17	8	–
Cookie Semi-Sweet Chocolate	1 (2.3 oz)	280	14	8	–
Cookie Semi-Sweet Chocolate & Walnuts	1 (2.3 oz)	310	16	8	–
Cookie White Chunk Macadamia	1 (2.3 oz)	310	17	9	–
Jumbo Cookie Snickerdoodle	1 (5 oz)	640	29	17	–
Nibbler Cookies	2 (0.9 oz)	110	5	3	–
Nibbler Cookies Chewy Chocolate Fudge	2 (0.9 oz)	110	5	4	–
Nibbler Cookies Cinnamon Sugar	2 (0.9 oz)	120	5	3	–
Nibbler Cookies Debra's Special	2 (0.9 oz)	100	5	2	–
Nibbler Cookies M&M's	2 (0.9 oz)	110	5	4	–
Nibbler Cookies Milk Chocolate	2 (0.9 oz)	110	5	3	–
Nibbler Cookies Milk Chocolate w/ Walnuts	2 (0.9 oz)	120	6	3	–
Nibbler Cookies Peanut Butter	2 (0.9 oz)	110	6	3	–
Nibbler Cookies Semi-Sweet Chocolate	2 (0.9 oz)	110	5	3	–
Nibbler Cookies Triple Chocolate	2 (0.9 oz)	110	6	3	–
Nibbler Cookies White Chunk Macadamia	2 (0.9 oz)	120	7	4	–

NATHAN'S

FOOD	PORTION	CALS	FAT	SAT FAT	TRANS FAT
¼ Pound Burger	1	537	30	12	–
¼ Pound Burger w/ Cheese	1	850	61	21	–
Bacon Cheeseburger	1	707	44	20	–
Cheesesteak Chicken	1 serv	565	19	10	–
Cheesesteak Original	1	741	43	19	–
Cheesesteak Supreme	1 serv	786	43	19	–

FOOD	PORTION	CALS	FAT	SAT FAT	TRANS FAT
Chicken Tender Pita	1	610	38	5	-
Chicken Tenders	3 pieces	512	37	5	-
Cole Slaw	1 serv	213	9	1	-
Corn Muffin	1	163	6	1	-
Famous Hot Dog	1	309	20	8	-
Fish N Chips	1 serv	1538	101	17	-
French Fries	1 reg	547	38	4	-
Hot Dog Nuggets	6 pieces	351	28	4	-
Hush Puppy	2 pieces	277	10	2	-
Onion Rings	1 sm	559	44	6	-
Platter Chicken Breast	1 serv	943	54	7	-
Platter Chicken Tender	1 serv	1301	83	10	-
Sandwich Chicken Tender	1	725	47	7	-
Sandwich Fish	1	469	20	4	-
Sandwich Grilled Chicken	1	524	29	5	-
Seafood Sampler	1 serv	3379	270	29	-
Shrimp N Chips	1 serv	2051	124	13	-
Super Burger	1	864	62	21	-

NEWPORT CREAMERY

Ice Cream Chocolate No Sugar Added	½ cup	110	3	-	-
Ice Cream Vanilla No Sugar Added	½ cup	100	3	-	-
Vanilla Yogurt	½ cup	120	3	-	-
Vanilla Yogurt Nonfat	½ cup	100	0	0	0

OLD SPAGHETTI FACTORY
CHILDREN'S MENU SELECTIONS

Grilled Cheese Sandwich	1 serv	360	22	8	-
Macaroni & Cheese	1 serv	350	9	5	-
Spaghetti w/ Tomato Sauce	1 serv	300	4	5	-
Spaghetti w/ Tomato Sauce & Meatballs	1 serv	440	13	4	-

DESSERTS

Caramel Turtle Pie	1 serv	660	29	15	-
Mud Pie	1 serv	680	32	17	-
New York Cheese Cake w/ Strawberry Topping	1 serv	690	40	24	-

MAIN MENU SELECTIONS

Baked Chicken	1 dinner serv	880	47	16	-

FOOD	PORTION	CALS	FAT	SAT FAT	TRANS FAT
Caesar Salad	1 sm	330	30	6	–
Caesar Salad Dinner Chicken	1 serv	1280	85	23	–
Chicken Marsala	1 dinner serv	960	44	24	–
Fettuccine Alfredo	1 dinner serv	1130	83	51	–
Fettuccine Chicken	1 dinner serv	960	56	33	–
Lasagne	1 dinner serv	630	33	15	–
Parmigiana Chicken	1 dinner serv	840	34	9	–
Parmigiana Eggplant	1 dinner serv	670	32	17	–
Pot Pourri	1 dinner serv	710	30	17	–
Ravioli Spinach & Cheese	1 dinner serv	480	15	7	–
Salmon Tuscany	1 dinner serv	680	43	18	–
Sandwich Meatball	1	860	41	15	–
Sandwich Sausage	1	730	40	14	–
Sandwich Tuscan Chicken	1	1060	60	12	–
Seafood Cheddar Melt	1 serv	790	42	14	–
Spaghetti w/ Clam Sauce	1 dinner serv	690	28	16	–
Spaghetti w/ Clam Sauce & Mizithra	1 dinner serv	960	54	33	–
Spaghetti w/ Meat & Clam Sauces	1 dinner serv	980	17	9	–
Spaghetti w/ Meat Sauce	1 dinner serv	470	5	1	–
Spaghetti w/ Meat Sauce & Mizithra	1 dinner serv	850	42	25	–
Spaghetti w/ Meat Sauce & Sausage	1 dinner serv	830	35	11	–
Spaghetti w/ Meatballs	1 dinner serv	840	33	12	–
Spaghetti w/ Mizithra	1 dinner serv	1010	64	40	–
Spaghetti w/ Mushroom & Clam Sauces	1 dinner serv	830	18	9	–
Spaghetti w/ Mushroom & Meat Sauces	1 dinner serv	460	6	1	–
Spaghetti w/ Mushroom Sauce	1 dinner serv	460	7	1	–
Spaghetti w/ Mushroom Sauce & Mizithra	1 dinner serv	850	43	25	–
Spaghetti w/ Tomato & Mizithra	1 dinner serv	840	42	25	–
Spaghetti w/ Tomato & Meat Sauces	1 dinner serv	460	5	1	–
Spaghetti w/ Tomato Sauce	1 dinner serv	440	5	1	–
Spaghetti w/ Tomato Sauce & Clam Sauce	1 dinner serv	560	17	9	–

FOOD	PORTION	CALS	FAT	SAT FAT	TRANS FAT
Starter Garlic Cheese Bread	1 serv	1220	85	21	–
Starter Meatballs	1 serv	910	61	22	–
Starter Sausage	1 serv	690	56	21	–
Starter Tortellini	1 serv	930	56	33	–
Tortellini Mortadella & Chicken	1 dinner serv	930	56	33	–
SOUPS					
Chicken Mulligatawny	1 serv	250	14	8	–
Chicken Orzo	1 serv	90	3	1	–
Clam Chowder	1 serv	380	29	18	–
Cream Of Broccoli	1 serv	220	12	7	–
Mediterranean White Bean	1 serv	150	6	1	–
Minestrone	1 serv	120	5	1	–

ON THE BORDER
CHILDREN'S MENU SELECTIONS

FOOD	PORTION	CALS	FAT	SAT FAT	TRANS FAT
Border Chicken Strips	1 serv	570	36	6	–
Corn Dog	1	320	21	5	–
Crispy Taco Mexican Dinner Beef	1 serv	740	31	12	–
Crispy Taco Mexican Dinner Chicken	1 serv	740	28	11	–
Hamburger	1	390	23	7	–
Nachos Bean & Cheese	1 serv	980	57	29	–
Nachos Cheese	1 serv	670	47	26	–
Quesadillas Chicken	1 serv	720	48	26	–
Sandwich Grilled Chicken	1	630	21	9	–
Soft Taco Mexican Dinner Beef	1 serv	840	35	14	–
Soft Taco Mexican Dinner Chicken	1 serv	750	27	11	–
Sundae w/ Chocolate Syrup	1 serv	300	13	8	–
Sundae w/ Strawberry Puree	1 serv	340	13	8	–
DESSERTS					
Border Brownie Sundae	1	440	25	12	–
Chocolate Turtle Empanadas	1 serv	1280	81	29	–
Dulce De Leche Cheesecake	1 serv	1160	72	39	–
Kahlua Ice Cream Pie	1 serv	850	44	17	–
Sizzling Apple Crisp	1 serv	960	36	19	–
Sopapillas	1 serv	1230	56	13	–
Vanilla Ice Cream	1 scoop	180	10	6	–

FOOD	PORTION	CALS	FAT	SAT FAT	TRANS FAT
MAIN MENU SELECTIONS					
Bacon Wrapped Shrimp	1 serv	730	62	18	–
Baja Chicken	1 serv	610	43	16	–
Bandera Sirloin	1 serv	640	43	17	–
Beans Black	1 serv	180	7	2	–
Beans Refried	1 serv	290	11	4	–
Black Bean & Corn Relish	1 serv	80	4	0	–
Border Chimichanga Fajita Chicken w/ Onions & Mushrooms	1 serv	1230	93	28	–
Border Chimichanga Ground Beef	1 serv	1310	98	31	–
Border Chimichanga Spicy Chicken	1 serv	1160	85	27	–
Border Sampler	1 serv	1940	120	56	–
Bordurrito Big Beef w/ Side Salad	1 serv	1600	103	21	–
Bordurrito Big Chicken w/ Side Salad	1 serv	1420	57	14	–
Burrito Beef	1 serv	1080	57	23	–
Burrito Chicken	1 serv	880	56	19	–
Burrito Three Sauce Fajita Chicken	1 serv	870	45	19	–
Burrito Three Sauce Fajita Steak	1 serv	1050	61	25	–
Carne Asada & Shrimp	1 serv	1040	74	29	–
Cheese Chile Relleno	1	880	61	23	–
Cheesy Pepper Jack Mashed Potatoes	1 serv	380	27	10	–
Chicken Flautas Appetizer	1 serv	970	66	17	–
Chile Con Queso	1 bowl	390	29	19	–
Chile Con Queso	1 cup	250	18	12	–
Corona Extra Dinner	1 serv	2040	128	44	–
Crispy Taco Beef	1	330	20	8	–
Crispy Taco Chicken	1	240	12	5	–
Crispy Taco Veggie	1	250	16	5	–
Dos XX Fish Tacos	1 serv	1590	113	25	–
Empanadas Beef	1	440	31	11	–
Empanadas Chicken	1	390	26	10	–
Empanadas Chicken	1 serv	1090	74	30	–

FOOD	PORTION	CALS	FAT	SAT FAT	TRANS FAT
Empanadas Ground Beef	1 serv	1150	81	30	–
Enchilada Beef	1	340	17	6	–
Enchilada Cheese & Onion	1	410	24	12	–
Enchilada Chicken	1	350	23	6	–
Fajitas 7 Pepper Steak	1 serv	910	62	24	–
Fajitas Blackened Chicken w/ Portobello Mushrooms	1 serv	640	29	13	–
Fajitas Carnitas	1 serv	830	62	29	–
Fajitas Chicken Con Queso	1 skillet	1130	82	53	–
Fajitas Grilled Vegetables w/ Portobello Mushrooms	1 serv	390	28	3	–
Fajitas Jalapeno BBQ Chicken	1 serv	760	32	15	–
Fajitas Mesquite Grilled Chicken	1 serv	440	18	3	–
Fajitas Mesquite Grilled Steak	1 serv	620	41	12	–
Fajitas Monterey Ranch Chicken	1 serv	840	21	17	–
Fajitas Shrimp	1 serv	750	63	18	–
Fajitas Ultimate	1 serv	1230	102	36	–
Firecracker Stuffed Jalapenos	1 serv	980	56	26	–
French Fries	1 serv	390	25	5	–
Grande Fajita Nachos Beef	1 serv	1970	127	54	–
Grande Fajita Nachos Chicken	1 serv	1890	113	49	–
Grande Fajita Nachos Combo	1 serv	1940	121	52	–
Guacamole	1 serv	130	10	1	–
Guacamole Live	1 serv	570	50	10	–
Margarita Chicken	1 serv	290	11	2	–
Mexican Rice	1 serv	220	6	2	–
Mexican Shrimp Scampi	1 serv	740	64	10	–
Pico Chicken & Shrimp	1 serv	730	51	17	–
Quesadillas Combo Fajita	1 serv	1450	96	49	–
Quesadillas Double Stacked Club	1 serv	1860	123	52	–
Quesadillas Fajita Chicken	1 serv	1430	91	46	–
Quesadillas Fajita Steak	1 serv	1530	107	52	–
Quesadillas Spinach & Mushroom	1 serv	1420	105	46	–
Ranchiladas	1 serv	1360	86	40	–
Red Chili Ribeye	1 serv	900	72	31	–
Salmon Mexican	1 serv	650	50	11	–

FOOD	PORTION	CALS	FAT	SAT FAT	TRANS FAT
Sandwich Chicken Blackened w/ French Fries	1 serv	1510	93	26	–
Sandwich Chicken Grilled w/ French Fries	1 serv	1430	92	25	–
Sauteed Shrimp	4	170	10	4	–
Shaken Margarita Shrimp Cocktail	1 serv	280	13	1	–
Shaken Margarita Shrimp Cocktail w/ Tortilla Chips	1 serv	780	40	8	–
Soft Taco Beef	1	340	19	8	–
Soft Taco Chicken	1	250	11	5	–
Soft Taco Veggie	1	210	9	4	–
Superior Dinner	1 serv	1350	85	33	–
Tamale	1	310	17	5	–
Tortilla Soup	1 bowl	350	22	9	–
Tortillas Corn	3	230	4	0	–
Tortillas Flour	3	300	9	2	–
Tres Enchilada Dinner Beef	1 serv	1010	52	18	–
Tres Enchilada Dinner Cheese	1 serv	1210	73	36	–
Tres Enchilada Dinner Chicken	1 serv	1040	68	19	–
Ultimate Loaded Queso	1 serv	900	59	31	–
Vegetables Grilled	1 serv	50	1	0	–
Vegetables Sauteed	1 serv	70	4	1	–
SALAD DRESSINGS AND SAUCES					
Chili Con Carne Sauce	1 serv (2 oz)	70	3	0	–
Chipotle Mayonnaise	1 serv (1 oz)	190	21	3	–
Dressing Chipotle Honey Mustard	1 serv (2 oz)	310	29	4	–
Dressing Ranch	1 serv (2 oz)	220	23	4	–
Dressing Smoked Jalapeno Vinaigrette	1 serv (2 oz)	230	22	3	–
Dressing Sweet Pepper Vinaigrette	1 serv (2 oz)	270	25	3	–
Dressing Fat Free Balsamic Vinaigrette	1 serv (2 oz)	50	0	0	0
Dressing Lo Fat Ranch	1 serv (2 oz)	110	6	1	–
Parrila Butter	1 serv (1 oz)	120	13	5	–
Pico De Gallo	1 scoop	20	1	0	–
Ranchero Sauce	1 serv (2 oz)	18	1	0	–
Salsa	1 serv (2 oz)	25	1	0	–

FOOD	PORTION	CALS	FAT	SAT FAT	TRANS FAT
Sour Cream	1 serv (2 oz)	140	14	2	–
SALADS					
Chopped Chicken w/ Dressing	1 serv	1330	89	34	–
Fiesta Blackened Chicken w/ Dressing	1 serv	1150	75	24	–
Fiesta Chicken w/ Dressing	1 serv	1140	74	23	–
Grande Taco Beef	1 serv	1450	102	37	–
Grande Taco Chicken	1 serv	1280	89	31	–
House	1 serv	170	10	4	–
Sizzling Fajita Chicken	1 serv	760	48	24	–
Sizzling Fajita Steak	1 serv	910	65	31	–
P.J. CHANG'S CHINA BISTRO					
Cantonese Scallops	1 serv	305	8	–	–
Chicken w/ Black Bean Sauce	1 serv	426	11	–	–
Pin Rice Noodles	1 serv	270	2	–	–
Vegetable Chow Fun	1 serv	677	18	–	–
PACIUGO GELATO					
Milk Base Amarena Black Cherry Swirl	1 scoop (3.5 oz)	160	4	3	0
Milk Base Banana Creme Pie	1 scoop (3.5 oz)	80	2	1	0
Milk Base Cheesecake	1 scoop (3.5 oz)	90	4	2	0
Milk Base Chocolate	1 scoop (3.5 oz)	80	3	2	0
Milk Base Chocolate Cookies'N Milk	1 scoop (3.5 oz)	90	3	2	0
Milk Base Coconut	1 scoop (3.5 oz)	80	3	2	0
Milk Base Coffee	1 scoop (3.5 oz)	75	3	2	0
Milk Base Fiordilatte	1 scoop (3.5 oz)	75	2	2	0
Milk Base French Vanilla Bean	1 scoop (3.5 oz)	80	3	2	0
Milk Base Green Tea	1 scoop (3.5 oz)	70	2	2	0
Milk Base Hazelnut	1 scoop (3.5 oz)	85	4	2	0
Milk Base Lemon Custard	1 scoop (3.5 oz)	75	3	3	0
Milk Base Mascarpone Chocolate Rum	1 scoop (3.5 oz)	95	5	3	0
Milk Base Pannacotta Wedding Cake	1 scoop (3.5 oz)	75	2	1	0
Milk Base Peppermint	1 scoop (3.5 oz)	75	2	1	0
Milk Base Rose	1 scoop (3.5 oz)	70	2	2	0
Milk Base Tiramisu	1 scoop (3.5 oz)	80	3	2	0
Milk Base Zabajone	1 scoop (3.5 oz)	80	3	2	0

FOOD	PORTION	CALS	FAT	SAT FAT	TRANS FAT
No Sugar Added Chocolate	1 scoop (3.5 oz)	28	1	1	0
No Sugar Added Mint	1 scoop (3.5 oz)	25	1	tr	0
No Sugar Added Mocha	1 scoop (3.5 oz)	28	1	1	0
No Sugar Added Strawberry Milk	1 scoop (3.5 oz)	23	1	tr	0
Soy Banana	1 scoop (3.5 oz)	40	2	tr	0
Soy Blueberry	1 scoop (3.5 oz)	40	2	tr	0
Soy Chocolate	1 scoop (3.5 oz)	38	2	1	0
Soy Coffee	1 scoop (3.5 oz)	35	2	tr	0
Soy Hazelnut	1 scoop (3.5 oz)	35	2	tr	0
Soy Strawberry	1 scoop (3.5 oz)	38	2	tr	0
Soy Wild Berries	1 scoop (3.5 oz)	40	2	tr	0
Water Base Blackberry	1 scoop (3.5 oz)	28	0	0	0
Water Base Ginger Lemon	1 scoop (3.5 oz)	25	0	0	0
Water Base Green Apple	1 scoop (3.5 oz)	28	0	0	0
Water Base Lemon Sage	1 scoop (3.5 oz)	25	0	0	0
Water Base Lychee	1 scoop (3.5 oz)	25	0	0	0
Water Base Orange Vidalia	1 scoop (3.5 oz)	25	0	0	0
Water Base Passion Fruit	1 scoop (3.5 oz)	23	0	0	0
Water Base Pineapple	1 scoop (3.5 oz)	28	0	0	0
Water Base Strawberry Port	1 scoop (3.5 oz)	25	0	0	0
Water Base Watermelon	1 scoop (3.5 oz)	25	0	0	0

PANDA EXPRESS
MAIN MENU SELECTIONS

FOOD	PORTION	CALS	FAT	SAT FAT	TRANS FAT
BBQ Pork	1 serv	350	19	7	–
Beef & Broccoli	1 serv	150	8	2	–
Beef w/ String Beans	1 serv	170	9	2	–
Black Pepper Chicken	1 serv	180	10	2	–
Chicken w/ Mushrooms	1 serv	130	7	2	–
Chicken w/ Potato	1 serv	220	11	2	–
Chicken w/ String Beans	1 serv	170	8	2	–
Egg Roll Chicken	1 (3 oz)	190	8	2	–
Fried Shrimp	6 pieces	260	12	3	–
Mandarin Chicken	1 serv	250	9	3	–
Mixed Vegetables	1 serv	70	3	1	–
Orange Chicken	1 serv	480	21	5	–
Spicy Chicken w/ Peanuts	1 serv	200	7	2	–
Spring Roll Veggie	1 (1.7 oz)	80	3	0	–
Steamed Rice	1 serv	330	1	0	–

FOOD	PORTION	CALS	FAT	SAT FAT	TRANS FAT
String Beans w/ Fried Tofu	1 serv	180	11	2	–
Sweet & Sour Chicken	1 serv	310	14	3	-
Sweet & Sour Pork	1 serv	410	30	7	–
Vegetable Chow Mein	1 serv	330	11	2	–
Vegetable Fried Rice	1 serv	390	12	3	–
SAUCES					
Hot	2 tsp	10	1	0	–
Hot Mustard	1 serv	18	0	0	0
Mandarin	1 serv	70	0	0	0
Soy	1 tbsp	16	0	0	0
Sweet & Sour	1 serv	60	0	0	0

PANERA BREAD
BAGELS AND SPREADS

FOOD	PORTION	CALS	FAT	SAT FAT	TRANS FAT
Bagel Asiago Cheese	1	330	5	3	–
Bagel Blueberry	1	320	2	0	–
Bagel Cinnamon Crunch	1	490	9	5	–
Bagel Dutch Apple & Raisin	1	340	3	0	–
Bagel Everything	1	290	2	0	–
Bagel French Toast	1	340	5	1	–
Bagel Mochachip Swirl	1	340	4	2	–
Bagel Nine Grain	1	290	1	0	–
Bagel Peanut Butter Crunch	1	400	6	3	–
Bagel Plain	1	280	1	0	–
Bagel Sesame	1	310	3	0	–
Cream Cheese Hazelnut Reduced Fat	1 serv (2 oz)	150	11	7	–
Cream Cheese Honey Walnut Reduced Fat	1 serv (2 oz)	150	11	7	–
Cream Cheese Mocha Reduced Fat	1 serv (2 oz)	160	11	30	–
Cream Cheese Plain	1 serv (2 oz)	190	18	12	–
Cream Cheese Plain Reduced Fat	1 serv (2 oz)	130	12	8	–
Cream Cheese Raspberry Reduced Fat	1 serv (2 oz)	120	10	7	–
Cream Cheese Smoked Salmon Reduced Fat	1 serv (2 oz)	120	10	6	–
Cream Cheese Sun Dried Tomato Reduced Fat	1 serv (2 oz)	140	11	7	–

FOOD	PORTION	CALS	FAT	SAT FAT	TRANS FAT
Cream Cheese Veggie Reduced Fat	1 serv (2 oz)	130	11	7	–
Hummus Roasted Garlic	1 serv (2 oz)	100	5	1	–
BEVERAGES					
Caffe Mocha	1 serv (11.5 oz)	360	16	55	–
Homestyle Lemonade	1 serv (16 oz)	80	0	0	0
Hot Chocolate	1 serv (11 oz)	350	15	10	–
IC Cappuccino Chip	1 serv (16 oz)	590	35	26	–
IC Caramel	1 serv (16 oz)	550	24	15	–
IC Honeydew Green Tea	1 serv (16 oz)	270	13	0	–
IC Mocha	1 serv (16 oz)	520	24	15	–
IC Spice	1 serv (16 oz)	470	22	13	–
Iced Green Tea	1 serv (16 oz)	60	0	0	0
Latte Caffe	1 serv (8.5 oz)	120	5	3	–
Latte Caramel	1 serv (11 oz)	400	16	9	–
Latte Chai Tea	1 serv (10 oz)	210	5	3	–
Latte House	1 serv (10.8 oz)	320	13	8	–
BREADS					
Artisan Country	1 slice	120	0	0	0
Artisan French	1 slice (2 oz)	110	0	0	0
Artisan Kalamata Olive	1 slice (2 oz)	140	2	0	–
Artisan Multigrain	1 slice (2 oz)	120	1	0	–
Artisan Raisin Pecan	1 slice (2 oz)	140	3	0	–
Artisan Sesame Semolina	1 slice (2 oz)	120	0	0	0
Artisan Stone Milled Rye	1 slice (2 oz)	110	0	0	0
Artisan Three Cheese	1 slice (2 oz)	120	2	1	–
Artisan Three Seed	1 slice	130	2	0	–
Ciabatta	1 (6 oz)	430	10	2	–
Cinnamon Raisin	1 slice (2 oz)	160	3	1	–
Focaccia Asiago Cheese	1 slice (2 oz)	150	6	2	–
Focaccia Basil Pesto	1 slice (2 oz)	150	6	2	–
Focaccia Rosemary & Onion	1 slice (2 oz)	140	5	1	–
French	1 slice (2 oz)	130	1	0	–
French Roll	1 (2.25 oz)	140	1	0	–
Holiday	1 slice (2 oz)	150	1	0	–
Honey Wheat	1 slice (2 oz)	140	3	1	–
Nine Grain	1 slice (2 oz)	150	3	1	–
Rye	1 slice (2 oz)	140	3	1	–
Sourdough	1 slice (2 oz)	120	0	0	0
Sourdough Roll	1 (2.5 oz)	160	0	0	0

FOOD	PORTION	CALS	FAT	SAT FAT	TRANS FAT
Sourdough Soup Bowl	1 serv (8 oz)	500	2	0	–
Sunflower	1 slice (2 oz)	160	5	1	–
Tomato Basil	1 slice (2 oz)	130	1	0	–
DESSERTS					
Bear Claw	1	380	21	11	–
Brownie Caramel Pecan	1	470	24	5	–
Brownie Chocolate Raspberry	1	370	18	5	–
Brownie Very Chocolate	1	460	22	5	–
Cinnamon Roll	1	560	26	12	–
Cobblestone	1	560	9	2	–
Coffee Cake Cherry Cheese	1	190	10	5	–
Cookie Chocolate Chipper	1	420	22	13	–
Cookie Chocolate Duet w/ Walnuts	1	410	25	17	–
Cookie Nutty Chocolate Chipper	1	440	26	12	–
Cookie Nutty Oatmeal Raisin	1	350	14	7	–
Cookie Shortbread	1	340	21	13	–
Croissant Apple	1	260	11	7	–
Croissant Cheese	1	300	16	10	–
Croissant Chocolate	1	440	23	13	–
Croissant French	1	265	15	9	–
Croissant Raspberry Cheese	1	280	13	8	–
Danish Apple	1	510	30	15	–
Danish Cheese	1	590	35	19	–
Danish Cherry	1	520	26	14	–
Danish Georgia Peach	1	580	30	15	–
Danish German Chocolate	1	770	46	24	–
Macaroon Chocolate Hazelnut	1	270	15	10	–
Mini Bundt Cake Carrot Walnut	1	430	21	3	–
Mini Bundt Cake Lemon Poppyseed	1	460	20	4	–
Mini Bundt Cake Pineapple Upside Down	1	450	20	8	–
Muffie Banana Nut	1	260	12	2	–
Muffie Chocolate Chip	1	240	10	3	–
Muffie Pumpkin	1	270	6	2	–
Muffin Banana Nut	1	470	20	3	–
Muffin Blueberry	1	450	15	3	–

FOOD	PORTION	CALS	FAT	SAT FAT	TRANS FAT
Muffin Chocolate Chip	1	540	22	8	–
Muffin Pumpkin	1	510	12	3	–
Muffin Low Fat Tripleberry	1	300	3	1	–
Pecan Roll	1	520	31	6	–
Scone Cinnamon Chip	1	560	27	16	–
Scone Orange	1	530	25	15	–
Strudel Apple Raisin	1	390	22	6	–
Strudel Cherry	1	400	24	6	–
SALADS					
Asian Sesame Chicken	1 serv	370	19	3	–
Caesar	1 serv	350	26	7	–
Caesar Grilled Chicken	1 serv	470	27	7	–
Classic Cafe	1 serv	380	36	5	–
Fandango	1 serv	400	28	7	–
Greek	1 serv	520	48	10	–
SANDWICHES					
Asiago Roast Beef	1	730	35	16	–
Bacon Turkey Bravo	1	770	28	9	–
Chicken Salad On Artisan Sesame Semolina	1	730	26	4	–
Chicken Salad On Nine Grain	1	640	29	5	–
Garden Veggie	1	570	23	7	–
Italian Combo	1	1050	54	18	–
Panini Coronado Carnitas	1	810	35	11	–
Panini Frontega Chicken	1	860	42	12	–
Panini Portobello & Mozzarella	1	650	29	10	–
Panini Turkey Artichoke	1	810	38	11	–
Peanut Butter & Jelly On French	1	450	15	3	–
Sierra Turkey	1	950	55	13	–
Smoked Ham On Artisan Stone Milled Rye	1	930	31	10	–
Smoked Ham On Rye	1	650	34	11	–
Smoked Turkey Breast On Artisan Country	1	590	16	2	–
Smoked Turkey On Sourdough	1	440	15	2	–
Tuna Salad On Artisan Multigrain	1	830	41	5	–
Tuna Salad On Honey Wheat	1	720	43	6	–
Turkey Fresco	1	580	17	5	–
Tuscan Chicken	1	950	56	10	–

FOOD	PORTION	CALS	FAT	SAT FAT	TRANS FAT
SOUPS					
Baked Potato	1 serv	260	16	8	–
Boston Clam Chowder	1 serv	210	11	6	–
Broccoli Cheddar	1 serv	230	16	9	–
Cream Of Chicken & Wild Rice	1 serv	200	12	6	–
Forest Mushroom	1 serv	140	7	4	–
French Onion	1 serv	220	10	5	–
Low Fat Chicken Noodle	1 serv	100	2	0	–
Low Fat Vegetarian Black Bean	1 serv	100	1	0	–
Low Fat Vegetarian Garden Vegetable	1 serv	90	1	0	–
Vegetarian Santa Fe Roasted Corn	1 serv	130	4	1	–
PAPA JOHN'S					
OTHER MENU SELECTIONS					
Bread Sticks	1 serv	140	2	0	–
Cheese Sticks	1 serv	180	8	3	–
Chickenstrips	1	83	4	1	–
Cinnapie	1 serv	114	6	1	–
PIZZA 14 INCH					
Original All The Meats	1/8 pie	405	20	7	–
Original BBQ Chicken & Bacon	1/8 pie	369	14	4	–
Original Cheese	1/8 pie	290	10	3	–
Original Chicken Alfredo	1/8 pie	310	12	4	–
Original Garden Fresh	1/8 pie	287	9	3	–
Original Hawaiian BBQ Chicken	1/8 pie	376	14	4	–
Original Pepperoni	1/8 pie	343	15	5	–
Original Sausage	1/8 pie	336	14	4	–
Original Spinach Alfredo	1/8 pie	303	12	5	–
Original The Works	1/8 pie	370	16	5	–
Thin Crust All The Meat	1/8 pie	371	24	7	–
Thin Crust BBQ Chicken & Bacon	1/8 pie	336	18	5	–
Thin Crust Cheese	1/8 pie	238	13	3	–
Thin Crust Chicken Alfredo	1/8 pie	276	15	5	–
Thin Crust Garden Fresh	1/8 pie	228	11	3	–
Thin Crust Hawaiian BBQ Chicken	1/8 pie	324	17	5	–

FOOD	PORTION	CALS	FAT	SAT FAT	TRANS FAT
Thin Crust Pepperoni	⅛ pie	294	18	5	–
Thin Crust Sausage	⅛ pie	303	18	5	–
Thin Crust Spinach Alfredo	⅛ pie	251	15	5	–
Thin Crust The Works	⅛ pie	315	18	5	–
SALAD DRESSINGS AND SAUCES					
BBQ Sauce	1 serv	48	0	0	0
Buffalo Sauce	1 serv	25	1	0	–
Cheese Sauce	1 serv	60	5	4	–
Garlic Sauce	1 serv	235	26	3	–
Honey Mustard Dressing	1 serv	170	19	3	–
Pizza Sauce	1 serv	25	2	0	–
Ranch Dressing	1 serv	140	14	3	–

PAPA MURPHY'S
PIZZA

FOOD	PORTION	CALS	FAT	SAT FAT	TRANS FAT
Deeper Dish Traditional	⅛ pie	440	24	10	–
Delite Large Cheese	¹⁄₁₀ pie	130	6	4	–
Delite Large Hawaiian	¹⁄₁₀ pie	140	7	4	–
Delite Large Meat	¹⁄₁₀ pie	190	12	5	–
Delite Large Pepperoni	¹⁄₁₀ pie	160	9	5	–
Delite Large Veggie	¹⁄₁₀ pie	150	8	4	–
Family Size Cheese	¹⁄₁₂ pie	270	10	5	–
Gourmet Family Size Chicken Garlic	¹⁄₁₂ pie	320	15	6	–
Gourmet Family Size Classic Italian	¹⁄₁₂ pie	360	19	8	–
Gourmet Family Size Veggie	¹⁄₁₂ pie	300	14	6	–
Papa's Family Size All Meat	¹⁄₁₂ pie	370	19	8	–
Papa's Family Size Cheese	¹⁄₁₂ pie	270	10	5	–
Papa's Family Size Cowboy	¹⁄₁₂ pie	370	19	7	–
Papa's Family Size Favorite	¹⁄₁₂ pie	380	20	8	–
Papa's Family Size Hawaiian	¹⁄₁₂ pie	290	11	5	–
Papa's Family Size Murphy's Combo	¹⁄₁₂ pie	480	20	7	–
Papa's Family Size Pepperoni	¹⁄₁₂ pie	310	15	7	–
Papa's Family Size Perfect	¹⁄₁₂ pie	300	13	6	–
Papa's Family Size Rancher	¹⁄₁₂ pie	330	15	7	–
Papa's Family Size Specialty	¹⁄₁₂ pie	340	17	6	–
Papa's Family Size Veggie Combo	¹⁄₁₂ pie	300	13	5	–

FOOD	PORTION	CALS	FAT	SAT FAT	TRANS FAT
Stuffed Big Murphy	⅛ pie	380	17	7	–
Stuffed Chicago Style	⅛ pie	370	16	7	–
SALADS					
Club	1 serv	190	21	8	–
Garden	1 serv	160	11	5	–
Italian	1 serv	220	17	6	–

PICCADILLY CAFETERIA
DESSERTS

FOOD	PORTION	CALS	FAT	SAT FAT	TRANS FAT
Gelatin Sugar Free	1 serv	0	0	0	0
Sugar Free Blueberry Pie	1 serv	314	17	5	–
Sugar Free Cherry Pie	1 serv	334	17	5	–
Sugar Free Chocolate Almond Pie	1 serv	611	44	34	–

MAIN MENU SELECTIONS

FOOD	PORTION	CALS	FAT	SAT FAT	TRANS FAT
Bass Blackened	1 serv	408	32	7	–
Bass Cajun Baked	1 serv	260	15	4	–
Bass Stuffed	1 serv	447	30	7	–
Beef Chopped Steak	1 serv	382	31	11	–
Beef Chopped Steak Fried	1 serv	225	12	4	–
Beef Roast Leg	1 sm serv	353	22	9	–
Broccoli Florets	1 serv	90	7	1	–
Broccoli w/ Cheese Sauce	1 serv	55	1	0	–
Brussels Sprouts	1 serv	92	6	1	–
Cabbage Steamed Bacon Seasoned	1 serv	108	8	3	–
Cabbage Steamed Buttered	1 serv	68	5	1	–
Catfish Filet Blackened	1 serv	523	43	8	–
Catfish Filet Cajun Baked	1 serv	401	28	6	–
Catfish Filet Stuffed	1 serv	561	41	8	–
Cauliflower Buttered	1 serv	73	4	1	–
Chicken Barbecued Quarters	1 serv	472	52	15	–
Chicken Grilled Breast	1 serv	345	21	5	–
Chicken Rotisserie Herb Dark Meat	1 serv	823	63	16	–
Chicken Rotisserie Herb White Meat	1 serv	602	32	9	–
Chicken Baked Cajun Boneless Breast	1 serv	428	27	6	–
Chicken Baked Quarters	1 serv	828	59	16	–

FOOD	PORTION	CALS	FAT	SAT FAT	TRANS FAT
Chicken Breast Italian Boneless Breast	1 serv	371	41	7	–
Chicken Breast Mesquite Smoke	1 serv	212	8	2	–
Chicken Breast Mesquite w/ BBQ Sauce	1 serv	240	9	3	–
Chicken Breast Southwestern	1 serv	315	35	14	–
Chicken Half Rotisserie Herb	1 serv	833	21	5	–
Corn	1 serv	125	6	1	–
Cottage Cheese	1 serv	117	5	3	–
Filet Mignon	1 (6 oz)	184	20	8	–
Green Beans	1 serv	136	11	4	–
Greens Collard Mustard Turnip	1 serv	135	10	4	–
Greens Turnip w/ Diced Turnips	1 serv	150	12	4	–
Grouper Filet Baked	1 piece (6 oz)	305	9	2	–
New York Strip	1 (10 oz)	871	71	26	–
Okra Creole	1 serv	77	4	2	–
Okra Fried	1 serv	240	13	4	–
Peas & Sugar Snap Mixed	1 serv	102	5	1	–
Pork Loin Marinated Boneless	1 serv	365	24	8	–
Pork Loin Roast Bone In	1 serv	373	13	5	–
Ribeye	1 (10 oz)	1038	91	34	–
Roast Beef	1 serv	481	30	13	–
Roll Parker House	1	147	5	1	–
Roll Whole Wheat	1	231	8	2	–
Shrimp Fried	1 serv	499	22	12	–
Tilapia Baked	1 serv	210	11	2	–
Tilapia Cajun Baked	1 serv	263	19	4	–
Trout Almondine Baked	1 lg serv	457	18	3	–
Trout Cajun Baked	1 lg serv	517	27	5	–
Trout Filet Baked	1 lg serv	464	19	4	–
Turkey Breast Carved	1 serv	302	11	3	–
Vegetables Mixed	1 serv	95	6	1	–
SALAD DRESSINGS AND TOPPINGS					
Au Jus	1 serv	6	0	0	0
Blue Cheese	2 tbsp	160	18	3	–
Cheese Sauce	2 oz	35	1	0	–
French	2 tbsp	130	13	2	–
Italian	2 tbsp	140	14	2	–
Ranch	2 tbsp	150	17	2	–

FOOD	PORTION	CALS	FAT	SAT FAT	TRANS FAT
Ranch Fat Free	2 tbsp	36	0	0	0
SALADS					
Asparagus & Tomato	1 serv	86	5	1	–
Caesar	1 serv	141	11	3	–
Cauilflower	1 serv	118	8	2	–
Chef	1 sm serv	146	9	4	–
Coleslaw Kosher Style	1 serv	140	13	2	–
Coleslaw Italian	1 serv	163	16	2	–
Combination	1 serv	63	3	1	–
Cucumber & Celery	1 serv	74	4	1	–
Cucumber & Tomato	1 serv	41	0	0	0
Cucumber Mix	1 serv	61	4	1	–
Cucumbers & Sour Cream	1 serv	90	7	4	–
Louisianne Bowl	1 serv	42	2	1	–
Mexican	1 serv	58	3	0	–
Piccadilly Bowl	1 serv	27	0	0	0
Piccadilly Fruit	1 serv	76	0	0	0
Shrimp Remoulade	1 serv	521	29	4	–
Spring Bowl	1 reg serv	24	0	0	0
Tomato Cucumber & Onion	1 serv	44	0	0	0
Vegetable Combo w/ Cherry Tomatoes	1 serv	66	4	0	–
SOUPS					
Gumbo Chicken & Sausage No Rice	1 serv	224	15	3	–
Gumbo Chicken No Rice	1 serv	89	2	1	–

PIZZA HUT
APPETIZERS

FOOD	PORTION	CALS	FAT	SAT FAT	TRANS FAT
Breadstick	1	150	6	1	tr
Breadstick Cheese	1	200	10	4	tr
Hot Wings	2 pieces	110	6	2	tr
Mild Wings	2 pieces	110	7	2	tr
BEVERAGES					
Diet Pepsi	1 med (14 oz)	0	0	0	0
Mountain Dew	1 med (14 oz)	190	0	0	0
Pepsi	1 med (14 oz)	180	0	0	0
DESSERTS					
Apple Pizza	1 slice	260	4	1	1
Cherry Pizza	1 slice	240	4	1	1
Cinnamon Sticks	2	170	5	1	tr

FOOD	PORTION	CALS	FAT	SAT FAT	TRANS FAT
PIZZA					
Fit 'N Delicious Diced Chicken Mushroom Jalapeno	1 med slice	170	5	2	tr
Fit 'N Delicious Diced Chicken Red Onion Green Pepper	1 med slice	170	5	2	tr
Fit 'N Delicious Diced Red Tomato Mushroom Jalapeno	1 med slice	150	4	2	tr
Fit 'N Delicious Green Pepper Red Onion Diced Red Tomato	1 med slice	150	4	2	tr
Fit 'N Delicious Ham Pineapple Diced Red Tomato	1 med slice	160	4	2	tr
Fit 'N Delicious Ham Red Onion Mushroom	1 med slice	160	5	2	tr
Hand Tossed Cheese	1 med slice	240	8	5	tr
Hand Tossed Chicken Supreme	1 med slice	230	6	3	tr
Hand Tossed Ham	1 med slice	220	6	3	tr
Hand Tossed Meat Lover's	1 med slice	300	13	6	1
Hand Tossed Pepperoni	1 med slice	250	9	5	tr
Hand Tossed Pepperoni Lover's	1 med slice	300	13	7	1
Hand Tossed Super Supreme	1 med slice	300	13	6	tr
Hand Tossed Supreme	1 med slice	270	11	5	1
Hand Tossed Veggie Lover's	1 med slice	220	6	3	tr
Pan Cheese	1 med slice	280	13	5	1
Pan Chicken Supreme	1 med slice	280	12	4	tr
Pan Ham	1 med slice	260	11	4	tr
Pan Meat Lover's	1 med slice	340	19	7	1
Pan Pepperoni	1 med slice	290	15	5	1
Pan Pepperoni Lover's	1 med slice	340	19	7	1
Pan Super Supreme	1 med slice	340	18	6	1
Pan Supreme	1 med slice	320	16	6	1
Pan Veggie Lover's	1 med slice	260	12	4	tr
Personal Pan Cheese	1 pie	630	27	12	1
Personal Pan Chicken Supreme	1 pie	620	23	9	1
Personal Pan Meat Lover's	1 pie	800	41	15	1
Personal Pan Pepperoni	1 pie	660	30	12	1
Personal Pan Pepperoni Lover's	1 pie	800	42	17	1
Personal Pan Super Supreme	1 pie	790	40	15	1
Personal Pan Supreme	1 pie	750	36	15	1
Personal Pan Veggie Lover's	1 pie	580	23	9	1
Stuffed Crust Cheese	1 lg slice	360	13	8	1

FOOD	PORTION	CALS	FAT	SAT FAT	TRANS FAT
Stuffed Crust Chicken Supreme	1 lg slice	380	13	7	1
Stuffed Crust Ham	1 lg slice	340	11	6	1
Stuffed Crust Meat Lover's	1 lg slice	450	21	10	1
Stuffed Crust Pepperoni	1 lg slice	370	15	8	1
Stuffed Crust Pepperoni Lover's	1 lg slice	420	19	10	1
Stuffed Crust Super Supreme	1 lg slice	440	20	9	1
Stuffed Crust Supreme	1 lg slice	400	16	8	1
Stuffed Crust Veggie Lover's	1 lg slice	360	14	7	1
Thin 'N Crispy Cheese	1 med slice	200	8	5	1
Thin 'N Crispy Chicken Supreme	1 med slice	200	7	4	1
Thin 'N Crispy Ham	1 med slice	180	6	3	1
Thin 'N Crispy Meat Lover's	1 med slice	270	14	6	1
Thin 'N Crispy Pepperoni	1 med slice	210	10	5	1
Thin 'N Crispy Pepperoni Lover's	1 med slice	260	14	7	1
Thin 'N Crispy Super Supreme	1 med slice	260	13	6	1
Thin 'N Crispy Supreme	1 med slice	240	11	5	1
Thin 'N Crispy Veggie Lover's	1 med slice	180	7	3	1
XL Full House Cheese	1 slice	280	12	6	1
XL Full House Chicken Supreme	1 slice	270	10	4	tr
XL Full House Ham	1 slice	260	10	4	tr
XL Full House Meat Lover's	1 slice	380	21	8	1
XL Full House Pepperoni	1 slice	290	13	5	tr
XL Full House Pepperoni Lover's	1 slice	310	15	6	1
XL Full House Super Supreme	1 slice	330	16	6	1
XL Full House Supreme	1 slice	310	15	6	1
XL Full House Veggie Lover's	1 slice	280	11	4	tr
SALAD DRESSINGS AND SAUCES					
Dipping Cup White Icing	1 serv	170	0	0	0
Dipping Sauce Breadstick	1 serv	45	0	0	0
Dipping Sauce Wing Blue Cheese	1 serv	230	24	5	1
Dipping Sauce Wing Ranch	1 serv	210	22	4	1
Dressing Caesar	2 tbsp	150	16	3	1
Dressing French	2 tbsp	140	11	2	1
Dressing Italian	2 tbsp	140	15	3	1
Dressing Ranch	2 tbsp	100	10	2	1

FOOD	PORTION	CALS	FAT	SAT FAT	TRANS FAT
Dressing Thousand Island	2 tbsp	110	9	2	1
Dressing Lite Italian	2 tbsp	60	5	1	tr
Dressing Lite Ranch	1 tbsp	70	7	2	tr

POLLO TROPICAL
DESSERTS

FOOD	PORTION	CALS	FAT	SAT FAT	TRANS FAT
Flan	1 serv (4 oz)	390	13	7	–
Key Lime	1 serv (3.9 oz)	210	9	5	–
Tres Leches	1 serv (5.4 oz)	410	9	0	–

MAIN MENU SELECTIONS

FOOD	PORTION	CALS	FAT	SAT FAT	TRANS FAT
Balsamic Tomato	1 combo	88	1	tr	–
Balsamic Tomato	1 sm	176	2	tr	–
Bananas Tropical	1 serv	437	11	2	–
Beef Skewers	1 (1 oz)	77	5	2	–
Black Beans	1 combo	90	3	0	–
Black Beans	1 sm	203	6	0	–
Boiled Yucca	1 combo	188	0	0	0
Boiled Yucca	1 sm	251	0	0	0
Caesar Salad	1 combo	130	11	2	–
Caesar Salad	1 sm	207	18	3	–
Chicken Boneless Breast	2 pieces	240	3	1	–
Chicken ¼ Dark Meat	1 serv	291	18	5	–
Chicken ¼ Dark Meat No Skin	1 serv	191	10	3	–
Chicken ¼ White Meat	1 serv	323	16	5	–
Chicken ¼ White Meat No Skin	1 serv	204	6	2	–
Chicken Caesar Salad	1 serv	669	41	8	–
Corn	1 combo	121	4	1	–
French Fries	1 sm	311	15	4	–
Ribs	¼ rack (2 oz)	200	15	7	–
Ribs	½ rack (4 oz)	400	31	13	–
Roast Pork	1 serv	392	23	11	–
Sandwich Chicken Caesar	1	881	34	7	–
Sandwich Grilled Chicken	1	827	24	3	–
Sandwich Roast Pork	1	773	26	9	–
Steak & Chicken Dark Meat	1 serv	437	28	9	–
TropiChop Chicken w/ Yellow Rice & Vegetables	1 serv	341	5	tr	–

FOOD	PORTION	CALS	FAT	SAT FAT	TRANS FAT
TropiChop Chicken w/ White Rice & Black Beans	1 serv	564	10	1	–
TropiChop Grilled Chicken Deluxe	1 serv	409	6	1	–
TropiChop Pork w/ White Rice & Black Beans	1 serv	714	23	7	–
TropiChop Pork w/ Yellow Rice & Vegetables	1 serv	480	21	6	–
TropiChop Rop Vieja	1 serv	618	17	3	–
TropiChop Shrimp Creole	1 serv	506	11	3	–
TropiChop Vegetarian	1 serv	580	13	1	–
TropiChop Max Chicken w/ Yellow Rice & Vegetables	1 serv	864	21	3	–
TropiChop Max Chicken w/ White Rice & Black Beans	1 serv	1117	27	5	–
TropiChop Max Grilled Chicken Deluxe	1 serv	753	11	1	–
TropiChop Max Pork w/ White Rice & Black Beans	1 serv	1273	50	15	–
TropiChop Max Pork w/ Yellow Rice & Vegetables	1 serv	1020	43	13	–
TropiChop Max Ropa Vieja	1 serv	1160	41	7	–
TropiChop Max Shrimp Creole	1 serv	102	29	7	–
TropiChop Max Vegetarian	1 serv	950	21	3	–
White Rice	1 combo	203	3	1	–
White Rice	1 sm	339	6	1	–
Wrap Chicken Ceasar	1	901	48	9	–
Wrap Chicken Classic	1	694	26	4	–
Wrap Curry Chicken	1	930	43	9	–
Wrap Steak	1	993	48	10	–
Yellow Rice w/ Vegetables	1 combo	163	3	0	–
Yellow Rice w/ Vegetables	1 sm	245	4	0	–
Yucatan Fries	1 serv	497	24	5	–
SALAD DRESSINGS AND SAUCES					
BBQ Sauce	1 serv (1.8 oz)	83	0	0	0
BBQ Sauce Guava	1 serv (1.8 oz)	83	0	0	0
Dressing Caesar	1 serv (1 oz)	161	17	3	–
Guacamole Sauce	1 serv (1.8 oz)	75	6	2	–
Mojo Sauce	1 serv (0.9 oz)	97	tr	1	–

FOOD	PORTION	CALS	FAT	SAT FAT	TRANS FAT
Mustard Curry Sauce	1 serv (1.8 oz)	265	30	8	–
Salsa	1 serv (1.8 oz)	8	0	0	0
SOUPS					
Caribbean Chicken	1 sm (8 oz)	121	2	tr	–
Tropical Shrimp	1 sm (8 oz)	134	3	1	–

POPEYES

FOOD	PORTION	CALS	FAT	SAT FAT	TRANS FAT
Buttermilk Biscuit	1	240	14	4	–
Cajun Rice	1 reg	180	7	3	–
Coleslaw	1 serv	230	17	17	–
Collard Greens	1 serv	50	2	1	–
Corn On The Cob	1	220	4	1	–
Etouffee Chicken	1 serv	223	6	6	–
Etouffee Crawfish	1 serv	200	7	1	–
French Fries	1 serv	261	12	5	–
Fried Catfish	1 serv	300	18	7	–
Fried Crawfish	1 serv	370	21	9	–
Green Beans	1 serv	40	1	0	–
Jambalaya Chicken Sausage	1 serv	257	13	3	–
Mashed Potatoes & Gravy	1 serv	120	4	2	–
Mashed Potatoes No Gravy	1 serv	100	3	1	–
Mild Breast	1	510	30	11	–
Mild Breast Skinless	1	280	11	5	–
Mild Leg	1	200	12	4	–
Mild Leg Skinless	1	110	5	2	–
Mild Strips	2	280	12	5	–
Mild Strips No Breading	2	200	8	4	–
Mild Thigh	1	390	27	9	–
Mild Thigh Skinless	1	210	14	5	–
Mild Wing	1	220	14	5	–
Mild Wing Skinless	1	130	7	3	–
Naked Chicken Strips	3	170	5	2	–
Popcorn Shrimp	1 serv	280	17	7	–
Red Beans & Rice	1 reg	340	19	6	–
Sandwich Catfish Fully Dressed	1	640	35	9	–
Sandwich Deluxe Tame w/ Mayo	1	728	39	9	–
Sandwich Deluxe Tame w/o Mayo	1	530	17	6	–

FOOD	PORTION	CALS	FAT	SAT FAT	TRANS FAT
Sandwich Shrimp Fully Dressed	1	740	40	10	–
Smothered Chicken	1 serv	210	8	2	–
Spicy Breast	1	530	31	11	–
Spicy Breast Skinless	1	290	12	5	–
Spicy Leg	1	190	11	4	–
Spicy Leg Skinless	1	120	8	2	–
Spicy Strips	2	310	14	6	–
Spicy Strips No Breading	2	190	7	3	–
Spicy Thigh	1	390	29	10	–
Spicy Thigh Skinless	1	200	13	5	–
Spicy Wing	1	220	15	5	–
Spicy Wing Skinless	1	140	9	3	–
Turnover Cinnamon Apple	1	250	10	3	–

QUIZNOS
COOKIES

FOOD	PORTION	CALS	FAT	SAT FAT	TRANS FAT
Dark Chocolate Chunk	1	380	15	8	0
Double Chocolate Chip	1	370	15	7	0
Oatmeal Raisin	1	340	11	5	0
Snickerdoodle	1	400	16	8	0

SANDWICHES

FOOD	PORTION	CALS	FAT	SAT FAT	TRANS FAT
Breakfast Bacon Egg & Cheddar	1	380	21	9	0
Breakfast Black Angus Steak & Cheddar	1 sm	330	13	6	0
Breakfast Egg & Cheddar	1	240	11	5	0
Breakfast Garden Vegetable w/ Cheddar	1	250	11	5	0
Breakfast Ham Egg & Cheddar	1	290	12	5	0
Deli Honey Ham & Swiss	1	260	4	1	0
Deli Oven Roasted Turkey & Cheese	1	250	4	1	0
Deli Roast Beef & Cheddar	1	230	4	1	0
Deli Tuna Melt	1	500	33	5	0
Sammie Alpine Chicken	1	200	6	2	0
Sammie Balsamic Chicken	1	170	4	1	0
Sammie Black Angus Steak	1	180	4	1	0
Sammie Bistro Steak Melt	1	180	4	1	0
Sammie Italiano	1	240	11	4	0

FOOD	PORTION	CALS	FAT	SAT FAT	TRANS FAT
Sammie Sonoma Turkey	1	160	4	1	0
Sub Baja Chicken w/ Bacon	1 sm	320	9	3	0
Sub Black Angus Steak On Rosemay Parmesan	1 sm	380	8	3	1
Sub Chicken Carbonara w/ Bacon	1 sm	360	10	3	0
Sub Classic Club w/ Bacon	1 sm	320	9	3	0
Sub Classic Italian	1 sm	360	15	5	0
Sub Honey Bacon Club	1 sm	320	9	3	0
Sub Honey Bourbon Chicken	1 sm	260	4	1	0
Sub Honey Mustard Chicken w/ Bacon	1 sm	330	9	3	0
Sub Mesquite Chicken w/ Bacon	1 sm	330	9	3	0
Sub Prime Rib Cheesesteak	1 sm	360	11	4	1
Sub Prime Rib & Peppercorn	1 sm	380	8	3	1
Sub Steakhouse Beef Dip	1 sm	260	6	2	0
Sub The Traditional	1 sm	260	5	1	0
Sub Turkey Bacon Guacamole	1 sm	360	12	4	0
Sub Turkey Ranch & Swiss	1 sm	250	4	1	0
Sub Tuscan Turkey On Rosemary Parmesan	1 sm	300	5	2	0
Sub Veggie	1 sm	270	8	2	0
SOUPS					
Bread Bowl Chili	1 serv	730	22	7	1
Bread Bowl Country French	1 serv	720	22	9	1
Broccoli Cheese	1 cup	150	10	5	1
Chicken Noodle	1 cup	130	3	1	0
Chili	1 cup	140	7	2	0

RANCH1
MAIN MENU SELECTIONS

FOOD	PORTION	CALS	FAT	SAT FAT	TRANS FAT
Baked Potato w/ Broccoli	1 serv	510	1	0	–
Baked Potato w/ Cheese	1 serv	790	25	12	–
Baked Potato w/ Chicken	1 serv	610	4	1	–
Chicken Tenders	1 serv	370	15	3	–
Fajita Grilled Chicken	1	330	16	7	–
Fruit Cup	1 serv	90	1	0	–
Hot Pasta Grilled Chicken	1 serv	590	10	2	–

FOOD	PORTION	CALS	FAT	SAT FAT	TRANS FAT
Platter Grilled Chicken & Vegetables	1 serv	790	7	2	–
Ranch Fries	1 lg	420	17	5	–
Ranch Fries	1 reg	350	14	5	–
Sandwich American Rancher	1	390	10	4	–
Sandwich Grilled Chicken Philly	1	450	14	5	–
Sandwich Ranch Classic	1	370	5	1	–
Sandwich Spicy Grilled Chicken	1	420	11	2	–
Sandwich Club	1	470	16	6	–
SALADS					
Gourmet Greens	1 serv	220	7	3	–
Gourmet Greens w/ Chicken	1 serv	350	11	4	–
Zesty Caesar	1 serv	180	3	2	–
Zesty Chicken Caesar	1 serv	290	6	2	–

RAX
MAIN MENU SELECTIONS

FOOD	PORTION	CALS	FAT	SAT FAT	TRANS FAT
Baked Potato	1	207	0	0	0
Baked Potato w/ Butter	1	306	11	–	–
Baked Potato w/ Cheese	1 serv	270	tr	–	–
Baked Potato w/ Cheese Bacon	1 serv	336	19	–	–
Baked Potato w/ Cheese Broccoli	1 serv	281	tr	–	–
Baked Potato w/ Sour Cream Topping	1 serv	257	4	–	–
BBC Sandwich	1	716	51	–	–
BBQ Beef Sandwich	1	399	20	–	–
Cheddar Melt	1	346	23	–	–
Deluxe Sandwich	1	521	34	–	–
Grilled Chicken Sandwich	1	526	33	–	–
Jr. Deluxe Sandwich	1	367	25	–	–
Mushroom Melt	1	599	37	–	–
Philly Melt	1	537	32	–	–
Regular Rax	1	388	22	–	–
Turkey Bacon Club	1	680	47	–	–
Turkey Sandwich	1	484	32	–	–
SALAD DRESSINGS					
1000 Island	1 serv	130	13	–	–

FOOD	PORTION	CALS	FAT	SAT FAT	TRANS FAT
Blue Cheese	1 serv	145	16	–	–
Buttermilk Ranch	1 serv	175	20	–	–
Catalina Fat Free	1 serv	32	0	0	0
Creamy Caesar	1 serv	140	15	–	–
Honey French	1 serv	140	5	–	–
Italian Fat Free	1 serv	12	0	0	0
Ranch Fat Free	1 serv	30	0	0	0
Vinaigrette	1 serv	30	2	–	–
SALADS					
Garden	1 serv	220	9	–	–
Grilled Chicken	1 serv	160	5	–	–
Side Salad	1 serv (19 oz)	40	4	–	–
SOUPS					
Chicken Noodle	1 serv	113	1	–	–
Chili	1 serv	158	9	–	–
Cream Of Broccoli	1 serv	95	4	–	–

RED LOBSTER
BEVERAGES

FOOD	PORTION	CALS	FAT	SAT FAT	TRANS FAT
Coffee	1 cup	0	0	0	0
Dannon Spring Water	1 glass	0	0	0	0
Diet Coke	1 serv	0	0	0	0
Hot Tea	1 cup	0	0	0	0
Iced Tea Unsweetened	1 glass	0	0	0	0
Lemonade Light	1 glass	5	0	0	0
Michelob Ultra	1 glass	95	0	–	0
Perrier Water	1 glass	0	0	0	0
Sutter Home Cabernet Sauvignon	1 glass	138	0	0	0
Sutter Home Chardonnay	1 glass	147	0	0	0
MAIN MENU SELECTIONS					
Baked Potato Plain	1	170	2	–	–
Baked Potato w/ Pico De Gallo Topping	1 serv	185	2	–	–
Cheddar Bay Biscuit	1	160	9	–	–
Fresh Buttered Vegetables	1 serv	143	12	–	–
Garden Salad	1 serv	52	2	–	–
Light House Broiled Flounder	1 serv	240	5	–	–
Light House Grilled Chicken	1 serv	527	14	–	–

FOOD	PORTION	CALS	FAT	SAT FAT	TRANS FAT
Light House Jumbo Shrimp Cocktail Dinner	1 serv	243	3	–	–
Light House King Crab Legs	1 serv	490	9	–	–
Light House Live Maine Lobster	1 serv	145	1	–	–
Light House Maine Lobster Tail	1 serv	104	5	–	–
Light House Rainbow Trout	1 lunch serv	273	14	–	–
Light House Rock Lobster Tail	1 serv	256	3	–	–
Light House Salmon	1 lunch serv	258	12	–	–
Light House Salmon	1 serv	578	31	–	–
Light House Snow Crab Legs	1 serv	262	5	–	–
Light House Tilapia	1 lunch serv	186	6	–	–
Light House Tilapia	1 serv	346	10	–	–
Seasoned Fresh Broccoli	1 serv	60	0	0	0
Shrimp Cocktail	1 jumbo	146	2	–	–
Wild Rice Pilaf	1 serv	208	5	–	–
SALAD DRESSINGS AND TOPPINGS					
Large Cocktail Sauce	1 serv	68	0	0	0
Lemon Wedge	1 serv	8	0	0	0
Melted Butter	1 serv	183	21	–	–
Red Wine Vinaigrette	1 serv	49	3	–	–
Topping Petite Shrimp	1 serv	30	1	–	–

RED MANGO

FOOD	PORTION	CALS	FAT	SAT FAT	TRANS FAT
Blenders Blueberry Moon	1 cup	150	2	1	0
Blenders Captain Berry	1 cup	140	1	0	0
Blenders Green Tea Blueberry	1 cup	130	0	0	0
Blenders Green Tea Honeydew	1 cup	130	0	0	0
Blenders Mango Island	1 cup	150	2	2	0
Blenders Pina Colada	1 cup	160	3	3	0
Blenders Tri-Berry	1 cup	130	0	0	0
Blenders Watermelon Breeze	1 cup	130	0	0	0
Frozen Yogurt All Flavors	½ cup	90	0	0	0

RITA'S

FOOD	PORTION	CALS	FAT	SAT FAT	TRANS FAT
Cream Ice	1 reg	312	4	3	–
Cream Ice Kids	1 serv	193	2	2	–
Custard	1 reg	385	21	14	–
Custard Kids	1 serv	285	15	11	–
Gelati w/ Chocolate Custard	1 reg	351	11	8	–
Gelati w/ Vanilla Custard	1 reg	120	13	9	–

FOOD	PORTION	CALS	FAT	SAT FAT	TRANS FAT
Gelati w/ Cream Ice w/ Chocolate Custard	1 reg	368	13	9	–
Gelati w/ Cream Ice w/ Vanilla Custard	1 reg	392	15	10	–
Ice	1 reg	263	0	0	0
Ice Kids	1 serv	165	0	0	0
Misto w/ Chocolate Custard	1 reg	409	7	5	–
Misto w/ Vanilla Custard	1 reg	420	7	5	–
Misto w/ Cream Ice w/ Chocolate Custard	1 reg	463	11	8	–
Misto w/ Cream Ice w/ Vanilla Custard	1 reg	473	12	8	–
Sugar Free Gelati w/ Chocolate Custard	1 reg	268	11	8	–
Sugar Free Gelati w/ Vanilla Custard	1 reg	288	13	9	–
Sugar Free Ice	1 reg	160	0	0	0
Sugar Free Ice Kids	1 serv	63	0	0	0
Sugar Free Misto w/ Chocolate Custard	1 reg	233	7	5	–
Sugar Free Misto w/ Vanilla Custard	1 reg	245	8	5	–

ROBEKS
FREEZES AND SHAKES

FOOD	PORTION	CALS	FAT	SAT FAT	TRANS FAT
800 Lb Gorilla	12 oz	375	9	–	–
Freeze Lemon	12 oz	279	2	–	–
Freeze Orange	12 oz	242	0	0	0
Shake Bananasplit	12 oz	302	0	0	0
Shake P-Nut Power	12 oz	422	18	–	–

SMOOTHIES

FOOD	PORTION	CALS	FAT	SAT FAT	TRANS FAT
Acai Energizer	12 oz	167	1	–	–
Awesome Acai	12 oz	183	1	–	–
Banzai Blueberry	12 oz	175	1	–	–
Berry Brilliance	12 oz	194	1	–	–
Big Wednesday	12 oz	172	1	–	–
Cardio Cooler	12 oz	215	1	–	–
Citrus Stinger	12 oz	194	1	–	–
Cranberry Quest	12 oz	173	0	–	0
Dr. Robeks	12 oz	181	1	–	–

FOOD	PORTION	CALS	FAT	SAT FAT	TRANS FAT
Guava Lava	12 oz	180	1	–	–
Hummingbird	12 oz	185	1	–	–
Infinite Orange	12 oz	181	0	0	0
Mahalo Mango	12 oz	174	1	–	–
Malibu Peach	12 oz	153	0	0	0
Outrageous Raspberry	12 oz	174	1	–	–
Passionfruit Cove	12 oz	168	1	–	–
Pina Koolada	12 oz	261	8	–	–
Polar Pineapple	12 oz	164	1	–	–
Pomegranate Passion	12 oz	196	0	0	0
Pomegranate Power	12 oz	211	0	0	0
Pro Arobek	12 oz	265	1	–	–
Raspberry Romance	12 oz	172	0	0	0
Robeks MuscleMax	12 oz	202	1	–	–
Robeks Rejuvenator	12 oz	193	1	–	–
South Pacific Squeeze	12 oz	188	1	–	–
Strawnana Berry	12 oz	179	0	0	0
Venice Burner	12 oz	231	1	–	–
Zen Berry	12 oz	190	1	–	–

RUBIO'S
MAIN MENU SELECTIONS

FOOD	PORTION	CALS	FAT	SAT FAT	TRANS FAT
Black Beans	1 serv	220	3	1	–
Burritos Baja Carne Asada	1	710	33	13	–
Burritos Baja Carnitas	1	660	30	12	–
Burritos Baja Chicken	1	640	28	9	–
Burritos Carne Asada Especial w/ Black Beans	1	970	37	10	–
Burritos Carne Asada Especial w/ Pinto Beans	1	950	38	10	–
Burritos Chicken Especial w/ Black Beans	1	920	32	7	–
Burritos Chicken Especial w/ Pinto Beans	1	900	32	7	–
Burritos Fish	1	780	41	8	–
Burritos HealthMex Chicken	1	520	11	2	–
Burritos HealthMex Veggie	1	470	8	1	–
Burritos Lobster	1	660	26	5	–
Burritos Mahi Mahi	1	630	30	9	–
Burritos Shrimp	1	650	25	7	–

FOOD	PORTION	CALS	FAT	SAT FAT	TRANS FAT
Carne Asada	1 serv	1430	87	31	–
Chips	1 serv	430	22	2	–
Grilled Grande Bowl Asada Black Beans	1 serv	770	37	12	–
Grilled Grande Bowl Asada Pinto Beans	1 serv	760	37	12	–
Grilled Grande Bowl Chicken Black Beans	1 serv	710	31	9	–
Grilled Grande Bowl Chicken Pinto Beans	1 serv	700	32	9	–
Guacamole	1 sm	170	16	3	–
Nachos Grande	1 serv	1270	79	27	–
Nachos Grande w/ Chicken	1 serv	1380	82	28	–
Pinto Beans	1 serv	190	3	2	–
Quesadillas Carne Asada	1	1010	61	30	–
Quesadillas Cheese	1	860	53	27	–
Quesadillas Grilled Chicken	1	860	56	28	–
Quesadillas Lobster	1	820	54	27	–
Quesadillas Shrimp	1	810	54	27	–
Roasted Chipotle	1 serv (1.5 oz)	10	0	0	0
Salsa Picante	1 serv (1.5 oz)	30	2	0	–
Salsa Regular	1 serv (1.5 oz)	15	0	0	0
Salsa Verde	1 serv (1.5 oz)	5	0	0	0
Tacos Carne Asada	1	220	8	3	–
Tacos Fish	1	310	18	3	–
Tacos Fish Especial	1	370	21	6	–
Tacos Grilled Chicken	1	300	16	4	–
Tacos Grilled Fish	1	310	16	5	–
Tacos HealthMex w/ Chicken	1	170	3	1	–
Taquitos	3	310	11	2	–
SALADS AND SALAD DRESSINGS					
Grilled Chicken Chopped Salad	1 serv	540	33	9	–
HealthMex Chicken	1 serv	220	4	1	–
Low Carb Chicken	1 serv	480	34	10	–
Serrano Grape Dressing	1 serv (1.3 oz)	10	0	0	0
RUBY TUESDAY'S					
Cajun Chicken Salad w/ Ranch Dressing	1 serv	636	46	–	–
Peppercorn Mushroom Sirloin	1 serv	947	57	–	–

FOOD	PORTION	CALS	FAT	SAT FAT	TRANS FAT

SALADWORKS
SALAD DRESSINGS

FOOD	PORTION	CALS	FAT	SAT FAT	TRANS FAT
Balsamic Vinaigrette	1 serv (2 oz)	192	17	2	–
Blue Cheese	1 serv (2 oz)	192	18	5	–
Creamy Italian	1 serv (2 oz)	232	22	3	–
Dijon Honey	1 serv	272	25	25	–
Fat Free Balsamic w/ Sundried Tomatoes	1 serv (2 oz)	28	0	0	0
French	1 serv (2 oz)	266	22	3	–
Herbal Ranch	1 serv (2 oz)	198	19	3	–
Italian Vinaigrette	1 serv (2 oz)	255	26	2	–
Lowfat Ranch	1 serv (2 oz)	34	1	0	–
Oriental Sesame	1 serv (2 oz)	147	6	0	–
Royal Caesar	1 serv (2 oz)	266	27	4	–
Russian	1 serv (2 oz)	221	21	3	–

SALADS

FOOD	PORTION	CALS	FAT	SAT FAT	TRANS FAT
B.L.T.	1 serv	262	24	11	–
Bently	1 serv	340	19	8	–
Caesar	1 serv	283	12	3	–
Caesar Chicken	1 serv	423	15	3	–
Caesar Shrimp	1 serv	350	12	3	–
Fiesta	1 serv	460	23	9	–
Garden	1 serv	58	1	0	–
Mandarin Chicken	1 serv	589	15	3	–
Newport	1 serv	184	7	1	–
Nicoise	1 serv	407	11	2	–
Spinach	1 serv	433	25	8	–
Tivoli	1 serv	563	27	11	–
Turkey Club	1 serv	720	19	5	–

SBARRO
DESSERTS

FOOD	PORTION	CALS	FAT	SAT FAT	TRANS FAT
Black Forest Cake	1 serv (4.6 oz)	480	24	–	–
Deluxe Carrot Cake	1 serv (5 oz)	540	29	–	–
Deluxe Cheese Cake	1 serv (5.7 oz)	560	40	–	–
Deluxe Milk Chocolate Cake	1 serv (4.3 oz)	490	25	–	–

MAIN MENU SELECTIONS

FOOD	PORTION	CALS	FAT	SAT FAT	TRANS FAT
Baked Ziti w/ Sauce	1 serv (14 oz)	700	41	–	–
Calzone Cheese	1 (12 oz)	770	28	–	–
Chicken Francese	1 serv (11 oz)	640	38	–	–

FOOD	PORTION	CALS	FAT	SAT FAT	TRANS FAT
Chicken Parmigiana	1 serv (11 oz)	520	22	–	–
Chicken Portofino	1 serv (12 oz)	730	48	–	–
Chicken Vesuvio	1 serv (11 oz)	690	43	–	–
Eggplant Rollatini w/ Cheese	1 serv (11 oz)	580	38	–	–
Garlic Roll	1 (2.2 oz)	170	5	–	–
Meat Lasagna	1 serv (13 oz)	650	37	–	–
Meatballs	1 serv (3.7 oz)	140	9	–	–
Mixed Vegetables	1 serv (7 oz)	190	15	–	–
Pasta Milano	1 serv (20 oz)	640	32	–	–
Pasta Rustica	1 serv (14 oz)	600	47	–	–
Penne Alla Vodka	1 serv (14 oz)	640	28	–	–
Penne w/ Sausage & Peppers	1 serv (14 oz)	710	49	–	–
Pizza Cheese	1 slice	460	13	–	–
Pizza Chicken Vegetable	1 slice	530	17	–	–
Pizza Fresh Tomato	1 slice	450	14	–	–
Pizza Mushroom	1 slice	460	14	–	–
Pizza Pepperoni	1 slice	730	37	–	–
Pizza Sausage	1 slice	670	31	–	–
Pizza Sauteed Spinach & Yellow Pepper	1 slice	670	24	–	–
Pizza Supreme	1 slice	630	27	–	–
Pizza White	1 slice	570	23	–	–
Pizza Gourmet Broccoli & Spinach	1 slice	720	28	–	–
Pizza Gourmet Cheese	1 slice	660	21	–	–
Pizza Gourmet Ham Pineapple & Bacon	1 slice	680	21	–	–
Pizza Gourmet Meat Delight	1 slice	780	29	–	–
Pizza Gourmet Mushroom	1 slice	610	20	–	–
Pizza Gourmet Mushroom & Spinach	1 slice	710	27	–	–
Pizza Gourmet Tomato & Basil	1 slice	700	25	–	–
Pizza Low Carb Cheese	1 slice	310	14	–	–
Pizza Low Carb Pepperoni	1 slice	420	14	–	–
Pizza Low Carb Sausage & Pepperoni	1 slice	560	35	–	–
Pizza Stuffed Pepperoni	1 slice	960	42	–	–
Pizza Stuffed Philly Cheesesteak	1 slice	830	33	–	–

FOOD	PORTION	CALS	FAT	SAT FAT	TRANS FAT
Pizza Stuffed Spinach & Broccoli	1 slice	790	34	–	–
Sausage & Peppers	1 serv (10 oz)	410	30	–	–
Spaghetti w/ Chicken Parmigiana	1 serv (15 oz)	930	36	–	–
Spaghetti w/ Chicken Francese	1 serv (15 oz)	800	37	–	–
Spaghetti w/ Chicken Vesuvio	1 serv (15 oz)	850	41	–	–
Spaghetti w/ Meatballs	1 serv (18 oz)	680	25	–	–
Spaghetti w/ Sauce	1 serv (20 oz)	820	28	–	–
Stromboli Pepperoni	1 (10 oz)	890	44	–	–
Stromboli Spinach Tomato & Broccoli	1 (10 oz)	680	24	–	–
SALADS					
Caesar	1 serv (8 oz)	80	5	–	–
Cucumber & Tomato	1 serv (8 oz)	130	11	–	–
Fruit Salad	1 serv (12 oz)	130	1	–	–
Greek	1 serv (8 oz)	60	5	–	–
Mixed Garden	1 serv (8 oz)	35	0	0	0
Pasta Primavera	1 serv (8 oz)	190	10	–	–
Stringbean & Tomato	1 serv (8 oz)	100	7	–	–

SEASON 52
CHILDREN'S MENU SELECTIONS

FOOD	PORTION	CALS	FAT	SAT FAT	TRANS FAT
Children's Chicken	1 serv	344	4	–	–
Children's Flatbread	1	468	18	–	–
Children's Pasta	1 serv	177	3	–	–
DESSERTS					
Boston Cream Pie	1 serv	188	7	–	–
Carrot Cake	1 serv	320	16	–	–
Chocolate & Peanut Butter Harlequin	1 serv	330	18	–	–
Fresh Spring Fruit	1 serv	35	0	0	0
Key Lime Pie	1 serv	283	13	–	–
Pecan Pie	1 serv	263	15	–	–
Sorbet w/ Fruit	1 serv	213	1	–	–
Strawberry Shortcake	1 serv	154	6	–	–
Strawberry Mango Cheesecake	1 serv	226	14	–	–
Toasted Almond Amaretto	1 serv	324	17	–	–
FLATBREADS					
Artichoke & Goat Cheese	1	469	18	–	–

FOOD	PORTION	CALS	FAT	SAT FAT	TRANS FAT
Garlic Chicken	1	474	16	–	–
Parmesan Crispbread	1	363	8	–	–
Spicy Shrimp	1	474	13	–	–
Steak & Mushroom	1	474	18	–	–
Tomato	1	460	17	–	–
MAIN MENU SELECTIONS					
Appetizer Goat Cheese Ravioli	1 serv	473	23	–	–
Appetizer Grilled Artichokes	1 serv	185	3	–	–
Appetizer Grilled Asparagus	1 serv	186	10	–	–
Appetizer Roasted Potato Wedges	1 serv	333	3	–	–
Appetizer Shrimp Cocktail	1 serv	221	2	–	–
Appetizer Shrimp Stuffed Mushrooms	1 serv	302	13	–	–
Appetizer Steak Skewers w/ Thai Salad	1 serv	438	15	–	–
Appetizer Steamed Mussels	1 serv	472	9	–	–
Cedar Salmon	1 serv	472	21	–	–
Chicken Boccone Pasta	1 serv	434	4	–	–
Chicken Breast	1 serv	403	5	–	–
Filet Mignon	1 serv	473	17	–	–
Grilled Rainbow Trout	1 serv	410	12	–	–
Grilled Scallops	1 serv	471	7	–	–
Pork Tenderloin	1 serv	392	12	–	–
Sandwich Chicken Breast	1	472	7	–	–
Sandwich Fresh Fish	1	437	6	–	–
Sandwich Grilled Steak	1	463	13	–	–
Sandwich Vegetable Stack	1	461	17	–	–
Shrimp Stuffed w/ Crab	1 serv	470	10	–	–
Soup Chicken Tortilla	1 serv (8 oz)	181	4	–	–
Soup Vegetable	1 serv (8 oz)	153	3	–	–
Spring Vegetable Plate	1 serv	465	11	–	–
Tuna w/o Soy Sauce	1 serv	175	1	–	–
Turkey Skewer	1 serv	404	4	–	–
Yellowfin Tuna	1 serv	466	3	–	–
SALADS					
Chicken Cobb	1 entree	474	21	–	–
Greek	1 entree	478	35	–	–
Mesclun Greens	1 side	315	15	–	–
Portobello & Romaine	1 entree	270	15	–	–

FOOD	PORTION	CALS	FAT	SAT FAT	TRANS FAT
Salmon	1 entree	470	26	–	–
Spinach	1 side	272	19	–	–
Spring Greens	1 side	240	18	–	–
Tabbouleh	1 side	417	16	–	–
Tomato & Blue Cheese Stack	1 side	352	25	–	–
SIZZLER					
Grilled Salmon w/ Broccoli	1 serv	393	19	5	–
Hibachi Chicken w/ Broccoli	1 serv	290	6	1	–
Petite Steak w/ Broccoli	1 serv	520	26	11	–

SKIPPER'S
CHILDREN'S MENU SELECTIONS

FOOD	PORTION	CALS	FAT	SAT FAT	TRANS FAT
Kids Catch Chicken Tenderloin + Chips & Kids Side	1 serv	560	11	4	–
Kids Catch Fish Bites + Chips & Kids Side	1 serv	490	15	8	–
Kids Catch Sandwich Grilled Cheese + Chips & Kids Side	1 serv	620	19	7	–
Kids Catch Shrimp + Chips & Kids Side	1 serv	520	11	3	–

MAIN MENU SELECTIONS

FOOD	PORTION	CALS	FAT	SAT FAT	TRANS FAT
Baked Potato Plain	1	210	0	0	0
Basket Chicken & Fish + Chips & Slaw	1 serv	620	27	9	–
Basket Chicken & Shrimp + Chips & Slaw	1 serv	760	25	5	–
Basket Chicken + Chips & Slaw	1 serv	730	25	7	–
Basket Clam Strips + Chips & Slaw	1 serv	890	34	6	–
Basket Clams & Fish + Chips & Slaw	1 serv	740	32	9	–
Basket Original Recipe Shrimp + Chips & Slaw	1 serv	800	25	4	–
Basket Popcorn Shrimp + Chips & Slaw	1 serv	750	25	5	–
Basket Prawn & Fish + Chips & Slaw	1 serv	730	41	10	–
Basket Prawn Seafood + Chips & Slaw	1 serv	720	40	7	–

FOOD	PORTION	CALS	FAT	SAT FAT	TRANS FAT
Basket Shrimp & Fish + Chips & Slaw	1 serv	650	27	8	–
Basket Shrimp Trio + Chips & Slaw	1 serv	1040	38	9	–
Clam Chowder	1 cup	120	8	0	–
Clam Strips	1 serv	270	6	1	–
Fish Bites + Chips & Slaw	6 pieces	490	17	4	–
French Fries	1 reg	180	6	2	–
Grilled Veggies	1 serv	35	0	0	0
Halibut + Chips & Slaw	1 serv	580	30	5	–
Homestyle Chicken Tenderloin	1 piece	190	2	2	–
Hush Puppies	3 pieces	240	9	2	–
Original Fish Fillet	1 piece	80	4	4	–
Original Fish + Chips & Slaw	2 pieces	510	29	11	–
Original Shrimp	9 pieces	220	2	0	–
Sandwich Fish + Chips & Slaw	1 serv	800	34	9	–
Sandwich Fried Chicken + Chips & Slaw	1	1260	49	15	–
Sandwich Grilled Chicken + Chips & Slaw	1	1070	50	13	–
Skipper's Platter + Chips & Slaw	1 serv	930	33	9	–
SALADS					
Caesar	1 sm	150	13	3	–
Caesar w/ Chicken	1 sm	340	17	4	–
Caesar w/ Salmon	1 sm	350	19	4	–
Green Salad w/o Dressing	1 sm	25	0	0	0

SMOOTHIE KING

FOOD	PORTION	CALS	FAT	SAT FAT	TRANS FAT
Activator Chocolate	1 (20 oz)	429	1	tr	–
Activator Strawberry	1 (20 oz)	559	1	tr	–
Activator Vanilla	1 (20 oz)	429	1	tr	–
Banana Boat	1 (20 oz)	520	14	8	–
Coconut Surprise	1 (20 oz)	457	6	2	–
Coffee Smoothies Amaretto	1 (20 oz)	118	tr	tr	–
Coffee Smoothies French Roast	1 (20 oz)	164	tr	tr	–
Coffee Smoothies French Vanilla	1 (20 oz)	118	tr	tr	–
Coffee Smoothies Hazelnut	1 (20 oz)	118	tr	tr	–
Coffee Smoothies Irish Creme	1 (20 oz)	118	tr	tr	–

FOOD	PORTION	CALS	FAT	SAT FAT	TRANS FAT
Coffee Smoothies Mocha	1 (20 oz)	206	1	tr	–
HeaterZ Banana Nut	1	400	22	–	–
HeaterZ Blueberry Muffin	1	370	26	–	–
HeaterZ Chocolate Peanut Butter Cup	1	380	13	–	–
HeaterZ Cinnamon Oatmeal Raisin	1	420	3	–	–
HeaterZ Coconut	1	440	13	–	–
HeaterZ Coffee Amaretto	1 (12 oz)	177	2	1	–
HeaterZ Coffee French Roast	1 (12 oz)	172	2	1	–
HeaterZ Coffee French Vanilla	1 (12 oz)	177	2	1	–
HeaterZ Coffee Hazelnut	1 (12 oz)	177	2	1	–
HeaterZ Coffee Irish Creme	1 (12 oz)	177	2	1	–
HeaterZ Coffee Mocha	1 (12 oz)	266	2	1	–
High Protein Almond Mocha	1 (20 oz)	402	13	2	–
High Protein Banana	1 (20 oz)	412	14	2	–
High Protein Chocolate	1 (20 oz)	401	13	2	–
High Protein Lemon	1 (20 oz)	390	13	2	–
High Protein Pineapple	1 (20 oz)	380	13	2	–
Hot Coffee Amaretto	1 (12 oz)	168	tr	tr	–
Hot Coffee French Roast	1 (12 oz)	164	tr	tr	–
Hot Coffee French Vanilla	1 (12 oz)	168	tr	tr	–
Hot Coffee Hazelnut	1 (12 oz)	168	tr	tr	–
Hot Coffee Irish Creme	1 (12 oz)	168	tr	tr	–
Hot Coffee Mocha	1 (12 oz)	209	1	tr	–
Iced Coffee Amaretto	1 (20 oz)	168	tr	tr	–
Iced Coffee French Roast	1 (20 oz)	164	tr	tr	–
Iced Coffee French Vanilla	1 (20 oz)	168	tr	tr	–
Iced Coffee Hazelnut	1 (20 oz)	168	tr	tr	–
Iced Coffee Irish Creme	1 (20 oz)	168	tr	tr	–
Iced Coffee Mocha	1 (20 oz)	209	1	tr	–
Kid Cup Berry Interesting	1	150	0	0	0
Kid Cup Choc-A-Laka	1	210	2	0	–
Kid Cup Gimmi-Grape	1	170	0	0	0
Kid Cup Smarti Tarti	1	150	0	0	0
Low Carb All Flavors	1 (20 oz)	225	6	3	–
Low Fat Angel Food	1 (20 oz)	330	1	tr	–
Low Fat Blackberry Dream	1 (20 oz)	343	tr	tr	–
Low Fat Caribbean Way	1 (20 oz)	392	tr	tr	–
Low Fat Celestial Cherry High	1 (20 oz)	285	tr	tr	–

FOOD	PORTION	CALS	FAT	SAT FAT	TRANS FAT
Low Fat Cherry Picker	1 (20 oz)	360	1	tr	–
Low Fat Cranberry Cooler	1 (20 oz)	538	tr	tr	–
Low Fat Cranberry Supreme	1 (20 oz)	577	1	tr	–
Low Fat Grape Expectations	1 (20 oz)	399	tr	tr	–
Low Fat Grape Expectations II	1 (20 oz)	529	tr	tr	–
Low Fat Healthy Apple	1 (20 oz)	380	2	1	–
Low Fat Immune Builder	1 (20 oz)	333	1	tr	–
Low Fat Instant Vigor	1 (20 oz)	359	1	tr	–
Low Fat Island Treat	1 (20 oz)	334	1	tr	–
Low Fat Lemon Twist Banana	1 (20 oz)	339	tr	tr	–
Low Fat Lemon Twist Strawberry	1 (20 oz)	399	tr	tr	–
Low Fat Light & Fluffy	1 (20 oz)	389	tr	tr	–
Low Fat Mangofest	1 (20 oz)	320	0	0	0
Low Fat Muscle Punch	1 (20 oz)	339	1	tr	–
Low Fat Muscle Punch Plus	1 (20 oz)	340	1	tr	–
Low Fat Orange Ka-BAM	1 (20 oz)	320	0	0	0
Low Fat Peach Slice	1 (20 oz)	341	tr	tr	–
Low Fat Peach Slice Plus	1 (20 oz)	471	tr	tr	–
Low Fat Pep Upper	1 (20 oz)	334	1	tr	–
Low Fat Pineapple Pleasure	1 (20 oz)	331	tr	tr	–
Low Fat Pineapple Surf	1 (20 oz)	440	1	0	–
Low Fat Raspberry Sunrise	1 (20 oz)	335	1	tr	–
Low Fat Strawberry Kiwi Breeze	1 (20 oz)	300	0	0	0
Low Fat Strawberry X-Treme	1 (20 oz)	370	0	0	0
Low Fat Youth Fountain	1 (20 oz)	267	tr	tr	–
Malts	1 (20 oz)	887	41	26	–
Mo'cuccino	1 (20 oz)	420	12	7	–
Peanut Power	1 (20 oz)	502	21	4	–
Peanut Power Plus Grape	1 (20 oz)	703	21	4	–
Peanut Power Plus Strawberry	1 (20 oz)	632	21	4	–
Pina Colada Island	1 (20 oz)	550	11	9	–
Power Punch	1 (20 oz)	430	1	tr	–
Power Punch Plus	1 (20 oz)	499	2	tr	–
Shakes	1 (20 oz)	875	41	25	–
Slim-N-Trim Chocolate	1 (20 oz)	270	2	1	–
Slim-N-Trim Orange Vanilla	1 (20 oz)	199	1	0	–
Slim-N-Trim Strawberry	1 (20 oz)	357	1	tr	–
Slim-N-Trim Vanilla	1 (20 oz)	227	1	tr	–

FOOD	PORTION	CALS	FAT	SAT FAT	TRANS FAT
Super Punch	1 (20 oz)	425	tr	tr	–
Super Punch Plus	1 (20 oz)	516	tr	tr	–
The Hulk Chocolate	1 (20 oz)	846	29	17	–
The Hulk Strawberry	1 (20 oz)	953	29	16	–
The Hulk Vanilla	1 (20 oz)	846	29	16	–
Yogurt D-Lite	1 (20 oz)	335	4	2	–

SONIC DRIVE-IN
ADD-ONS

FOOD	PORTION	CALS	FAT	SAT FAT	TRANS FAT
Bacon	1 serv (0.5 oz)	80	7	3	–
Cheddar Cheese Shredded	1 serv (1 oz)	104	9	6	–
Cheese	1 serv (0.7 oz)	70	6	4	–
Chili	1 serv (1 oz)	52	4	2	–
Cone Coat Chocolate	1 serv (1 oz)	143	8	7	–
Green Chilies	1 serv (1 oz)	10	0	0	0
Hickory Barbecue Sauce	1 serv (1 oz)	41	0	0	0
Honey Mustard Dressing	1 serv (1.1 oz)	110	9	1	–
Jalapenos Nachos Sliced	1 serv (1 oz)	5	0	0	0
Malt	1 serv (1 oz)	104	1	0	–
Maraschino Cherry	1 serv (8 g)	10	0	0	0
Marinara Sauce	1 serv (1 oz)	15	0	0	0
Ranch Dressing	1 serv (1 oz)	147	16	2	–
Slaw	1 serv (0.9 oz)	45	3	0	–
Sweet Pickle Relish	1 serv (1.1 oz)	40	0	0	0
Syrup Blue Coconut	1 serv (1 oz)	65	0	0	0
Syrup Cherry	1 serv (1 oz)	64	0	0	0
Syrup Chocolate	1 serv (1 oz)	74	0	0	0
Syrup Grape	1 serv (1 oz)	63	0	0	0
Syrup Vanilla	1 serv (1 oz)	61	0	0	0
Syrup Watermelon	1 serv (1 oz)	71	0	0	0
Thousand Island Dressing	1 serv (1 oz)	150	15	2	–
Topping Pineapple	1 serv (1.5 oz)	108	0	0	0
Topping Strawberry	1 serv (1 oz)	101	4	3	–
Topping Strawberry	1 serv (1.2 oz)	38	0	0	0

BEVERAGES

FOOD	PORTION	CALS	FAT	SAT FAT	TRANS FAT
Barq's Root Beer	1 sm	160	0	0	0
Barq's Root Beer	1 lg	333	0	0	0
Coca-Cola	1 sm	139	0	0	0
Coca-Cola	1 lg	291	0	0	0
Diet Coca-Cola	1 sm	1	0	0	0

FOOD	PORTION	CALS	FAT	SAT FAT	TRANS FAT
Diet Coca-Cola	1 lg	3	0	0	0
Diet Sprite	1 sm	4	0	0	0
Diet Sprite	1 lg	8	0	0	0
Dr Pepper	1 sm	144	0	0	0
Dr Pepper	1 lg	300	0	0	0
Float or Flurry Blue Coconut Slush	1 reg	424	12	12	–
Limeade	1 sm	143	0	0	0
Limeade	1 lg	303	0	0	0
Limeade Cherry	1 sm	169	0	0	0
Limeade Cherry	1 lg	361	0	0	0
Limeade Strawberry	1 sm	172	0	0	0
Limeade Strawberry	1 lg	341	0	0	0
Slush Blue Coconut	1 lg	521	0	0	0
Slush Watermelon	1 lg	526	0	0	0
Sprite	1 sm	138	0	0	0
Sprite	1 lg	288	0	0	0
BREAKFAST SELECTIONS					
Breakfast Burrito	1	731	47	22	–
Fruit Taquitos	1 serv	302	7	1	–
Sunrise	1 lg	368	0	0	0
Sunrise	1 reg	224	0	0	0
Toaster Bacon Egg & Cheese	1	500	20	11	–
Toaster Ham Egg & Cheese	1	436	19	7	–
Toaster Sausage Egg & Cheese	1	570	36	14	–
DESSERTS					
Banana Split	1 serv	467	11	10	–
Chocolate Covered Shake Banana	1 reg	625	25	23	–
Chocolate Covered Shake Cherry	1 reg	587	24	23	–
Chocolate Covered Shake Peanut Butter	1 reg	678	34	25	–
Chocolate Covered Shake Strawberry	1 reg	608	24	23	–
Cream Pie Shake Banana	1 reg	775	27	21	–
Cream Pie Shake Chocolate	1 reg	795	27	21	–
Cream Pie Shake Coconut	1 reg	721	26	21	–
Dish Of Vanilla	1 serv	265	11	11	–
Float Or Flurry Cherry Slush	1 reg	421	12	12	–

FOOD	PORTION	CALS	FAT	SAT FAT	TRANS FAT
Float Or Flurry Coca-Cola	1 reg	379	12	12	–
Float Or Flurry Dr Pepper	1 reg	377	12	12	–
Float Or Flurry Grape Slush	1 reg	423	12	12	–
Float Or Flurry Orange Slush	1 reg	422	12	12	–
Float Or Flurry Rootbeer	1 reg	386	12	12	–
Float Or Flurry Watermelon Slush	1 reg	427	12	12	–
Ice Cream Cone	1	285	11	11	–
Shake Banana	1 reg	508	18	18	–
Shake Chocolate	1 reg	564	18	18	–
Shake Pineapple	1 reg	615	18	18	–
Shake Strawberry	1 reg	510	18	18	–
Shake Vanilla	1 reg	454	18	18	–
Sonic Blast Butterfinger	1 reg	636	26	23	–
Sonic Blast M&M's	1 reg	641	27	24	–
Sonic Blast Oreo	1 reg	638	27	21	–
Sonic Blast Reese's	1 reg	658	30	23	–
Sundae Chocolate	1 serv	362	11	11	–
Sundae Hot Fudge	1 serv	392	15	15	–
Sundae Pineapple	1 serv	399	11	11	–
Sundae Strawberry	1 serv	322	11	11	–
MAIN MENU SELECTIONS					
Ched'R'Peppers	1 serv	256	12	5	–
Cheese Fries	1 lg	322	19	6	–
Cheese Fries	1 reg	265	17	6	–
Cheese Tater Tots	1 reg	329	22	7	–
Cheese Tater Tots	1 lg	435	27	8	–
Chicken Strip Dinner	1 serv	749	32	5	–
Chicken Strip Snack	1 serv	272	13	2	–
Chicken Strips	2	184	9	1	–
Chili Cheese Fries	1 lg	357	22	7	–
Chili Cheese Fries	1 reg	299	19	6	–
Chili Cheese Tater Tots	1 reg	363	25	7	–
Chili Cheese Tater Tots	1 lg	547	36	11	–
Corn Dog	1	262	17	5	–
Extra Long Coney Cheese	1	666	42	17	–
Extra Long Coney Plain	1	483	27	10	–
French Fries	1 lg	252	13	2	–
French Fries	1 reg	195	11	2	–
Fritos Chili Pie	1 serv	611	44	13	–

FOOD	PORTION	CALS	FAT	SAT FAT	TRANS FAT
Hot Dog Plain	1	262	16	5	–
Jr. Burger	1	353	21	6	–
Mozzarella Sticks	1 serv	382	19	11	–
No. 1 Hamburger	1	577	36	7	–
No. 1 Sonic Cheeseburger	1	647	42	11	–
No. 2 Hamburger	1	481	25	5	–
No. 2 Sonic Cheeseburger	1	551	31	9	–
Onion Rings	1 lg	507	35	7	–
Onion Rings	1 reg	331	23	5	–
Regular Coney Cheese	1	366	24	10	–
Regular Coney Plain	1	262	16	5	–
Sandwich Breaded Chicken	1	582	23	4	–
Sandwich Country Fried Steak	1	748	47	12	–
Sandwich Grilled Chicken	1	343	13	2	–
SuperSonic No. 1	1	929	66	19	–
SuperSonic No. 2	1	839	56	17	–
SuperSonic Onion Rings	1 serv	706	10	1	–
SuperSonic Tots	1 serv	485	28	5	–
SuperSonic Fries	1 serv	358	18	3	–
Tater Tots	1 lg	365	21	4	–
Tater Tots	1 reg	259	16	3	–
Toaster Sandwich Bacon Cheddar Burger	1	675	38	11	–
Toaster Sandwich BLT	1	581	41	9	–
Toaster Sandwich Chicken Club	1	675	29	8	–
Toaster Sandwich Country Fried Steak	1	708	45	11	–
Toaster Sandwich Grilled Cheese	1	282	12	5	–
Wrap Chicken Strip	1	574	29	5	–
Wrap Grilled Chicken	1	539	27	5	–
Wrap w/o Ranch Chicken Strip	1	428	13	2	–
Wrap w/o Ranch Grilled Chicken	1	393	12	3	–

SOUPLANTATION
BREADS AND MUFFINS

FOOD	PORTION	CALS	FAT	SAT FAT	TRANS FAT
Bread Indian Grain Low Fat	1 slice	200	2	0	–
Bread Low Fat Sourdough	1 slice	150	1	0	–
Cornbread Buttermilk Low Fat	1 piece	140	2	0	–

FOOD	PORTION	CALS	FAT	SAT FAT	TRANS FAT
Focaccia Big Hearth Pizza	1	140	6	2	–
Focaccia Bruschetta	1 piece	130	6	2	–
Focaccia Pepperoni	1 piece	160	7	3	–
Focaccia Roasted Potato	1 piece	150	6	2	–
Focaccia Sauteed Vegetables	1 piece	150	7	2	–
Focaccia Tomatillo	1 piece	140	6	2	–
Focaccia Low Fat Garlic Parmesan	1 piece	100	3	0	–
Muffin Apple Cinnamon Bran 96% Fat Free	1	80	1	0	–
Muffin Apple Raisin	1	150	7	1	–
Muffin Banana Nut	1	150	7	1	–
Muffin Big Blue Blueberry	1	310	12	2	–
Muffin Black Forest	1	230	9	2	–
Muffin Cappuccino Chip	1	160	4	2	–
Muffin Caribbean Key Lime	1	170	6	1	–
Muffin Cherry Nut	1	150	7	1	–
Muffin Chocolate Brownie	1	170	8	2	–
Muffin Chocolate Chip	1	170	8	2	–
Muffin Country Blackberry	1	170	6	2	–
Muffin French Quarter Praline	1	290	15	2	–
Muffin Georgia Peach Poppyseed	1	150	6	1	–
Muffin Lemon	1	140	4	1	–
Muffin Macadamia Nut Spice	1	220	9	2	–
Muffin Maple Walnut	1	230	10	2	–
Muffin Nutty Peanut Butter	1	170	8	1	–
Muffin Pumpkin Raisin	1 piece	150	6	1	–
Muffin Strawberry Buttermilk	1	140	6	1	–
Muffin Sweet Orange & Cranberry	1	200	7	1	–
Muffin Taffy Apple	1	160	6	1	–
Muffin Tropical Papaya Coconut	1	180	7	2	–
Muffin Zucchini Nut	1	150	7	1	–
Muffin 96% Fat Free Cranberry Orange Bran	1	80	1	0	–
Muffin 96% Fat Free Fruit Medley Bran	1	80	1	0	–
Muffin Low Fat Chile Corn	1	140	3	1	–

FOOD	PORTION	CALS	FAT	SAT FAT	TRANS FAT
DESSERTS					
Cobbler Apple	½ cup	350	10	2	–
Cobbler Blissful Blueberry	½ cup	380	10	2	–
Cobbler Cherry	½ cup	340	10	2	–
Cobbler Cranberry Apple	½ cup	370	10	2	–
Cobbler Peach	½ cup	360	10	2	–
Cookie Chocolate Chip	1 sm	70	3	1	–
Fat Free Apple Medley	½ cup	70	0	0	0
Fat Free Banana Royale	½ cup	80	0	0	0
Fat Free Frozen Yogurt Chocolate	½ cup	95	0	0	0
Jell-O Fat Free All Flavors	½ cup	80	0	0	0
Jell-O Fat Free Sugar Free All Flavors	½ cup	10	0	0	0
Pudding Banana	½ cup	160	4	0	–
Pudding Vanilla	½ cup	140	4	0	–
Pudding Low Fat Butterscotch	½ cup	140	3	0	–
Pudding Low Fat Chocolate	½ cup	140	3	0	–
Pudding Low Fat Rice	½ cup	110	2	1	–
Soft Serve Reduced Fat Vanilla	½ cup	140	4	3	–
Tapioca Low Fat	½ cup	140	3	0	–
MAIN MENU SELECTIONS					
Alfredo Broccoli w/ Basil	1 cup	380	17	8	–
Alfredo Fettuccine	1 cup	390	18	10	–
Alfredo Four Cheese	1 cup	390	13	7	–
Alfredo Roasted Garlic & Asiago	1 cup	330	11	6	–
Alfredo Roasted Mushroom w/ Rosemary	1 cup	380	14	8	–
Alfredo Southwestern	1 cup	350	16	9	–
Beef Stroganoff	1 cup	340	21	11	–
Carbonara Pasta	1 cup	280	8	4	–
Chili Arizona	1 cup	220	8	4	–
Chili Longhorn Beef	1 cup	190	6	3	–
Chili Rock N' Mole	1 cup	240	13	5	–
Chili Santa Fe Black Bean Low Fat	1 cup	190	3	0	–
Chili Texas Red	1 cup	240	8	4	–
Chili Three Bean Turkey Low Fat	1 cup	140	3	1	–

FOOD	PORTION	CALS	FAT	SAT FAT	TRANS FAT
Chili Vegetarian	1 cup	150	3	0	–
Chili Cheatin' Heart	1 cup	300	19	5	–
Chili Deep Kettle House Low Fat	1 cup	230	3	2	–
Creamy Herb Chicken	1 cup	310	17	8	–
Creamy Pepper Jack	1 cup	290	15	6	–
Garden Vegetable w/ Italian Sausage	1 cup	300	10	3	–
Garden Vegetable w/ Meatballs	1 cup	270	7	3	–
Greek Mediterranean	1 cup	290	8	3	–
Italian Vegetable Beef	1 cup	270	6	2	–
Italian Sausage w/ Red Pepper Puree	1 cup	250	10	4	–
Lemon Cream & Asparagus	1 cup	230	9	2	–
Linguini w/ Clam Sauce	1 cup	380	10	5	–
Low Fat Oriental Green Bean & Noodle	1 cup	240	3	0	–
Macaroni & Cheese	1 cup	260	6	3	–
Nutty Mushroom	1 cup	390	20	9	–
Pasta Florentine	1 cup	360	10	4	–
Penne Arrabbiatta	1 cup	340	10	6	–
Pesto Cilantro Lime	1 cup	370	21	3	–
Roasted Eggplant Marinara	1 cup	340	10	6	–
Smoked Salmon & Dill	1 cup	360	16	8	–
Tuscany Sausage w/ Capers & Olives	1 cup	240	10	4	–
Vegetable Ragu	1 cup	250	5	2	–
Vegetarian Marinara w/ Basil	1 cup	260	4	2	–
Walnut Pesto	1 cup	310	9	3	–
SALAD DRESSINGS					
Bacon	2 tbsp	120	11	2	–
Balsamic Vinaigrette	1 tbsp	180	19	2	–
Basil Vinaigrette	2 tbsp	160	17	1	–
Blue Cheese	1 tbsp	140	14	3	–
Creamy Italian	2 tbsp	120	13	2	–
Honey Mustard	2 tbsp	150	13	2	–
Honey Mustard Fat Free	2 tbsp	45	0	0	0
Italian Fat Free	2 tbsp	20	0	0	0
Kahlena French	2 tbsp	120	9	2	–

FOOD	PORTION	CALS	FAT	SAT FAT	TRANS FAT
Parmesan Pepper Cream	2 tbsp	160	17	3	–
Ranch	2 tbsp	130	13	2	–
Ranch Fat Free	2 tbsp	50	0	0	0
Reduced Calorie Cucumber	2 tbsp	80	7	1	–
Roasted Garlic	2 tbsp	140	14	2	–
Thousand Island	2 tbsp	110	11	2	–
SALADS					
Ambrosia w/ Coconut	½ cup	170	6	3	–
Antipasto w/ Peppered Salami	1 cup	140	10	3	–
Artichoke Rice	½ cup	160	8	1	–
Aunt Doris' Red Pepper Slaw Fat Free	½ cup	70	0	0	0
Baja Bean & Cilantro Low Fat	½ cup	180	3	0	–
Bartlett Pear & Walnut	1 cup	180	12	2	–
BBQ Julienne Chopped	1 cup	190	10	2	–
BBQ Smokehouse w/ Bacon & Peanuts	1 cup	190	10	3	–
Caesar Asiago	1 cup	190	14	2	–
California Cobb	1 cup	180	8	2	–
Cape Cod Spinach w/ Walnuts	1 cup	170	14	2	–
Carrot Ginger w/ Herb Vinaigrette	½ cup	150	12	1	–
Carrot Raisin Low Fat	½ cup	90	3	0	–
Chicken Tortilla	1 cup	180	10	3	–
Chinese Krab	½ cup	160	8	1	–
Citrus Noodle w/ Snow Peas	½ cup	140	6	1	–
Country French w/ Bacon	1 cup	210	18	6	–
Ensalada Azteca	1 cup	130	9	3	–
Field Corn & Very Wild Rice	½ cup	170	9	1	–
Greek	1 cup	120	9	3	–
Greek Couscous w/ Feta	½ cup	170	9	1	–
Italian Garden Vegetable	½ cup	110	8	1	–
Italian Sub Salad w/ Turkey & Salami	1 cup	260	17	6	–
Italian White Bean	½ cup	140	5	0	–
Joan's Blue BLT	1 cup	250	16	5	–
Joan's Broccoli Madness	½ cup	180	14	3	–
Lemon Rice w/ Cashews	½ cup	160	7	2	–
Mandarin Noodles w/ Broccoli Low Fat	½ cup	120	3	0	–

FOOD	PORTION	CALS	FAT	SAT FAT	TRANS FAT
Mandarin Shells w/ Almonds	½ cup	120	3	0	–
Mandarin Spinach w/ Caramelized Walnuts	1 cup	170	11	1	–
Marinated Summer Vegetables Fat Free	½ cup	80	0	0	0
Mediterranean	1 cup	150	11	2	–
Monterey Blue w/ Peanuts	1 cup	200	12	4	–
Moroccan Marinated Vegetables Low Fat	½ cup	90	3	0	–
Old Fashioned Macaroni Salad w/ Ham	½ cup	180	11	2	–
Oriental Ginger Slaw w/ Krab Low Fat	½ cup	70	3	0	–
Penne w/ Chicken In Citrus Vinaigrette Low Fat	½ cup	130	3	0	–
Pesto Orzo w/ Pinenuts	1 cup	220	17	3	–
Pesto Pasta	½ cup	160	7	1	–
Pineapple Coconut Slaw	½ cup	150	10	3	–
Poppyseed Coleslaw	½ cup	120	9	1	–
Potato BBQ	½ cup	160	8	1	–
Potato Dijon w/ Garlic Dill Vinaigrette	½ cup	150	12	1	–
Potato German	½ cup	120	3	1	–
Potato Jalapeno	½ cup	140	5	1	–
Potato Picnic	½ cup	150	7	1	–
Potato Southern Dill Low Fat	½ cup	120	3	2	–
Ragin' Cajun	1 cup	200	14	2	–
Ranch House BLT Salad w/ Turkey	1 cup	180	11	4	–
Red Potato & Tomato	½ cup	120	10	2	–
Roasted Vegetables w/ Feta & Olives	1 cup	140	11	2	–
Roasted Potato Salad w/ Chipotle Chili Vinaigrette	½ cup	140	6	1	–
Roma Tomatoes Mozzarella & Basil	1 cup	120	9	2	–
San Francisco Herb Rice	½ cup	170	5	2	–
Shrimp & Seafood	½ cup	200	11	2	–
Smoked Turkey & Spinach w/ Almonds	1 cup	190	10	2	–

FOOD	PORTION	CALS	FAT	SAT FAT	TRANS FAT
Sonoma Spinach w/ Honey Dijon Vinaigrette	1 cup	210	14	3	–
Southern Black-Eyed Peas	½ cup	130	6	0	–
Southwestern Rice & Beans	½ cup	90	3	0	–
Spiced Pecans & Roasted Vegetables	1 cup	180	11	3	–
Spicy Southwestern Pasta Low Fat	½ cup	130	3	0	–
Spinach Gorgonzola w/ Spiced Pecans	1 cup	210	19	4	–
Strawberry Fields w/ Caramelized Walnuts	1 cup	130	8	1	–
Summer Barley w/ Black Beans Low Fat	½ cup	110	3	0	–
Summer Lemon w/ Spiced Pecans	1 cup	220	15	3	–
Thai Noodle w/ Peanut Sauce	½ cup	170	8	1	–
Three Bean Marinade	½ cup	170	6	1	–
Tomato Cucumber Marinade	½ cup	80	5	0	–
Traditional Spinach w/ Bacon	1 cup	160	11	4	–
Tuna Tarragon	½ cup	240	14	2	–
Turkey Chutney Pasta	½ cup	230	9	2	–
Watercress & Orange	1 cup	90	4	1	–
Wild Rice & Chicken	½ cup	300	22	5	–
Won Ton Chicken Happiness	1 cup	150	8	1	–
Zesty Tortellini	½ cup	190	15	2	–
SOUPS					
Albino Bean Chicken	1 cup	190	6	3	–
Albondigas Locas	1 cup	210	10	4	–
Autumn Root Vegetable w/ Wild Rice	1 cup	80	0	0	0
Baked Potato & Cheese w/ Bacon	1 cup	290	18	10	–
Be Wild With Mushroom	1 cup	220	16	9	–
Big Chunk Chicken Noodle Low Fat	1 cup	160	3	2	–
Black Bean Sausage Fling	1 cup	350	23	11	–
Black Bean & Chorizo	1 cup	230	9	3	–
Bombay Lentil Low Fat	1 cup	160	3	2	–
Broc On	1 cup	220	18	11	–

FOOD	PORTION	CALS	FAT	SAT FAT	TRANS FAT
Broccoli Cheese	1 cup	280	20	11	–
Butternut Squash	1 cup	140	6	4	–
Cheese Stuffed Cappelletti	1 cup	130	4	2	–
Chesapeake Corn Chowder	1 cup	280	16	8	–
Chicken Got Smoked	1 cup	350	21	14	–
Chicken Tortilla w/ Jalapeno Chiles & Tomatoes Low Fat	1 cup	100	3	1	–
Chunky Potato Cheese w/ Thyme	1 cup	210	10	6	–
Classical French Onion	1 cup	130	5	2	–
Classical Minestrone Low Fat	1 cup	120	2	0	–
Classical Shrimp Bisque	1 cup	240	16	7	–
Country Corn & Red Potato Chowder	1 cup	160	6	3	–
Cream Of Broccoli	1 cup	210	15	6	–
Cream Of Chicken	1 cup	260	18	9	–
Cream Of Mushroom	1 cup	290	21	8	–
Cream Of Rosemary Potato	1 cup	270	19	10	–
Creamy Vegetable Chowder	1 cup	200	10	4	–
Devotion To The Ocean	1 cup	220	12	7	–
El Paso Lime & Chicken	1 cup	160	4	1	–
Field Of Creams Cauliflower w/ Cheese	1 cup	260	20	9	–
Field Of Creams Celery	1 cup	210	15	7	–
Field Of Creams Spinach	1 cup	280	22	10	–
Field Of Creams Tomato Basil	1 cup	220	15	7	–
Fire Roasted Green Chili & Corn Chowder	1 cup	230	14	6	–
Garden Fresh Vegetable Low Fat	1 cup	110	1	0	–
Garlic Kickin Roasted Chicken	1 cup	140	6	3	–
Hungarian Vegetable Low Fat	1 cup	120	2	0	–
Irish Potato Leek	1 cup	250	15	7	–
Living On The Veg	1 cup	90	1	0	–
Manhattan Clam Chowder	1 cup	130	4	1	–
Mulligatawny	1 cup	210	12	5	–
Navy Bean w/ Ham	1 cup	340	10	4	–
Neighbor Joe's Gumbo	1 cup	280	8	3	–
Posole	1 cup	150	6	2	–
Ratatouille Provencale Fat Free	1 cup	110	0	0	0

FOOD	PORTION	CALS	FAT	SAT FAT	TRANS FAT
Roasted Mushroom w/ Sage	1 cup	320	25	11	–
Spicy Sausage & Pasta	1 cup	310	12	5	–
Split Pea w/ Ham	1 cup	350	10	4	–
Tomato Chipotle Bisque	1 cup	240	16	8	–
Tomato Parmesan & Vegetables Low Fat	1 cup	120	3	1	–
Toot Your Horn For Crab & Corn	1 cup	290	20	12	–
Vegetarian Lentils & Brown Rice Low Fat	1 cup	130	1	0	–
Yankee Clipper Clam Chowder w/ Bacon	1 cup	330	20	10	–

SOUTHERN TSUNAMI SUSHI BAR
SALADS

FOOD	PORTION	CALS	FAT	SAT FAT	TRANS FAT
Calamari	1 serv (4 oz)	148	3	0	–
Edamame	1 serv (4 oz)	124	7	1	–
Harusame	1 serv (5 oz)	148	2	0	–
Seabreeze	1 serv (4 oz)	113	3	1	–

SUSHI

FOOD	PORTION	CALS	FAT	SAT FAT	TRANS FAT
California Roll	1 (0.8 oz)	31	1	tr	–
Cream Cheese Roll w/ Salmon	1 piece (0.8 oz)	43	2	1	–
Crunchy Shrimp Roll	1 piece (0.9 oz)	42	2	tr	–
Dragon Roll	1 piece (0.8 oz)	42	2	tr	–
Freshwater Eel Roll	1 piece (0.8 oz)	41	1	tr	–
Green Horseradish	1 tsp	7	0	0	0
Inari	1 piece (1.9 oz)	105	2	tr	–
Nigiri Cuttlefish	1 piece (1 oz)	42	1	1	–
Nigiri Egg Cake	1 piece (1.4 oz)	73	1	0	–
Nigiri Fish Roe	1 piece (1.4 oz)	61	1	0	–
Nigiri Fresh Salmon	1 piece (1.3 oz)	68	1	0	–
Nigiri Fresh Water Eel	1 piece (1.6 oz)	108	5	1	–
Nigiri Octopus	1 piece (1.1 oz)	57	1	0	–
Nigiri Sea Eel	1 piece (1.6 oz)	90	3	1	–
Nigiri Shrimp	1 piece (1.1 oz)	44	1	1	–
Nigiri Smoked Salmon	1 piece (1.3 oz)	68	1	0	–
Nigiri Tilapia	1 piece (1.2 oz)	49	1	1	–
Nigiri Tuna	1 piece (1.3 oz)	60	0	0	–
Nigiri Yellowtail	1 piece (1.2 oz)	54	1	0	–
Ocean Crab Roll	1 piece (0.8 oz)	33	1	tr	–

FOOD	PORTION	CALS	FAT	SAT FAT	TRANS FAT
Orange Roll	1 piece (0.8 oz)	32	1	tr	–
Pickled Ginger	1 tbsp	9	0	0	0
Rainbow Roll	1 piece (1 oz)	41	1	tr	–
Sea Eel Roll	1 piece (0.8 oz)	36	1	tr	–
Soy Sauce	1 pkg	16	0	0	0
Spicy Roll Salmon	1 piece (0.8 oz)	40	1	tr	–
Spicy Roll Shrimp	1 piece (0.8 oz)	31	1	tr	–
Spicy Roll Tuna	1 piece (0.8 oz)	37	1	tr	–
Tempura Roll	1 piece (0.9 oz)	44	1	0	–
Tofu Roll	1 piece (0.8 oz)	27	tr	tr	–
Tsunami Roll Crab & Fish Roe	1 piece (0.8 oz)	39	1	tr	–

STARBUCKS
BAKED SELECTIONS

FOOD	PORTION	CALS	FAT	SAT FAT	TRANS FAT
Apple Fritter	1	480	22	10	0
Bagel French Toast	1	280	1	0	0
Bagel Multigrain	1	280	3	0	0
Bagel Plain	1	280	0	0	0
Bar Cranberry Bliss	1	320	16	9	0
Bar Toffee Almond	1	400	19	8	0
Brownie Espresso	1	340	19	8	0
Cinnamon Roll	1	470	26	11	0
Cocoa Crispy Square	1	420	17	7	0
Cookie Chocolate Chunk	1	420	20	13	0
Cookie Coffee Ginger	1	470	18	11	1
Cookie Penguin	1	370	18	11	0
Cookie Rainbow	1	420	19	12	0
Cookies Mini Black & White	2	240	12	1	0
Croissant Butter	1	370	23	15	0
Doughnut Glazed	1	490	23	9	0
Loaf Banana Nut	1 serv	470	24	10	0
Loaf Iced Lemon	1 serv	500	18	9	0
Loaf Marble	1 serv	410	22	10	0
Loaf Pumpkin	1 serv	380	14	2	0
Mallorca Sweet Bread	1	420	24	11	0
Muffin Blueberry	1	310	11	3	0
Muffin Pumpkin Cream Cheese	1	490	24	6	0
Muffin Reduced Fat Chocolate	1	290	5	4	0
Muffin Walnut Bran	1	430	18	2	0

FOOD	PORTION	CALS	FAT	SAT FAT	TRANS FAT
Reduced Fat Coffee Cake Banana Chocolate Chip	1	390	8	5	0
Reduced Fat Coffee Cake Blueberry	1 serv	320	6	5	0
Reduced Fat Coffee Cake Cinnamon Swirl	1 serv	290	4	3	0
Reduced Fat Coffee Cake Pumpkin Chocolate Chip	1	300	6	3	0
Rustic Apple Tart	1	190	5	2	0
Scone Blueberry	1	480	22	12	1
Scone Cran Apple Crumb	1	490	20	11	1
Scone Raspberry	1	470	21	12	1
BEVERAGES					
Apple Juice	1 grande	250	0	0	0
Cafe Americano	1 grande	15	0	0	0
Cafe Au Lait Nonfat Milk	1 grande	70	0	0	0
Caffe Mocha No Whip Nonfat Milk	1 grande	220	3	1	0
Caffe Mocha Whip Nonfat Milk	1 grande	290	10	5	0
Cappuccino Nonfat Milk	1 grande	80	0	0	0
Caramel Macchiato Nonfat Milk	1 grande	190	1	1	0
Caramel Apple Cider Whip	1 grande	380	8	5	0
Caramel Apple Spice No Whip	1 grande	310	tr	0	0
Chocolate Milk Nonfat	1 grande	280	3	1	0
Cinnamon Dolce Creme No Whip Nonfat Milk	1 grande	220	0	0	0
Cinnamon Dolce Whip Nonfat Milk	1 grande	290	7	5	0
Coffee Of The Week	1 grande	5	tr	0	0
Coffee Of The Week Decaf	1 grande	5	0	0	0
Frappuccino Blended Coffee Cafe Vanilla No Whip Nonfat Milk	1 grande	310	3	2	0
Frappuccino Blended Coffee Cafe Vanilla No Whip Soy	1 grande	310	3	2	0
Frappuccino Blended Coffee Cafe Vanilla Whip Nonfat Milk	1 grande	430	14	9	0
Frappuccino Blended Coffee Cafe Vanilla Whip Soy	1 grande	430	14	9	0

FOOD	PORTION	CALS	FAT	SAT FAT	TRANS FAT
Frappuccino Blended Coffee Caramel No Whip Nonfat Milk	1 grande	270	4	3	0
Frappuccino Blended Coffee Caramel No Whip Soy	1 grande	270	4	3	0
Frappuccino Blended Coffee Caramel Whip Soy	1 grande	380	15	9	0
Frappuccino Blended Coffee Cinnamon Dolce No Whip Nonfat Milk	1 grande	260	3	2	0
Frappuccino Blended Coffee Cinnamon Dolce No Whip Soy	1 grande	260	3	2	0
Frappuccino Blended Coffee Cinnamon Dolce Whip Soy	1 grande	370	14	9	0
Frappuccino Blended Coffee Expresso Nonfat Milk	1 grande	190	3	2	0
Frappuccino Blended Coffee Expresso Nonfat Milk	1 grande	240	3	2	0
Frappuccino Blended Coffee Java Chip No Whip Nonfat Milk	1 grande	340	8	5	0
Frappuccino Blended Coffee Java Chip No Whip Soy	1 grande	190	3	2	0
Frappuccino Blended Coffee Java Chip Whip Nonfat Milk	1 grande	460	19	12	1
Frappuccino Blended Coffee Java Chip Whip Soy	1 grande	460	19	12	1
Frappuccino Blended Coffee Mocha No Whip Nonfat Milk	1 grande	260	4	2	0
Frappuccino Blended Coffee Mocha No Whip Soy	1 grande	260	4	2	0
Frappuccino Blended Coffee Mocha Whip Nonfat Milk	1 grande	380	15	9	0
Frappuccino Blended Coffee Pumpkin Spice No Whip Nonfat Milk	1 grande	290	4	2	0
Frappuccino Blended Coffee Pumpkin Spice No Whip Soy	1 grande	290	4	2	0

FOOD	PORTION	CALS	FAT	SAT FAT	TRANS FAT
Frappuccino Blended Coffee Pumpkin Spice Whip Nonfat Milk	1 grande	400	15	9	0
Frappuccino Blended Coffee Pumpkin Spice Whip Soy	1 grande	400	15	9	0
Frappuccino Blended Coffee Whip Nonfat Milk	1 grande	370	14	9	0
Frappuccino Blended Coffee White Chocolate Mocha No Whip Nonfat Milk	1 grande	300	5	3	0
Frappuccino Blended Coffee White Chocolate Mocha No Whip Soy	1 grande	300	5	3	0
Frappuccino Blended Coffee White Chocolate Mocha Whip Nonfat Milk	1 grande	410	16	10	0
Frappuccino Blended Coffee White Chocolate Mocha Whip Soy	1 grande	410	16	10	0
Frappuccino Blended Creme Tazo Chai No Whip Nonfat Milk	1 grande	330	2	0	0
Frappuccino Blended Creme Tazo Chai Whip Nonfat Milk	1 grande	570	15	9	0
Frappuccino Blended Creme Vanilla Bean No Whip Nonfat Milk	1 grande	350	3	0	0
Frappuccino Blended Creme Vanilla Bean Whip Nonfat Milk	1 grande	470	14	7	0
Frappuccino Light Blended Coffee Cafe Vanilla Nonfat Milk	1 grande	190	1	0	0
Frappuccino Light Blended Coffee Caramel	1 grande	160	2	0	0
Frappuccino Light Blended Coffee Cinnamon Dolce Nonfat Milk	1 grande	140	1	0	0
Frappuccino Light Blended Coffee Java Chip Nonfat Milk	1 grande	200	5	3	0
Frappuccino Light Blended Coffee Mocha Nonfat Milk	1 grande	140	1	0	0

FOOD	PORTION	CALS	FAT	SAT FAT	TRANS FAT
Frappuccino Light Blended Coffee Nonfat Milk	1 grande	130	1	0	0
Frappuccino Light Blended Coffee Pumpkin Spice Nonfat Milk	1 grande	150	1	0	0
Frappuccino Light Blended Creme Double Chocolaty Chip Whip Nonfat Milk	1 grande	510	19	11	0
Frappuccino Light Blended Creme Pumpkin Spice No Whip Nonfat Milk	1 grande	360	3	0	0
Frappuccino Light Blended Creme Pumpkin Spice Whip Nonfat Milk	1 grande	470	13	7	0
Frappuccino Light Blended Creme Tazo Green Tea No Whip Nonfat Milk	1 grande	380	3	0	0
Frappuccino Light Blended Creme Tazo Green Tea Whip Nonfat Milk	1 grande	440	13	7	0
Frappuccino Light Blended Creme Tazo Green Tea Whip Nonfat Milk	1 grande	490	14	7	0
Frappaccino Light Blended Creme White Chocolate No Whip Nonfat Milk	1 grande	480	7	4	0
Frappuccino Light Blended Creme White Chocolate Whip Nonfat Milk	1 grande	610	19	12	0
Frappuccino Light Expresso Nonfat Milk	1 grande	110	1	0	0
Hot Chocolate No Whip Nonfat Milk	1 grande	240	3	1	0
Hot Chocolate Whip Nonfat Milk	1 grande	320	10	5	0
Iced Brewed Coffee	1 grande	90	0	0	0
Iced Cafe Mocha Whip Nonfat Milk	1 grande	290	14	7	0
Iced Caffe Americano	1 grande	15	0	0	0
Iced Caffe Latte Nonfat Milk	1 grande	90	0	0	0

FOOD	PORTION	CALS	FAT	SAT FAT	TRANS FAT
Iced Caffe Mocha No Whip Nonfat Milk	1 grande	170	3	0	0
Iced Caramel Macchiato Nonfat Milk	1 grande	190	2	1	0
Iced Latte Pumpkin Spice No Whip Nonfat Milk	1 grande	220	0	0	0
Iced Latte Pumpkin Spice Whip Nonfat Milk	1 grande	330	11	7	0
Iced Latte Skinny Cinnamon Dolce No Whip Nonfat Milk	1 grande	80	0	0	0
Iced Latte Sugar Free Flavored Syrup Nonfat Milk	1 grande	80	0	0	0
Iced Latte Syrup Flavored Nonfat Milk	1 grande	160	0	0	0
Iced Latte Vanilla Nonfat Milk	1 grande	160	0	0	0
Iced Peppermint White Chocolate Mocha No Whip Nonfat Milk	1 grande	370	6	5	0
Iced Peppermint White Chocolate Mocha Whip Nonfat Milk	1 grande	490	17	11	0
Iced Tazo Latte Black Tea Nonfat Milk	1 grande	170	0	0	0
Iced Tazo Latte Black Tea Soy	1 grande	200	3	0	0
Iced Tazo Latte Chai Nonfat Milk	1 grande	200	0	0	0
Iced Tazo Latte Green Tea Nonfat Milk	1 grande	220	5	0	0
Iced Tazo Latte Green Tea Soy	1 grande	260	4	1	0
Iced Tazo Latte Red Tea	1 grande	200	3	0	0
Iced Tazo Latte Red Tea Nonfat Milk	1 grande	170	0	0	0
Iced White Chocolate Mocha No Whip Nonfat Milk	1 grande	310	6	5	0
Iced White Chocolate Mocha Whip Nonfat Milk	1 grande	430	17	11	0
Latte Caffe Nonfat Milk	1 grande	130	5	0	0
Latte Cinnamon Dolce No Whip Nonfat Milk	1 grande	210	0	0	0

FOOD	PORTION	CALS	FAT	SAT FAT	TRANS FAT
Latte Cinnamon Dolce w/ Sugar Free Syrup Nonfat Milk	1 grande	130	0	0	0
Latte Cinnamon Dolce Whip Nonfat Milk	1 grande	280	7	5	0
Latte Pumpkin Spice No Whip Nonfat Milk	1 grande	260	0	0	0
Latte Pumpkin Spice Whip Nonfat Milk	1 grande	330	7	5	0
Latte Skinny Caramel No Whip Nonfat Milk	1 grande	130	0	0	0
Latte Skinny Cinnamon Dolce No Whip Nonfat Milk	1 grande	130	0	0	0
Latte Skinny Cinnamon Dolce No Whip Nonfat Milk	1 grande	130	0	0	9
Latte Skinny Hazelnut No Whip Nonfat Milk	1 grande	130	0	0	0
Latte Skinny Vanilla No Whip Nonfat Milk	1 grande	130	0	0	0
Latte Syrup Flavored Nonfat Milk	1 grande	200	0	0	0
Milk Nonfat	1 grande	180	0	0	0
Peppermint White Chocolate Mocha No Whip Nonfat Milk	1 grande	420	6	5	0
Peppermint White Chocolate Mocha Whip Nonfat Milk	1 grande	490	13	9	0
Pumpkin Spice Creme No Whip Nonfat Milk	1 grande	270	0	0	0
Pumpkin Spice Creme Whip Nonfat Milk	1 grande	340	7	5	0
Shaken Black Iced Tea & Lemonade	1 grande	130	0	0	0
Shaken White Iced Tea Blueberry	1 grande	80	0	0	0
Steamed Apple Juice	1 grande	230	0	0	0
Tazo Black Shaken Iced Tea & Lemonade	1 grande	130	0	0	0
Tazo Chai Latte Iced Tea Soy	1 grande	230	3	0	0
Tazo Chai Latte Nonfat Milk	1 grande	200	0	0	0
Tazo Chai Latte Soy	1 grande	230	3	0	0

FOOD	PORTION	CALS	FAT	SAT FAT	TRANS FAT
Tazo Latte Black Tea Soy	1 grande	190	3	0	0
Tazo Latte Green Tea Soy	1 grande	220	3	0	0
Tazo Latte Black Tea Nonfat Milk	1 grande	170	0	0	0
Tazo Latte Green Tea Nonfat Milk	1 grande	200	0	0	0
Tazo Latte Red Tea Nonfat Milk	1 grande	170	0	0	0
Tazo Latte Red Tea Soy	1 grande	190	3	0	0
Tazo Shaken Iced Tea Green	1 grande	80	0	0	0
Tazo Shaken Iced Tea Green & Lemonade	1 grande	130	0	0	0
Tazo Shaken Iced Tea Orange Passion	1 grande	70	0	0	0
Tazo Shaken Iced Tea Passion	1 grande	80	0	0	0
Tazo Shaken Iced Tea Passion & Lemonade	1 grande	130	0	0	0
Tazo Tea	1 grande	0	0	0	0
Vanilla Creme Whip Nonfat Milk	1 grande	270	7	5	0
Vanilla Creme No Whip Nonfat Milk	1 grande	200	0	0	0
White Chocolate Mocha No Whip Nonfat Milk	1 grande	360	6	5	0
White Chocolate Mocha Whip Nonfat Milk	1 grande	430	13	9	0
SALADS					
Fiesta	1 (9.4 oz)	320	10	2	0
Fruit & Cheese Plate	1 (8.6 oz)	400	20	10	0
Vegetable Vinaigrette	1 (10.7 oz)	310	15	4	0
SANDWICHES					
Breakfast Wrap Bacon Avocado Aged Cheddar & Egg	1	380	24	10	0
Breakfast Wrap Spinach Roasted Tomato Feta & Egg	1	240	10	4	0
Club Chicken Cheddar Bacon w/ Mayo	1	480	18	6	0
Club Turkey & Avocado	1	390	19	5	0
Egg Salad On Multigrain	1	470	21	5	0
Turkey & Swiss w/ Mayo	1	310	13	5	0

FOOD	PORTION	CALS	FAT	SAT FAT	TRANS FAT
TOPPINGS					
Caramel	1 tbsp	15	1	0	0
Chocolate	1 tsp	5	0	0	0
Flavored Sugar Free Syrup	1 pump	0	0	0	0
Flavored Syrup	1 pump	20	0	0	0
Mocha Syrup	1 pump	25	1	0	0
Sprinkles	1 serv	0	0	0	0
STEAK ESCAPE					
BEVERAGES					
Coca-Cola	12 oz	110	0	0	0
Coca-Cola	44 oz	430	0	0	0
Diet Coke	12 oz	0	0	0	0
Diet Coke	44 oz	0	0	0	0
Hi-C Fruit Punch	12 oz	116	0	0	0
Hi-C Fruit Punch	44 oz	452	0	0	0
Lemonade	12 oz	126	0	0	0
Lemonade	44 oz	488	0	0	0
Sprite	12 oz	110	0	0	0
Sprite	44 oz	430	0	0	0
CHILDREN'S MENU SELECTIONS					
Kids Fries	1 serv	249	13	–	–
Kids Tenders	2 pieces	240	11	–	–
Sandwich Chicken	1	205	7	–	–
Sandwich Ham	1	183	1	–	–
Sandwich Steak	1	210	3	–	–
Sandwich Turkey	1	183	1	–	–
MAIN MENU SELECTIONS					
12 Inch Sandwich Grand Cobbler	1	680	4	–	–
12 Inch Sandwich Grand Escape	1	776	12	–	–
12 Inch Sandwich Grandest Chicken	1	770	10	–	–
12 Inch Sandwich Great Escape	1	776	12	–	–
12 Inch Sandwich Hambrosia	1	684	4	–	–
12 Inch Sandwich Ragin' Cajun	1	756	10	–	–
12 Inch Sandwich Turkey Club	1	675	4	–	–
12 Inch Sandwich Vegetarian	1	524	2	–	–

FOOD	PORTION	CALS	FAT	SAT FAT	TRANS FAT
12 Inch Sandwich Wild West BBQ	1	841	12	–	–
7 Inch Sandwich Grand Cobbler	1	380	2	–	–
7 Inch Sandwich Grand Escape	1	435	6	–	–
7 Inch Sandwich Grandest Chicken	1	425	5	–	–
7 Inch Sandwich Great Escape	1	428	6	–	–
7 Inch Sandwich Hambrosia	1	382	2	–	–
7 Inch Sandwich Ragin' Cajun	1	418	5	–	–
7 Inch Sandwich Turkey Club	1	390	2	–	–
7 Inch Sandwich Vegetarian	1	302	1	–	–
7 Inch Sandwich Wild West BBQ	1	469	6	–	–
Fries	1 serv (12 oz)	498	26	–	–
Fries	1 serv (32 oz)	996	52	–	–
Fries Loaded Bacon & Cheddar	1 serv	905	44	–	–
Fries Loaded Ranch & Bacon	1 serv	1044	71	–	–
Smashed Potatoes Loaded Bacon & Cheddar	1 serv	636	26	–	–
Smashed Potatoes Loaded Ranch & Bacon	1 serv	692	34	–	–
Smashed Potatoes Plain	1 serv	246	0	–	0
Smashed Potatoes w/ Chicken	1 serv	318	4	–	–
Smashed Potatoes w/ Ham	1 serv	336	2	–	–
Smashed Potatoes w/ Steak	1 serv	391	5	–	–
Smashed Potatoes w/ Turkey	1 serv	336	2	–	–
SALAD DRESSINGS AND TOPPINGS					
American Cheese	1 slice	101	9	–	–
Bacon	1 serv (1 oz)	80	7	–	–
BBQ Sauce	1 serv (1 oz)	40	0	0	0
Black Olives	1 serv (1 oz)	32	3	–	–
Brown Mustard	1 serv (1 oz)	0	0	0	0
Cheddar Cheese	1 slice	116	9	–	–
Dressing Italian	1 serv (0.5 oz)	51	5	–	–
Dressing Ranch	1 serv (0.5 oz)	83	9	–	–
Lettuce	1 serv (1 oz)	2	0	0	0
Margarine	1 serv (1 oz)	203	23	–	–
Mayonnaise	1 serv (1 oz)	101	11	–	–
Peppers Jalapeno	1 serv (1.5 oz)	11	0	–	0

FOOD	PORTION	CALS	FAT	SAT FAT	TRANS FAT
Peppers Mild	1 serv (1.5 oz)	11	0	0	0
Provolone Cheese	1 slice	80	6	–	–
Sour Cream	1 serv (1 oz)	61	6	–	–
Swiss Cheese	1 slice	100	8	–	–
Tomatoes	1 serv (2 oz)	24	0	0	0
SALADS					
Grilled Salad w/ Chicken	1 serv	175	5	–	–
Grilled Salad w/ Ham	1 serv	130	2	–	–
Grilled Salad w/ Steak	1 serv	185	6	–	–
Grilled Salad w/ Turkey	1 serv	130	2	–	–
Side	1 serv	40	5	–	–

SUBWAY
ADD-ONS AND SALAD DRESSINGS

FOOD	PORTION	CALS	FAT	SAT FAT	TRANS FAT
American Cheese	1 serv (0.4 oz)	40	4	2	0
Bacon Strips	2	45	4	2	0
Banana Pepper Slices	3	0	0	0	0
Cheddar	1 serv (0.5 oz)	60	5	3	0
Fat Free Italian	1 serv (2 oz)	35	0	0	0
Fat Free Red Wine Vinaigrette	1 serv (0.7 oz)	30	0	0	0
Jalapeno Pepper Slices	3	<5	0	0	0
Mayonnaise	1 tbsp	110	12	2	0
Mayonnaise Light	1 tbsp	50	5	1	0
Monterey Cheddar Shredded	1 serv (0.5 oz)	50	5	3	0
Mustard Yellow or Deli	2 tsp	5	0	0	0
Olive Oil Blend	1 tsp	45	5	0	0
Pepperjack Cheese	1 serv (0.5 oz)	50	4	3	0
Provolone	1 serv (0.5 oz)	50	4	2	0
Ranch	1 serv (2 oz)	320	35	6	1
Ranch	1.5 tbsp	120	13	2	0
Red Wine Vinaigrette	1 serv (2 oz)	80	1	0	0
Sauce Chipotle Southwest	1.5 tbsp	100	10	2	0
Sauce Fat Free Honey Mustard	1.5 tbsp	30	0	0	0
Sauce Fat Free Sweet Onion	1.5 tbsp	40	0	0	0
Swiss	1 serv (0.5 oz)	50	5	3	0
Vinegar	1 tsp	0	0	0	0
BREADS					
6 Inch Italian	6 in	200	2	1	0
Hearty Italian	6 in	220	2	1	0
Honey Oat	6 in	250	4	1	0

FOOD	PORTION	CALS	FAT	SAT FAT	TRANS FAT
Italian Herb & Cheese	6 in	250	5	3	0
Italian White	1 mini	140	2	1	0
Moneterey Cheddar	6 in	240	5	3	0
Parmesan Oregano Bread	6 in	220	3	1	0
Wheat	1 mini	140	2	1	0
Wheat	6 in	200	3	1	0
Wrap	1	190	5	1	0
DESSERTS					
Apple Slices	1 pkg	35	0	0	0
Cookie Chocolate Chip	1	210	10	6	0
Cookie Chocolate Chip w/ M&M's	1 (1.6 oz)	210	10	5	0
Cookie Chocolate Chunk	1	220	10	5	0
Cookie Double Chocolate Chip	1 (1.6 oz)	210	10	5	0
Cookie Oatmeal Raisin	1	200	8	4	0
Cookie Peanut Butter	1	220	12	5	0
Cookie Sugar	1	220	12	6	0
Cookie White Chip Macadamia Nut	1	220	11	5	0
Raisins	1 pkg	150	0	0	0
SALADS					
Ham w/o Dressing & Croutons	1 serv	120	3	1	0
Oven Roasted Chicken Breast w/o Dressing & Croutons	1 serv	140	3	1	0
Roast Beef w/o Dressing & Croutons	1 serv	120	3	2	0
Subway Club w/o Dressing & Croutons	1 serv	150	4	2	0
Sweet Onion Chicken Teriyaki w/o Dressing & Croutons	1 serv	210	3	1	0
Turkey Breast	1 serv	110	3	1	0
Turkey Breast & Ham w/o Dressing & Croutons	1 serv	120	3	1	0
Veggie Delight w/o Dressing & Croutons	1 serv	60	1	0	0
SANDWICHES					
6 Inch Chicken & Bacon Ranch	1	580	30	11	1
6 Inch Cold Cut Combo	1	410	17	7	1
6 Inch Double Stacked Cold Cut Combo	1	550	28	10	1

FOOD	PORTION	CALS	FAT	SAT FAT	TRANS FAT
6 Inch Double Stacked Italian BMT	1	630	35	14	0
6 Inch Double Stacked Steak & Cheese	1	540	18	8	1
6 Inch Double Stacked Subway Club	1	420	8	4	0
6 Inch Double Stacked Sweet Onion Chicken Teriyaki	1	480	7	2	0
6 Inch Double Stacked Turkey Breast	1	330	5	2	0
6 Inch Ham	1	290	5	2	0
6 Inch Italian BMT	1	450	21	8	0
6 Inch Meatball Marinara	1	560	24	11	1
6 Inch Oven Roasted Chicken Breast	1	310	5	2	0
6 Inch Roast Beef	1	290	5	2	0
6 Inch Spicy Italian	1	480	25	9	0
6 Inch Steak & Cheese	1	400	12	6	1
6 Inch Subway Club	1	320	6	2	0
6 Inch Subway Melt	1	380	12	5	0
6 Inch Sweet Onion Chicken Teriyaki	1	370	5	2	0
6 Inch Tuna	1	530	31	7	1
6 Inch Turkey Breast	1	280	5	2	0
6 Inch Turkey Breast & Ham	1	290	5	2	0
6 Inch Veggie Delite	1	230	3	1	0
Breakfast Cheese & Egg	1	317	15	5	–
Mini Sub Ham	1	180	3	1	0
Mini Sub Roast Beef	1	190	4	2	0
Mini Sub Tuna w/ Cheese	1	320	18	5	0
Mini Sub Turkey Breast	1	190	3	1	0
Softwich Santa Fe Turkey	1	520	10	4	0
TACO BELL					
Border Bowl Southwest Steak	1 serv	600	24	6	1
Border Bowl Zesty Chicken	1 serv	640	35	6	1
Border Bowl Zesty Chicken w/o Dressing	1 serv	440	15	3	1
Burrito 7 Layer	1	490	18	7	1
Burrito Bean	1	350	9	4	1

FOOD	PORTION	CALS	FAT	SAT FAT	TRANS FAT
Burrito Chili Cheese	1	370	16	8	1
Burrito Grilled Stuft Chicken	1	640	23	7	1
Burrito Supreme Beef	1	420	17	8	1
Burrito ½ Lb Beef & Potato	1	530	23	7	1
Burrito ½ Lb Combo Beef	1	440	18	7	1
Burrito Fiesta Chicken	1	360	10	4	0
Burrito Fiesta Steak	1	370	13	5	0
Burrito Stuft Grilled Steak	1	630	25	8	1
Burrito Supreme Chicken	1	400	13	6	1
Burrito Supreme Steak	1	390	14	6	1
Chalupa Baja Beef	1	410	27	6	0
Chalupa Baja Chicken	1	390	23	4	0
Chalupa Baja Steak	1	390	24	5	0
Chalupa Nacho Cheese Beef	1	370	22	5	2
Chalupa Nacho Cheese Chicken	1	360	18	3	1
Chalupa Nacho Cheese Steak	1	340	19	4	2
Chalupa Supreme Beef	1	380	20	7	1
Chalupa Supreme Chicken	1	360	20	5	0
Chalupa Supreme Steak	1	360	21	8	0
Cheesy Fiesta Potatoes	1 serv	290	17	4	2
Cheesy Fiesta Potatoes	1 serv	290	17	4	2
Cinnamon Twists	1 serv	170	7	0	0
Crunchwrap Supreme	1	560	24	8	2
Crunchwrap Supreme Spicy Chicken	1	540	24	8	2
Crunchy Taco	1	170	25	4	0
Crunchy Taco Supreme	1	210	10	4	1
Empanada Caramel Apple	1	290	14	3	2
Enchirito Beef	1	360	17	8	1
Enchirito Chicken	1	340	13	7	1
Fresco Border Bowl Zesty Chicken w/o Dressing	1 serv	350	8	2	0
Fresco Burrito Bean	1	330	7	3	1
Fresco Burrito Fiesta Chicken	1	330	8	3	0
Fresco Burrito Supreme Chicken	1	330	8	3	0
Fresco Burrito Supreme Steak	1	330	8	3	1
Fresco Crunchy Taco	1	150	8	3	0
Fresco Soft Taco Grilled Steak	1	160	5	2	0

FOOD	PORTION	CALS	FAT	SAT FAT	TRANS FAT
Fresco Soft Taco Ranchero Chicken	1	170	4	2	0
Fresco Soft Taco Beef	1	180	2	3	0
Gordita Baja Beef	1	340	19	5	0
Gordita Baja Chicken	1	320	16	4	0
Gordita Baja Steak	1	320	17	4	0
Gordita Nacho Cheese Beef	1	300	14	4	2
Gordita Nacho Cheese Chicken	1	280	11	3	1
Gordita Nacho Cheese Steak	1	270	12	3	1
Gordita Supreme Beef	1	310	16	6	1
Gordita Supreme Chicken	1	290	12	5	0
Gordita Supreme Steak	1	290	13	5	0
Guacamole Side	1 serv	70	5	1	0
Mexican Pizza	1	530	30	8	1
Mexican Rice	1 serv	180	7	3	0
MexiMelt	1 serv	260	14	7	1
Nacho Supreme	1 serv	440	26	7	2
Nachos	1 serv	330	21	4	2
Nachos Bellgrande	1 serv	770	44	9	3
Pintos 'n Cheese	1 serv	160	6	3	1
Quesadilla Cheese	1	470	26	12	1
Quesadilla Chicken	1	520	28	12	1
Quesadilla Steak	1	520	28	13	1
Salsa Side	1 serv	15	0	0	0
Soft Taco Grande	1	430	20	8	2
Soft Taco Grilled Steak	1	270	16	5	0
Soft Taco Ranchero Chicken	1	270	14	4	0
Soft Taco Supreme Beef	1	250	13	6	1
Sour Cream Side	1 serv	80	7	5	0
Taco Double Decker	1	320	13	5	1
Taco Double Decker Supreme	1	370	17	7	1
Taco Spicy Chicken	1	170	8	2	0
Taco Salad Express	1	610	32	10	2
Taco Salad Fiesta	1	840	45	11	2
Taco Salad Fiesta Chicken	1	790	38	8	1
Taco Salad Fiesta Chicken w/o Shell	1	430	18	6	1
Taco Salad w/o Shell Fiesta	1	470	24	10	2
Taquitos Grilled Chicken	1 serv	310	11	5	0
Taquitos Steak Grilled	1 serv	310	11	5	0
Tostada	1	240	10	4	1

FOOD	PORTION	CALS	FAT	SAT FAT	TRANS FAT
TACO CABANA					
Black Beans	1 serv (4 oz)	111	tr	–	–
Borracho Beans	1 serv (4 oz)	108	3	–	–
Breakfast Taco Bacon & Egg	1	246	12	–	–
Breakfast Taco Barbacoa	1	307	15	–	–
Breakfast Taco Chorizo & Egg	1	248	12	–	–
Breakfast Taco Potato & Egg	1	234	10	–	–
Burrito Bean & Cheese	1	710	27	–	–
Burrito Beef	1	653	24	–	–
Burrito Black Bean	1	559	11	–	–
Burrito Chicken	1	665	26	–	–
Calabacita	1 serv (4 oz)	78	5	–	–
Chips	1 serv (2 oz)	285	14	–	–
Elotes	1	220	11	–	–
Fajitas Beef	1 serv (4 oz)	245	12	–	–
Fajitas Chicken Dark	1 serv (4 oz)	236	11	–	–
Fajitas Chicken White	1 serv (4 oz)	191	6	–	–
Grilled Chicken Dark	1 serv (4.5 oz)	298	18	–	–
Grilled Chicken Dark No Skin	1 serv (3.4 oz)	170	7	–	–
Grilled Chicken White	1 serv (5 oz)	295	14	–	–
Grilled Chicken White No Skin	1 serv (3.8 oz)	167	3	–	–
Guacamole	1 serv (1 oz)	48	4	–	–
Queso	1 serv (3 oz)	184	12	–	–
Refried Beans	1 serv (4 oz)	171	6	–	–
Sour Cream	1 serv (1 oz)	57	5	–	–
Spanish Rice	1 serv (4 oz)	181	5	–	–
Taco Bean & Cheese	1	292	12	–	–
Taco Black Bean	1	216	5	–	–
Taco Carne Guisada	1	202	8	–	–
Taco Crispy Beef	1	148	7	–	–
Taco Soft Chicken	1	217	9	–	–
Tortilla Corn	1 (6 in)	70	1	–	–
Tortilla Flour	1 (6 in)	129	3	–	–
Tortilla Soup	1 sm	249	8	–	–
Tortilla Soup	1 lg	371	13	–	–
TACO JOHN'S					
DESSERTS					
Apple Grande	1 serv	240	9	3	–
Choco Taco	1 serv	300	15	7	–

FOOD	PORTION	CALS	FAT	SAT FAT	TRANS FAT
Churro	1 serv	230	11	2	–
Cinnamon Mini Swirl	1 piece	10	0	0	0
MAIN MENU SELECTIONS					
Burrito Bean	1	380	12	5	–
Burrito Beefy	1	430	20	9	–
Burrito Chicken & Potato	1	460	19	7	–
Burrito Combination	1	400	16	7	–
Burrito Meat & Potato	1	490	23	8	–
Burrito Super	1	450	20	9	–
Crispy Taco	1 serv	180	10	4	–
Mexican Rice	1 serv	250	5	1	–
Nachos	1 serv	380	23	6	–
Potato Olés	1 sm	440	26	6	–
Potato Olés	1 lg	790	47	11	–
Potato Olés Bravo	1 serv	580	36	11	–
Potato Olés Super	1 serv	980	62	22	–
Potato Olés w/ Nacho Cheese	1 serv	550	35	10	–
Quesadilla Cheese	1	480	28	15	–
Quesadilla Chicken	1	540	29	15	–
Refried Beans	1 serv	400	14	5	–
Sierra Taco Beef	1	430	23	8	–
Sierra Taco Chicken	1	390	17	5	–
Softshell Taco	1	220	10	5	–
Softshell Taco Chicken	1	190	6	3	–
Super Nachos	1 serv	830	51	17	–
Super Nachos Chicken	1 serv	780	45	15	–
Taco Bravo	1 serv	340	14	5	–
Taco Burger	1	280	12	5	–
Texas Chili	1 serv	270	12	6	–
SALAD DRESSINGS AND TOPPINGS					
Bacon Ranch Dressing	1 serv (3 oz)	250	19	3	–
Barbecue Sauce	1 serv (2 oz)	70	0	0	0
Chipotle Cream Sauce	1 serv (3 oz)	450	45	9	–
Creamy Italian Dressing	1 serv (3 oz)	260	29	5	–
Guacamole	1 serv (2 oz)	90	9	3	–
Hot Sauce	1 serv (1 oz)	5	0	0	0
House Dressing	1 serv (3 oz)	140	15	2	–
Jalapenos	1 serv (2 oz)	15	1	0	–
Mild Sauce	1 serv (1 oz)	5	0	0	0
Nacho Cheese	1 serv (3 oz)	120	9	4	–

FOOD	PORTION	CALS	FAT	SAT FAT	TRANS FAT
Pico De Gallo	1 serv (2 oz)	15	0	0	0
Ranch Dressing	1 serv (3 oz)	280	31	5	–
Salsa	1 serv (2 oz)	20	0	0	0
Sour Cream	1 serv (2 oz)	120	12	7	–
Super Hot Sauce	1 serv (1 oz)	10	0	0	0
SALADS					
Chicken Festiva w/o Dressing	1 serv	400	23	10	–
Chicken Taco w/o Dressing	1	530	27	11	–
Side w/o Dressing	1 serv	80	5	2	–
Taco w/o Dressing	1 serv	580	32	13	–

TACOTIME
DESSERTS

FOOD	PORTION	CALS	FAT	SAT FAT	TRANS FAT
Churro Plain	1 (1.5 oz)	205	15	3	3
Churro w/ Cinnamon & Sugar	1 (2 oz)	245	15	3	3
Crustos	1 serv	294	6	1	0
Empanada Apple	1 (4 oz)	234	7	1	0
Empanada Cherry	1 (4 oz)	240	7	1	0
Empanada Pumpkin	1 (4 oz)	256	8	1	0
MAIN MENU SELECTIONS					
Burrito Big Juan Seasoned Ground Beef	1 (13 oz)	651	28	12	1
Burrito Big Juan Shredded Beef	1 (13 oz)	633	25	12	1
Burrito Big Juan Chicken	1 (13 oz)	594	19	10	1
Burrito Casita Chicken	1 (12 oz)	494	18	10	1
Burrito Casita Seasoned Ground Beef	1 (12 oz)	552	25	13	1
Burrito Casita Shredded Beef	1 (12 oz)	533	25	13	1
Burrito Chicken & Black Bean	1 (10 oz)	478	16	6	0
Burrito Chicken BLT	1 (10 oz)	721	41	11	0
Burrito Chicken Ranchero	1 (10.8 oz)	654	32	10	0
Burrito Crisp Chicken	1 (5.5 oz)	336	10	1	0
Burrito Crisp Meat	1 (5.8 oz)	450	22	7	0
Burrito Crisp Pinto Bean	1 (6 oz)	394	16	4	1
Burrito Soft Meat	1 (6.7 oz)	426	16	7	0
Burrito Soft Pinto Bean	1 (6.7 oz)	377	11	5	1
Burrito Veggie	1 (11 oz)	534	18	7	1
Cheddar Fries	1 sm (6 oz)	374	26	8	6
Cheddar Melt	1 (2.8 oz)	250	12	7	0
Mexi-Fries	1 sm (5 oz)	290	19	4	6

FOOD	PORTION	CALS	FAT	SAT FAT	TRANS FAT
Mexi-Rice	1 serv (4 oz)	87	1	0	0
Nachos Grande	1 serv (16.5 oz)	1132	57	24	1
Refritos w/ Chips	1 serv (7 oz)	304	11	6	2
Refritos w/o Chips	1 serv (6.7 oz)	285	11	6	2
Stuffed Fries	1 sm (5 oz)	321	7	6	5
Taco Crisp Seasoned Ground Beef	1 (4.3 oz)	225	12	5	0
Taco Super Soft Chicken	1 (11 oz)	540	18	10	1
Taco Super Soft Seasoned Ground Beef	1 (11 oz)	598	25	12	1
Taco Super Soft Shredded Beef	1 (11 oz)	579	25	12	1
Taco Value Soft	1 (5.3 oz)	314	13	6	0
Taco ½ Lb Shredded Beef	1 (9 oz)	440	18	9	0
Taco ½ Lb Soft Chicken	1 (9 oz)	401	11	6	0
Taco ½ Lb Soft Seasoned Ground Beef	1 (9 oz)	459	18	8	0
Taco Chips	1 serv (2 oz)	150	3	0	0
SALAD DRESSINGS AND TOPPINGS					
Cheddar Cheese Milk	1 serv (2 oz)	223	18	12	0
Dressing Chipotle Ranch	1 serv (1 oz)	165	18	3	0
Dressing Ranch	1 serv (1 oz)	181	20	3	0
Dressing Thousand Island	1 serv (1 oz)	132	12	2	0
Guacamole	1 serv (1 oz)	50	5	1	0
Salsa Nuevo	1 serv (1 oz)	8	0	0	0
Salsa Verde	1 serv (1 oz)	6	0	0	0
Sour Cream	1 serv (1.5 oz)	85	7	5	0
SALADS					
Taco Chicken	1 reg (9.2 oz)	351	15	5	0
Taco Seasoned Ground Beef	1 reg (7.8 oz)	396	23	8	0
Taco Shredded Beef	1 reg (7.8 oz)	377	22	8	0
Tostada Delight Chicken	1 (10.5 oz)	565	29	14	1
Tostada Delight Seasoned Ground Beef	1 (10.5 oz)	623	36	16	1
Tostada Delight Shredded Beef	1 (10.5 oz)	604	36	16	1
TASTI D-LITE					
Vanilla	1 sm (4 oz)	40	tr	–	–

FOOD	PORTION	CALS	FAT	SAT FAT	TRANS FAT
TCBY					
FROZEN YOGURT AND SORBET					
Hand Scooped Butter Pecan Perfection	½ cup	110	5	2	0
Hand Scooped Chocolate Chocolate Swirl	½ cup	120	4	2	0
Hand Scooped Chocolate Chunk Cookie Dough	½ cup	160	6	3	0
Hand Scooped Cookies & Cream	½ cup	140	4	3	1
Hand Scooped Cotton Candy	½ cup	120	4	2	0
Hand Scooped Mint Chocolate Chunk	½ cup	140	5	4	0
Hand Scooped Mocha Almond	½ cup	150	5	2	0
Hand Scooped No Sugar Added Chocolate Chocolate Swirl	½ cup	90	1	0	0
Hand Scooped No Sugar Added Vanilla	½ cup	80	1	0	0
Hand Scooped No Sugar Added Vanilla Fudge Brownie	½ cup	100	2	2	0
Hand Scooped Pralines & Cream	½ cup	140	5	2	0
Hand Scooped Psychedelic Sorbet	½ cup	290	0	0	0
Hand Scooped Rainbow Cream	½ cup	120	4	2	0
Hand Scooped Rocky Road	½ cup	220	7	4	0
Hand Scooped Strawberries & Cream	½ cup	120	3	2	0
Hand Scooped Vanilla Chocolate Chunk	½ cup	140	5	4	0
Hand Scooped Vanilla Bean	½ cup	120	4	2	0
Soft Serve Frozen Yogurt All Flavors 96% Fat Free	½ cup	140	3	2	–
Soft Serve Frozen Yogurt All Flavors Nonfat	½ cup	110	0	0	0
Soft Serve Frozen Yogurt All Flavors Nonfat No Sugar Added	½ cup	90	0	0	0
Soft Serve Frozen Yogurt Low Carb	½ cup	110	7	5	–

FOOD	PORTION	CALS	FAT	SAT FAT	TRANS FAT
Soft Serve Sorbet All Flavors Nonfat Nondairy	½ cup	100	0	0	0
SMOOTHIES					
Berrylicious	1 (16 oz)	290	3	2	0
Black 'N Blueberry	1 (16 oz)	280	3	2	0
Mando Mango	1 (16 oz)	310	3	2	0
Mango Tango	1 (16 oz)	330	3	2	0
Mangolada	1 (16 oz)	340	6	5	0
Pina Paradise	1 (16 oz)	350	12	9	0
Pink Pineapple	1 (16 oz)	340	9	7	0
Straight Up Strawberry	1 (16 oz)	280	4	2	0
Strawberry Bonanza	1 (16 oz)	320	4	2	0
Strawberry Fling	1 (16 oz)	340	3	2	0

TIM HORTONS
BAKED SELECTIONS

FOOD	PORTION	CALS	FAT	SAT FAT	TRANS FAT
Bagel Blueberry	1	270	1	0	0
Bagel Cinnamon Raisin	1	270	1	0	0
Bagel Everything	1	280	2	0	0
Bagel Flax Seed	1	290	5	1	0
Bagel Onion	1	260	2	0	0
Bagel Plain	1	260	2	0	0
Bagel Poppy Seed	1	270	2	0	0
Bagel Sesame Seed	1	270	3	0	0
Bagel Sun Dried Tomato	1	310	4	1	0
Bagel Twelve Grain	1	330	9	1	0
Cinnamon Roll Frosted	1	470	25	12	1
Cinnamon Roll Glazed	1	420	23	11	0
Cookie Caramel Chocolate Pecan	1	230	11	5	0
Cookie Chocolate Chip	1	230	9	6	0
Cookie Oatmeal Raisin Spice	1	220	8	5	0
Cookie Peanut Butter Chocolate Chunk	1	260	15	7	0
Cookie Triple Chocolate	1	250	13	8	0
Cookie White Chocolate Macadamia Nut	1	240	12	6	0
Croissant Butter	1	340	18	5	5
Croissant Cheese	1	370	20	7	5
Danish Chocolate	1	430	24	9	0

FOOD	PORTION	CALS	FAT	SAT FAT	TRANS FAT
Danish Maple Pecan	1	380	20	7	0
Danish Cherry Cheese	1	330	13	6	0
Donut Apple Fritter	1	300	11	5	0
Donut Chocolate Dip	1	210	9	4	0
Donut Chocolate Glazed	1	260	10	5	0
Donut Honey Dip	1	210	8	4	0
Donut Honey Stick	1	280	15	5	–
Donut Maple Dip	1	210	8	4	0
Donut Old Fashion Glazed	1	320	19	9	0
Donut Old Fashion Plain	1	260	19	9	0
Donut Sour Cream Plain	1	270	17	8	0
Donut Walnut Crunch	1	360	23	10	0
Donut Filled Angel Cream	1	310	13	5	2
Donut Filled Blueberry	1	230	8	4	0
Donut Filled Boston Cream	1	250	9	4	0
Donut Filled Canadian Maple	1	260	9	4	0
Donut Filled Strawberry	1	230	8	4	0
Honey Cruller	1	320	19	9	0
Muffin Blueberry	1	330	11	2	0
Muffin Blueberry Bran	1	300	10	1	0
Muffin Carrot Wheat	1	400	19	3	0
Muffin Chocolate Chip	1	430	16	5	0
Muffin Cranberry Blueberry Bran	1	290	10	2	0
Muffin Cranberry Fruit	1	350	12	2	0
Muffin Fruit Explosion	1	360	11	2	0
Muffin Raisin Bran	1	360	10	2	0
Muffin Strawberry Sensation	1	350	11	2	0
Muffin Low Fat Blueberry	1	290	3	1	0
Muffin Low Fat Cranberry	1	290	3	1	0
Tea Biscuit Plain	1	250	9	2	0
Tea Biscuit Raisin	1	290	10	2	0
Timbits Apple Fritter	1	50	2	1	0
Timbits Chocolate Glazed	1	70	3	1	0
Timbits Old Fashion Plain	1	70	5	3	0
Timbits Filled Banana Cream	1	60	2	1	0
Timbits Filled Lemon	1	60	2	1	0
Timbits Filled Strawberry	1	60	2	1	0
Timbits Filled Strawberry	1	60	2	1	0

FOOD	PORTION	CALS	FAT	SAT FAT	TRANS FAT
BEVERAGES					
Cafe Mocha	1 (10 oz)	160	7	6	0
Cappuccino Iced	1 (12 oz)	300	15	8	0
Coffee Decaffeinated + Sugar & Cream	1 (10 oz)	75	4	2	0
Coffee + Sugar & Cream	1 (10 oz)	75	4	2	0
English Toffee	1 (10 oz)	220	6	5	0
Flavor Shot	1 serv	5	0	0	0
French Vanilla	1 (10 oz)	240	7	7	0
Hot Chocolate	1 (10 oz)	240	6	5	0
Hot Smoothie	1 (10 oz)	260	10	9	0
Iced Cappuccino w/ Milk	1 (12 oz)	180	2	1	0
Tea + Sugar & Milk	1 (10 oz)	50	1	0	0
CREAM CHEESE					
Garden Vegetable	1.5 oz	120	11	7	1
Light Plain	1.5 oz	60	5	4	0
Plain	1.5 oz	130	12	7	1
Strawberry	1.5 oz	120	10	6	1
SANDWICHES					
B.L.T.	1	450	18	5	0
Breakfast Bacon Egg Cheese	1	410	25	17	0
Breakfast Egg Cheese	1	360	21	15	0
Breakfast Sausage Egg Cheese	1	520	37	21	0
Chicken Salad Salad	1	380	9	1	0
Egg Salad	1	390	13	3	0
Ham & Swiss	1	440	12	5	0
Toasted Chicken Club	1	460	7	3	0
Turkey Breast	1	390	5	2	0
SOUPS					
Beef Stew	1 serv (10 oz)	236	8	3	0
Chicken Noodle	1 serv (10 oz)	120	2	1	0
Chili	1 serv (10 oz)	300	16	6	0
Country Field Mushroom	1 serv (10 oz)	150	3	2	0
Cream Of Broccoli	1 serv (10 oz)	160	9	4	0
Hearty Vegetable	1 serv (10 oz)	70	0	0	0
Minestrone	1 serv (10 oz)	120	3	0	0
Potato Bacon	1 serv (10 oz)	180	6	2	1
Split Pea w/ Ham	1 serv (10 oz)	150	3	3	0
Turkey Rice	1 serv (10 oz)	120	2	0	0
Vegetable Beef Barley	1 serv (10 oz)	110	2	0	0

FOOD	PORTION	CALS	FAT	SAT FAT	TRANS FAT
YOGURT					
Low Fat Creamy Vanilla w/ Berries	1 (6 oz)	160	3	2	0
Low Fat Strawberry w/ Berries	1 (6 oz)	150	3	2	0
T.J. CINNAMONS					
Chocolate Twist	1	250	12	4	0
Cinnamon Twist	1	280	14	5	4
Mocha Chill w/ Whipped Cream	1 (12.5 oz)	306	7	4	0
Mocha Chill w/o Whipped Cream	1 (12.5 oz)	264	4	2	tr
Original Roll w/o Icing	1	507	10	4	0
Pecan Sticky Bun	1	688	22	5	0
TJ Icing	1 serv (1 oz)	117	5	2	1
TOGO'S					
SALAD DRESSINGS					
1000 Island	1 serv (2.3 oz)	231	22	–	–
Caesar	1 serv (2.3 oz)	241	23	–	–
Oriental	1 serv (2.3 oz)	221	14	–	–
Ranch	1 serv (2.3 oz)	321	33	–	–
Reduced Calorie Italian	1 serv (2.3 oz)	60	5	–	–
Reduced Calorie Ranch	1 serv (2.3 oz)	191	16	–	–
SALADS					
Caesar Salad	1 serv	471	31	–	–
Garden Salad	1 serv	256	10	–	–
Oriental Salad	1 serv	499	21	–	–
Potato Salad	1 serv (4 oz)	215	13	–	–
Taco Salad	1 serv	943	59	–	–
SANDWICHES					
Albacore Tuna	1 sm	701	30	–	–
Avocado & Turkey	1 sm	675	28	–	–
Avocado Cucumber & Alfalfa Sprouts	1 sm	637	28	–	–
Bar-B-Q Beef	1 sm	724	22	–	–
California Roasted Chicken	1 sm	510	15	–	–
Cheese Swiss American Provolone	1 sm	859	46	–	–
Chunky Chicken Salad	1 sm	636	26	–	–
Egg Salad w/ Cheese	1 sm	728	35	–	–

FOOD	PORTION	CALS	FAT	SAT FAT	TRANS FAT
Ham & Cheese	1 sm	661	26	–	–
Hot Pastrami	1 sm	705	26	–	–
Hummus	1 sm	668	21	–	–
Italian Salami & Cheese	1 sm	770	33	–	–
Italian Salami Capicolla Mortadella Cotto & Provolone	1 sm	736	32	–	–
Meatballs w/ Pizza Sauce & Parmesan	1 sm	707	28	–	–
Pastrami Reuben	1 sm	875	45	–	–
Roast Beef Hot & Cold	1 sm	552	11	–	–
Turkey & Cranberry	1 sm	623	13	–	–
Turkey & Bacon Club	1 sm	667	26	–	–
Turkey & Cheese	1 sm	638	23	–	–
Turkey & Ham w/ Cheese	1 sm	670	25	–	–

WENDY'S
BEVERAGES

FOOD	PORTION	CALS	FAT	SAT FAT	TRANS FAT
Chocolate Milk 1%	8 oz	170	3	2	0
Coca-Cola	1 med (12 oz)	140	0	0	0
Dasani Water	1 bottle	0	0	0	0
Diet Coke	1 med (11 oz)	0	0	0	0
Frosty	1 sm (8 oz)	330	8	5	0
Milk 2%	8 oz	120	5	3	0
Sprite	1 med (12 oz)	130	0	0	0

CHILDREN'S MENU SELECTIONS

FOOD	PORTION	CALS	FAT	SAT FAT	TRANS FAT
French Fries	1 serv (3.2 oz)	280	14	3	4
Kid's Meal Cheeseburger	1	320	13	6	1
Kid's Meal Ham & Cheese	1 serv	240	6	3	0
Kid's Meal Hamburger	1	270	9	4	1
Kid's Meal Turkey & Cheese	1 serv	250	6	3	0
Kid's Meal Chicken Nuggets	4 pieces	180	11	3	2

SALAD DRESSINGS AND TOPPINGS

FOOD	PORTION	CALS	FAT	SAT FAT	TRANS FAT
Ancho Chipotle Ranch	1 pkg	110	10	2	0
Blue Cheese	1 pkg	260	27	5	0
Buttery Best Spread	1 pkg	50	6	1	0
Caesar	1 pkg	120	13	3	0
Cheddar Cheese Shredded	2 tbsp	70	6	4	0
Creamy Ranch	1 pkg	230	23	4	0
Creamy Ranch Reduced Fat	1 pkg	100	8	2	0
Crispy Noodles	1 pkg	60	2	0	0

FOOD	PORTION	CALS	FAT	SAT FAT	TRANS FAT
Croutons Homestyle Garlic	1 pkg	70	3	0	0
Dipping Sauce Deli Honey Mustard	1 pkg	170	16	3	0
Dipping Sauce Heartland Ranch	1 pkg	200	22	4	0
Dipping Sauce Spicy Southwest Chipotle	1 pkg	150	15	3	0
Dipping Sauce Sweet & Sour Hawaiian	1 pkg	70	0	0	0
Dipping Sauce Wild Buffalo Ranch	1 pkg	180	19	3	0
French Fat Free	1 pkg	80	0	0	0
Granola Topping	1 pkg	110	5	1	0
Honey Mustard	1 pkg	280	26	4	0
Honey Mustard Low Fat	1 pkg	110	3	0	0
Hot Chili Seasoning	1 pkg	5	0	0	0
Italian Vinaigrette	1 pkg	140	12	2	0
Ketchup	1 tsp	7	0	0	0
Mayonnaise	1 tsp	30	3	1	0
Mustard	½ tsp	5	0	0	0
Nuggets Sauce Barbeque	1 pkg	45	0	0	0
Nuggets Sauce Honey Mustard	1 pkg	130	12	2	0
Nuggets Sauce Sweet & Sour	1 pkg	50	0	0	0
Oriental Sesame	1 pkg	190	11	2	0
Roasted Almonds	1 pkg	130	11	1	0
Saltines	2	25	1	0	0
Sour Cream Reduced Fat	1 pkg	45	4	3	0
Thousand Island	1 pkg	260	25	4	0
Tortilla Strips	1 pkg	110	5	1	0
SALADS					
Caesar Chicken w/o Dressing & Croutons	1 serv	180	5	3	0
Ceasar Side Salad w/o Dressing & Croutons	1 serv	70	5	2	0
Chicken BLT w/o Dressing & Croutons	1 serv	340	18	9	0
Mandarin Chicken w/o Dressing	1 serv	170	2	1	0
Side Salad w/o Dressing	1	35	0	0	0
Southwest Taco w/o Dressing Tortilla Strip & Sour Cream	1 serv	440	22	12	1

FOOD	PORTION	CALS	FAT	SAT FAT	TRANS FAT
SANDWICHES AND SIDES					
Baked Potato Plain	1	270	0	0	0
Baked Potato w/ Sour Cream & Chives	1 serv	320	4	3	0
Big Bacon Classic	1	580	29	12	2
Chicken Nuggets	5 pieces	220	14	3	2
Chili	1 sm (8 oz)	220	6	3	0
Classic Single w/ Everything	1	420	19	7	1
French Fries	1 med (5 oz)	440	21	4	5
Frescata Black Forest Ham & Swiss	1	480	20	6	0
Frescata Club	1	440	16	4	0
Frescata Roasted Turkey & Basil Pesto	1	420	16	3	0
Frescata Roasted Turkey & Swiss	1	490	21	7	0
Hamburger	1	280	9	4	1
Homestyle Chicken Strips	3 pieces	410	18	4	3
Jr. Bacon Cheeseburger	1	370	17	7	1
Jr. BBQ Cheeseburger	1	330	13	6	1
Jr. Cheeseburger	1	320	13	6	1
Jr. Cheeseburger Deluxe	1	360	16	6	1
Mandarin Orange Cup	1 serv	80	0	0	0
Sandwich Crispy Chicken	1	380	15	3	2
Sandwich Spicy Chicken Fillet	1	510	19	4	2
Sandwich Ultimate Chicken Grill	1	360	7	2	0
Yogurt Low Fat Strawberry	1 pkg	140	2	1	0
WETZEL'S PRETZELS					
Original w/ Butter	1	320	4	–	–
Original w/o Butter	1	280	1	–	–
WHATABURGER					
BEVERAGES					
Barq's Root Beet	1 sm (16 oz)	220	0	0	0
Cherry Coke	1 sm (16 oz)	210	0	0	0
Coca-Cola	1 sm (16 oz)	207	0	0	0
Coffee	1 sm (8 oz)	5	0	0	0
Coffee Decaf	1 sm (8 oz)	5	0	0	0
Diet Coke	1 sm (16 oz)	0	0	0	0

FOOD	PORTION	CALS	FAT	SAT FAT	TRANS FAT
Dr Pepper	1 sm (16 oz)	190	0	0	0
Fanta Orange	1 sm (16 oz)	210	0	0	0
Fanta Strawberry	1 sm (16 oz)	230	0	0	0
Fanta Strawberry	1 sm (16 oz)	230	0	0	0
Iced Tea Sweetened	1 (34 oz)	430	0	0	0
Iced Tea Unsweetened	1 sm (19 oz)	0	0	0	0
Lemonade Hi-C Poppin' Pink	1 sm (16 oz)	200	0	0	0
Malt Chocolate	1 sm (16 oz)	670	15	11	0
Malt Strawberry	1 sm (16 oz)	670	15	10	0
Malt Vanilla	1 sm (16 oz)	600	17	12	0
Milk Reduced Fat	8 oz	120	5	3	0
Orange Juice Tropicana	1 (10 oz)	140	0	0	0
Powerade Fruit Punch	1 sm (16 oz)	130	0	0	0
Shake Chocolate	1 sm (16 oz)	630	16	11	0
Shake Strawberry	1 sm (16 oz)	630	16	11	0
Shake Vanilla	1 sm (16 oz)	560	17	12	0
Sprite	1 sm (16 oz)	200	0	0	0
CHILDREN'S MENU SELECTIONS					
Kid's Meal Chicken Strips	1 serv	770	51	10	8
Kid's Meal Justaburger	1 serv	570	29	9	5
DESSERTS					
Apple Pie A La Mode	1 serv	520	20	9	3
Apple Pie Hot	1	230	11	3	3
Cinnamon Roll	1	400	7	2	1
Cookie Chocolate Chunk	1 (2 oz)	230	11	7	0
Cookie White Chocolate Chunk Macadamia	1 (2 oz)	250	14	8	0
Peach Pie A La Mode	1 serv	570	23	11	1
MAIN MENU SELECTIONS					
Biscuit	1	300	17	8	0
Biscuit Honey Butter Chicken	1	610	38	12	2
Biscuit Sandwich Bacon Egg & Cheese	1	500	32	14	0
Biscuit Sandwich Egg & Cheese	1	450	28	13	0
Biscuit Sandwich Sausage Egg & Cheese	1	690	49	21	0
Biscuit w/ Bacon	1	355	20	10	0
Biscuit w/ Gravy	1	530	36	14	5
Biscuit w/ Sausage	1	540	37	17	0
Breakfast Platter w/ Bacon	1 serv	730	45	16	4

FOOD	PORTION	CALS	FAT	SAT FAT	TRANS FAT
Breakfast Platter w/ Sausage	1 serv	930	62	23	4
Breakfast On A Bun w/ Bacon	1	380	22	7	0
Breakfast On A Bun w/ Sausage	1	570	39	15	0
Chicken Strip w/ Gravy	4	840	54	9	5
Chicken Strips	1	200	12	2	1
French Fries	1 sm	260	13	4	5
Gravy White Peppered	1 serv	60	5	1	3
Hashbrown Sticks	4	200	12	3	4
Justaburger	1	329	16	6	0
Onion Rings	1 med	420	28	13	0
Pancakes Plain	1 serv	580	8	2	3
Pancakes w/ Bacon	1 serv	630	12	3	3
Pancakes w/ Sausage	1 serv	820	20	10	3
Sandwich Chicken Strip Honey BBQ	1	1110	59	15	2
Sandwich Chicken Strip Junior Honey BBQ	1	720	41	12	1
Sandwich Egg	1	330	18	6	0
Sandwich Grilled Chicken	1	450	18	4	0
Sandwich Grilled Chicken	1	450	18	4	0
Taquito Sausage & Egg	1	410	24	8	0
Taquito w/ Bacon & Egg	1	370	21	7	0
Taquito w/ Bacon Egg & Cheese	1	420	24	9	0
Taquito w/ Potato & Egg	1	430	23	7	2
Taquito w/ Potato Egg & Cheese	1	470	27	9	2
Taquito w/ Sausage Egg & Cheese	1	450	28	11	0
Texas Toast	1 slice	180	8	1	0
Whataburger	1	640	32	10	0
Whataburger Double Meat	1	890	51	18	1
Whataburger Jr.	1	330	16	6	0
Whataburger Triple Meat	1	1140	70	26	1
Whataburger w/ Bacon & Cheese	1	800	45	17	1
Whatacatch	1	480	30	6	1
Whatacatch Dinner	1 serv	1095	92	19	11
Whatachick'n	1	530	20	4	1
SALADS					
Chicken Strips	1 serv	570	38	7	3

FOOD	PORTION	CALS	FAT	SAT FAT	TRANS FAT
Garden Salad	1	60	0	0	0
Grilled Chicken	1 serv	230	7	2	0

WHITE CASTLE
BEVERAGES

Barq's Red Cream Soda	1 sm (21 oz)	260	0	0	0
Barq's Root Beer	1 sm (21 oz)	250	0	0	0
Coca-Cola	1 sm (21 oz)	220	0	0	0
Coffee Black	1 sm (12 oz)	<5	0	0	0
Crave Cooler Coke	1 sm (21 oz)	150	0	0	0
Diet Coke	1 sm (21 oz)	0	0	0	0
Fanta Orange	1 sm (21 oz)	240	0	0	0
Hi-C Flashing Fruit Punch	1 sm (21 oz)	240	0	0	0
Hot Chocolate	1 sm (12 oz)	220	6	1	3
Hot Tea	1 sm (12 oz)	0	0	0	0
Ice Tea Unsweetened	1 sm (21 oz)	0	0	0	0
Iced Tea Sweetened w/ Lemon	1 sm (16 oz)	170	0	0	0
Iced Tea Sweetened w/ Lemon	1 sm (21 oz)	170	0	0	0
Lemonade Raspberry	1 sm (21 oz)	290	0	0	0
Pibb Xtra	1 sm (21 oz)	220	0	0	0
Powerade Mountain Blast	1 sm (21 oz)	140	0	0	0
Sprite	1 sm (21 oz)	220	0	0	0

MAIN MENU SELECTIONS

Cheeseburger	1	170	9	4	1
Cheeseburger Bacon	1	200	11	5	1
Cheeseburger Bacon Double	1	370	22	10	2
Cheeseburger Double	1	300	17	8	2
Cheeseburger Jalapeno	1	180	10	5	1
Cheeseburger Jalapeno Double	1	320	19	9	2
Chicken Rings	6	210	23	5	4
Clam Strips	1 reg	250	22	4	6
Fish Nibblers	1 reg	280	16	4	0
French Fries	1 reg	310	15	3	4
Mozzarella Cheese Sticks	3	250	14	6	2
Onion Chips	1 reg	480	23	4	5
Sandwich Chicken Breast w/ Cheese	1	200	8	3	2
Sandwich Chicken Ring	1	180	8	2	2

FOOD	PORTION	CALS	FAT	SAT FAT	TRANS FAT
Sandwich Chicken Ring w/ Cheese	1	200	10	3	2
Sandwich Fish w/ Cheese	1	180	8	3	3
White Castle	1	140	7	3	1
White Castle Double	1	250	13	5	1
SAUCES AND SPREADS					
Dressing Ranch	1 serv (1 oz)	150	17	3	0
Ketchup	1 pkg	10	0	0	0
Lemon Juice	1 pkg	0	0	0	0
Mayonnaise	1 pkg	60	7	1	0
Sauce BBQ	1 serv (1 oz)	35	1	0	0
Sauce Hot	1 pkg	0	0	0	0
Sauce Marinara	1 serv (1 oz)	15	0	0	0
Sauce Seafood	1 serv (1 oz)	30	0	0	0
Sauce Tartar	1 pkg	30	3	0	0
Sauce Zesty Zing	1 serv (1 oz)	110	11	2	0
Sauce Fat Free Honey Mustard	1 serv (1 oz)	50	0	0	0

WINCHELL'S DONUTS

FOOD	PORTION	CALS	FAT	SAT FAT	TRANS FAT
Chocolate Bar	1	240	16	–	4
Chocolate Round	1	240	16	–	4
Chocolate Twist	1	240	16	–	0
Croissant	1	260	17	–	7
Glazed Round	1	230	15	–	4
Glazed Twist	1	230	15	–	4
Iced Chocolate	1	230	15	–	5
Traditional	1	215	14	–	4

ZOUP!
DESSERTS

FOOD	PORTION	CALS	FAT	SAT FAT	TRANS FAT
Cookie Chocolate Chunk	1	410	19	–	–
Cookie Peanut Butter	1	420	21	–	–
SANDWICHES					
Pesto Three Cheese	1	720	42	–	–
Tuna Melt	1	600	23	–	–
Wrap American Farm	½	435	29	–	–
Wrap Asian	½	615	33	–	–
Wrap Chicken Caesar	½	505	19	–	–
Wrap Greek	½	485	33	–	–
Wrap Tuna	½	365	13	–	–

FOOD	PORTION	CALS	FAT	SAT FAT	TRANS FAT
SOUPS					
Chicken & Dumplings	1 serv (8 oz)	130	3	–	–
Chicken Potpie	1 serv (8 oz)	200	8	–	–
Italian Wedding w/ Turkey Meatballs	1 serv (8 oz)	120	4	–	–
Jamaican Bay Gumbo	1 (8 oz)	140	3	–	–
Lobster Bisque	1 serv (8 oz)	260	18	–	–
Pepper Steak	1 (8 oz)	160	6	–	–
Potato Cheddar	1 serv (8 oz)	210	13	–	–
Sesame Noodle Bowl	1 serv (8 oz)	80	3	–	–
Shrimp & Crawfish Etouffee	1 (8 oz)	130	4	–	–
Sicilian Pizza	1 serv (8 oz)	150	7	–	–
Spicy Crab & Rice	1 serv (8 oz)	110	2	–	–
Turkey Chili	1 (8 oz)	120	2	–	–
Wild Mushroom Barley	1 (8 oz)	108	3	–	–

THE CALORIE COUNTER
4th Edition

Diet trends may come and go,
but one thing is certain: calories count!

Wherever you turn, people are talking about calories. Eat too many and you gain weight. Eat fewer and you lose it. Move your body and you burn calories faster and lose weight quicker.

The Calorie Counter, 4th Edition, is the most comprehensive calorie counter in the marketplace:

- Calorie counts for more than 20,000 foods— more than 50% of the food counts new or revised.
- Expanded categories with new and revised generic foods.
- More than 600 take-out foods.
- 97 regional and national restaurant chains listed, with more than 5,000 menu choices.
- Introductory text expanded, revised, and updated.
- Website and email access to the authors. Got questions? Get answers at www.TheNutritionExperts.com.

A weight-loss guide that won't let you down!

THE CHOLESTEROL COUNTER
7th Edition

Your lifestyle choices can significantly improve your health!

Small, consistent changes in the way you eat and live can help reduce your cholesterol levels and lower your risk for heart disease, stroke, certain kinds of cancer, and dementia. Nationally known nutritionists Annette Natow and Jo-Ann Heslin help you make good choices each time you sit down to eat, and they explain the latest scientific research on evaluating and treating high cholesterol in terms you can understand and apply to your life right now. This totally rewritten and expanded 7th edition of *The Cholesterol Counter* includes:

- Cholesterol, fiber, calories, and portion sizes for more than 20,000 foods and more than 100 national and regional restaurant chains.
- An individual risk-assessment quiz.
- Worksheets, tables, and tips to easily keep track of your daily cholesterol intake.
- The importance of fiber and cholesterol-lowering "superfoods" in your diet.

THE DIABETES CARBOHYDRATE & CALORIE COUNTER
3rd Edition

What can I eat now that I have diabetes?

Whether you're newly diagnosed or trying to fine-tune your diabetes management, Natow and Heslin help you to use carbohydrate counting to plan meals that will keep your blood sugar down and help you control complications. The more you know about diabetes, the better you can take care of yourself and the healthier you will be. This thoroughly revised, easy-to-use counter presents the most up-to-the-minute information for the person with diabetes.

- More than 11,000 food listings, including calorie, carbohydrate, sugar, and fat counts.
- Counts for generic, brand name, take-out, and restaurant foods.
- Worksheets, tips, and tools to help you manage your diabetes.
- Up-to-date information on carbs, sugar, fiber, sweeteners, the glycemic index—and how to use each in meal planning.
- Recommendations for individualizing weight loss goals.

An essential reference for people living with diabetes.